B. S. Drasc

GERMFREE RESEARCH

RESEARCH
Biological Effect of
Gnotobiotic Environments

ACADEMIC PRESS RAPID MANUSCRIPT REPRODUCTION

Proceedings of
the IVth International Symposium on Germfree Research
Held in New Orleans, Louisiana, April, 1972

GERMFREE RESEARCH

Biological Effect of Gnotobiotic Environments

EDITED BY

JAMES B. HENEGHAN

Departments of Surgery and Physiology
Louisiana State University Medical Center
New Orleans, Louisiana

ACADEMIC PRESS   New York and London 1973

ACADEMIC PRESS, INC.
111 Fifth Avenue, New York, New York 10003

United Kingdom Edition published by
ACADEMIC PRESS, INC. (LONDON) LTD.
24/28 Oval Road, London NW1

Library of Congress Cataloging in Publication Data

International Symposium on Germfree Research, 4th,
    New Orleans, 1972.
    Germfree research.

    1. Germfree life--Congresses. I. Heneghan,
James B., ed. II. Title. [DNLM: 1. Germ-free
life--Congresses. W3 IN918M 1972. WNLM: [QY 50
I601g 1972]]
QH324.4.I48 1972   616.01'0724   72-88372
ISBN 0-12-340650-1

CONTENTS

Section I. Introduction

Section II. Gnotobiotic Technology in Clinical Medicine

CONTENTS

CONTENTS

Section VI. Nutrition and Metabolism

CONTENTS

CONTENTS

CONTENTS

CONTENTS

Section XII. Gnotobiotic Technology

xiv

FOREWORD

It is a privilege to prepare a Foreword for the Proceedings of the IVth International Symposium on Germfree Research for which the Department of Surgery of the Louisiana State University School of Medicine was pleased to act as host. It seems appropriate that some background might be given to explain the role of a Department of Surgery in such an endeavor.

The Germfree Laboratories of our Department came into existence as an extension of an experimental study of strangulation intestinal obstruction, which had been a long-standing research interest of ours. Earlier work had indicated that the gastrointestinal flora played a key role in the fatal outcome of animals — and probably of humans — with strangulation intestinal obstruction. In spite of the significant improvement in survival with appropriate antibiotic therapy, there still remained some unanswered questions for which the germfree animal seemed to be an ideal tool to obtain the necessary data. In 1961, after one of our residents, Dr. C. Edward Floyd, had obtained some basic technical data through a visit to the Lobund Laboratories of the University of Notre Dame, we embarked on a small program using guinea pigs. Our initial efforts were not successful, and after a short time — and with too little knowledge to know that we couldn't do what we were attempting to do! — we switched to dogs, and have occupied a large portion of our time, effort, and space with studies in gnotobiotic dogs ever since.

In 1962, Dr. James B. Heneghan joined us as Director of the Germfree Laboratories in the Department of Surgery, after receiving the first Ph.D offered by the University of Notre Dame for graduate work in the germfree field. The activities at L.S.U. have expanded greatly since then, due to his constant attention to the problems of germfree work, and to the expanding interest of a number of others in the Department of Surgery.

As our own interests in germfree work expanded, it became apparent that there were a number of other institutions working in similar areas, and that closer contact with these would be valuable to all. We have been happy to participate in both national and international meetings since then, and have thought that these major meetings served many useful purposes. The natural attractions of New Orleans for either a national or an international meeting made it obvious that we might hope to host a meeting at some time, but we thought it might be presumptuous to offer our own facilities when we were such relative newcomers to the field. We were thus highly honored and flattered when we were considered as the site for the IVth International Symposium on Germfree Research, and immediately began to try to find the necessary funds to sponsor such a meeting. The initial response to a request for such funding was quite disappointing, but the subsequent response of both national and other organizations was such as to make the meeting possible and, we believe, successful.

To this meeting came leaders of germfree research from all over the world, with representatives from 13 different countries actively participating in the meeting. This in itself is an accomplishment for which we are most gratified. The opportunity to show our colleagues from other parts of the world our City, our Medical Center, our Department of Surgery, and our Germfree Laboratories was an opportunity for which we are properly grateful. We hope those who came enjoyed and profited from the meetings as much as we did. We hope they left with a good impression of our Laboratories, Department, University, City, and Country — if so, the meeting will have served the major purpose of all international meetings — to prove that people can communicate peacefully with people.

With that hope in mind, we view these Proceedings of the IVth International Symposium on Germfree Research and give credit to the major force in their presentation, Dr. James B. Heneghan.

Isidore Cohn, Jr.
Professor and Chairman
Department of Surgery

PREFACE

Germfree research has evolved out of its technological era and is rapidly being employed in many diverse areas of biological research. This is emphasized by the variety of the 97 papers which were presented during the IVth International Symposium on Germfree Research in New Orleans on April 16 − 20, 1972. Representatives from 13 different countries contributed to the scientific program with topics as broad as: the application of germfree techniques in human medicine and the effects of this treatment on patients; advances in germfree plant research; techniques for rearing germfree baboons and germfree snails; and the use of germfree techniques to evaluate samples of lunar material. Thus, germfree research which started as an extremely esoteric basic research tool has now continued its scientific evolution to a point where the technology can be applied to practical problems, such as: protection of immune deficient patients, reduction of post-operative wound infection, immunological aspects of cancer, allergic diseases, cholesterol metabolism and heart disease, and nutrition and food utilization.

Following a world-wide appeal for abstracts, 97 participants were selected to deliver papers at the symposium, including 12 leaders in the field of germfree research who presented position papers in their particular area of interest. The assistance of the following members of the organizing committee was a significant factor in the success of the symposium: Marie E. Coates, Isidore Cohn, Jr., Hendrick Eyssen, Henry L. Foster, Helmut A. Gordon, Richard A. Griesemer, Bengt Gustafsson, Shogo Sasaki, Bernard S. Wostmann and Charles E. Yale.

On behalf of the organizing committee and of all the scientists engaged in germfree research, we wish to express our gratitude to those agencies whose major financial support has made this symposium possible: Animal Resources Branch, Division of Research Resources, National Institutes of Health; American Cancer Society; Institute of Laboratory Animal Resources, National Academy of Sciences; Association for Gnotobiotics; Charles River Breeding Laboratories, Inc.; Louisiana State University School of Dentistry; and Laboratory Animal Breeders Association. In addition we are grateful for the use of the auditoriums and facilities of the L.S.U. School of Medicine, L.S.U. School of Dentistry and the Veterans Administration Hospital.

A special note of thanks goes to the following colleagues who served as chairpersons of sessions during the symposium and then edited the papers presented in their sessions: P. Bealmear, R. J. Fitzgerald, H. A. Gordon, C. E. Miller, E. A. Mirand, B. P. Phillips, M. Pollard, S. Rovin, D. Savage, M. Wagner, R. B. Wescott, R. Wilson, B. S. Wostmann, and C. E. Yale.

In the enormous task of preparation of the proceedings, the assistance of the following individuals was greatly appreciated. The typing of the manuscripts into "camera ready" copy was efficiently performed by Mary Louise Laney of Studio/Comp of New Orleans. Her professional efforts were a significant factor in meeting our publication deadline. Proofreading was carried out by Helen L. Heneghan, Linda Thompson and Daniel Dessauer.

The social program was centered around a Social Hour at the Terrace Suite of the Jung Hotel and a Banquet in the Grand Ballroom of the Royal Orleans Hotel, which was highlighted by New Orleans Jazz provided by the Louis Cottrell Preservation Hall Jazz Band. The Social Hour was made possible by the financial assistance of the commercial exhibitors.

I wish to express my appreciation to the participants and authors of the IVth International Symposium on Germfree Research. I thank them for their cooperation and patience with the "traffic light," many deadlines, and especially for their adherence to the "6-book-page" limitation on their papers. In this regard, any reader of these proceedings who does not find sufficient detail in the area of his interest should contact the author directly.

To my wife, Helen, goes my thanks for the following: directing the Ladies Program, typing the grant applications and reports; organizing the abstracts, papers, and other material related to the symposium; answering the mountains of correspondence; and finally for encouraging me to complete this seemingly endless task. In retrospect I feel that she actually deserves the title co-chairman and co-editor of the symposium. In addition, I acknowledge the effect these activities have had on our family life and assure our sons, Jimmy and Mike, that as this proceedings goes to press they will again have "full-time" parents.

Finally I hope that both the scientific and social interchange which we have experienced during the New Orleans meeting will have a positive lasting effect on our lives and I hope to see everyone again at the next symposium in Stockholm in 1975.

James B. Heneghan

GERMFREE RESEARCH

Biological Effect of Gnotobiotic Environments

SECTION I

INTRODUCTION

GERMFREE RESEARCH: A NEW APPROACH IN MICRO-ECOLOGY

James B. Heneghan
Departments of Surgery and Physiology
Louisiana State University Medical Center
New Orleans, Louisiana 70112, U.S.A.

Introduction

For most laymen and scientists, the words environment and ecology evoke nightmares: the toxic effects of chemical pollution, the bio-behavioral disturbances caused by overcrowding or automated work, the pathologic consequences of exposure to intense and unnatural stimuli, and thousands of other real and imagined threats to mankind's existence on this planet in the 21st century. Although this concern is based on the holistic "spaceship-earth" concept, which is centered around the finite nature of our physical environment, similar problems exist at the micro-environmental level and have equally important micro-ecological effects on the intact survival of individuals. By employing closed microbial environments, germfree research seeks to understand and control the complex interrelationships between the microbial flora and the host and between the various elements of the flora. In this manner germfree research attempts to do more than establish simple cause and effect relationships; it seeks to define the positive and negative feedback loops which exist in the host-flora and inter-flora relationships – a microbiocybernetics.

The purpose of this paper is to summarize the present status of germfree* research and the use of gnotobiotic** environments in the study of

---

* ** Terminology

"Gnotobiotic: A word derived from the Greek "gnotos" and "biota" meaning known flora and fauna. *Gnotobiote* (Gnotobiotic animal): one of an animal stock or strain derived by aseptic cesarean section (or sterile hatching of eggs) which are reared and continuously maintained with germfree techniques under isolator conditions and in which the composition of any associated fauna and flora, if present, is fully defined by accepted current methodology. *Germfree animal* (axenic animal): A gnotobiote which is free from all demonstrable associated forms of life including bacteria, viruses, fungi, protozoa and other saprophytic or parasitic forms." (Source: Gnotobiotes, Institute of Laboratory Animal Resources, International Standard Book No. 0-309-01858-7, National Academy of Science, Washington, D.C.).

micro-ecology. This is not a review paper but rather it points to trends and attempts to predict future directions in: Clinical Gnotobiotics; General Applied Gnotobiotics; Interpretation of the Characteristics of Germfree Life; and Gnotobiotic Technology.

Clinical Gnotobiotics

The use of germfree technology to create gnotobiotic environments for clinical medicine has been centered around two major applications: surgical isolators to prevent post-operative wound infection and reverse isolation units to protect immune-deficient patients. The use of barrier systems and massive antibiotics to control the microbiological environments of hospital patients causes significant alterations in the micro-ecological host-parasite relationships. The complexity of these micro-environments is only beginning to be understood.

Surgical Environments. One of the first applications of gnotobiotic environments to clinical medicine was the use of flexible film isolators to reduce post-operative wound infection in lengthy surgical procedures where the risk of wound infection is high. Plastic isolators, while they exert absolute control of both air-borne and contact exogenous microorganisms, present difficulties in operative techniques. On the other hand, laminar air flow surgical suites, which offer a technical facility comparable to the conventional operating room, tend to control only air-borne contamination. Since each approach has clear cut advantages and disadvantages, an equal effort should be applied to develop and evaluate both technologies.

Germfree animal experimentation in the future should be directed towards quantitating the numbers of microorganisms necessary to produce post-operative infection under controlled conditions.

Patient Environments. Progress in maintaining gnotobiotic environments for hospital patient care can be summarized as follows: 1) germfree infants have been obtained by cesarean section and by antibiotic decontamination; 2) two infants have been maintained in germfree isolators for periods of up to 2½ years; 3) no insurmountable obstacles or untoward effects have been observed in these infants at the present time; and 4) germfree isolators simple enough for parents to care for their infants at home are under development. For the first time the effects of gnotobiotic isolation are being studied on the following parameters of human patient status: fecal bile acids, sugar absorption, psychological development, and hemorrhagic complications during treatment for leukemia.

Future experimentation should be directed towards the development of improved: patient isolation systems, antibiotic decontamination procedures, recolonization techniques, and measurements of physiological and psychological changes due to microbial environmental control.

General Applied Gnotobiotics

A substantial part of germfree research has been and will continue to be centered around experimentation based on the "clean-environment" concept. In such experimental situations the gnotobiotic animal provides information on host response without the variable influence of the "normal" microbial flora. Although such research is utilized to study very important aspects of health and disease, the conclusions reached must be interpreted with regard to recent evidence which indicates that the germfree animal is not simply a conventional animal minus a flora. The absence of a flora results in a variety of direct and indirect alterations in the micro-environment, some of which are local and others generalized — all of which may influence the experimental results. This is why more research is necessary to understand the germfree animal as a research tool.

Oncology. Studies on carcinogenesis in gnotobiotic rodents can be summarized as follows: 1) some spontaneous murine hematopoietic neoplasms are seriously affected by the absence of a conventional microbial environment, whereas, non-hematopoietic tumors are not; 2) the data obtained following the introduction of chemical carcinogens in germfree and conventional mice are conflicting and the effects of the microbial environment awaits further clarification; 3) oncogenic viruses have not been demonstrated in germfree rats as they have been in all germfree mouse strains following whole-body x-irradiation; and 4) germfree rats do develop spontaneous neoplasms, both benign and malignant, and attempts to compare the incidences between germfree and conventional rats must await additional data. Finding viral carcinogens in all germfree mice supports the existence of the vertical transmission of these oncogenes. On the other hand, some investigators feel that the failure to demonstrate viral material in germfree rats attacks the theory of the universal viral etiology of cancer; others argue that the viruses are there but have not been found.

Recent studies in germfree mice have supported the value of maintaining a gnotobiotic state during treatment for leukemia. Germfree AKR mice which develop spontaneous leukemia tolerated larger doses of cyclophosphamide than the conventional controls; they also exhibited longer survival.

Thus the continued use of gnotobiotic environments in patient care and in research provides another weapon in the fight to eliminate cancer as one of the three leading causes of death in the U.S.A.

Dental Research. Current germfree dental research on the traditional studies of the role of the flora in tooth decay is centered around the causes of the adherent properties of the oral flora and the prevention of caries by immunization. A new trend is evident however, in the increased emphasis placed on studies of the oral microbial flora in periodontal disease. Two new germfree animal models which develop periodontal disease spontaneously have been

5

described: germfree rice rats and germfree beagles. Studies of the natural history of periodontal disease in these hosts should provide valuable information on the role of the oral flora in its etiology, and thus help to reduce the threat of periodontal disease which is the major cause of tooth loss in people over 20 years of age.

Microbiology. Present emphasis in the field of microbiology is centered around attempts to establish a "normal" microbial flora in germfree animals in an effort to understand the complex micro-ecological relationships between microbes themselves and between the microbes and their hosts. As a result of histological examination of the colon and cecum of mice, a dense layer of microorganisms in the mucous layer around the epithelium has been demonstrated; these fusiform organisms are strict anaerobes which may outnumber the other components of the "normal" microbial flora by a factor as large as 1,000. In the past, these organisms were not discovered by standard culture techniques because of their extreme sensitivity to oxygen. Attempts to establish these strict anaerobes in gnotobiotic animals as monocontaminants have been unsuccessful thus far; however, a recent report has described the successful implantation of one of these strict anaerobes in gnotobiotic animals previously contaminated with *Staphylococcus aureus*.

Since the widespread use of broad spectrum antibiotics in clinical medicine has produced a variety of resistant strains of microorganisms, the development of a kanamycin resistant *Serratia marcescens* has been experimentally produced and studied in gnotobiotic mice.

Recently decontamination has taken on a new meaning and emphasis in the germfree field. Combinations of non-absorbable antibiotics are fed to patients and experimental animals in quantities which suppress organisms normally cultured in their feces. The observation that this procedure can produce "germfree" patients and experimental animals, if they are maintained in a gnotobiotic environment, awaits further confirmation; nevertheless, subjects so treated tend to exhibit some of the same micro-ecological relationships as normal germfree animals. There are two major stimuli for this work: 1) the need to reduce to a minimum the endogenous and potentially pathogenic organisms of isolated patients and 2) an economical way to change any conventional animal into a "germfree" animal.

Nutrition. Due to the nutritional problems inherent in sterilizing the diets necessary to rear germfree animals, nutritional studies have been in the forefront of germfree research from its beginning. Now that many of the problems of hand-rearing gnotobiotic mammals have been solved and second generation animals obtained, carefully controlled nutritional and metabolic studies are able to define the qualitative and quantitative requirements in the absence of a microflora.

The micro-chemical environment presented to the intestinal epithelium for nutrient absorption has three inputs: 1) chemicals in the diet; 2) chemicals of host origin; and 3) chemicals derived by the intestinal microbial flora. Also the flora may not only synthesize *de novo* substances but also may alter substances of dietary or host origin. The advantages of gnotobiotic environments in establishing the precise nature of these micro-chemical relationships are obvious.

There is considerable interest in the development of chemically defined liquid diets which can be filter sterilized in order to obtain a germfree animal with the lowest possible antigenic stimulation. Further efforts in the quest for an "antigen-free" animal model will probably be directed towards reducing endogenous antigenic stimuli.

Germfree animals and gnotobiotic techniques have been used to control trace element contamination and thereby are playing a role in determining which trace elements are necessary for life.

Interpretation of the Characteristics of Germfree Life

As alluded to previously, the germfree animal is much more than a conventional animal minus its flora. Indeed, the absence of a microbial flora may produce many complex micro-ecological changes in the germfree animal which make interpretation of the results more difficult and signal the need for increased experimentation to understand the germfree animal as a research tool.

One of the oldest anomalies found in germfree rodents is the enlarged cecum; in fact, it was first observed in the original investigations of Nuttal and Thierfelder in 1895 and is still a common finding. In an effort to explain cecal enlargement, the reduced weight of the heart, the lower total blood volume, the decreased cardiac output, and the other possibly related characteristics of the germfree rodent, the intestinal contents of germfree and conventional rodents were examined in detail and certain endogenous depressant substances isolated. It is postulated that these bioactive substances are inactivated by the "normal" intestinal flora and are thus prevented from exerting their effects in conventional animals. When confirmed this may provide one of the first examples of a synergistic micro-chemical environmental relationship between the host and flora.

The germfree animal's cecum is filled with very liquid contents and the animals also exhibit a chronic mild diarrhea. This retention of water in the lower portion of the gastrointestinal tract of germfree rats is probably due to: 1) unabsorbable negatively charged macromolecules which increase the colloid osmotic pressure and 2) the virtual absence of chloride ions which prevent water absorption coupled to the active absorption of Na^+.

Two other basic alterations in gastrointestinal function observed in

7

germfree animals compared to conventional are: 1) increased intestinal transit time and 2) decreased epithelial cell turnover. The mechanisms responsible for these fundamental difference brought about by the absence of an intestinal flora have not been determined and provide fertile ground for future investigations.

Gnotobiotic Technology

The list of species successfully reared under gnotobiotic environments continues to grow; recent reports have described the techniques for rearing germfree dogs, baboons, snails and hamsters. Although SPF hamster colonies have been established it appears as though the goal of a germfree hamster still remains elusive.

With the depletion of world food supplies and ever increasing population, the application of germfree technology and the use of gnotobiotic environments to study the growth of plants appears to be rising. A recent report deals with the effects of bacterial growth and nitrogen metabolism in gnotobiotic ensilages of three species of plants. In addition, the technological advancements in the growth of germfree plants have allowed scientists at the Manned Spacecraft Center to evaluate the effects of lunar material on the growth of gnotobiotic plants.

While it is true that germfree research has passed successfully out of its technological development era, the techniques presently employed must be improved and simplified. One very important future requirement is the continued development and universal application of a standard technology for rearing germfree animals. The initial efforts in this area have been carried out by the Subcommittee on Standards for Gnotobiotes, Institute of Laboratory Animal Resources, National Academy of Sciences.

Summary

The present national and international concern about our environment and the ecological relationships which preserve it has developed rapidly during the past 10 years. On the other hand modern germfree research through the application of gnotobiotic environments has been in the forefront of micro-ecological research for over 25 years; therefore, germfree research is not a new approach in micro-ecology as the title implies, but rather, its role in environmental science has not been emphasized in the past. Thus germfree research will play an important role in the effort to assure mankind enough seats on his spaceship planet in the 21st century.

THOUGHTS ON THE ROLE OF GNOTOBIOTICS
IN CLINICAL MEDICINE

Keynote Address*

Wallace E. Herrell, M.D. **
445 Central Avenue
Northfield, Illinois 60093, U.S.A.

I am keenly aware of the honor you do me by asking me to come here. When your Organizing Committee invited me to deliver the keynote address, I accepted with some trepidation for the simple reason that my investigative activities have not been in the field of gnotobiotic research. However, I have devoted most of my professional life to the experimental and clinical use of chemotherapeutic and antibiotic agents in the treatment of infectious disease, a field of endeavor which, in my opinion, is closely related to your work.

Permit me to say that I find many similarities between the early days of antibiotic research and gnotobiotic research. For example, I note with considerable interest the comments published by Gordon and Pesti in their excellent review entitled "The Gnotobiotic Animal as a Tool in the Study of Host Microbial Relationships," which recently appeared in *Bacteriological Reviews.* According to them, the concept of gnotobiotic experimentation is credited to Pasteur. They also pointed out that while this is correct in the microbic sense, the need to work with pure systems in biologic experimentation (namely, the growth of plants in "sterile" soil) could be traced farther back. I was interested to note that Pasteur outlined the actual gnotobiotic experiment, but he speculated that, on elimination of microbial associates such as is the case in the germfree experiment, life of the animal host would be impossible. As further indicated by Gordon and Pesti, however, Metchnikoff and others held the opposite view − that microbes were antagonistic to the well-being of the host. I assume therefore from my reading that there was considerable activity in this field before the final proof that normal life is indeed possible in the absence

*4th International Symposium on Germfree Research, New Orleans, Louisiana, April 17, 1972.

**Professor of Clinical Medicine, University of Kentucky; Editor-in-Chief, Clinical Medicine and Medical Digest Publications.

of germs. This proof came about as a result of the epoch-making studies reported from the Lobund Laboratories at Notre Dame in the 1940s.

Permit me now to comment on the rather interesting similarity with regard to the early days of research in antibiotics which many associate with the work of Fleming, who in 1929 described penicillin which was finally isolated in pure form 11 years later (1940) by the group of investigators at Oxford headed by Florey. Meanwhile, in 1938 Dubos isolated tyrothricin from *Bacillus brevis.* If one looks at the record, he will find that as long ago as 1877 Pasteur and Joubert were aware that certain airborne organisms inhibited the growth of the anthrax bacillus, and they even suggested that the phenomenon, which they referred to as "antibiosis," might be used in the treatment of certain infections. It was subsequently well established that these products elaborated by the antagonistic microbes have definite chemical and biologic properties. Here, therefore, is the origin of what later was to be named "antibiotics," a term actually derived from the word "antibiosis." The term antibiotic was suggested by Waksman a little over 50 years after the work by Pasteur and Joubert.

The first antibiotic to be described was isolated in 1899 by Emmerich and Loew. It was derived from *Pseudomonas aeruginosa* and was given the name "pyocyanase" by them. They also suggested its local use for therapy of anthrax and diptheria because of its marked antibacterial activity against both of these organisms.

Is it not interesting that the concept of gnotobiotic experimentation came about in 1885, yet its big moment, if you will accept the expression, occurred in the 1940s. Likewise, the phenomenon of antibiosis was first suggested in 1877, yet the big moment for antibiotics also occurred in 1940 when penicillin was first isolated in a form suitable for intramuscular injection.

In our early studies on antibiotics my colleagues and I made use of a research tool which in my opinion can in some ways be compared with your research tool. I refer to the use of the tissue culture method which my colleague, Dorothy Heilman, and I used in 1938 in our first studies with gramicidin, and shortly thereafter, penicillin. With the use of the tissue culture media we were able to learn a great deal with our very limited supply of gramicidin and penicillin. In fact, with only a few milligrams of the antibiotic we were able to learn much. It was in our tissue culture studies that we established the fact that gramicidin was hemolytic and would therefore never be suitable for systemic use. Shortly thereafter, using this method, we were able with only a few milligrams to establish the fact that penicillin was not only bactericidal but at the same time nonhemolytic, and indeed extraordinarily nontoxic for tissues. For example, penicillin in antibacterial amounts was found not to interfere with the growth and migration of tissue elements such as lymphocytes, fibroblasts, or macrophages. Our conviction in 1938 that the tissue culture technique was of value in microbiology was ultimately justified since it turned out to be a tool of such importance in the ultimate development of the vaccine for poliomyelitis.

When supplies of penicillin were more plentiful we progressed from the tissue culture studies to the use of penicillin in the treatment of infections in experimental animals such as mice, hamsters, and guinea pigs. With guinea pigs we ran into a problem which is, in my opinion, related to gnotobiotic research. In 1943 during a study of experimental leptospirosis in guinea pigs, F. R. Heilman and I attempted to treat these animals with penicillin. We discovered much to our surprise that young guinea pigs, including the controls, who received from 1,000 to 5,000 units of penicillin daily frequently died after several days. Death was preceded for a day or two by a state of apathy, anorexia, loss of weight, ruffled fur, and rectal temperatures at the lower limits of normal. Examination of these animals revealed only a state of generalized vasodilatation. This occurred with penicillin including calcium as well as sodium penicillin from four different sources. In sections of the brain, liver, and kidneys the only significant finding was markedly dilated capillaries throughout the tissues. Since the normal bacterial intestinal flora of the guinea pig is predominantly Gram-positive, we suspected that penicillin must have secondarily interfered with this flora and thereby with the metabolism of certain substances essential to the health of these animals. However, to this day I am unable to explain this observation which we published in 1943. I relate this observation at this time, however, for two reasons. First, I have always been grateful that the Food and Drug Administration was not as active in 1943 as today because I feel sure that, had they known that as little as 1,000 to 5,000 units of penicillin would kill normal healthy young guinea pigs, this remarkable therapeutic agent may have never received an effective new drug application. The second reason I mentioned this observation is to indicate that I suspect that our explanation of this phenomenon in guinea pigs was not correct since your germfree guinea pigs seem to do very well upon i.p. administration of penicillin. If it has not already been done I would hope that one of you would follow up those studies and give germfree guinea pigs 5,000 units of penicillin daily in an attempt to explain this toxic effect. If such studies have been done I have not seen the reports. If they have been done in germfree guinea pigs and I have missed the published report, I apologize for parading my ignorance.

I must now address my remarks to the problem of the possible role of gnotobiotic research in clinical medicine, as I see the matter. Let me first say that it is my conviction that your germfree studies not only have already made but will continue to make some monumental contributions to the care and treatment of some important diseases in man. In fact, it is my conviction that gnotobiotic research may have some clinical application in nearly every medical specialty and sub-specialty ranging from pediatrics to geriatrics.

11

WALLACE E. HERRELL

Immunologic Deficiency States

The first clinical situation I propose to discuss is the role of gnotobiotic research in immunologic deficiency states — namely agammaglobulinemia and hypogammaglobulinemia. It was my great pleasure to hear the report by Dietrich and his colleagues presented at the Eleventh Interscience Conference on Antimicrobial Agents and Chemotherapy in Atlantic City, October 1971. It seemed to me clearly evident from the report of the German investigators that the plastic isolator modeled after those used for germfree animals can be used with success in clinical situations and, when combined with the use of antibiotics, these patients might even be rendered germfree in the true sense of the word. This would be the first induction of the germfree state in man, and it is my opinion that medical history will deal kindly with these studies. The fact that these children developed normally, except for their immune systems, is of tremendous interest. As I recall, a thymic transplant had failed but it is not inconceivable that at a later date a transplantation of fetal thymus could again be attempted. I was pleased to note from your program that you will be hearing more from these same investigators concerning these studies.

Permit me to suggest that there is another relatively new category of immune defect which deserves the attention of those of you in gnotobiotic research. I refer to the so-called granulomatous disease of children first described by Bridges and his colleagues. The most consistent features of this disease include an elevated gammaglobulin, leukocytosis, anemia, an elevated sedimentation rate, and severe chronic infections. In this interesting situation there is no demonstrable disturbance in their ability to form circulating antibodies. The Minneapolis, Minnesota investigators have now clearly shown that the defect here is a lack of the ability of the leukocytes to destroy both Gram-positive and Gram-negative microbes in spite of the fact that these leukocytes are capable of ingesting these organisms. As I have indicated, this condition bears no resemblance to the situation in patients with hypogammaglobulinemia. What I am suggesting is that here is another clinical situation in which it would be profitable to examine the induction of a germfree state since many of those children succumb to chronic infections. One might keep them alive and germfree while further studies on the intracellular defect are carried out and development of methods to correct or control the defect continued.

Amyloidosis

It would appear that gnotobiotic research may contribute to our knowledge of another disease, namely, amyloidosis, which not infrequently occurs in multiple myeloma and Hodgkin's disease as well as in certain chronic infections. Those of us in clinical medicine have heretofore also considered amyloidosis a consequence of chronic suppurative infections such as osteo-

12

myelitis, tuberculosis, and other chronic infections.

I note with considerable interest that disseminated amyloidosis has been observed by Anderson in select colonies of germfree mice. In his report in the October 1971 issue of the *American Journal of Pathology* he observed that amyloidosis occurred in a significant number of germfree mice and therefore in the absence of any inciting inflammatory process. He suggested that deficient or defective immunoglobulin production might trigger amyloid production in experimental and clinical situations known to be predisposed to this disease. Thus, these select colonies of germfree mice would appear to be the experimental counterpart of adult-onset agammaglobulinemia. If insufficient production of gammaglobulin per se is responsible for amyloidosis in these patients, then this does indeed suggest a possible therapeutic approach in the treatment of patients prone to develop this disease. We could probably supply these patients with gammaglobulin in an effort to prevent amyloidosis.

Leukemia, Lymphomas, and Other Malignancies

It is my conviction that there is another area in clinical medicine where gnotobiotic research is destined to play an important role, and that is in connection with the treatment of leukemia, multiple myeloma, the lymphomas, and other malignant diseases.

It is a well-established fact that these patients are prone to infections and that this susceptibility is especially evident in those with granulocytopenia and in those who receive intensive chemotherapy, irradiation, and steroids which are immunosuppressive. These patients are especially prone to become victims of Gram-negative bacteremia. The most commonly isolated organism is *Pseudomonas aeruginosa* and less frequently, *Escherichia coli, Klebsiella pneumoniae,* Proteus, *Serratia marcescens,* and bacteroides. Furthermore, death comes swiftly and often before antibacterial therapy can be used effectively: of those with Pseudomonas bacteremia, 50 per cent die within 72 hours of the initial positive blood culture. Aside from the control of infections in these patients there is possibly another large dividend to be gained from gnotobiotic research. For example, by providing a germfree state one should be able to give even larger doses of X-ray and chemotherapy as well as the other immunosuppressive agents and thereby hopefully arrive at *curative* rather than *suppressive* doses of these agents. Personally I consider this one of the most exciting aspects of gnotobiotic research in clinical medicine. It is my conviction therefore that in the future we should attempt to establish the germfree environment *before* and not *after* initiating therapy in these patients.

Gastroenterology

Gastroenterology is another clinical field in which gnotobiotic research has a tremendous potential. Consider for example the problem of hepatic coma which is associated with a marked elevation of blood ammonia. Since the bacterial flora of the gastrointestinal tract probably supplies the bacterial enzymes involved in converting urea to ammonia, this is the basis for the use of neomycin and other antibiotics which have been used in the treatment of cirrhosis, especially in those patients with decompensated liver disease with impending coma.

Intestinal amebiasis is another clinical situation in which your germfree studies have established for a fact something that we in clinical medicine have postulated for some time. For example, we have known that the broad-spectrum antibiotics were of value in the treatment of intestinal amebiasis; however, they are of no value in the treatment of amebic abscesses of the liver. We therefore postulated that the reason for the effectiveness of antibiotics in intestinal amebiasis was associated with the fact that by removing the bacterial flora we deprived the ameba of its source of nutrition and therefore the ameba failed to survive. Gnotobiotic research, it would appear, has settled the matter. I refer to the study in germfree guinea pigs (Phillips *et al.*) in which it was found that intracecal seeding with *Entamoeba histolytica* failed to induce severe enteritis which under similar conditions occurs in conventional animals. Conversely, when the animals were exposed to the combination of ameba plus bacteria these lesions did develop. In other words, what was nothing more than a suspicion or clinical impression on our part is now a fact, thanks to germfree research.

Aside from the study of many enteric infections, gnotobiotic research will, in my opinion, continue to make substantial contributions to our knowledge of gastrointestinal physiology and metabolism, both normal and abnormal. Further, with this research tool, it is my belief that you may solve another important clinical problem, namely, the mechanism involved in the development of diarrhea which is often a troublesome situation associated with the use of some antibiotics which are otherwise important in clinical medicine.

Nephrology

Another area in which gnotobiotic research may play an important role is in nephrology. The germfree studies of uremia are tremendously important. I note that it has been observed that blood urea nitrogen remained much lower in some studies in germfree than in conventional animals. In the presence of uremia in man other problems commonly encountered are intestinal ulcerations and hemorrhage. I was interested to note that some investigators have reported that these ulcerations were not observed in germfree animals. Since uremia and infections, as well as gastrointestinal hemorrhage, are so important in patients with nephrosis and nephritis, it seems only reasonable to suggest that these patients should, if possible, be placed in a germfree environment in the hope that reparative processes would occur since, as is well known, many of these patients will go into remission, even those who are suffering with acute as well as chronic renal disease. In children with nephrosis one of the real hazards is bacterial infection such as pneumonia, septicemia, or peritonitis, especially pneumococcal peritonitis.

The observation that in kidney trauma germfree animals were found to have a longer survival than conventional controls suggests that this may be another possible area for clinical investigation.

Transplantation and Open Heart Surgery

It seems safe to say that in no area of clinical medicine are things moving faster than in the area of cardiac and renal transplantation as well as in the field of open heart surgery. Now that you in gnotobiotic research have shown that by using plastic film isolators one can provide a local germfree environment without great expense, these techniques could and most certainly should be added to the surgical management of those patients.

Large numbers of patients are now being operated on to replace diseased and damaged cardiac valves. At the same time, the medical literature is full of reports which reveal that these prosthetic valves have been successfully inserted; unfortunately, not long thereafter a bacterial infection may develop in the newly implanted valves. While we have had considerable success following the use of intensive antibacterial therapy in treating bacterial endocarditis in general, I can tell you that bacterial endocarditis developing in the prosthesis is much more difficult to treat, and the mortality and morbidity are extremely high. What I am suggesting is that these patients should also be placed in a germfree environment in an effort to reduce the incidence of this unfortunate complication which may occur following an otherwise successful surgical procedure.

Burns

I need not remind you that, aside from fluid and electrolyte loss, shock and infection pose the greatest problems in the successful care of the severely burned patient. I would therefore suggest that here is another clinical situation in which gnotobiotic research offers a great deal in our search for improved methods of treatment of burns.

Geriatrics

The field of geriatrics is a rapidly expanding branch of medicine, and much still needs to be done in this area. Hopefully, gnotobiotic research will supply us with some information in connection with degenerative processes associated with aging and hopefully will provide some clues which may help in our effort to increase the life span.

15

Miscellaneous

There are many other areas in clinical medicine where gnotobiotic research has and will continue to make substantial contributions in clinical medicine but time does not permit a complete discussion of all of them. One area does, however, deserve mention – the importance of gnotobiotic research in the study of dental caries and periodontal disease. In my opinion, gnotobiotic research will also play an important role in veterinary medicine, including studies on animal nutrition and growth.

Some Observations and Suggestions

Permit me to make some observations and suggestions. First of all, most great contributions in science and medicine have come from individuals working more or less alone, as in the case of my great friend, Alexander Fleming. As he so aptly stated in his address at the Mayo Foundation in 1945, "A team is fine when you have something to go on, but a team is the worst possible way of starting out to find something brand new." Between the time of his original discovery and the success of the Oxford team, he tried to interest others, namely, a chemist in a neighboring institution but, as Fleming put it, the chemist got stuck because the bacteriologist in his institution would not cooperate. So it turns out years later that "the Oxford people . . . had something to go on and extended the work and showed that penicillin was good stuff." I would suggest that you in gnotobiotic research, many of whom I suspect have worked alone, have now reached a point in time when a team approach is important. I mean that you now need integration. There must be more integration between the gnotobiotic researcher, the microbiologist, the pathologist, and the clinician. In other words, a team effort is now needed. The successful use of antibiotics in clinical medicine resulted from close collaborative efforts between clinicians and microbiologists.

The second matter concerns the suggestion that I have made concerning the need to immediately initiate extensive use of these germfree programs in many areas of clinical medicine. I well realize that this involves more than simply buying a batch of plastic isolators and starting in business. To accomplish this will, of course, involve facilities for proper feeding and nursing care by personnel properly trained in these techniques, but it is my conviction that it can be done. This will require the team effort. I can already hear hospital administrators cry about the additional cost of hospital care, but my answer is simply this: we already have very elaborate and extremely expensive special units such as intensive care units, coronary care units, dialysis units, and others in all of our well-equipped, modern hospitals. Why therefore should we not have germfree units? If we can spend billions of dollars getting to the moon to find out among other things that it is germfree, why not spend a few million on the germfree programs? Let me hasten to say that I am not opposed to the space program. In fact, I know of few, if any, true scientists who are.

The third matter is in another area. As I understand it, you have a European, an American, and also a Japanese society for gnotobiotic research, but you do not have an official publication of any society nor do you have an international journal of gnotobiotic research. It seems to me that such a publication would serve a useful purpose, especially if the journal carried reports which deal with possible applications of gnotobiotic research in clinical medicine. I presume there are valid reasons both for and against the creation of such a publication and that you have or will give thought to the matter.

The fourth of my observations and suggestions concerns the matter of some of the antibacterial and antifungal agents. I note that in your germfree studies you have used a variety of combinations of antibacterial agents including bacitracin, streptomycin, vancomycin, and gentamicin, usually combined with the antifungal agent, nystatin. You might wish to look at some of the newer antifungal agents which are now available and which are also suitable for administration by the oral route. These include: 1) the new amphotericin B preparation suitable for oral use which has a broad spectrum and is highly active against *Candida albicans* and other pathogenic fungi; 2) hamycin, another antifungal agent suitable for oral use and which is inhibitory for *Blastomyces dermatitidis, Histoplasma capsulatum, Cryptococcus neoformans,* and *Candida albicans;* and 3) 5-fluorocytosine, another antifungal agent which is active against a number of pathogenic fungi including *Candida albicans* and *Cryptococcus neoformans.*

You are at this time writing your names in the annals of medical history and you are doing so with indelible ink. May I repeat what I said at the start — I appreciate the honor you do me by asking me to come here, and I thank you for your kind attention.

SECTION II

GNOTOBIOTIC TECHNOLOGY IN CLINICAL MEDICINE

GERMFREE TECHNOLOGY IN CLINICAL MEDICINE: PRODUCTION AND MAINTENANCE OF GNOTOBIOTIC STATES IN MAN

M. Dietrich, T. M. Fliedner and *D. Krieger*
Center for Internal Medicine and Pediatrics, Division of Hematology
and Center for Basic Clinical Research, Division of Clinical Physiology,
University of Ulm, Ulm Germany

Introduction

In man, states of high susceptibility to infection may occur temporarily. This is true for bone marrow deficiencies, whether primary due to hematological disorders or secondary to treatment by ionizing radiation or chemotherapeutics, for severe burns, for defects of the immune competence, whether congenital or due to immune suppression after organ transplantation. In children and in adults these phases cannot be controlled completely by usual therapeutic measures.

For a few years germfree techniques have been adapted for clinical use in order to prevent infection in states described above. The purpose of such a prophylactic therapy is to prevent infection by exogenous germs but also by potential pathogens of the patient's own microflora.

The achievement and maintenance of a germfree or gnotobiotic state respectively by the means of complete isolation and decontamination of the endogenous microflora by antibiotics may enable the medical team to attempt all promising treatments of the underlying disease such as transplantation of thymus or bone marrow without the threat of complicating infection or pronounced secondary disease.

Methods

Patients studied. Twenty adult patients suffering from AL (Acute Myelocytic, Acute Undifferentiated Leukemia, Acute Erythroleukemia) have been isolated and 15 of them decontaminated in 25 treatment periods of 20-86 days.

Non-identical male twins with a congenital combined immune deficiency, previously described as lymphopenic hypogammaglobulinemia, have been treated by means of gnotobiotic care from the age of 4 weeks on. The infants were suffering from a severe hemorrhagic enteritis and a putrid skin infection.

Microbiology. During the time of observation sampling has been done from different sites regularly two times a week: external ear, nose, oral cavity, groin, anus, back, umbilicus, axilla, toes, preputium, urine, and feces. The isolator and the introduced items have been tested microbiologically in irregular intervals: gloves, locks, plastic walls, drugs, alimentation, brushes, etc.

For quantitation of the intestinal microbes, a fecal sample of 0.5 g was mixed with 4.5 g brain-heart-infusion and serially diluted. At the same time the samples were incubated in thioglycollate (for anaerobic culturing) as well as on plates (for aerobic and anaerobic culturing). The anaerobic culturing was done in evacuated anaerobic jars as described by Lerche and Reuter (1).

The following media were used: Endoagar of MacConkey No. 3, Enterococci confirmatory agar, S 110 Staph. (Chapman), Sabouraud-Glucose agar, tomato juice agar, Clostridial reinforced agar and Fortner plate.

The bacteria to be given to the infants for the implantation of a "normal" intestinal microflora were received from other laboratories (Bifidobacteria: courtesy of Dr. Schuler-Malyoth, Starnberg, and *Bacteroides vulgatis:* courtesy of Prof. Werner, Bonn) and from the fecal flora from a healthy donor.

The bacterial strains were separated by culturing on plates and stored in liquid nitrogen as well as a sample of the fecal specimen. The inoculated bifidobacteria were given in milk. The bacteroides that have been cultured in thioglycollate have been applied in that medium orally (+ milk) and rectally. The aerobic bacteria have been given in 0.9% sodium chloride.

The sensitivity to antibiotics of each single bacterial strain was tested by agar diffusion test.

Gnotobiotic care for isolation. The reverse isolation of the adults took place in an isolation system of Life Island type and in an Ulm Isolated Bed System (Fig. 1). Prior to the isolation period, the isolators were sterilized by a 2% solution of peracetic acid and tested for sterility. All items to be introduced in the systems were sterilized by autoclaving, sterilization by ethylene oxide or surface disinfection by peracetic acid or glutaraldehyde. This included the daily meals and beverages, but tablets, pills and other oral drugs could not be sterilized. The isolation barrier was maintained by ultraviolet light locks for the exchange of items and by ultra high efficiency air filter systems.

The isolation of the infants took place in plastic isolation systems constructed analogous to isolators used for the care of germfree animals (in collaboration with von Stenglin, Metall u. Plastik, Radolfzell, Germany). Each system consists of a maintenance and a storage isolator. They are made of polyvinylchloride (PVC) and placed on mobile tables of aluminum. Each isolator has its independent air filter system to provide sterile air. The storage isolator has an entry port to which an autoclaved drum can be attached for loading the isolator with sterile items. Three neoprene gloves are attached to work inside the isolator. The isolator itself is connected to the maintaining isolation system by a

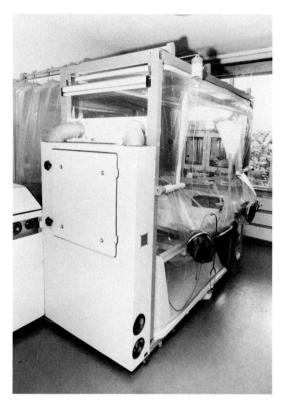

FIG. 1. Ulm Isolated Bed System. View of the completely tight isolator with a solid framework allowing unhindered visual communication.

plastic tunnel of 0.7 m. This tunnel can be locked from both sides so that the isolators can be separated and one of them used as transport isolator. The living room for the baby is 0.75 m high, 0.7 m wide and 1.5 m long for the first year of life, and 1.0 m high for the second year of life. Five neoprene gloves allow manipulations within the isolator. The outlet port is built so that used outgoing material is passed into a dip tank filled with phenol after being wrapped in a plastic bag. This germicidal trap enables the attending personnel to withdraw all items from the isolation system very quickly so that blood specimen etc. can be obtained without important delay of time. Infusions are performed by leading a tubing set through the germicidal trap. The isolation system for the age above 2 years until approximately 5 years consists of a larger bed isolator, storage isolator and a playground with dimensions of 2 m high, 2.5 m wide and 3 m long. Seven neoprene gloves are attached to the playground so that the infant can be caught from the outside in every situation.

23

Gnotobiotic care in decontamination. The decontamination therapy of the adults, applied throughout the isolation period, consisted of daily bathing with TEGO tenside (Cl_2-H_{25}-NH-C_2H_4-NH-CH_2-COOH), a surface disinfecting agent, inhalation of neomycin sulfate, bacitracin and nystatin, the treatment of the oral cavity with hexetidine and a combination of non-absorbable antimicrobial agents (BANEPON: Bacitracin 160,000 units, neomycin sulfate 3.0 g, polymixin B 200 mg and nystatin 6 mio units/day). This antibiotic regimen has been given up to 9 weeks and to a total dose of 207.0 g neomycin sulfate, 13.8 g polymyxin B, 11 mio units bacitracin and 414 mio units nystatin without limiting side effects.

The following regimen had been instituted to decontaminate the two infants: Surface disinfecting agents were used to clean the skin. The TEGO compound used may cause microtraumatic lesions. Therefore the bath with TEGO 103 S was followed by a bath with sterile water and the application of sterile baby oil.

Antibiotic ointments and sprays (neomycin, bacitracin, gentamycin) were applied to treat ear, nose, throat and prepuce.

Absorbable antibiotics were given to eliminate bacteria in places not to be treated locally (ampicillin).

Non-absorbable antibiotics to eliminate the intestinal microflora were given, including fungistatics, to prevent fungal overgrowth (neomycin sulfate, polymyxin E and nystatin).

Results

In the adult patients the decontamination treatment resulted in a markedly decreased variety of the microbial flora as indicated by discovering only one or occasionally two microbes in the samples. A large number of the swabs and the fecal and urine specimens have been sterile when cultured microbiologically. Of 378 skin swabs 177 (47%) and of 226 fecal samples 164 (73%) did not show any bacterial growth. Whereas 99% of the skin swabs remained negative for fungal growth, 124 of 226 (55%) of the fecal samples contained *Candida species.* Only 5 of 73 (7%) of swabs of the oral cavity remained negative for bacterial growth. The findings suggest that only elimination of a number of bacterial strains occurs under the non-resorbable antibiotic treatment, but "germfree states" or bacteria- and fungi-free states, respectively, could not be observed. These findings correspond with the results of other investigators. However, of 728 evaluated observation days only on 110 (15%) was the body temperature above 38°C. The susceptibility to infection could be characterized by granulocytopenia below 1500/μl on 635 of 728 evaluated days (87%) and below 500/μl on 398 days (55%). Though this study was not controlled by a randomized group, the incidences of infection seemed to be low compared with the experience of leukemia treatment on the normal ward. The survival rate 30 days after the discontinuation of the gnotobiotic care was 76% (19 of 25 treatments). But so far by the applied antibiotic regimen, germfree states could not be achieved and mono- or di-flora occurred in those cases in which bacteria had been resistant to all antibiotics available. This led to the fatal event of one of the patients due to a monoassociation of an aerobacter resistant to all antibiotics except gentamycin sulfate, which was not available as nonresorbable agent.

This means that the decontamination procedures in adults are not yet optimal and can cause hazardous shifting of the microflora, thus eventually resulting in adverse effects. Retrospectively controlled patient studies (2) and the described comparatively high survival rate indicate that gnotobiotic care may offer definite advantages. However, more studies have to be executed by randomizing the patient groups in advance as it is performed by the E.O.R.T.C. (European Organization for Research on Treatment of Cancer) Gnotobiotic Project Group (3). Better results have been achieved in the infants characterized above regarding the elimination of microbes.

Eight weeks after the decontamination, *Escherichia coli* interm. from urine or feces of E. R. and *Aerobacter aerogenes* from urine of W. R. could be cultured, thus demonstrating the suppression of the microbial flora but only partial elimination.

After 8 months of decontamination in E. R., the following microbes could be cultured occasionally: *Candida albicans, Staphylococcus epidermidis,* and enterobacter (trignotophoric state). In W. R., *Klebsiella sp.* and *S. epidermidis* could be cultured rarely (dignotophoric state). When microbes could be cultured under the suppression by antibiotics, they were mostly found in throat, feces, and urine in both children. The antibiotic regimen has been changed, therefore. Gentamycin sulfate and nystatin have been given as nonabsorbable antimicrobial agents. Ampicillin and Dicloxacillin completed the antibiotic therapy (Table I).

In child W. R., only at the plastic wall of his isolator, *S. epidermidis* could be cultured twice during 15 consecutive weeks. This finding can be explained by accidental contamination of the swabs outside the isolation system. The antibiotic regimen was then discontinued, whereas the fungistatic nystatin was still given. One week after the discontinuation of the antibiotics, two spore-forming bacilli, *B. macerans* and *B. polymyxa,* could be cultured on skin, urine and feces. At the same time these spore-forming bacilli could be detected in the nystatin compound that was obviously contaminated by the producer. The nystatin was then discontinued and no fungal growth observed afterwards. To attempt the elimination of the spore-forming bacilli, further antibiotic therapy was given consisting of gentamycin sulfate. However, the said bacilli could be cultured occasionally under this suppressive therapy. In 9 of 77 urine samples (12%) and in 9 of 72 fecal samples (13%) the spore-forming bacilli were found.

25

TABLE I.

	Absorbable antibiotics	Days	Daily dose	Total dose
E. R.	Ampicillin	252	1.5 g	378.0 g
	Dicloxacillin	252	1.0 g	252.0 g
	Clotrimacole	28	1.0 g	28.0 g
W. R.	Ampicillin	63	1.8 g	113.4 g
	Dicloxacillin	63	1.2 g	75.6 g
	Nonabsorbable anti-microbial agents			
E. R.	Gentamycin sulfate	462	500-2000 mg	349.5 g
	Nystatin	436	3.0-4.0 Mio	1.64^9 I.U.
W. R.	Gentamycin sulfate	252	500 mg	126.0 g
	Nystatin	82	2.3 Mio	0.18×10^9 I.U.

In child E. R., all microbes could be eliminated except *Enterobacter sp.*, appearing on the plates in two colony types, and *C. albicans.* These germs could be cultured from the fecal samples only occasionally. Thus, suppression was evident and the lack of signs of infection indicated satisfying control by the antibiotic treatment.

At the end of the decontamination therapy in both infants a dignoto-phoric state was achieved after a temporary "germfree state" (bacteria- and fungi-.free) of child W. R. After the improvement of the immune system of both infants (4) it was decided to reconstitute a "normal intestinal flora" before termination of isolation in order to control any unforeseen event. To minimize the unknown risk, the inoculation of the bacteria was performed step by step, so that any possible emerging infection by the implanted bacteria could be treated by antibiotics elected on the basis of previously known sensitivity tests.

Two strains of bifidobacteria and subsequently single bacterial strains were inoculated in child W. R., each after an interval of observation. Bifidobacteria (No. 11A and L3) were given for one week at the quantity of 1×10^6 and subsequently of 1×10^{10} each for two weeks. After an observation period of five months during which the stable colonization of the bifidobacteria was followed up, *B. vulgatis* (BM 137) were given in thioglycollate in the number of 2×10^6 by oral route as well as by rectal implantation. Four months after the successful implantation of the *Bacteroides sp.*, *E. coli* were given by oral and rectal implantation of 2×10^6 bacteria. Two weeks later *S. faecalis* was implanted by oral and rectal application of 2×10^6 bacteria and 2 weeks later followed by the implantation of *S. epidermidis* also by oral and rectal application of 2×10^6. One week later a 1.0 g fecal specimen, obtained from a

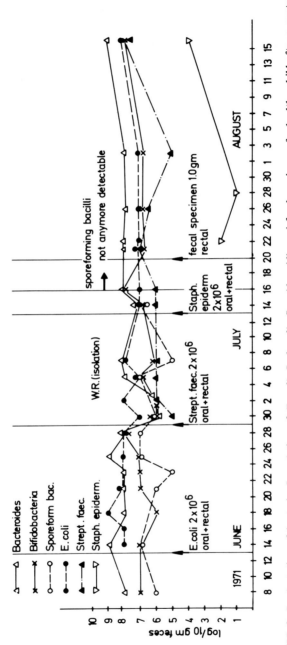

FIG. 2. Implantation of bacteria. Inoculation of *E. coli, S. faecalis, S. epidermidis,* and fecal specimen of a healthy child after a penta-gnotophoric state has been reached (two strains of bifido bacteria, two strains of spore-forming bacilli and bacteroides).

healthy child, was implanted rectally (Fig. 2).

After the discontinuation of the antibiotics in the dignotophoric E. R., a fecal specimen of child W. R. was implanted, when W. R. had been associated with bacteroides, bifidobacteria and spore-forming bacilli. Two weeks later, 2×10^6 S. faecalis and 2×10^6 E. coli were given rectally, followed by the implantation of 2×10^6 of S. epidermidis and 1 week later followed by the implantation of 1.0 g fecal specimen of a healthy child.

All the implanted bacteria have been colonized successfully. There were no direct signs of microbial interaction except that the spore-forming bacilli in both children could not be detected any more after the implantation of S. epidermidis and C. albicans has never been detected in the feces of E. R. after an anaerobic and subsequently an aerobic microflora had been implanted. Furthermore, the implantation of Bacteroides sp., Bifidobacteria sp., S. faecalis and E. coli did not seem to have any adverse or enhancing effect on the number of those microorganisms per g feces, that had been colonized already.

After the release from the isolation to the ordinary environment the follow-up of the intestinal microflora for two months showed a stable composition. Occasionally new bacteria could be found in W. R.: C. albicans and Staphylococcus aureus. In child E. R., changes of the microflora occurred more rapidly and the following microbes have been detected in the intestinal flora during 3 months: Citrobacter freundii, Proteus sp., and hemolytic E. coli. The microflora of the oral cavity was immediately changing its composition by several strains of bacteria usually found in the throat that have been acquired in the ordinary environment.

The isolation techniques have been proven satisfactory for the purpose of prevention of contamination in both adults and children (5). Two sources of possible contamination had not been eliminated: oral drugs or other drugs contaminated by the producer and possibly necessary transfusions of blood or blood contents that are associated with microorganisms in case of a bacteremia (viremia, fungemia) of the donor or in case of the contamination by processing of the transfused blood, i.e. to obtain platelets (6).

Summary

After a training session of only a few hours, nurses, doctors, physical therapists and other personnel in the hospital have been able to treat babies in such an isolated environment. During the time of confinement the physical development of the infants has been almost within normal limits. Despite a 2½ year life in a hospital environment and approximately the same time in isolation without the skin contact these infants did not show the severe psychological problems of hospitalized children. Never before has it been reported that human beings can live without an intestinal microflora and with sterile nutrition for such a long time, as described here. Germfree states could be observed for short periods of only days in babies that have been delivered germfree (7, 8).

From the microbiological observations it may be assumed that child W. R. could be decontaminated and kept bacteria- and fungi-free for some time. Knowing the fact that children with combined immune deficiency are highly susceptible to viral infection, it may be concluded that these children were virus-free also, since there were no signs of viral infection during the whole period of confinement in isolation.

The reconventionalization of the children was planned in such a way that each step of this procedure could be controlled strictly. It was felt that the composition of a "normal microflora" in the intestinal tract of the children, after being reconventionalized, should be able to compete with transitory organisms and thus protect against infection by potential pathogens. In addition to the main flora of the anaerobic *Bacteroides sp.* and *Bifidobacteria sp.* and the obligatory aerobic bacteria *E. coli* and *S. faecalis, S. epidermidis* was chosen because it is occasionally detected in the feces but definitely obligatory in the skin flora of healthy individuals (9, 10).

The inoculation of the single bacteria step by step showed successful colonization, whether given each alone or 2-4 species in combination, given orally (bifidobacteria), or orally and rectally, or rectally alone.

Host-microbial relationships are difficult to evaluate in human beings. In fact, only under gnotobiotic conditions conclusions may be drawn from microbiological and physiological investigations. Only few data are available from animal or *in vitro* experiments (11-14). These data suggest a large variety of specific effects of microbes on the host's physiology. But, perhaps none of these findings may be of significance for the human situation because they are achieved in different species, under different alimentation and, most important, in exgermfree, after the microbial association, gnotophoric animals. There are not any experiments done in this regard to our knowledge. So far, significant signs of interaction could not be seen in the described children which could be attributed to the gnotophoric states.

References

1. Lerche, M., and Reuter, G., *Zbl. Bakt. I., Abt. Orig. 179:* 354 (1960).
2. Bodey, G. P., Gehan, E. A., Freireich, E. J., and Frei, E. II, *Amer. Med. Sci. 262:* 138 (1971).
3. E.O.R.T.C. Gnotobiotic Project Group, Europ. J. Cancer, (In Press).
4. Flad, H. D., Genscher, U., Dietrich, M., Trepel, U., Teller, W., and Fliedner, T. M., *Acta Paed. Scand.,* (In Preparation).
5. Dietrich, M., Meyer, H., Krieger, D., Genscher, U., and Fliedner, T. M., *Europ. J. Clin. Biol. Res.,* (In Press).
6. Buchholz, D. H., Young, V. M., Friedman, N. R., Reilley, J. A., and Mardiney, M. R., *New Engl. J. Med. 282:* 433 (1971).

7. Van der Waaij, D., Germfree Delivery (Film), Gnotobiotic Club, London, England, October 10, 1968.
8. Barnes, R. D., Fairweather, D. V., Reynolds, E. O., Tuffrey, M. and Holliday, J., *J. Obstet. Gyn. Brit. Commonw. 75:* 689 (1968).
9. Haenel, H., *Amer. J. Clin. Nutr. 23:* 1433 (1970).
10. Somerville, D. A., *Br. J. Derm. 81:* 248 (1969).
11. Hentges, D. J., *Amer. J. Clin. Nutr. 23:* 1451 (1970).
12. Luckey, T. D., *Amer. J. Clin. Nutr. 23:* 1533 (1970).
13. Schaedler, R. W., Dubos, R., and Costello, R., *J. Exptl. Med. 122:* 77 (1965).
14. Tanami, J., *J. Chiba Med. Soc. 35:* 1 (1959).

PATIENT ISOLATORS DESIGNED IN THE NETHERLANDS

D. van der Waaij
Radiobiological Institute TNO, 151 Lange Kleiweg,
Rijswijk (Z. H.), The Netherlands

J. M. Vossen
Department of Pediatrics, University Hospital,
Leiden, The Netherlands

and

C. Korthals Altes
Sophia Children's Hospital, Rotterdam, The Netherlands

Introduction

Patients require protective isolation under certain circumstances, e.g., when the immune defense capacity is impaired. This isolation, however, often involves "imprisonment" for a number of weeks. This means that consideration must be given to making this period of confinement as tolerable as possible while at the same time maintaining a protective environment. In order to meet these provisions, three aspects were of major concern when the present system was designed. These were: 1) bacteriological, 2) nursing and medical care, and 3) psychological.

Methods

Bacteriological Aspects. 1) The isolator must be safe and must prevent contact or aerogenic contamination; 2) it must be easily cleaned and sterilized; 3) a simple device is required for the introduction of sterile materials and for the removal of used or soiled items; 4) there must be two interconnected chambers in order to accomplish proper decontamination of the patient (1); 5) a bath tub should be included for bathing and for skin disinfection of the patient; 6) there should be toilet facilities for the elimination and removal of body wastes; 7) the cleaning and sterilization of the isolator during patient occupancy should be accomplished with little difficulty. The possibility must be provided to move the patient to one of the two chambers while these operations were in progress and then to switch back so that the just occupied chamber could receive the same

31

treatment (Figs. 1 and 2); and 8) there must be the possibility for direct isolation, if patients who under immune suppressives become contagious.

Nursing and Medical Care. The design of the system should be such that as few demands as possible are made on the nursing and medical personnel. This is the most expensive aspect of patient isolation; therefore, the amount of labor involved should be kept to a minimum. The patient must be easily accessible from at least two sides. It must be possible to quickly transfer materials into and out of the isolator. The necessary medical treatment should be accomplished with as few impediments as is possible.

Psychological Aspects. In order that the patient remain in "contact" with the outside environment, there should be a clear view to all sides. There should be, however, the possibility of complete privacy when desired. A telephone, radio, and television which may be controlled from the inside should be present. The blowers of the isolator should have a low noise level and there should be no wind effect. The design of the isolator should be such that family and other

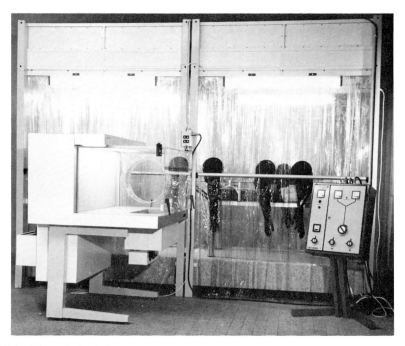

FIG. 1. View of the isolator. Note the cross-flow cabinet used for the introduction of presterilized materials, which is closed by a double hinged flap. Also can be seen the plastic drapes and the neoprene gloves. The horizontal bar is meant to prevent the patient from falling out of the unit. These bars can be removed very easily by lifting, before patient handling and bedmaking, by means of the neoprene gloves.

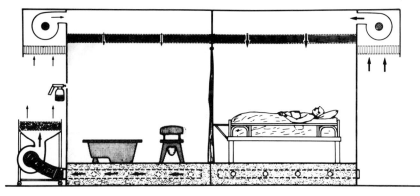

FIG. 2. Schematic diagram showing the situation in the isolator during peracetic acid sterilization. The tubing system in the platform of the sprayed compartment is connected to a sodalime-blower unit (at the left hand side of the isolator) for suction and neutralization of peracetic acid fumes.

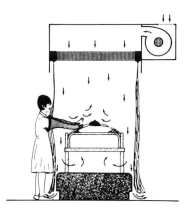

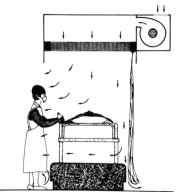

FIG. 3. Diagram showing the situation when the isolator is used with the drapes closed.

FIG. 4. Diagram showing the air pattern when the isolator is used with the drapes opened. The blower speed is previously increased so as to keep the air velocity at 0.5 m/sec in the opening.

visitors may come close enough to permit private conversations. If for psychological or other reasons the patient can no longer tolerate the situation, there should be means provided for exit at any time. In other words, the patient should not feel involuntarily enclosed.

Type of Isolator: Down-Flow or Cross-Flow? Because of the psychological and nursing aspects, in particular, it was felt that an attempt should be made to use the laminar flow (L.F.) type of isolation system. This would open up the possibility of having "open communication" with the patient when required. The patient would be more readily accessible than in a plastic enclosure (2-6). It

33

was difficult to make the choice between the down-flow (7) and cross-flow mechanisms (8-10), but the down-flow system was adopted. This seemed the safest for a number of reasons (11), including the following: 1) air turbulences caused by the patient remain confined to the inside of the isolator when created at more than 20 cm from the opening; 2) extreme low noise level when the unit is used closed; 3) the isolator could be of such dimensions that every spot could be reached from the outside; and 4) for contagious patients, two-directional protection could be more readily provided. That is, the patient could be more easily protected from the environment and personnel and vice versa (Fig. 5).

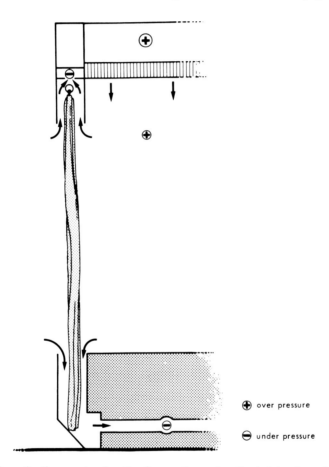

FIG. 5. Schematic diagram showing the flow pattern when the isolator is used for two directional isolation. The tubing system in the platform as well as the perforated tube just above the rails suspending the drapes are in this situation connected to a blower-filter unit which maintains an underpressure in the tubes.

Results

The Down-Flow Isolation System as adopted is depicted in Figures 1 through 4.

Bacteriological Testing. Before actual use by patients, the units are tested for safety by aerosolization of 10^4 *Escherichia coli* cells per m^3 of air both inside and outside of the isolator. When sprayed inside, no cells should be detected in the outside environment and vice versa. This is determined by slit-sampling and settling plates containing the appropriate culture medium.

Isolation of Babies (Congenital Combined Immunological Deficiencies). For babies, we prefer a larger cross-flow cabinet equipped with a double-hinged flap with gloves (12). Here again the flap permits, when closed, reduction of air volume, which leads to a reduction of noise and prevents dehydration of the baby. The low activity level and small dimensions of young babies makes the use of a cross-flow cabinet possible.

Transportation of the baby to the X-ray room, for example, is performed in a rigid type of isolator which is otherwise permanently connected to the cross-flow unit by means of a 60 cm diameter rigid tube. When the child is in the cabinet, the transport isolator is used for the storage of items. In the cabinets, larger items, which should be avoided, will strongly disturb the flow pattern. Older babies that move violently also may cause air turbulences when the flap is

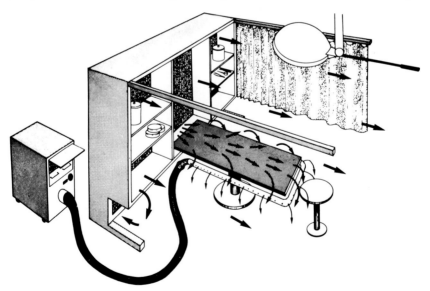

FIG. 6. Diagram showing the flow pattern of the mobile cross-flow unit, which also exists during surgery. When the surgical team disturbs the horizontal air flow, the protective air stream above the patient remains uninfluenced.

opened. Therefore, these should be isolated in a down-flow isolator. The interior of these cabinets is also sterilizable by peracetic acid.

Mobile Surgical Laminar Flow Unit. To make surgical operation of an isolated patient possible again, protection from airborne contamination during surgery, which was sought in the application of L.F. Down-Flow systems, had to be discarded since they have a very high sedimentation index (13), while cross-flow systems operated with an air velocity of 0.5 m/sec have an extremely low sedimentation index. Therefore, a cross-flow device was constructed (Fig. 6). To minimize air turbulences by the surgical team standing along both long sides of the table, a U-formed canal is attached 30 cm beneath the surface of the table. The canal is perforated and connected to a blower unit which supplies it with sterile air which is blown out of the perforations at an angle of 30° downward. This sucks air from above the table, preventing contaminated air from rising to the table surface.

The cross-flow unit is maintained at an air velocity of 0.50 m/sec during operation.

References

1. van der Waaij, D., de Vries, J. M., and Lekkerkerk, J. E. C., in "Infections and Immunosuppression in Sub-Human Primates," Munksgaard, Copenhagen, (1970).
2. Barnes, R. D., Tuffery, M., and Cook, R., *Lancet 1:* 622 (1968).
3. Bodey, G. P., Hart, J. Freireich, E. J., and Frei, E., *Cancer 22:* 1018 (1968).
4. Levitan, A. A., and Perry, S. *Amer. J. Med. 44:* 234 (1968).
5. Meindersma, T. E., and van der Waaij, D., *Fol. Med. Neerland. 11:* 76 (1968).
6. Schwarts, S. A., and Perry, S., *J.A.M.A. 197:* 105 (1966).
7. Huszar, R. J., *J.A.M.A. 207:* 549 (1969).
8. Bodey, G. P., Freireich, E. J., and Frei, E., *Cancer 24:* 972 (1969).
9. Lidwell, O. M., and Towers, A. G., *J. Hyg. Camb. 67:* 95 (1969).
10. Solberg, C. O., Matsen, J. M., Versley, D., Wheeler, D. J., Good, R. A., and Meuwissen, H. J., *Appl. Microbiol. 21:* 209 (1971).
11. van der Waaij, D., and Andreas, A. H., *J. Hyg. Camb. 69:* 83 (1971).
12. de Koning, J., van der Waaij, D., Vossen, J. M., Versprille, A., and Dooren, L. J., *Maandschr. Kindergeneesk. 38:* 1 (1970).
13. Blowers, R., and Crew, B., *J. Hyg. Camb. 58:* 427 (1960).

A SIMPLIFIED PLASTIC FLEXIBLE FILM ISOLATOR SYSTEM FOR THE GERMFREE DELIVERY AND MAINTENANCE OF INFANTS WITH IMMUNE DEFICIENCY

Raphael Wilson, Mary Ann South and *L. Russell Malinak*
The Baylor College of Medicine, Houston, Texas 77025

and

Alexander R. Lawton, Max D. Cooper and *Charles E. Flowers Jr.*
The University of Alabama Medical Center
Birmingham, Alabama 35233, U.S.A.

Introduction

The few germfree deliveries of human infants performed to date have employed highly technical equipment requiring specially trained personnel (1). They have also necessitated extensive modifications of routine medical and nursing procedures, and have involved high cost. All of these deliveries with the exception of the first one (2) were made in situations in which there was a high probability that the newborn would be immune-deficient. With the increased awareness of immune deficiency disease in infants, it is desirable to have a simplified and less costly system for delivering babies germfree when the likelihood of congenital immune deficiency is great and for maintaining them under germfree or gnotobiotic conditions until their immunological competence can be evaluated and appropriate treatment applied if a deficiency is present. Such a system has been devised and was used in 1970 in Birmingham and in 1971 in Houston. In both cases there was a history of immune deficiency and death among infants previously born to the presenting pregnant females.

Methods

The basic isolator system consists of two polyvinyl flexible film units comparable to those designed by Trexler for germfree animals (3). One unit, called the crib isolator, houses the baby and is connected by a sterile plastic sleeve to a second unit, called the supply isolator, where materials needed for the routine care of the child are stored (Fig. 1). A similar system was first used in Germany for the treatment of immune deficient twins (4). The original crib

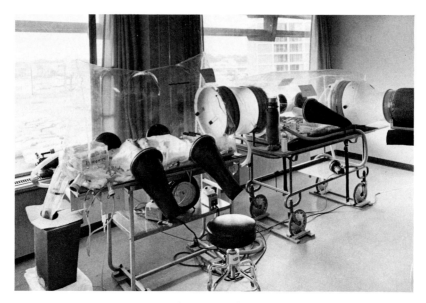

FIG. 1. Flexible film isolator system for the germfree delivery and maintenance of infants with immune deficiency.

isolator was fitted with separate filters for air and oxygen mounted under the isolator to reduce the number of possible obstructions to attending personnel. A stethoscope is fixed in the wall of the isolator through a nipple. Two extra nipples are provided to accommodate intravenous equipment and leads for monitoring instruments if they are needed. At the end of the crib isolator is a dunk tank to facilitate the rapid removal of laboratory specimens, empty formula bottles and food jars, soiled diapers and linens, etc.

The supply isolator has an air supply independent of the crib isolator. The doors or caps between the crib and supply isolators are normally in place although the two units remain connected by the sterile sleeve. This is aimed at preventing the contamination of both isolators if an accident should occur with one of them. The supply isolator has two 18-inch doors, one to connect to the crib isolator and the other to supply cylinders. Supplies are sterilized by either steam or ethylene oxide, depending on their nature, in the filter wrapped fenestrated cylinders now common in the germfree research laboratory. Formula and baby foods are commercially available as sterile preparations; so they are not re-sterilized. Instead, the containers are introduced into the supply isolator from cylinders exposed to ethylene oxide to sterilize the exterior surfaces of the bottles and jars from which the labels have been removed.

To perform the germfree deliveries, the preparation of the operating rooms, the patients, and the surgical teams was made in the routine manner with an intensification of precautions to minimize the chance of airborne and contact contamination of the infants in the operating room. A primary low transverse Cesarean section was performed in the usual way and the infant was placed immediately after clamping and cutting the cord into the sterile crib isolator which contained resuscitation equipment and other items ordinarily available in the operating room for the emergency care of newborns. As soon as the attending pediatricians were satisfied with the baby's status, the isolator was removed from the operating room and taken to the nursery, where it was connected to the supply isolator.

Beginning at this time, the babies were attended by the nurses usually on duty in this section of the hospital who had been given an hour's instruction in the operation of the isolators. Procedures such as roentgenology and the collecting of blood and other laboratory specimens were performed by hospital personnel regularly assigned to such tasks. All reported minimal inconvenience of working in the system (Fig. 2).

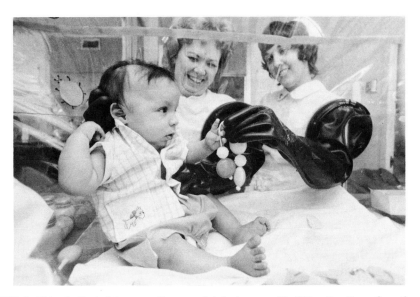

FIG. 2. The plastic isolator permits normal infant care with little alteration of routine procedures.

The success of the system, of course, is measured in microbiological terms. The monitoring consists of taking cultures twice weekly of feces, nose, throat, various skin sites, the isolator gloves and walls, and formula and food. These are incubated aerobically and anaerobically. Where applicable, direct smears are made and stained.

Results

The Birmingham baby remained germfree during the one week it was isolated, at the end of which time it was removed from the isolator, since it had been determined that the baby did not have an immune deficiency. The Houston baby, though, proved to have severe combined immune deficiency and has been in isolation now for seven months. Soon after birth, he became contaminated with *Alcaligenes faecalis* (Fig. 3). The dunk tank was the suspected source of contamination, since *A. faecalis* was cultured from the disinfecting solution, which had an erroneously low concentration of the disinfectant.

To decontaminate the baby, colimycin was administered orally, but without success, in spite of the fact that it was effective *in vitro* against *A. faecalis*. This failure was attributed to the use of an intravenous preparation, colistin methane sulfonate, selected to be given orally since its sterility was more certain than the oral preparation, colistin sulfate. However, this form needs to be activated by tissue hydrolysis and is ineffective unless given intravenously. Gentamicin then replaced colistin and the contaminant quickly disappeared.

Several weeks later, *Staphylococcus epidermidis* was cultured from the baby. This contaminant was traced to small pinhole breaks in the gloves. A course of treatment with gentamicin and then with kanamycin failed to eradicate this contaminant. Since no infection was present and the organism did not seem to present a threat to the baby, no further efforts were made immediately to eliminate it. In January, a *Clostridium sp.* was detected in the cultures. No defects in the isolator were identified, and the source of this organism is undetermined.

Prior to doing a skin graft in March to evaluate cellular immunity, it was decided that the elimination of both of these organisms was desirable. Procaine penicillin, highly effective against them both, was given orally. Within a few weeks, the organisms were no longer detectable, although the level of penicillin in the gut was low as a result of acid destruction. After several weeks, the penicillin was discontinued. Subsequently, however, both organisms have reappeared, and the baby has again been placed on penicillin. In the meantime, the relative merits of the germfree vs. a gnotobiotic state are being weighed.

The ease with which hospital personnel adapted to caring for the baby in the isolator led us to consider the feasibility of transferring the units to the parents' home. The parents were judged capable of attending the baby at home, although neither has a medical or technical background. The psychological advantages of being at home were believed great for both the baby and the family.

Consequently, the baby was sent home first on a five-day trial visit at Thanksgiving. Since this visit went very well, a longer visit of two weeks was made at Christmas. A third visit at home of two and a half weeks was terminated

40

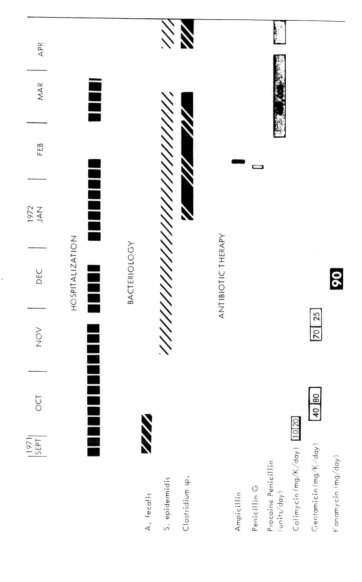

FIG. 3. The microbiological and antibiotic therapy record of an immune-deficient child during the first seven months of isolation.

41

only because we wanted to hospitalize the baby while skin grafting was done to determine his cellular immunity. At the same time he was transferred into a larger isolator to accommodate his increased physical activity.

He went home again before Easter and is still there after one month. To date he has spent a little more than a third of his life at home. Once a week technicians go to the home to draw blood, take microbiological cultures, transfer supplies into the isolator, and remove soiled and used items. His presence at home has not been disruptive to family life and has been no heavy burden on the parents.

The baby is being observed closely by two groups interested in his psychological development. Both groups agree that the child is progressing normally, is a happy baby, and has suffered no ill effects to date from his isolation. The length of his stay in the isolator is uncertain at present. It is hoped that during the coming year he will spontaneously develop immune competence. If he does not, a plan for supplying him with immune capability will be developed.

Conclusion

It is concluded that plastic flexible film isolators are practical in the delivery and maintenance of infants with immune deficiency. They provide a system than can be employed in any well equipped general hospital without great expense, elaborate procedures, or highly specialized personnel. They also make it possible to transport an immune-deficient child home without compromising the barrier, and thus minimizing the psychological effects of prolonged hospitalization.

Acknowledgements

Supported in part by U.S.P.H.S. Grants RR 3212, AI 08227, K4 AI 238230, CA 12093, K6 CA 14219, and CA 03367.

The authors are sincerely grateful to George Cassady, Paul Kincade, and Douglas Martin at the University of Alabama Medical Center, and to Lucien Landry, Ellen Hunt, and Anthony Mastromarino at the Baylor College of Medicine for their valuable assistance and cooperation.

References

1. Barnes, R. D., in "Germfree Biology: Experimental and Clinical Aspects," (E. A. Mirand and N. Back, eds.), Plenum Press, New York, p. 45, (1969).
2. Alpert, S., Gray, J., Romney, S., and Levenson, S. M., *Lancet 1:* 841 (1969).
3. Trexler, P. C., and Reynolds, L. I., *Appl. Microbiol. 5:* 406 (1957).
4. Flad, H. D., Genscher, U., Dietrich, M., Krieger, D., Trepel, F. W., Hochapfel, G., Teller, W., and Fliedner, T. M., *Rev. Europ. Etudes Clin. Biol. 16:* 328 (1971).

BIOMEDICAL APPLICATIONS OF LAMINAR AIRFLOW

L. L. Coriell and *G. J. McGarrity*
Institute for Medical Research
Camden, New Jersey 08103, U.S.A.

and

W. S. Blakemore
The Graduate Hospital
Philadelphia, Pennsylvania, U. S. A.

Introduction

The two objectives of the present study were: 1) to determine the relative efficacy of different flow rates on removal of particulate airborne contaminants, and 2) to describe a new laminar flow rack and cage system for isolation of laboratory mice.

Methods

Flow rate studies were performed in an 6 x 10 ft. room in which the entire ceiling is made of high efficiency particular air (HEPA) filters capable of removing 99.97% of particles 0.3 microns in diameter. The vertical velocity of the filtered air can be varied from 10 to 100 fpm and the air leaves the room through exhaust grills near the floor on two sides of the room. Ninety percent of the air is recirculated and cooling coils are included for temperature control.

Aerosols of latex particles or of T3 bacteriophage were generated with a Schoeffel nebulizer placed in the center of the room at a height of three feet and samples were collected three feet upstream or three feet laterally at velocities of 10, 12, 18, 26, 37, 49, 53, 67, and 72 fpm. Latex particles with a diameter of 1.0 micron were counted with an electronic particle counter (Dynac) which samples 0.1 ft^3 air per minute. T3 bacteriophage suspensions having a titer of approximately 10^{10} PFU/ml when nebulized provided many particles less than 1.0 micron as determined by Andersen samplers. In the present studies phage aerosols were sampled with all glass impingers (AGI-4) and assayed by standard techniques.

Results

Figure 1 illustrates results from sampling of latex aerosols upstream of the nebulizer. The curve is the average of four tests. With static air in the room the particulate counts averaged 5×10^5 per cubic foot of air. With a vertical air flow rate of 10 fpm the particle count was reduced one log, at 20 fpm 3 logs, and at 30 fpm 4 logs or 99.99%.

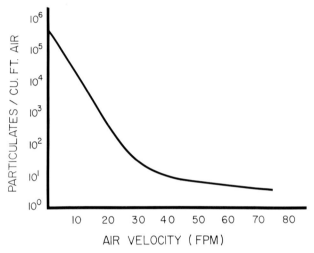

FIG. 1. Effect of air velocity on upstream diffusion of latex aerosols generated with a Schoeffel nebulizer.

In tests in which the sampler was located three feet lateral to the nebulizer the curve was even steeper and better than 4 log reduction of particulates was achieved at a vertical flow rate of 20 feet per minute (Fig. 2). These results are obtained with massive contamination by means of a nebulized aerosol of latex particles which makes it possible to obtain fairly reproducible results.

The efficiency of various flow rates were also observed during a routine microbiological procedure. Thirty-two bacterial settling plates were exposed around the periphery of a table on which a technician assayed T3 *Escherichia coli* bacteriophage. This required preparation of serial dilutions of phage and preparation of pour plates. Each assay required approximately 30 minutes. The number of viable particulates collected on the settling plates in different air velocities was recorded and averages of five separate tests were as follows: the average number of viable airborne particles sedimenting onto 32 TSA plates was 2.23 per hour when the fans were not in operation. With the vertical air flow at 10 fpm the average plaques were reduced 7-fold to 0.35 where it remained for air flows of 18, 26, and 37 fpm. That these organisms were sedimenting during the test and not when the plates were being handled at the beginning and end of

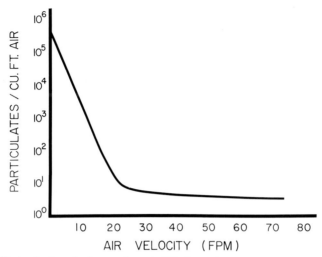

FIG. 2. Effect of air velocity on lateral diffusion of latex aerosols generated with a Schoeffel nebulizer.

the test period was established by additional control plates that were opened only at the beginning and at the end of the test period.

Engineering Studies. Possible drawbacks to use of laminar airflow include cost, noise, control of temperature and bulkiness of equipment. We have studied some of these parameters in the variable flow room. With increased air velocity the operating cost of the current used to move the air at 72 fpm is approximately twice the cost at 10 fpm (56 vs 28 cents per day). With the recirculation of 90 percent of the air the temperature rise must be controlled by passing the air over a cooling coil, otherwise the room temperature increases about 3½°F for each 10 fpm increment of air flow rate. The noise level with zero air velocity was 45 decibels (dB) on the A scale, and this increased to 52 dB at 10 fpm, 56 dB at 18 fpm, 61 dB at 26 fpm, 67 dB at 49 fpm, 71 dB at 60 fpm and 74 dB at 72 fpm.

A laminar airflow hood for housing laboratory rodents (Anigard Hood, Baker Co., Sanford, Maine) has been designed and tested (Fig. 3). The hood incorporates HEPA filtration, a variable air velocity inside the hood of 25 to 40 fpm, automatic watering, and an air curtain of 160-210 fpm at the front opening, which restricts the passage of aerosols into and out of the hood. Eight cages, without bedding, are positioned inside the hood on lazy susan bearings for easy access. Feces and urine drop through the open cages to a collecting pan and are washed away by an automatic flushing device.

The effectiveness of the air curtain was determined by Andersen and Reyniers bacterial air samplers, AGI-4 samplers and by housing specific pathogen-free mice. Studies conducted in an animal room during cage cleaning

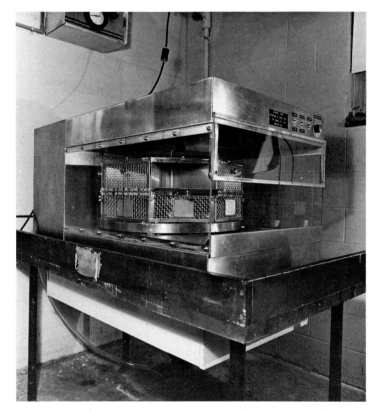

FIG. 3. Laminar flow hood for housing laboratory mice to prevent airborne spread of infection and to permit manipulation of the mice without removing them from the hood.

showed 108 CFU/ft^3 air in the laboratory and 1.3 CFU/ft^3 air inside the hood, an 83-fold reduction (average of 6 tests). The efficiency of the air curtain was greater than 99.99% in restricting T3 bacteriophage aerosols generated with a DeVilbiss nebulizer in 13 tests as shown in Table I.

The hood offers an effective method of housing infected animals and animals hypersusceptible to infection. The advantages of this mouse cage are as follows: It protects animals from airborne spread of infection from other animals in the same room. Watering and cage cleaning are automatic, and manipulation, inoculation, or examination of mice can be made without removing them from the laminar flow environment.

Conclusions

There have been many reports in the literature recommending the use of laminar flow rooms and cabinets for use in hospitals, research laboratories and

TABLE I. Bacteriophage Tests of the Anigard Hood

T3 phage nebulized 2 inches outside hood opening.
Sampling carried out 2 inches *inside* the hood.

Experiment	PFU/ft^3*	
	Laminar Flow Off	Laminar Flow On
1	1.5×10^4	0
2	1.1×10^4	0
3	3.2×10^4	0
4	3.2×10^4	0
5	1.5×10^4	0
6	3.2×10^3	0

*PFU/ft^3 = plaque forming units per cubic foot of air.

T3 phage nebulized inside the hood.
Sampling 2 inches *outside* the hood opening.

Experiment	Off	On
1	2.7×10^6	1.5×10^1
2	2.0×10^7	6.3×10^2
3	4.8×10^6	0
4	5.5×10^5	0
5	3.3×10^5	1.5×10^1
6	8.0×10^3	0
7	1.0×10^5	0

animal care rooms. Our studies indicate that in at least some areas use of the conventionally employed flow rate of 100 fpm is unnecessary and inefficient in terms of cost-effectiveness. More studies are needed on the basic design and performance of these systems for different applications and on their clinical significance in reducing infection.

Acknowledgements

The authors wish to thank Judi Sarama, Vicky Ammen, and Mary Federico for technical assistance.

These studies were supported by a grant from the John A. Hartford Foundation, General Research Support Grant FR-5582 from the National Institutes of Health, and Grant-in-Aid Contract N-43 from the State of New Jersey.

EVALUATIVE STUDY OF PATIENTS WITH ACUTE LEUKEMIA UNDER GNOTOBIOTIC CONDITIONS BY THE GNOTOBIOTIC PROJECT GROUP OF THE EUROPEAN ORGANIZATION FOR RESEARCH ON TREATMENT OF CANCER (E.O.R.T.C.)

D. van der Waaij
Radiobiological Institute TNO, Lange Kleiweg 151,
Rijswijk (Z. H.), The Netherlands

and

M. Dietrich
Hamatologische Abteilung, University of Ulm,
79 Ulm/Donau, West Germany

Introduction

Prevention of infections in patients with a decreased immune capacity, in general, has become urgent and has developed into a new branch of medicine: Clinical Gnotobiology. The two most important subjects of investigation in Clinical Gnotobiology are: 1) **Microbiological isolation of the patient**, in order to prevent contamination with microorganisms which are pathogenic for the patient (**exogenous infection**), and 2) **Bacteriological decontamination** of the patient to prevent **endogenous infections** resulting from (potentially) pathogenic microorganisms belonging to the patients own microflora.

In order to facilitate the efficient development of this new discipline in Western Europe, international cooperation was deemed necessary. For this purpose the Gnotobiotic Project Group was formed 4 years ago.

A prospective study on randomized patient groups seemed to be necessary to evaluate the efficiency of both isolation techniques and decontamination procedures (1). A certain minimum number of patients is required to obtain statistically significant data. Most centers in Europe, with only one or two beds for protective isolation, are not able to carry out such an investigation except on a long-term basis. The Gnotobiotic Project Group makes it possible to obtain the required data within a much shorter period.

Objectives

The objectives of the study are: 1) to investigate the validity of the use of

49

an isolation system to protect patients who are highly susceptible to infections; and 2) to evaluate and compare the efficiency of the systemic antibiotic treatment as a **curative measure** versus antibiotic decontamination of the digestive tract as a **preventive** type of **treatment**.

The groups of patients to be studied by the E.O.R.T.C. Gnotobiotic Project Group are listed in Table I. It was decided to confine the present study

TABLE I. Patient groups to be admitted to the evaluative study:

a) Acute leukemias
b) Chronic leukemia with bone-marrow deficiencies
c) Bone-marrow aplasias
d) Lymphoreticular malignancies
e) Solid tumors
f) Congenital immune deficiencies
g) Bone-marrow transplantations
h) Organ transplantations
i) Burns

to patients with Acute Leukemia because of their frequency in the various units within the Gnotobiotic Project Group and the mostly limited phase of increased susceptibility during remission-induction therapy.

Included in the study are patients undergoing chemotherapy for induction of remission. These patients are randomized on the basis of: 1) age (2 to 15, 16 to 40, and 41 to 60 years of age); 2) presence or absence of infection on admission, and 3) clinical history of the patient – 1, 2, or more induction therapy phases. Excluded are patients with psychological or psychiatric contra-indications, with renal failure (creatine clearance less than 60 ml/min/body surface), and with ages below 2 or above 60 years.

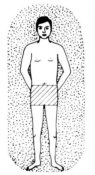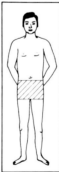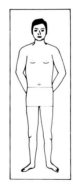

FIG. 1. Schematic representation of the three groups to which the patients are allocated randomly: (I) No isolation; (II) Protective isolation; (III) Protective isolation plus antibiotic decontamination.

During the screening phase, the criteria for admission are collected and reported to the Admissions Bureau of the **Statistical Center** in Ulm. After the randomization of the patient, this information is teletyped, and the admission phase begins. The patients are allocated by the Statistical Center randomly to three groups (Fig. 1): 1) treatment on the normal ward under standard hospital conditions, i.e., microorganisms are present in the environment and in the patient; 2) the second group receives treatment in isolation. This is accomplished either in a so-called ultra-clean ward or in a system for strict isolation (laminar airflow or plastic isolator). 3) The third group is treated under the same conditions as the second, but in combination with antibiotic decontamination of the digestive tract.

The decontamination and recontamination procedures are left to the discretion of the attending physician.

Criteria for Adequate Isolation

As a result of experimental findings in animals, the Project Group agreed that the **occurrence of new colonizations by potentially pathogenic (and actually pathogenic) species during isolation** should be investigated in the patients included in the study. New colonizations should not occur in an isolated patient when the barrier is intact. The newly colonizing species may be relatively non-pathogenic in a given case, but one cannot predict which species are going to colonize the patient.

The effect of isolation on the course of the disease in patients with a low defense capacity is expressed by the number of days that the patient suffers from exogenous infections. A day of infection is defined as each day with: a) **positive blood cultures**, whether correlated or not with increased body temperature; b) **clinical signs of infection** confirmed by bacteriological culturing; and c) **fever of unknown origin**, with clinical signs of infection (afterwards, correlation can be sought with one of the virus antigens selected).

The possible benefit of antibiotic decontamination for the patients with low defense capacity is investigated by the frequency of infections caused by endogenous microorganisms, i.e., those also isolated during the inventory on admission. The over-all number of days with infections is compared in the three groups.

Criterion for Adequate Antibiotic Decontamination

The efficiency of the various techniques for antibiotic decontamination in use is expressed by the number of samples (feces and throat swabs) that are negative for pathogenic and potentially pathogenic microbes.

Central Service Laboratories

Even if the isolation facilities are deemed adequate, routine monitoring of the patients' microflora is necessary. This involves culturing and typing for pathogenic and potentially pathogenic microorganisms, viruses, and parasites. It is quite a laborious task and not all laboratories have the personnel or facilities to perform the necessary tests. For the collection of valid data and to assure that patients receive maximum benefit, it is desirable that the various isolation systems in current use in Europe be compared as to certain parameters. In view of this, it was decided that identification of potentially pathogenic micro-organisms should be performed in central service laboratories (Fig. 2). Three such centers are now in operation: a Typing Center for Bacteriology, in Rijswijk, The Netherlands; one for Virology, in Brussels, Belgium; and one for Parasitology, in Nijmegen, The Netherlands.

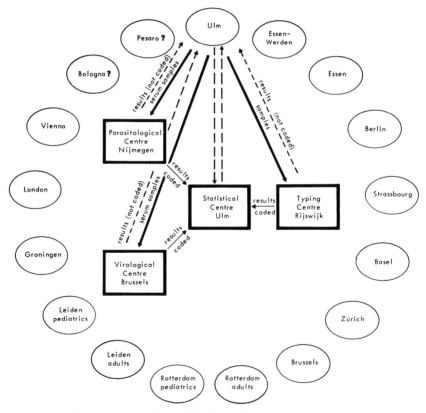

FIG. 2. Relationships among the participating units and the Central Service Centers. In this schematic representation, attention is focused on one Unit (Ulm).

Operation of the Typing Centers

Oral washings, fecal material, and isolates from infections from patients included in the study are routinely shipped in liquid nitrogen containers to the Typing Center at Rijswijk for bacteriological typing. There the samples are processed for typing of *Staphylococcus aureus, Pseudomonas aeruginosa,* and all *Enterobacteriaceae species.* The latter is accomplished by biotyping (2). Serum samples are mailed to the Parasitological and Virological Centers for the determination of antibody titers against *Pneumocytes carinii, Toxoplasma gondii*, and various **virus antigens** such as **cytomegalic** virus, **Herpes** virus, **measles** virus, and **respiratory** viruses. The role of the Statistical Center involves evaluation of results in addition to randomization of patients.

Clinical and Experimental Cooperation

The members of this Project Group are clinicians as well as scientists working with experimental animals. It is the general opinion of the Group that, particularly in antibiotic decontamination, which is still in the experimental phase, cooperation between basic researchers and clinical groups has to be very close.

Observations made by the clinicians can be investigated in experimental animal models, and data obtained in animal research can be considered in the patients' treatment immediately. It is known from work with germfree animals that many physiological mechanisms are different in a gnotobiote. A number of experiments have demonstrated that changes in decontaminated animals are similar to those seen in decontaminated patients.

Subgroups

A number of **subgroups** within the Gnotobiotic Project Group were formed to investigate certain problems more thoroughly. These include "psychological aspects of isolation," "virological infections in isolated patients," "epidemiological problems," and "tests to study the immune capacity of the patients as an indication for isolation." In this way, optimal use is made of the research facilities available in the participating units.

Especially in these subgroups, a close cooperation between basic research and clinical investigation exists.

References

1. "The Protocol of the Gnotobiotic Project Group," *Europ. J. Cancer 8:* 367 (1972).
2. van der Waaij, D., Vossen, J. M., and Speltie, T. M., *J. Hyg., Camb. 70:* 1 (1972).

A GAUNTLET ISOLATOR FOR HIP ARTHROPLASTY

P. C. Trexler
Royal Veterinary College, London

and

M. F. Pilcher
Bethnal Green Hospital, London, England

Introduction

Total hip replacement offers enormous benefits to the patient with disabling osteoarthritis of the hip. Unfortunately, the incidence of infection following this procedure is unacceptably high in many centers, and the result of such infection is nothing short of disastrous. Charnley (1) has developed a system consisting of a sterile enclosure within the theater and a "body exhaust" system for the operating team. However, this is a fairly expensive installation and would not necessarily be acceptable to other surgeons using a busy general theater.

A flexible film isolator for use in human surgery was described by Levenson *et al.* (2, 3). This isolator has been used routinely for a great variety of surgical procedures. However, it is rather expensive, so has not gained wide acceptance. While the half-suits used for the surgical team greatly assist in the freedom of movement within the sterile area, they do add to the expense of fabrication and require ventilation and communication apparatus for personnel.

Simpler gauntlet isolators have been used for human surgery (4, 5). These isolators are quite similar to those used for operating on animals, but have not been integrated with operating theater routines. The movements of the surgical team are restricted by the gauntlets, and light reflected from the plastic surface is somewhat annoying.

The objective of the study reported is to develop a means for providing a sterile site for complicated surgical procedures, such as total hip replacement, while integrating well with theater routines and at a cost in materials and effort commensurate with benefits obtained. It seemed to us that the gauntlet isolator was the method of choice, particularly because of its successful development as a means for obtaining the large farm animals in a gnotobiotic state (6).

Results

Soft, flexible polyvinyl chloride film 0.004 in. thick is used to fabricate operating chambers approximately 11 ft long and 17 ft in circumference. View areas for the surgical team are made of pressed polished film approximately 0.01 in. thick. Full-length sleeves made of P.V.C. film with a frosty surface accommodate the surgeon, two assistants, and a scrub nurse in the operating chamber, and a circulating nurse at the supply station at the foot-end of the isolator. The supply-end of the isolator is placed on a special trolley, 24 in x 56 in, which supports the filters and provides a work space for instruments and supplies.

The chamber is strapped to the patient at the site of the incision. A standard Vi-drape forms a portion of the floor of the isolator and provides a seal with the skin of the patient. Two filters, 17 in. in diameter, with three layers of F. M. 004 filter media, are in the roof at the supply-end of the isolator and provide approximately 150 c.f.m. sterile air. The air is exhausted through a collapsed sleeve, 12 in. in diameter, made of flexible P.V.C. film, which serves to maintain sufficient air pressure in the chamber to keep it inflated but soft enough to permit movement by the surgical team. The entire isolator is placed within polyethylene bags and is then sterilized by gamma radiation before it is introduced into the theater.

Instruments and many of the autoclavable supplies are introduced into the isolator from a drum 16 in. in diameter and 20 in. long, by a "split-seam" process as described by Levenson (3). Non-autoclavable supplies and additional instruments are introduced through a 8 in. diameter vertical opening in the floor of the supply-end of the isolator through a cone of sterile air emerging at a velocity of about 300 f.p.m.

The isolators are supplied with gloves only at the supply station. The remaining sleeves are blind. Surgical gloves with rigid cuff support rings for the remainder of the team are introduced either in the drum or through the vertical entry port. The supply nurse places the support rings in the glove-cuffs and then passes the appropriate glove into the plastic sleeves. The glove is moved into place by a circulating nurse and is retained by a rubber O ring and tape applied on the outside. The blind end of the sleeve is cut off just before use, to present a sterile glove. Punctured gloves are readily changed by partially withdrawing the old glove, and placing a new glove over the old cuff and support ring. The hand is then withdrawn and the old glove is cut off to present the new glove.

During the course of this development work, 7 Charnley-type operations (1) were performed. Considerable time was spent in preparing the theater for the operation, but this can obviously be reduced with practice and the use of uniform apparatus and procedures.

Conclusions

The use of gauntlet-type isolators appears to be feasible for complex operations such as total hip replacement. A satisfactory isolator design and procedures have been developed. Clinical trials are being organized.

Acknowledgements

This work has been supported in part by contract with the National Research Development Corporation and Vickers Medical Engineering Ltd.

References

1. Charnley, J., *Brit. J. Surg. 51:* 195 (1964).
2. Levenson, S. M., Trexler, P. C., Malm, O. J., Horowitz, R. E., and Moncrief, W. H., *Surg. Forum 11:* 303 (1960).
3. Levenson, S. M., Trexler, P. C., LaConte, M. L., and Palaski, E., *Amer. J. Surg. 107:* 710 (1964).
4. Landy, J., *J. Arkansas Med. Soc. 57:* 503 (1961).
5. Hashimoto, Y., Sakakibara, K., Mori, K., Sakakibara, B., Washiju, T., and Takahashi, H., in "Advances in Germfree Research and Gnotobiology," Iliffe Books, Ltd., London, p. 364, (1968).
6. Trexler, P. C., *Vet. Record 88:* 15 (1971).

BIOTYPING OF ENTEROBACTERIACEAE: A METHOD TO DETERMINE THE EFFICACY OF THE BARRIER FUNCTION OF ISOLATION UNITS

J. Dankert
Laboratory of Medical Microbiology
University of Groningen, Groningen, The Netherlands

Introduction

Patients with reduced defense capacities are prone to infections. These infections are caused by either endogenous or exogenous (potentially) pathogenic microorganisms.

In order to eliminate the risk of contamination, these susceptible patients are maintained under protective isolation conditions. The barrier of isolation depends on the type of isolation facility, the precautions taken, and the colonization resistance of the (isolated) patients (1).

Renal transplant patients show a decreased defense mechanism due to surgical procedures and immunosuppressive therapy. Renal transplantation patients treated in a reverse isolation unit show a low infection rate (2). Isolation can be effective, since others report a high incidence of infection (3-5).

To determine the efficacy of the barrier function of isolation units, all isolation precautions should be tested and the colonization resistance of the patients should be known (Figure 1). The colonization resistance is influenced by antibiotic therapy (1). As a consequence of failure of the barrier, contamination of the isolation facility as well as the patient may occur. To determine the adequacy of isolation, the effect of various contamination levels that passed the barrier and the colonization resistance of the patient is expressed in the number of contaminations and the frequency of occurrence of colonizations. Colonizations should be prevented, since they imply potential infection.

The acquisition of *Staphylococcus aureus* was used to determine the efficacy of an ultra-clean isolation unit (6). In our unit, this method could not be applied, since the staff members who harbored this microorganism were treated before exposure to the patients and examined regularly. The patients were also treated for the elimination of this microorganism. In this paper, the results of a study of the efficacy of the barrier function by means of biotyping of Enterobacteriaceae are presented.

Barrier Function: Prevention of Infection

Unit	Patient	Consequence of failure
Ventilation	Colonization resistance	Contamination
Cleaning technique	and antibiotic therapy	Colonization
Nursing organization		Infection
and technique		
Sterilization		
instruments		
foods		
other items		

FIG. 1. Outline of principal factors which influence the effectiveness of an isolation unit.

Materials and Methods

Patients. The study was done during the period from September 1971 till February 1972. During this period, 6 patients received kidney allografts in the Surgery Department of the University Hospital. They were all studied during their stay in the isolation unit in the Department of Medicine of the University Hospital. The age of recipients ranged from 16 to 43 years.

Immunosuppressive therapy consisted of azathioprine, 50 mg, and prednisone, 100 mg, daily. Two of the patients received antilymphocytic globulin (A.L.G.) twice.

Antimicrobial therapy consisted of oral administration of ampicillin (1-2 g daily) for 10 days. Afterwards 2 patients received sulfathiozole (3 g daily) orally, 3 patients were treated orally with trimethoprim (160 mg daily) and sulfamethoxazol (800 mg daily), and 1 patient received nalidixin acid (2 g daily).

Controls. As controls, 4 patients who were not isolated received antibiotics and 2 patients received antibiotics at home. Furthermore, 4 volunteers, not having received antimicrobial therapy during the last year, served as healthy controls.

Isolation unit. The isolation unit facility was an "ultra-clean" isolation unit. The unit consisted of 4 patients' rooms (Fig. 2). Rooms (45 m^3) were ventilated with 800 to 900 m^3 of air per hour. The filtered air (American Air Filter Company, Unipack) was blown into the unit under overpressure. The air was exhausted through the entry lock of the patient rooms. The air was humidified by means of steam; the air temperature was 24°C $\pm$ 2°C. Twice a day the entire ward was disinfected with an 0.3% (g/v) solution of paratoluol-sulphon-chloramid-Na in water. Items, such as the radio and the television, were disinfected with 0.5% (v/v) chlorhexidin in 70% (v/v) ethanol. Other isolation unit procedures were of the common type (7, 8).

Sampling patients. Immediately after admittance in the isolation ward,

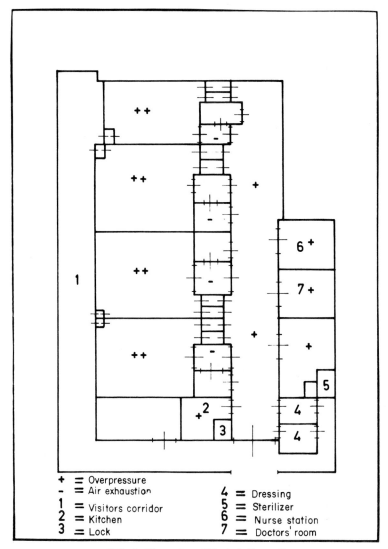

FIG. 2. Floor plan of the isolation unit.

rectal and nasal swabs were taken. A sample of feces was processed weekly.

Isolation room. Each room was swabbed at various sites once a week. During one hour 9 settling plates (blood agar) were exposed in each room.

Staff. Each member was swabbed before the first entrance.

Processing of fecal samples. The feces were serially diluted up to 10^{-12} in phosphate-buffered meat broth, pH 7.1. Of every dilution step, a loopful was

TABLE I. Tests Used In Biotyping Enterobacteriaceae

Serial code number	Test	Serial code number	Test
1	xylose	11	dulcitol
2	maltose	12	ornithine decarboxyl.
3	rahmnose	13	lysine decarboxyl.
4	mannitol	14	H_2S
5	arabinose	15	urease
6	sorbitol	16	citrate
7	lactose	17	inositol
8	indol	18	adonitol
9	sucrose	19	raffinose
10	salicine		

Code number 1-7, 9-11, 17-19:	carbohydrate 1% in meat broth, phenol red 0.2% in saline, pH 7.1 − 7.2
12, 13:	Moeller medium (Difco)
8:	Bacto tryptone (Difco)
14	Broth containing ferric citrate and sodium thiosulfate
15:	Modifica Bacto urea broth (Difco)
16:	Koser medium (Oxoid, Ltd.)

inoculated on blood agar, MacConkey agar, aesculine-azide-bile agar, acetamide agar, Baird-Parker medium, and Sabouraud agar (Oxoid, Ltd.). From every MacConkey agar, 8 to 14 colonies were picked up for further pure culturing.

Biotyping. The procedure was performed in sterile microtrays with 8 x 12 cups (0.2 ml per cup). Cups were filled under strictly aseptic conditions in a laminar flow cabinet. The liquid media used were mentioned in Table I. Filled trays were incubated overnight in order to test sterility. Of the suspension, processed as mentioned, one drop was pipetted into each cup of the test series. The test was read after 24 hours of incubation at 37°C. Coding of biotypes was binominar (9).

Results

To evaluate the efficacy of the barrier function of an isolation unit, an inventory of fecal aerobic flora of each patient was made at admittance to the isolation room. Species and biotypes of Enterobacteriaceae not found in the inventory phase during isolatin were designated as contaminants. Biotypes recovered twice or more frequently were considered to colonize the patient. Species such as *Enterococcus, Pseudomonas aeruginosa, Staphylococcus,* and

Candida were, if isolated, found in all cases in the inventory phase as well as in subsequent samples. The typing results of a representative individual out of each group are shown in Figure 3.

The colonization pattern of the renal transplantation patient (Figure 3) shows, in the inventory phase, 7 biotypes, of which two could be isolated during

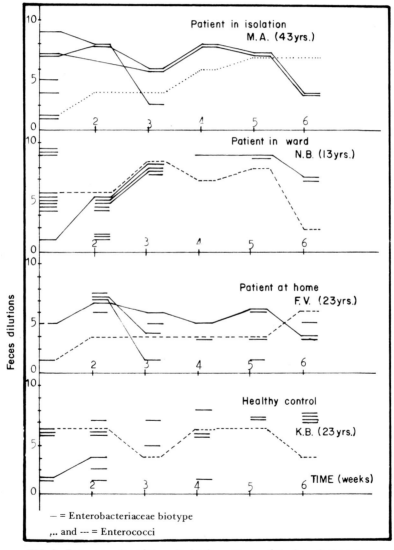

FIG. 3. Four examples of the colonization patterns of the intestinal tract.

the entire isolation period. This patient received sulfathiazole. After the isolation period, the patient was treated in a ward. The same 2 biotypes could be isolated in the first 2 weeks.

The patient shown in Figure 3, receiving antibiotics under open ward conditions, was treated with neomycin, orally. In the inventory phase, 11

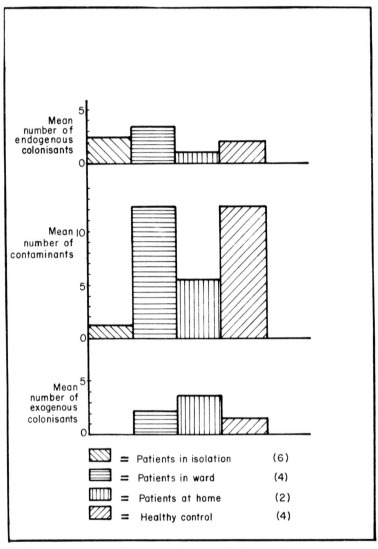

FIG. 4. The mean numbers of contaminants and colonizants of Enterobacteriaceae in the intestinal tract during a six-week period.

biotypes could be isolated. After the first sample, the antimicrobial therapy was started. The endogenous colonizant disappeared in the course of 3 weeks of therapy. Only 1 exogenous colonizant remained present during the investigation period. This biotype was resistant for neomycin.

The patient treated with antimicrobial therapy at home received a high dose of penicillin i.m. She was already under investigation for 3 weeks and remained colonized with 1 biotype. Twice, new contaminants were isolated. After penicillin treatment, 4 new biotypes were detected in the feces. Two of these colonized the patient for a longer period.

The healthy control had 1 endogenous colonizant, no exogenous colonizants, and every week between 2 and 5 contaminants.

The results of the biotyping of Enterobacteriaceae present in the feces of patients and healthy controls are shown in Figure 4. All categories show similar number of endogenous colonizations. The number of contaminants in the intestinal tract was a tenth as much in renal transplant patients as in patients receiving antibiotics in wards and in healthy controls. Exogenous colonizants were not found in the isolated patients.

The source of the contaminations which occurred in all rooms of the unit could not be detected; there was no evidence of cross-contamination. The microbiological monitoring of the ventilation system, the cleaning and nursing techniques, and the effect of sterilization procedures showed a high percentage of sterile samples (Table II).

TABLE II. Microbiological Evaluation of the Isolation Unit

	No. of samples	Sterile Samples (%)	Samples containing potential pathogens (%)
Air	198	33	4
Surfaces	345	50	6
Sinks	92	66	16
Furniture	69	64	6
Staff	52	10	38
Instruments	102	92	0
Food	92	45	1

The (potential) pathogens belonged predominantly to the *Enterobacteriacea species*. In addition, *P. aeruginosa*, other *Pseudomonas species*, and *Achromobacter* and *Alcaligenes species* were isolated.

Biotyping of the Enterobacteriaceae isolated from the room showed frequently that the intestinal tract of the patient might be the source of these bacteria. Only on 3 occasions could a biotype not be traced in this way. In 1 instance, *P. aeruginosa* was isolated from the room. This type could not be isolated either from any other site of the room or from any patient's material.

Discussion

The incidence of infection in renal transplantation patients is high (4). This is found in patients maintained in protective isolation (10) as well as in patients treated without barrier nursing (3, 5). On the other hand, the rate of infection in patients protected in an isolation unit with an effective barrier is low (2).

In our study, one patient suffered from an endogenous fungal infection (mucormycosis) during treatment in isolation. Colonization with exogenous microorganisms did not occur in the renal transplantation patients involved in this study. A small number of contaminations with Enterobacteriaceae biotyes, however, was found. In all contaminations, biotypes were found in a concentration of 10^4 per gram of feces or less. This may indicate that the patients were exposed to low numbers of bacteria.

The low colonization resistance in renal transplantation patients treated with immunosuppressives and antibiotics seems to be comparable to that of other patients who received only antibiotics. The number of endogenous colonizations with Enterobacteriaceae biotypes was similar in the two groups. The antimicrobial therapy increases the colonization resistance for sensitive bacterial species, but decreases the colonization resistance for resistant strains.

The colonization of the intestinal tract appeared to be continued in 5 renal transplantation patients during treatment under open ward conditions following release from the isolation unit. The mean number of contaminations with Enterobacteriaceae biotypes in the first 2 weeks was 3 times as high as in the isolation unit. The same number of contaminations in a 2-week period was found in the intestinal tract of patients who received only antibiotics and were maintained under open-ward conditions.

By determining the contaminations and the exogenous colonizations with potentially pathogenic Gram-negative rods, the potential chance of infection can be investigated. In view of the findings described, we feel that biotyping of Enterobacteriaceae isolated from feces of patients in an isolation unit seems to be a valuable tool to determine the efficacy of the barrier function of an isolation unit.

Summary

The efficacy of the barrier function of an "ultra-clean" isolation unit has been studied. The precautions taken have been monitored and the colonization of the intestinal tract of renal transplantation patients has been determined in comparison with three control groups: patients treated with antibiotics under open ward conditions; patients treated similarly at home; and healthy persons.

A high percentage of the samples taken from the unit and different items was sterile. Enterobacteriaceae species were biotyped by means of 19 liquid media. A small number of contaminations in the intestinal tract of renal transplantation patients could be found. Exogenous colonization did not occur, in contrast with the three control groups mentioned.

Acknowledgements

This study was carried out with the technical assistance of Mr. K. Beenakker. We also thank the medical and nursing staff of the isolation unit for their valuable cooperation.

References

1. van der Waaij, D., Berghuis-de Vries, J. M., and Lekkerkerk-van der Wees, J. E. C., *J. Hyg., Camb., 69:* 405 (1971).
2. van der Waaij, D., and Vossen, J. M., *J. Hyg., Camb.,* (Submitted for Publication).
3. Rifkind, D., Marchioro, T. L., Waddell, W. R., and Starzl, T. E., *J.A.M.A. 189:* 397 (1964).
4. McDonald, J. C., Ritchey, R. J., Fuselier, P. F., Lindsey, E. S., and McCracken, B. H., *Surg. 70:* 189 (1971).
5. Burgos-Calderon, R., Pankey, G. A., and Figueroa, J. E., *Surg. 70:* 334 (1971).
6. Andrews, H. J., and Bagshawe, K. D., *J. Hyg., Camb., 64:* 501 (1966).
7. Woodruff, M. F. A., Robson, J. S., McWhirter, R., Nolan, B., Wilson, T. I., Lambie, A. T., William, J. M., and MacDonald, M. K., *Brit. J. Urol. 34:* 3 (1962).
8. Bagshawe, K. D., *Brit. Med. J. 2:* 871 (1964).
9. van der Waaij, D., Vossen, J. M., and Speltie, T., *J. Hyg. Camb.,* (In Press).
10. Woodruff, M. F. A., Nolan, B., Robson, J. S., and MacDonald, M. K., *Lancet 1:* 6 (1969).

SECTION III

EFFECT OF GNOTOBIOTIC ENVIRONMENT ON ISOLATED PATIENTS

INVESTIGATION OF BEHAVIOR OF LEUKEMIA PATIENTS TREATED IN GERMFREE ISOLATORS

K. Köhle, C. Simons, M. Dietrich, A. Durner
Departments of Psychosomatic Medicine, Hematology,
Clinical Physiology and Psychotherapy,
University of Ulm, Ulm, Germany

Introduction

Besides organizational and financial difficulties, the introduction of gnotobiotic methods in clinical treatment is also hindered by psychological resistance. The treatment of patients in isolated-bed systems has a very great influence on the social interactive processes of the doctor/nursing staff/patient/ relatives (2, 3, 4, 5), and considerable adaptability is required of all concerned. Resistance on the part of the nurses and doctors, as well as psychological complications arising in the patients, have occasionally led to treatments being terminated, thus presenting psychological medicine a challenge to investigate these interactive processes and to work on the resulting conflicts together with those concerned.

Methods

Within a period of three years we investigated 20 patients with acute leukemia during 25 treatment periods in isolated-bed-systems (Life Island, Ulm Bed). The total treatment time was 944 days, the average time of isolation was 37.8 days. Before commencing treatment, all patients were informed about the diagnosis and prognosis of leukemia, as well as the rational and experimental aspects of the isolation treatment; participation in the treatment program was voluntary.

All patients were given the following psychological examination before treatment was commenced: interviews with the patient and closest relative, psychological test-evaluation, and the social circumstances were ascertained. Documentation of the course of treatment was made with the aid of Holland's depression/anxiety questionnaire; daily interviews enabled continuous observation of the patient and at the same time supporting psychotherapy. Once a week interactionally centered group discussions were carried out with the nursing team. A social worker was available to work on psychosocial problems.

Results

Behavior patterns relating specifically to disease or isolation are methodically difficult to separate, owing to the quantity of effective factors. The investigation of a suitably large control group of conservatively treated patients has not yet been completed. First of all descriptively typical behavior patterns of the patients and their effect on the nurse/doctor interactive processes are calculated.

The confrontation with the leukemia diagnosis, the course of the disease and also the side effects of the treatment alarms the patient and gives him a feeling of insecurity; his self confidence is undermined and states of depression ensue. Processes of adjustment and resistance occur in phases between the poles of denying and accepting the illness (6). As maintaining communication with the patient is the chief therapeutic aim, a differentiated investigation must be made into the phases of resistance specifically related to communication requirements, and frank information about the course of the disease is essential (6).

The isolation treatment leads to the patient becoming totally dependent upon the doctors and nurses; the patient loses his accustomed autonomy and he is forced into a process of regression which results in relationship analogous to that of parents/child. The treatment situation is however contradictory: In spite of his dependence and forced passivity, the ability to cooperate actively is also demanded of the patient, and he finds it difficult to adapt to both. In the emotional sphere the diminishing autonomy leads to fear and a reduced self confidence which results in reactive depression. The struggle to restore autonomy as well as the extensive frustration of many gratifications results in aggression. However, it is inhibited due to fear of being rejected, as the doctor and nurses are at the same time rescuers and captors. A characteristic "aggressive dependency" relationship ensues. This aggressive dependency can be elucidated by the advice given by an extremely compliant patient to his successor: the only way of enduring the isolator being to boss the nurses around. The increased aggressive emotional state during the course of the treatment can be clarified by the retesting results of the Rorschach-test: 3 patients in the isolator showed a marked increase in aggression, specifically in destructiveness. In 3 control patients no such change could be perceived. Two typical adjustment strategies which are dependent upon the patient's personality structure are to be found in this situation:

1) The dependence is accepted as temporary and necessary for the treatment of the disease. The intensive care by the nurses and doctors is experienced positively as being analogous to the care of the child by its parents. The regression takes place in the service of the ego; the patient is able to be confident. His own self-confidence increases through an idealization of the medical and nursing staff and a partial identification with the same. One

casuistic example of this: Before the beginning of treatment the patient dreams that he sees behind the isolator a music band at his place of work playing to welcome him, and left and right of the isolator were funeral processions, recognized as symbolizing death. During the treatment he dreamt of a lottery prize which he used to build the resident physician an enormous center for gnotobiotic treatment, administered by himself. In the interaction, the patient's positive attitude causes the medical and nursing staff to be rewarded for their efforts. The communication with this patient is undisturbed.

2) If the dependence cannot be accepted, a withdrawal in contact relationship often occurs. In isolation the appearance of individual autonomy is retained. If oral traits determine the behavior, offers by doctor and nurses will be rejected. These often experience feelings of guilt, at first increasing their offers, then also withdrawing, feeling disappointed. Where anal behavior traits are dominant, the medical and nursing staff will be kept in suspense, thus demonstrating their own strength of will through keeping others waiting. Possible effects are irritation and aggression on the part of the personnel. The restoration of autonomy at a lower level of functioning or also allowing for regressive ways of communication, overcomes fear and depression. If these behavioral strategies fail, fear can lead to psychosomatic symptoms or else find expression in direct panic. The more unstable the psychological balance has been before the onset of the disease, the easier it will be for the ego-functions to decompensate under the stress of the isolator treatment. The stress is also increased because of the cessation of previous social compensatory possibilities. Thus a patient who had for months only been able to maintain the interactive balance with his wife through constant mutual suicide threats, already showed depersonalization symptoms after the first day in the isolator. In the forced dependence he was first able to express similar threats to the doctors and nurses during an attack of febrile delirium. Aggressive resistance is aided moreover by the familiar defense mechanisms, of which projection (e.g. suspicions of poisoning after the patient's disappointment about his own impotence) and displacement (third parties on whom the patient is not dependent, such as the isolated-bed system or the food, are criticized instead of the doctor and nurses) play particularly important roles. It is of therapeutic importance to understand that the negative reactions of the patient in the interaction express his attempt to master the situation and result from a "negative transference" of emotions, which existed in a similar restricted situation in early childhood in relation to his parents. This comprehension can be achieved by working together with the patient; it excludes the vexation of the doctors or nurses themselves, and enables the maintainance of an intensive working alliance. This relationship is strengthened by special gratifications such as in the choice of food and so on. Of help is a relationship of the patient with a person upon whom he is not directly dependent; thus it is very much easier to produce, express and work at aggressive

impulses during our psycho-therapeutic interviews.

When the isolation treatment is of short duration, the effects of sensorial deprivation and social isolation only play a small role. Using the Rorschach-test we found in comparison to the control patients no increase in movement responses when motor activity is restricted, as in the corresponding experimental situations (1). A prolonged confinement to a constant environment, an extended reduction of social contacts, and the immobilization all result in a decline in outside interests and a restriction in enthusiasm for interaction with the personnel. This leads to social withdrawal, depression and apathy.

The narcissistic withdrawal of libido to the patient's own body accelerates hypochondriacal behavior patterns and the rise of psychosomatic complaints. The personnel often respond to this withdrawal with helplessness and perplexity about possiblities to stimulate the patient's interest, and finally this is also followed by a rather more indifferent withdrawal. A complete grasp of the course as well as a fixed time for the possible termination of the isolation is therapeutically important for the patient. Contact with the outside world can be improved by the use of the telephone and by visits from the relatives. Outside stimuli can be increased by television, newspapers, etc. being available. Physiotherapy is particularly important because of the restricted possibilities for muscular activity.

Psychological complications. We attribute the surprisingly low incidence of more serious psychological complications to the extreme tendency toward social adaptation in the personality of leukemia patients, to the choice of suitable patients, and to the intensive care. None of the 25 treatment periods had to be terminated prematurely because of psychiatric complications. The psychiatric complications and the psychological reactions are shown in Table I. Serious symptoms were mainly induced by complications of the somatic course of the disease, in particular by high fever and pain. Figures 1 and 2 show examples of the development of anxiety and depression in relation to the course of the fever. Depressive reactions and communication impairments increase with the length of stay in the isolator, which is partly to be attributed to the increased incidence of somatic complications and partly to the growth of psychological strain caused by the length of illness and the stay in the isolator.

Out of 33 patients selected at random, only one appeared unsuitable for the isolation treatment. This 53 year old woman had suffered since childhood from deafness and was also for neurotic reasons incapable of cooperation. A febrile delirium which began on the second day of conservative treatment confirmed our doubts.

Principally all patients should be excluded from the isolation treatment who either reject the treatment themselves, or who because of low intelligence or physical impairment are not capable of sufficient cooperation; that is to say,

TABLE I. Psychiatric Complications and Psychological Reactions During 25 Isolation
Treatment Periods of Patients Suffering from Acute Leukemia

		Treatment Periods	%
Psychosis	Delirium	3	12
	_ _ _ _ _ _ _ _		
	Depersonalization	1	4
Severe Anxiety States		4	16
Urgent Wish to Leave Isolator		4	16
Psychomatic Symptoms and/or Hypochondriac Complaints		5	20
Reactive Depressive States		13	52
Suicidal Tendency		2	8
Temporary Withdrawal Breaking Off of Communication		11	44
Ability or Willingness to Cooperate Impaired		11	44

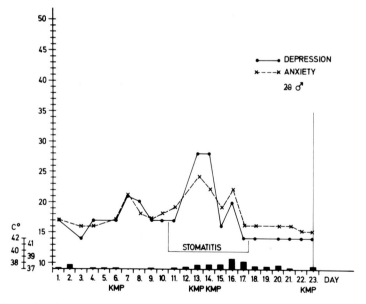

FIG. 1. Anxiety-depression scale adapted from J. F. Holland (5). Depression and anxiety as
a consequence of somatic complication (stomatitis, fever).

75

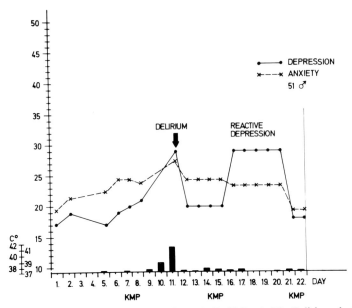

FIG. 2. Anxiety-depression scale adapted from J. F. Holland (5). Delirium during high fever, followed by a phase of reactive depression.

patients who in their case histories show a tendency to psychiatric clinical syndromes.

Conclusions

During the gnotobiotic treatment of 20 leukemia patients, which led to 25 treatment periods in isolated-bed systems, serious psychopathological disorders occurred in our therapeutic setting surprisingly seldom. Various adjustment strategies of the patients led to heavy burdens on the nursing staff. The task of a psychosomatic specialist in the team of medical and nursing staff is first and foremost handling these problems of interaction. Besides this, his participation in the identification of psychologically unsuitable patients, and in the care of patients with psychiatric complications is necessary. Systematic supportive psychotherapy of the patients has proved to us to be valuable — but does not seem to be absolutely necessary as a minimum requirement.

Acknowledgement

Supported by Deutsche Forschungsgemeinschaft, Bad Godesberg; and Werner-Reimers-Stiftung, Bad Homburg.

References

1. Benedick, M. R., and Klopfer, W. G., *J. project. Techniques 28:* 261 (1964).

2. Burke, L., Acute leukemia task force, Subcommittee on patient protection, N.I.H., Bethesda, Md., (Feb. 1967).
3. Holland, J. F., Acute leukemia: psychological aspects of treatment, Boerhave Course Cytostatic Seminars, Leyden, Holland, (Sept. 1970).
4. Holland, J. F., Marris, S., Plumb, M., Tuttolemundo, A., and Yates, J., *Abstr. Vol. XIII,* Int. Congress Hematology, Munchen, p. 358, (1970).
5. Köhle, K., Simons, C., Weidlich, S., Dietrich, M., and Durner, A., *Psychother. Psychosom. 19:* 85 (1971).
6. Kubler-Ross, E., "On death and dying," Macmillan, New York, (1969).

FECAL BILE ACIDS AND NEUTRAL STEROLS OF GNOTOBIOTIC, ANTIBIOTIC FED NORMAL, AND NORMAL HUMAN CHILDREN

Thomas F. Kellogg
Department of Biochemistry, Mississippi State University,
State College, Mississippi 39762, U.S.A.

Introduction

The effect of a normal intestinal microflora on fecal neutral sterols and bile acids has been investigated in a number of experimental animals. The general conclusions (1, 2) were that the intestinal microflora is responsible for an increase in both the kinds and amounts of fecal bile acids and neutral sterols excreted as compared to either germfree subjects or subjects fed high levels of antibiotics. The studies reported in this paper extend the observations to include human subjects and show that oral antibiotic administration to a conventional child renders his fecal bile acids and neutral sterols virtually identical to those of gnotobiotic children.

Methods

Fecal samples were collected and stored in an equal weight of methanol. The samples were collected from patients in the University of Ulm Germany Medical School, and mailed to our laboratory for analysis. The details of the two gnotobiotic children's history and maintenance have been published elsewhere. Subject E.R. had had no fecal microorganisms detectable for approximately three months prior to sampling but was found to be contaminated with a bacterium of the Klebsiella-aerobacter group and *Candida albicans*. Subject W.R. was contaminated with a sporeformer. With the above exceptions both subjects were free of all other microbiological association as shown by standard microbiological examination of feces, skin, and body orifices. The antibiotic fed normal child was receiving 4 x 0.5 g oxacillin daily *per os*. Both this child and the normal child were hospitalized in an open ward and were similar in age to the gnotobiotic children. The fecal neutral sterols were analyzed by the methods of Miettinen *et. al.* (3). The methods of Grundy *et. al.* (4) were employed for the fecal bile acid assay. The bile acid conjugates were separated on TLC using the system S-VIII of Hofmann (5).

Results

The two gnotobiotic children's fecal C_{27} neutral sterols were 100% cholesterol; no 5-β neutral sterols could be detected. The antibiotic fed child excreted 95% cholesterol, 4% coprostanol, and a trace (less than 0.1%) of coprostanone. The normal child fed a similar diet excreted 42.2% cholesterol, 55.5% coprostanol, and 2.0% coprostanone. These results are summarized in Table I.

TABLE I. Fecal Endogenous Neutral Sterols of Gnotobiotic, Antibiotic Fed Normal, and Normal Human Children

Status	Percent of Total Fecal Endogenous N.S.		
	Cholesterol	**Coprostanol**	**Coprostanone**
Gnotobiotic (E.R.)	100	0	0
Gnotobiotic (W.R.)	100	0	0
Normal + oxacillin	95	4	0.1
Normal	42.2	55.5	2.0

The fecal bile acids of the gnotobiotic and antibiotic fed children were conjugated with glycine. The normal child's bile acids were non-conjugated. After hydrolysis the fecal bile acids were analyzed by TLC and GLC. The results of this analysis are given in Table II.

TABLE II. Fecal Bile Acids of Gnotobiotic, Antibiotic Fed Normal, and Normal Human Children

Status	Percent of Total Fecal Bile Acids			Cholic
	Lithocholic	**Chenodeoxycholic**	**Deoxycholic**	**Cholic**
Gnotobiotic (E.R.)	0	35	0	61*
Gnotobiotic (W.R.)	0	48	0	44
Normal + oxacillin	0	50	0	35
Normal	27	0	70	0

*Only the major bile acid components are reported. Minor unidentified components are the difference between amounts reported and 100%.

Discussion

These studies show that gnotobiotic human subjects are comparable to germfree experimental laboratory animals (6) as regards the absence of 5-β neutral sterols, deconjugated bile acids, and 7-dehydroxy bile acids in their feces. A free living human subject given proper doses and type of antibiotics will closely resemble a gnotobiotic subject in their qualitative fecal bile acid and neutral sterol excretion. These studies suggest the possibility of studying the effects of microbiological modification of fecal steroids and the dietary interaction with it (1) directly by using antibiotic fed and non-antibiotic fed free living human subjects.

Quantitative studies must be carried out in a situation where intake of dietary sterol and nutrient intake can be controlled or at least monitored.

Acknowledgement

This investigation was supported by PHS Research Grant No. HL-14525 from National Heart and Lung Institute.

References

1. Kellogg, T. F., *Fed. Proc. 30:* 1808 (1971).
2. Kellogg, T. F., in "The Bile Acids Vol. II," (D. Kritchevsky, and P. Nair, eds.), Plenum Press, N.Y., (In Press).
3. Miettinen, T. A., Ahrens, E. H. Jr., and Grundy, S. M., *J. Lipid Res. 6:* 411 (1965).
4. Grundy, S. M., Ahrens, E. H. Jr., and Miettinen, T. A., *J. Lipid Res. 6:* 397 (1965).
5. Hofmann, A. F., in "New Biochemical Separations," (L. J. Morris and T. James, eds.), Van Nostrand, London, p. 261 (1964).

DIFFERENCES IN ABSORPTION OF ACTIVELY ABSORBED SUGAR IN "GNOTOBIOTIC PATIENTS"

K. Rommel, M. Dietrich, R. Böhmer, R. Binder
Center for Internal Medicine and Pediatrics
Department for Hematology, Department for Clinical Pathology
and
Center for Basic Clinical Research, Department for Clinical Physiology
University of Ulm, Ulm, Germany

Introduction

Theoretical as well as practical aspects of the absorptive capacity for the alimentation of gnotobiotic patients suggested a study on absorption in three patient groups: 1) patients in isolation and during antibiotic decontamination, and cytostatic therapy, 2) patients in isolation and during cytostatic therapy, and 3) patients with cytostatic therapy alone in the ordinary environment.

Methods

Planning the study we were confronted above all with the following theoretical and practical difficulties: 1) There are many conflicting results about malabsorption induced by neomycin. 2) Typical methods of measuring absorption as small intestinal perfusion or biopsies of the small intestinal mucosa were technically impossible to perform. Investigations of feces do not solely reflect the activities of the small intestine. 3) Endoscopic studies could not be performed due to the kind and severity of the disease as well as its treatment.

The procedure that we used to calculate the intestinal absorption is based upon the simple pragmatic analysis of the blood level by using the DOST law of the corresponding areas. The observed concentrations in the blood have been plotted in a diagram versus the time — in our case: two hours. The blood level diagram also can be analyzed by hybrid computers. The methods used are easy to perform, therefore, only the use of the law on corresponding areas is described in more detail.

The supposition of the mathematical procedure to find the kinetic values is that the blood level of an orally given substance is a function of the processes which the substance undergoes on its way to the blood stream, as well as in the blood stream.

The planimetry of the area below the curve of the blood concentration is performed by a polarplanimeter for the oral as well as for the intravenous tests.

The percentage of the relations of the areas corresponds with the rate of absorption.

Generally the percentage of absorbed dosage of a substance can be expressed by the following equation:

$$(1) \quad P\ (D_a/D_{iv}) \ = \ \frac{F_a}{F_{iv}}\ .\ 100$$

or expressed in weight units:

$$(2) \quad D_a \ = \ \frac{F_a}{F_{iv}}\ .\ D_{iv}$$

Symbols

D_a = "absorbed moiety," present in blood
D_{iv} = moiety, present in blood after i.v. injection of the test substance
F_a = area measured after oral intake of test substance
F_{iv} = area measured after i.v. injection of test substance

Results

So far 5 patients have been investigated during isolation, decontamination and cytostatic therapy, 2 patients in isolation and cytostatic therapy without decontamination and 4 patients with cytostatic therapy alone, without isolation and decontamination. These patients suffered from acute myelocytic and undifferentiated leukemia. They were randomized to the different groups by a statistical center during an evaluative study of the protective effect of isolation systems and decontamination of the European Organization for Research on Therapy of Cancer (E.O.R.T.C.) gnotobiotic project group. The group of decontaminated patients received a daily antibiotic regimen of: 3.0 g neomycin sulfate, 200 mg polymyxin B and 160,000 units bacitracin and 6 Mio Units nystatin, all nonabsorbable antibiotics. The cytotoxic treatment consisted of cytoxin arabinoside or daunorubicin, vincristin and prednisone in combination. The isolation took place in a plastic isolation system ("Life Island" and in an "Ulm isolated bed" system). The longest treatment period of this program was 85 days, the shortest 20 days. Analyses of the blood concentration were done after the intake of galactose — an actively absorbed hexose. The excretion of xylose in the urine was measured during 5 hours after the administration of xylose. The concentrations of xylose in the blood have not been measured in order to reduce the number of venipunctures.

We found a significant reduction of the xylose excretion during the treatment of patients by cytotoxic therapy under gnotobiotic conditions, i.e., isolation and antibiotic decontamination. The largest decrease of the xylose excretion in this group was 95%. After the decontamination of the described treatment procedures and the reconventionalization the excretion of xylose was normalized.

This finding corresponds well with the results of a decreased xylose absorption after neomycin sulfate obtained by other investigators in patients and animals.

The excretion of xylose in patients receiving cytostatic therapy without isolation and decontamination and the other group with cytostatic treatment alone was not significantly altered during the course of treatment.

In contrast, the absorption of galactose evidently was not influenced by the decontamination therapy when compared to the results of the xylose absorption.

These findings should be considered with the fact in mind that both sugars are absorbed actively, even though xylose is absorbed at a much slower rate. Whereas xylose is a pentose, galactose belongs to the hexoses. The carrier of galactose is identical with the carrier of glucose. Glucose, however, has a higher affinity for this carrier.

Considering that the primary monosaccharides are of relatively small relevance for alimentation, it seems to be interesting to investigate also the digestion of maltose and perhaps also saccharose for theoretical as well as practical purposes. The monosaccharides originating from disaccharides are absorbed in the mucosal cell by a different energy-independent transport mechanism.

Currently, our group is investigating these problems in an experimental model using conventional, decontaminated ex-conventional and germfree rats and the method of small intestinal perfusion.

Acknowledgement

Research supported by the Deutsche Forsuchungsgemeinschaft.

References

1. Dost, F. H., *Grundlagen der Pharmakokinetik Georg-Thieme-Verlag*, Stuttgart (1968).
2. Rommel, K., in "Biochemische und klinische Aspekte der Zucker-absorption," (K. Rommel and P. H. Clodi, eds.), F. K. Schattauer Verlag, Stuttgart-New York, (1970).

USE OF A SURGICAL ISOLATOR FOR MAJOR SURGERY: INFLUENCE ON WOUND CONTAMINATION AND POSTOPERATIVE WOUND INFECTIONS

Seymour Alpert
Department of Surgery

Theodore Salzman
Departments of Medicine and Microbiology and Immunology

Catherine Sullivan, Carla Palmer, and *Stanley M. Levenson*
Department of Surgery
Albert Einstein College of Medicine
Bronx, New York 10461, U.S.A.

Introduction

Wound infection is an all too common secondary disease which complicates major surgery, affects some one million five hundred thousand patients yearly and adds some ten billion dollars in additional expense for the patients affected in the United States (1).

The incidence of wound infection varies greatly from hospital to hospital as exemplified in a 1967 study of the effectiveness of ultra-violet light in the operating room (2). Table I taken from that publication indicates the incidence of postoperative wound infections as related to potential bacterial contamination of the wound during operation. Clean contaminated wounds (the group which interests us most from the point of view of this discussion) were defined as those occurring in patients in which either the bronchus, gastrointestinal tract, genito-urinary tract or oro-pharyngeal cavity were entered but without unusual contamination. The incidence of wound infection in this group was 10.4% for the five institutes reporting but varied from about 8% to 22%.

Although there are a large number of variables (including the local and systemic "resistance" of the patient) involved in the pathway to an infected wound, the presence of an infecting organism is, of course, a must. Various techniques have been used during the last 80-90 years to try to break the wound infection cycle by eliminating or destroying the infecting organism. No attempt will be made to review these here; discussion may be found elsewhere (3-6). The approach used in our study was directed at the mechanical separation of the

TABLE I. Incidence of Postoperative Wound Infection

Type of case	No. of Wounds	% Infections
Refined-clean	6,656	3.3
Other clean	5,034	7.4
Clean-contaminated	2,589	10.4
Contaminated	681	16.3
Dirty	581	28.6
Not classified	72	8.3
Total	15,613	7.4

wound from exogenous environmental sources. The technology involved is partly spin-off and partly second generation development of germfree animal research (7-16).

Materials and Methods

Our surgical isolator, in the design of which Trexler played a major role, is a large plastic bag hung like a shower curtain (Fig. 1). It is pre-packaged and pre-sterilized (Fig. 2). The operative site is prepped and attached to the isolator by means of a sterile adhesive drape incorporated into the bottom wall of the isolator. The patient is entirely outside the sterile internal environment (Fig. 3).

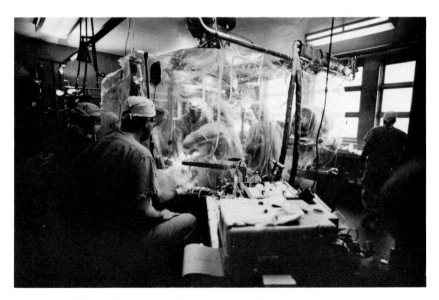

FIG. 1. View of operation in progress with the surgical isolator.

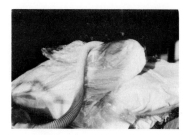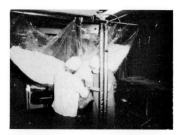

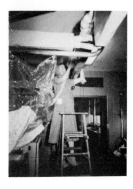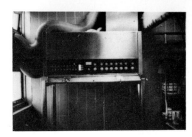

FIG. 2. Upper left: Appearance of surgical isolator on its removal from storage box. Isolator was folded, packaged and sterilized with ethylene oxide. Upper right: Nurses hanging the surgical isolator to frame. Lower left: Nurse inserting air filter into air supply duct. Lower right: Consol used to regulate air supply to isolator and surgical team. Consol also houses electronic communication system.

The surgical team is incorporated into the wall of the isolator in half suits. The mobility of the plastic wall allows adequate movement for all surgical manipulations. Thus, once the incision is made, it is exposed only to sterile air and gloves, wall, and equipment within the isolator (Fig. 4).

Our study groups to date consist of one hundred and thirty-one patients operated by the surgical isolator technique and one hundred and twenty-eight in the conventional operating room environment. Except for the operative environment, the patients in both groups were studied and managed in an identical manner; this included the type of skin preparation prior to operation, and the application of an adhesive plastic sheet to the operative field of the patients operated on in the conventional operating room.

The types of operations performed are listed in Table II. The patients were on the wards of the Jacobi Hospital, Bronx Municipal Hospital Center and were cared for pre- and postoperatively in identical ways. The patients in both groups were cared for by the same physicians and nurses. The selection of patients was random, but not according to a preplanned scheme so simultaneousness was not attempted or achieved in all cases. The gastrointestinal surgery consisted of the

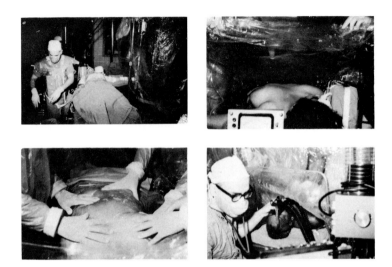

FIG. 3. Upper left: Preparation of operative site of patient about to undergo laparotomy. Surgeon wearing special vest for distribution of air supply. Upper right: Patient being placed under a surgical isolator after skin has been prepped. Lower left: Bottom of isolator being attached to skin of abdomen and chest. Lower right: Operation in progress. Note the free access anesthesiologist has to patient's head.

usual sorts of cases, including gastrectomies, colectomies and cholecystectomies. The gynecologic surgery was mostly hysterectomies, and the urologic surgery kidney transplants. The category "Others" contained clean cases such as various portal decompression procedures, splenectomy, orthopedic procedures, and herniorrhaphies.

All operative procedures performed with the isolator technique were carried out readily. Neither the surgeons, nurses, nor anesthesiologists experienced any difficulties.

Extensive microbiologic testing was done before, during and after surgery. Preoperative cultures of the oro-pharynx, urine, stool and skin of the proposed operative site were taken. The skin was again cultured after the final prepping of the operative site. The interior of the isolator and its air were cultured and the conventional rooms were cultured with fallout plates placed at various points as well as air samples. The cultures of the operative sites were taken sequentially, that is, the various layers of the incision as it was being made, the depth of the wound, the surface and cut edge of a viscus, and in reverse during closure. This procedure allowed for discovery not only of the total cases contaminated but gave evidence of first bacterial contamination and its likely source. Postoperatively all patients were followed clinically, the wounds examined and photographed while the patient was in the hospital and in our outpatient followup clinics. Any wound exudate and drainage were smeared and cultured.

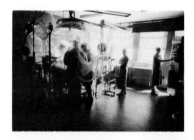

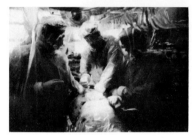
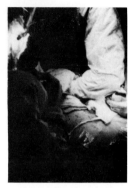

FIG. 4. Upper: Operation with surgical isolator in progress. Lower left and right: Close up views of operation in progress to show half suits and ease of activities of surgeon.

Positive bacterial cultures were obtained at all stages of surgery for both groups.

Results and Discussion

When all cases are reviewed the incidence of contamination for each stage can be seen to be greater for patients operated in the conventional environment than in the surgical isolator (Table III). When only clean-contaminated cases, a somewhat more homogeneous group, is examined, the same differences are evident. The most striking difference is the incidence of contamination at incision, 23% for the conventional group and 7% for the isolator group (Table

TABLE II. Types of Operations

	Isolator	Conventional
Gastrointestinal	76	90
Gynecologic	13	21
Urologic	1	2
Others	41	15
Total	131	128

TABLE III. Incidence of Contamination

	Incision		Depth of Wound		Closure	
	All Cases					
Isolator	11/130	(8%)	63/129	(49%)	55/127	(43%)
Conventional	28/128	(22%)	104/128	(81%)	103/128	(80%)
	Clean-Contaminated Cases					
Isolator	6/86	(7%)	49/86	(57%)	41/85	(48%)
Conventional	25/107	(23%)	92/107	(86%)	88/107	(82%)

III). It seems that even in the short period of time required to make an incision, the conventional environment adds a large load of contamination to the wound.

Table IV compares contamination rates in the two groups before and after a viscus is entered. The time factor before cutting a viscus is longer than for making the incision only. Here a huge difference in bacterial contamination, 9% for isolator cases and 43% for conventional cases, is demonstrated. The added bacterial load to wound contamination consequent to cutting a viscus is evident. Analysis of fairly homogenous groups of patients, that is, patients undergoing cholecystectomies, some with and some without exploration of the common duct, is also shown in Table IV. Again a very striking difference in environmental contribution to wound contamination is seen, 2.4% for isolator cases and 41% for conventional cases, up to the point the cystic duct was cut. Again the added contamination consequent to cutting a viscus is demonstrated.

The commonest bacterial species found by far in all the patients of both the isolator and conventional groups was coagulase negative Staphylococcus. Coagulase positive Staphylococcus appeared infrequently, less than 5% of all positive cultures. The coliforms as a group were present in approximately 10% of all positive cultures. The details of these findings are to be published elsewhere.

There were no wound infections in the clean cases. *Table V shows the wound infection rates for clean-contaminated cases in both the isolator and conventional group, 3.5% and 9.4% respectively.* The 10.4% incidence for

TABLE IV. Contamination Before and After Cutting A Viscus

	Before	After
	All clean-contaminated cases	
Isolator	8/86 (9%)	57/86 (66%)
Conventional	46/107 (43%)	100/107 (93%)
	Cholecystectomies, with and without exploration of the common bile duct	
Isolator	1/44 (2.3%)	20/44 (49%)
Conventional	18/44 (41%)	39/44 (89%)

TABLE V. Incidence of Wound Infection
All Clean-Contaminated Cases

	No. of Cases	Percentage
Isolator	3/86	3.5%
Conventional	10/107	9.4%
Ann. Surg. 1967 (2)	270/2589	10.4%

patients in this category as reported in the ultra-violet study already alluded to (2) is presented for baseline comparison.

Finally, the organisms producing the wound infection for the conventional group are shown in Table VI. In 3 of the 10 cases, we could not identify a specific source of contamination — thus during operation, the offending bacterial species was not cultured, although other species of bacteria were isolated during the course of surgery. In the other 7 cases, the bacterial species causing the wound infection had been cultured during operation and the sites at which they were first cultured are listed.

Table VI also lists similar information for the isolator cases and the same

TABLE VI. Wound Infection

Operation	Organism	Source
Conventional Cases — Infecting Bacteria		
Myomectomy	Aerobacter, Proteus	Unknown
Cholecystectomy	Pseudomonas	Unknown
Choledochojejunostomy & gastrojejunostomy	Aerobacter	CBD, stomach small bowel
Hysterectomy	Proteus	vagina
Jejunostomy	E. coli	incision
Cholecystectomy, gastroenterostomy	Proteus	gall bladder stomach
Cholecystectomy & CBDE	E. coli	gall bladder
Cholecystectomy & CBDE	Proteus	gall bladder
Hemicolectomy	E. coli	bowel
Hemicolectomy	E. coli	bowel
Cholecystectomy	E. coli	gall bladder
Cholecystectomy	Staph. coag. pos.	Unknown
Isolator Cases — Infecting Bacteria		
Hemigastrectomy & vagotomy	Staph. coag. pos.	Unknown
Cholecystectomy & antrectomy	Proteus	cut cystic duct
Cholecystectomy & CBDE	Coliforms	gall bladder

comments hold for the single "unknown" source and the 2 "known" sources. It is evident that the usual sources of bacteria producing a wound infection in the clean-contaminated category of cases is a cut viscus.

Conclusions

The surgical isolator is a practical operative tool which readily reduces considerably the environmental source of wound contamination during operation. The isolator is a valuable clinical investigative tool for studying the sources of wound contamination.

Most wound infections, in patients undergoing major abdominal surgery, clean-contaminated cases, can be traced to bactera derived from a cut viscus.

The use of the isolator is associated in some way not yet understood with a significant reduction in wound infection rates.

Acknowledgements

Supported in part by N.I.H. Grants AM-05664 (Germfree Program), FR-66 (General Clinical Research Center — Acute), and 5-K5-GM-14,208 (Research Career Award, S.M.L.).

References

1. Altemeier, W. A., and Levenson, S. M., *J. Trauma 10:* 1084 (1970).
2. National Research Council Committee of Trauma Report, Published in Annals of Surgery Supplement Issue (1967).
3. Williams, R. E. O., Blowers, R., Garrod, L. P., Shooter, R. A., in "Hospital Infection, Causes and Prevention," The Year Book Publishers, Inc., Chicago, (1960).
4. Meleney, F. L., in "Clinical Aspects and Treatment of Surgical Infections," W. B. Saunders, Co. (1949).
5. Howe, C. W., Mozden, P. J., *S. Clin. North America 43:* 859 (1963).
6. MacLeod, C. M., Cluff, L. E., *Bact. Rev. 24:* 1 (1960).
7. Levenson, S. M., Trexler, P. C., Malm, O. J., Horowitz, R. E., and Moncrief, *Surgical Forum 11:* 306 (1960).
8. Levenson, S. M., Trexler, P. C., Malm, O. J., LaConte, M., Horowitz, R. E., and Moncrief, W. H., *Am. J. Surg. 104:* 891 (1962).
9. Trexler, P. C., and Levenson, S. M., *Proc. Gnotobiote Workshop and Symposium,* p. 13, (1963).
10. Levenson, S. M., Trexler, P. C., LaConte, M., Pulaski, E. J., *Am. J. Surg. 107:* 710 (1964).
11. Levenson, S. M., Del Guercio, L. R. M., LaDuke, M., Kranz, P., Johnston, J., Alpert, S., and Salzman, T., in "Research in Burns," E. & S. Livingstone Ltds., London, (1966).
12. Kranz, P., Levenson, S. M., and LaDuke, M., *ASHRAE J. 3:* 37 (1965).
13. Alpert, S., Salzman, T., Del Guercio, L. R. M., Levenson, S. M., LaDuke, M., and Johnston, M., *Surgical Forum 17:* 78 (1966).
14. LaDuke, M., Hrynus, G. W., Johnston, M., Alpert, S., and Levenson, S. M., *Am. J. Nursing 67:* 72 (1967).

15. Dinerman, M., Johnston, M., Clark, J., Salzman, T., Alpert, S., and Levenson, S. M., *Assoc. Operating Room Nurses Journal*, p. 35, (1968).
16. Alpert, S., Salzman, T., Sullivan, C., Palmer, C., and Levenson, S. M., *Surgical Forum* *22:* 65 (1971).

CLINICAL EXPERIENCE WITH THE CONTROL OF THE MICROFLORA

J. M. Vossen and *L. J. Dooren*
Dept. of Pediatrics, University Hospital, Leiden, The Netherlands

and

D. van der Waaij
Radiobiological Institute TNO, Rijswijk, The Netherlands

Introduction

Since the end of 1968, four infants suffering from severe combined immunodeficiency (C.I.D.) were admitted to the pediatric department of the University Hospital of Leiden. Without immunologic reconstitution by bone marrow transplantation (B.M.T), these infants almost invariably die from infections before their first birthday. They were maintained in protective isolation in a laminar cross-flow bench, modified for nursing of infants. After isolation the microflora of the infants was inventoried, and if indicated gastrointestinal decontamination (G.I.D.) was undertaken to prevent endogenous infectious complications.

Materials and Methods

1. Strict reverse isolation in a laminar cross-flow bench. An industrial laminar cross-flow bench was modified for the purpose of adequate nursing of infants. The working table was raised and its depth was enlarged, as well as the perspex side walls. The ceiling was extended by a perspex hood. The front side could be closed, approximately 95% of the outflow opening (spatial) by means of a double hinged perspex flap to reduce further the risk of airborne contamination. Several neoprene gloves were fitted in this flap to make manipulations inside the bench possible when the flap was closed. Blower speed was made adjustable by means of a variac. This made it possible to decrease the airflow in the bench considerably when the flap was closed, at the same time reducing the noise level and the risk of dehydration of the patient. One of the perspex side walls was provided with a 45 cm diameter cylindrical sluice. This made a connection of the bench with a rigid plastic isolator possible. The latter was designed for transportation of the infant, e.g. to the X-ray department. It was also used as a storage isolator and for temporary stay of the infant; e.g. in case of sterilization of the interior of the laminar flow isolator. Optimal climatologic conditions in the interior of the laminar flow isolator could be attained by airconditioning the cubicle in which it was localized. The interior of the bench as well as the bed were sterilized by spraying with a 2% peracetic acid solution. All food, beverages, items and drugs were sterilized before being introduced into the isolator through the open front. A sterile vitamin preparation was given as well to compensate for the low vitamin content of sterilized meals. Sterilization was done preferably by autoclaving, and otherwise either by ethylene oxide sterilization or by filtering through Millipore filters. Presterilized disposable materials were used whenever possible. All handling of the patient was done either through the closed front by means of neoprene gloves, or through the open front by personnel dressed with face mask, cap, sterilized gown and sterilized gloves. Technical data of the laminar cross flow bench, as well as the nursing techniques used are described in detail elsewhere (1).

2. **Microbiological monitoring.** The endogenous microflora of the infants was inventoried during the first week of strict reverse isolation. To this end, samples of feces and urine, and swabs from nose, oropharynx, ears, axillae, groins, prepuce/vagina and infected sites on the skin were collected three times. During the rest of the isolation period the same samples were taken twice or three times a week. All swabs were moistened with sterile brain heart infusion (B.H.I. Oxoid) broth before sampling. The swabs and the feces (and the urine) were cultured qualitatively on several media under standard aerobic and anaerobic conditions. Isolation of viruses and serologic investigation for the presence of specific antivirus antibodies were performed only on clinical indication. Identification of bacteria, yeasts and fungi isolated was performed down to the species level, whenever possible, by routine bacteriologic methods. Attention was paid only to pathogenic and potentially pathogenic micro-organisms (2). No systematic search nor identification of the anaerobic flora was made. Typing of *Staphylococcus aureus* was performed by the phage typing technique (3), of *Pseudomonas aeruginosa* by the pyocine typing method (4), and of Enterobacteriaceae by way of a "biotyping" method (5, 6, 7). Especially the typing of the ubiquitous Enterobacteriaceae provides a valuable tool to study the efficacy of the reverse isolation procedures.

In patients undergoing G.I.D. more frequent samples of the feces were examined by Gram staining. If this slide revealed the presence of bacteria, the feces were cultured quantitatively. For this purpose they were serially diluted in B.H.I. broth. In case the Gram stain was negative, a 1:10 dilution of feces in B.H.I. broth was made. After centrifugation the supernatant was passed through a 0.45μ Seitz filter. The filter disk was washed three times with sterile B.H.I. broth, after which it was cultured in B.H.I. agar (2).

3. Antibiotic decontamination and control of the microflora. In three of the four infants the initial inventory of the endogenous microflora revealed the presence of microorganisms with a rather high potential pathogenicity and/or with an unfavorable sensitivity pattern for antimicrobial drugs. This formed the indication for G.I.D. with a combination of two nonabsorbable antibiotics and an antimycotic drug according to the method described elsewhere (8). Skin disinfection by way of daily bathing in 0.5% chlorhexidine in water for 15 min. was performed whenever the clinical condition of the patient allowed it.

In case the decontamination was successful, i.e. in case no more microorganisms could be isolated during a period of at least 2 weeks, the administration of nonabsorbable antibiotics was discontinued. Three days later recontamination by rectal implantation of an apathogenic microflora was performed. A selected human fecal flora without viruses, yeasts, fungi and parasites and free of aerobic bacteria was administered to germfree mice and established a normal colonization resistance (9) in these mice. It proved to be apathogenic after lethal irradiation of these mice. This anaerobic apathogenic fecal flora (A.A.F.F.) was implanted rectally on three consecutive days in one of the decontaminated infants.

Results

For the sake of simplicity the microbiological findings from different sites of the patients were compiled into three regions: (1) the naso-oro-pharyngeal region, (2) the feces and (3) the skin. Only "colonizing" potentially pathogenic (p.p.) microorganisms were taken into consideration, i.e. every p.p. microbial species isolated at least twice out of 4 consecutive samples. Four infants with severe combined immunodeficiency (J.M., G.W., G.C. and Y.D.) were kept in strict reverse isolation during a period of 345 days in total. Apart from one transient colonization by an exogenous microorganism, probably originating from contaminated food, no other exogenous colonizations have been detected.

G.I.D. was successful as demonstrated by extensive culturing of the feces. With the exception of one infant (G.C.–Fig. 1) the endogenous microflora of the two other regions could be greatly reduced but not eliminated by the decontamination procedures. A few microbial species persisted on ulcerative infected skin and/or mucosal lesions. Microbiological data of the first two patients (J.M. and G.W.) are described elsewhere more extensively (2). Fig. 1 shows the microbiological data of the third patient (G.C.) and demonstrates the successful elimination of the endogenous microflora by the decontamination procedure. Fig. 2 presents the results of serial quantitative cultures of the feces of the same patient. From day 25 after the recontamination with A.A.F.F., two of the six initially isolated *E. coli* biotypes reappeared in the feces in concentration of $10^9 - 10^{10}$ per gram of feces. Later on *Staphylococcus albus* was also isolated. Both species were present in other regions (Fig. 1). This rather

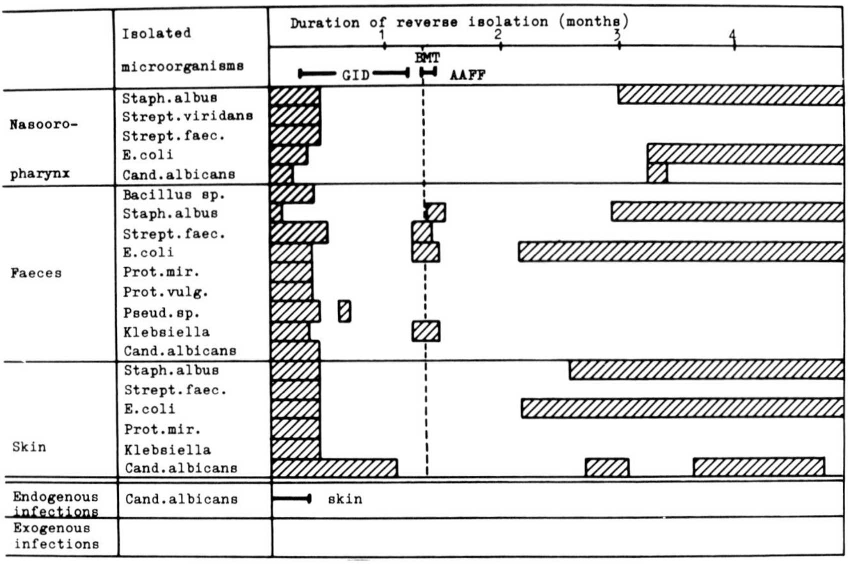

Isolated microorganisms
Duration of reverse isolation (months)
1
2
3
4
BMT
GID
AAFF
Nasooro-pharynx
Staph.albus
Strept.viridans
Strept.faec.
E.coli
Cand.albicans
Faeces
Bacillus sp.
Staph.albus
Strept.faec.
E.coli
Prot.mir.
Prot.vulg.
Pseud.sp.
Klebsiella
Cand.albicans
Skin
Staph.albus
Strept.faec.
E.coli
Prot.mir.
Klebsiella
Cand.albicans
Endogenous infections
Cand.albicans
skin
Exogenous infections

FIG. 1. Microbiological results of patient G.C., male, age 3½ months, severe combined immunodeficiency.

R.I.
G.I.D.
A.A.F.F.
B.M.T.
D.
log. M.O./g F.
S.F.
E.C.
P.S.
K
S.Al.
Ps.S.
(C.A.)
(B.S.)
(E.C., K., S.F., S. Al.)*
E.C.
S. Al.
S.F.
K.
P.V.
-35
-30
-25
-5
0
5
25
30
35
40
50
55
109
121
268
Time in days

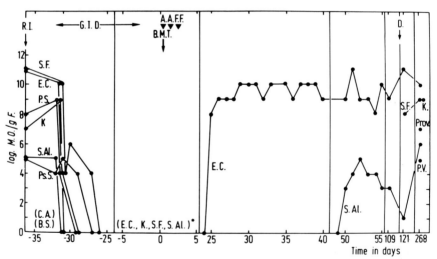

FIG. 2. Feces cultures: quantitative results (patient G.C.) log. M.O./g.F: log. of number of microorganisms per g feces. ( )*: less than 10^2 microorganisms per g feces. R.I.: reverse isolation. D: discharge.

high fecal concentration of Enterobacteriaceae is also found in normal infants during several weeks after birth (Van der Waaij, unpublished data) and may at least partially be due to the milk diet (10).

Apart from a slight bowel distension and a mild degree of nausea and vomiting, an increase in diarrhea, which was already present in these patients, became a troublesome complication of antibiotic decontamination. Whereas no biochemical disturbance could be demonstrated without G.I.D. (Fig. 3) or

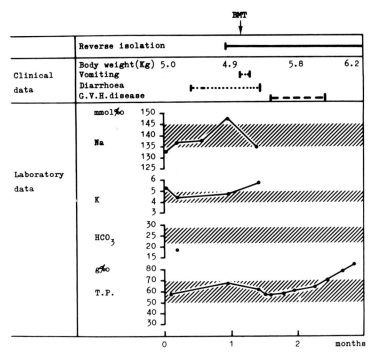

FIG. 3. Clinical and chemical laboratory data of patient J.M., male, age 5 months, severe combined immunodeficiency.

before G.I.D., severe diarrhea resulting in hypoelectrolytemic dehydration and acidosis (Figs. 4, 5 and 6) required intravenous fluid therapy in the three infants during G.I.D. Threatening cardiac decompensation in all three infants made rapid intravenous restoration of potassium necessary. The hypocalcemia in patient G.C. (Fig. 5) led to tetanic convulsions which could only be stopped after intravenous calcium administration. Oral calcium load in this patient resulted in a loss of the administered calcium in the feces, no rise of the calcium excretion in the urine and no rise of the low serum calcium level. An excess in the urinary excretion of other electrolytes was not found either. Recontamination with A.A.F.F. in patient G.C. resulted in normal stool within 48 hours and restoration of water and electrolyte balance within one week. The total

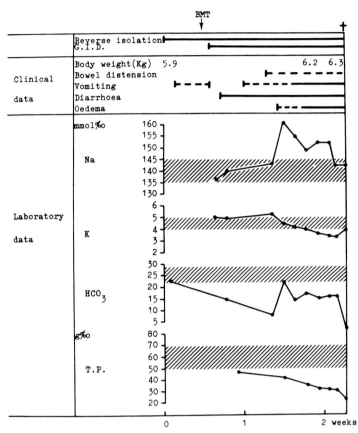

FIG. 4. Clinical and chemical laboratory data of patient G.W., male, age 9 months, severe combined immunodeficiency.

protein level (T.P.) in the serum of patients G.W. (Fig. 4) and Y.D. (Fig. 6) decreased progressively, resulting in generalized edema.

Two patients, J.M. and G.C., are in good health now after complete immunologic reconstitution following bone marrow transplantation. Patient G.W. died from *Pneumocystis carinii* pneumonia; at autopsy no microorganisms were cultured from spleen, liver, kidneys and lungs. In patient Y.D. a multiple resistant salmonella (Dublin), which already colonized the infant prior to isolation, caused recurrent bacteremia and was the ultimate cause of death.

Comments and Conclusions

Strict reverse isolation using laminar flow technique and appropriate nursing procedures proved to be effective in preventing exogenous microbial

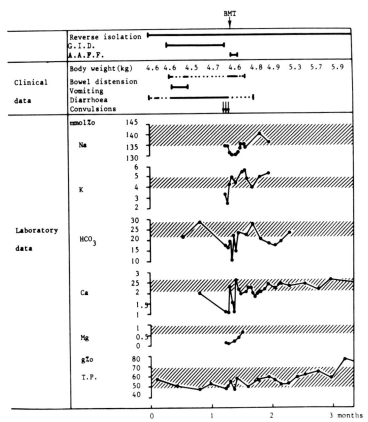

FIG. 5. Clinical and chemical laboratory data of patient G.C., male, age 3½ months, severe combined immunodeficiency.

colonization. In our opinion G.I.D. is indicated in case a potentially dangerous endogenous microflora is found in the initial inventory. This is especially true when an extreme loss of defense capacity against bacterial invasion from the digestive tract can be expected; e.g. in the case of graft versus host (G.V.H.) disease after bone marrow transplantation. Animal experiments favor the hypothesis that elimination of the microbial flora might mitigate the pathology of G.V.H. disease (11). It should be noted that strict reverse isolation and antibiotic decontamination are preventive measures and in that sense are of no value in patients with clinical infections which cannot be eradicated by other treatments. Endogenous microorganisms propagating by the intracellular route or residing there, e.g. viruses and parasites, cannot be eliminated by antibiotic decontamination.

Attention should be paid to the adverse effects seen after G.I.D. in these infants. Bowel distension (well known in germfree animals and correlated with

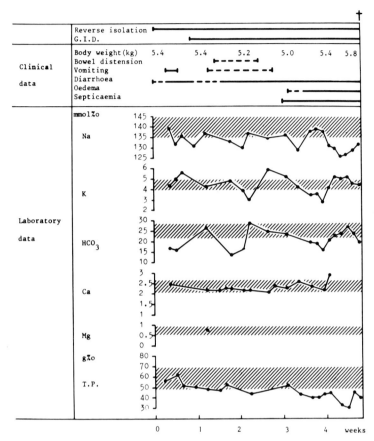

FIG. 6. Clinical and chemical laboratory data of patient Y.D., male, age 8 months, severe combined immunodeficiency.

the presence of a bioactive substance in the gut (12)) as well as vomiting (most probably due to local irritation by the antibiotics) are usually mild complications. Diarrhea on the other hand may result in severe loss of water and electrolytes, especially in infants with severe G.I.D., in whom loose stool, malabsorption and failure to thrive are already the rule. Two mechanisms could cause these disturbances: (1) the elimination of the microflora and in that way the preservation of a hypothetical substance called "water absorption inhibitor" (13) which is normally destroyed by the intestinal microflora. This may decrease water absorption and electrolyte absorption simultaneously, as far as the latter is attributable to solvent drag. The colonic secretion of potassium into the watery luminal content most probably accounts for the severe potassium deficiency seen in these patients. (2) The antibiotics administered orally may have a toxic effect on the intestinal mucosa blocking the active transport mechanism of some electrolytes, e.g. calcium, and leading to intestinal loss of proteins. Neomycin is known to produce such a malabsorption after oral administration (14). The toxic effect on distant organs after absorption and the neuromuscular blocking effect after massive aspiration of the aminoglucoside antibiotics need no further comment (15). Daily monitoring of the serum level of these antibiotics is indicated.

Recolonization of the digestive tract with an apathogenic anaerobic fecal flora after successful decontamination seems the obvious policy to circumvent the adverse effects of antibiotic decontamination and to prevent endogenous infection as well. More research is necessary to find a proper method for decontamination and to maintain an adequate intake of water, electrolytes and calories during that period. The colonization resistant flora of the intestinal tract still needs to be elucidated.

References

1. Koning, J. de, Waaij, D. van der, Vossen, J. M., Versprille, A., and Dooren, L. J., *Maandschr. Kindergeneesk. 38:* 1 (1970).
2. Vossen, J. M., and Waaij, D. van der, *Eur. J. Clin. Biol. Research,* (In Press).
3. Blair, J. E., and Williams, R. E. O., *Bull. W.H.O. 24:* 771 (1961).
4. Gillies, R. R., and Govan, J. R. W., *J. Path. Bact. 91:* 339 (1966).
5. Bettelheim, K. A., and Taylor, R. J., *J. Med. Microbiol. 2:* 225 (1969).
6. Waaij, D. van der, and Kal, H. B., *TNO Nieuws 26:* 567 (1971).
7. Dankert, J., in "Germfree Research: Biological Effect of Gnotobiotic Environments," (J. B. Heneghan, ed.), Academic Press, New York, p. 59, (1973).
8. Waaij, D. van der, Vries, J. M. de, and Lekkerkerk, J. E. C., in "Infections and Immunosuppression in Subhuman Primates," Munksgaard, Copenhagen, p. 21, (1970).
9. Waaij, D. van der, Berghuis-de Vries, J. M., and Lekkerkerk-van der Wees, J. E. C., *J. Hyg. Camb. 69:* 405 (1971).
10. Lee, A., Gordon, J., Lee, Ch. J., and Dubos, R., *J. Exp. Med. 133:* 339 (1971).
11. Jones, J. M., Wilson, R., and Bealmear, P. M., *Radiat. Res. 45:* 577 (1971).
12. Gordon, H. A., *Nature 205:* 571 (1965).
13. Csaky, T. Z., in "The Germ-free Animal in Research," (M. E. Coates, ed.), p. 151, (1968).
14. Hayman, H., Fisher, C. J., Duggan, K. C., Rubert, M. W., and Faloon, W. W., *Gastroenterology 47:* 161 (1964).
15. Yow, M. D., and Yow, E. M., *Ped. Clin. N. Amer. 8:* 1043 (1961).

CONTROLLED TRIAL OF PROPHYLAXIS OF INFECTIONS FROM EXOGENOUS AND ENDOGENOUS MICROORGANISMS

Jerome W. Yates and *James F. Holland*
Roswell Park Memorial Institute
Buffalo, New York 14003, U.S.A.

Introduction

Since the advent of platelet transfusions to control hemorrhage, infection has become the major complication in acute leukemia patients receiving chemotherapy. Improved antibiotics and chemotherapy have only minimally altered morbidity and mortality from infection (1). Prophylaxis from infection using elaborate isolator systems for control of ambient contamination along with topical and enteric antimicrobial agents for endogenous suppression have been reported effective in reducing infection in these patients (2, 3). Substantial alterations in remission rate or survival primarily attributable to these environmental manipulations have not been found.

The intuitive assumption that patient isolation and endogenous flora suppression will contribute significantly to a reduction of infection remains to be proved. A prospective randomized study was therefore designed and executed to examine the relative effectiveness of barrier isolation utilizing high efficiency particulate air (H.E.P.A.) filtration and oral nonabsorbable antibiotics for gut flora suppression in an attempt to achieve a reduction in the number and severity of infections.

Methods

Acute myelocytic leukemia patients receiving cancer chemotherapy were selected as a homogenous high risk group. Patients were randomly allocated to: 1) conventional open ward care without antibiotics; 2) standard "reverse isolation" with antibiotics; 3) an isolator without antibiotics; or 4) an isolator with antibiotics. Patients receiving antibiotics (gentamicin, vancomycin and nystatin) for gut flora suppression also received mouthwash, douche and topical antimicrobial agents for the suppression of surface microflora. All isolator patients received a sterile diet, whereas only 9 of 22 in reverse isolation received a sterile diet. The remaining 13 were given foods found to have a relatively low bacterial count.

107

An air-conditioned area separate from the ward was constructed to house the isolators, nursing station, dietary kitchen, bacteriology laboratory and sterilizer room. Isolator patients were cared for by nurses assigned only to the unit while physicians attended both ward and isolator patients.

Four types of total barrier patient isolators were used for this study: 1) a cylindrical plastic tent isolator (Life Island, Mark V, Matthews Research, Alexandria, Va.); 2) a box-shaped plastic tent with H.E.P.A. filtration (Plysu Industrial Limited, Woburn Sands, England); 3) a single occupancy vertical laminar air flow room (VLAF); and 4) a double occupancy VLAF isolator (American Sterilizer Company, Erie, Pa.). Figure 1 illustrates personnel attending a patient in a half suit and full suit in the double occupancy VLAF isolator. Patient access was achieved using bedside gauntlets, half suits, and full suits, all of which were made as extensions of the walls of the isolators. Isolator material was between the patient and attendant or visiting personnel at all times.

Airborne isolator contamination was measured using an Anderson Air Sampler (Anderson Air Sampler, Salt Lake City, Utah), Rodac (replicate organism detection and counting) plates and settling plates. Patient cleanliness was assessed using quantitative body surface cultures obtained in a systematic sampling of total surface on various segments of the patient. Stools were cultured aerobically and anaerobically while aerobic quantitative cultures were obtained from the urine, mouthwash and douche.

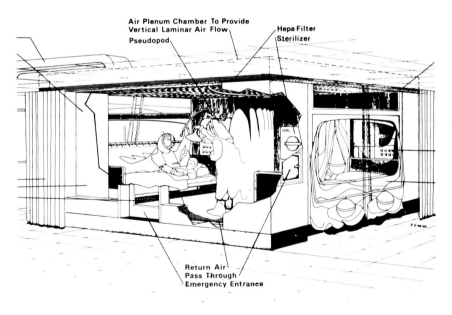

FIG. 1. Diagram of Single Occupancy Vertical Laminar Air Flow Room.

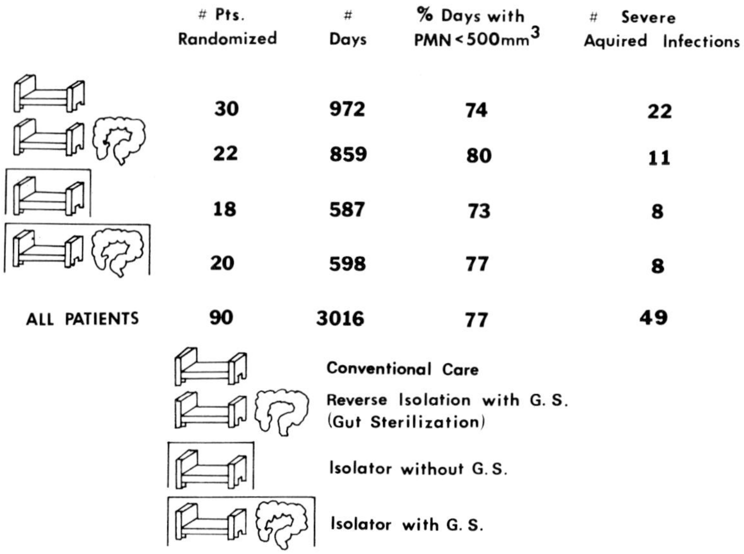

	# Pts. Randomized	# Days	% Days with PMN $<500mm^3$	# Severe Aquired Infections
	30	972	74	22
	22	859	80	11
	18	587	73	8
	20	598	77	8
ALL PATIENTS	90	3016	77	49

Conventional Care

Reverse Isolation with G. S. (Gut Sterilization)

Isolator without G. S.

Isolator with G. S.

FIG. 2. Number of severe acquired infections in patients treated with conventional care, reverse isolation with gut sterilization (G.S.), isolator without G.S., and isolator with G.S.

Results

A total of 90 randomizations involving patients ranging in age from 17 to 78 was conducted over a period of 34 months (Fig. 2). Fourteen patients were randomized two or three times, always to options including only those unoccupied during previous periods of isolator study. Patients unwilling to accept isolation or considered unsuitable for psychological reasons for isolation were excluded from randomization. Those leukopenic from their disease or expected to be leukopenic as a result of chemotherapy were randomly allocated to one of the four groups. They remained on study until they: 1) were removed because of psychological difficulty (3 patients); 2) developed complications from gut sterilization (1 patient); 3) achieved an absolute granulocyte count of $500/mm^3$ and were expected to attain remission ; or 4) approached imminent death. The evaluation of the outcome of those individuals whose isolation was compassionately terminated because of impending death was done as if they had died on study.

Patients infected at the time of their randomization (clinical, x-ray or bacteriologic evidence of infection for which antibiotic therapy was given) were found to have a significantly higher death rate than those entering the study uninfected. Also patients who had previously received anti-leukemic therapy were less likely to die during their study period than those receiving chemotherapy for the first time. Other studies where only previously treated

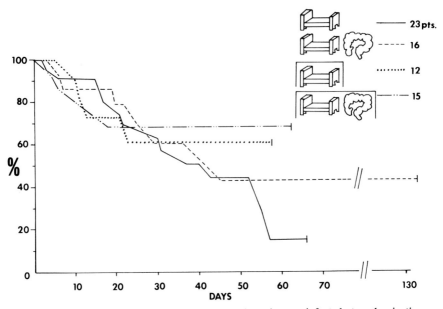

FIG. 3. Rate of acquisition of severe infections in patients uninfected at randomization.

and/or those uninfected were selected for placement in isolators biased results because these patients enjoy a better prognosis for immediate survival. Both patient isolation and enteric and surface antimicrobial agents do produce a reduction of culturable ambient and patient contamination. Airborne contamination is less by two log orders in the isolators when compared to a ward room. The use of nonabsorbable oral antibiotics yields a greater percentage of sterile (no recoverable organisms in cultures) in stool cultures (56% versus 2%). The 2% sterile stools occurring in patients not receiving oral nonabsorbable antibiotics were the result of systemic antibiotic therapy.

An analysis, by using life table techniques, of the comparative rate of

	SEPSIS	MOUTH + PHARNYX	LUNGS	MISC.
	5	7	8	2
	4	2	4	1
	4	0	1	3
	1	0	3	4

FIG. 4. The type of severe acquired infections in patients (Legend: see Figure 2).

acquisition of severe infection in patients uninfected at randomization can be seen in Fig. 3. Protection from the acquisition of severe infections was apparent in isolator patients only after day 23. In non-isolator patients, 11 severe infections were acquired after day 23 and 6 of these involved the respiratory tract. Fig. 4 illustrates the type of severe infections encountered in the study patients. There is a suggestion that some protection may be afforded by the isolators and/or the sterile diets against oropharyngeal infections.

Patients were independently randomized for chemotherapy regardless of study allocation. Because of the prognostic bias introduced by infection at the time of randomization, an analysis on only uninfected patients and their fate was accomplished (Fig. 5). Isolator patients not receiving antibiotics suppressing gut flora fared better than the other three groups. There was little difference in either the remission rate or the death rate of the other three groups. Patient survival was directly related to attaining remission. The deletion in the analysis of those patients having received what might retrospectively be considered inferior chemotherapy failed to alter these results. As seen in Fig. 2, all patients spent approximately 75% of their days on study with granulocyte counts less than 500/mm^3 indicating comparable chemotherapeutic-induced leukopenia.

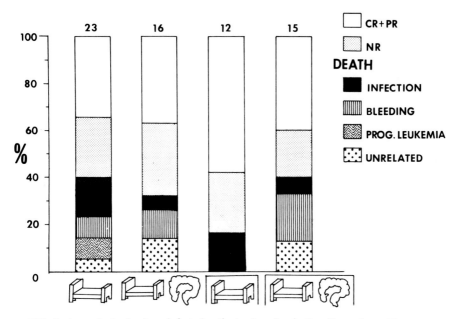

FIG. 5. An analysis of only uninfected patients at randomization (Legend: see Figure 2).

Summary and Conclusions

Although elaborate patient isolator systems can reduce ambient contamination, and gut flora suppressing antibiotics appear to reduce enteric contamination, a significant reduction of infectious morbidity and mortality among patients subjected to these environmental manipulations has not resulted. A reduction in the number of pseudomonas infections among isolator patients was found, though with evaluation the numbers were not significant. There appears to be some protection from upper and lower respiratory tract infections among isolator patients. Fewer deaths directly attributable to infection have occurred in those receiving oral nonabsorbable antibiotics (Fig. 5). No substantial explanation for the best remission rate occurring in those patients isolated and not receiving gut sterilization antibiotics is apparent, but possibly is related to the small sample studied.

Antimicrobial therapy and the use of patient isolators both appear to provide some benefit to patients with compromised host defenses. A better delineation of these beneficial effects through the continued study of supportive techniques should be accomplished.

Acknowledgement

This investigation was supported by the United States Public Health Service Grant No. CA-10044 from the National Cancer Institute.

References

1. Frei, E., Levin, R. H., Bodey, G. P., Morse, E. E., and Freireich, E. J., *Cancer Res. 25:* 1511 (1965).
2. Siegel, S., Henderson, E., Perry, S., and Levine, A., Abstract No. 49, *Blood 38:* 803 (1971).
3. Bodey, G. P., Gehan, E. A., and Freireich, E. J., *Proc. Am. Soc. Clin. Oncology,* (1971).

SECTION IV

CARCINOGENESIS IN GNOTOBIOTIC ENVIRONMENTS

CARCINOGENESIS IN GNOTOBIOTIC RODENTS

H. E. Walburg, Jr.
Biology Division, Oak Ridge National Laboratory
Oak Ridge, Tennessee 37830, U.S.A.

Introduction

Although it was clear from early studies on the pathogenesis of neoplasia in gnotobiotic animals that tumors could be induced by chemical carcinogens and oncogenic viruses, casual observation of relatively young germfree (GF) mice suggested that these animals were less susceptible to development of spontaneous neoplasia than their conventional (CONV) counterparts (1). Nonetheless, spontaneous tumors in GF mice were reported by Ward in 1961 (2) and were repeatedly confirmed thereafter (see ref 3). Neoplasms have also been induced by radiation in GF mice (4, 5). As more animals were examined at advanced ages, a greater number of spontaneous tumors was observed. These observations were qualitative in nature and suggested that gnotobiotic animals are capable of developing tumors in response to radiation, oncogenic viruses, and chemicals and in addition develop spontaneous tumors in many different tissues.

Recent Results

Recently, attempts have been made to quantitate both the development of spontaneous neoplasms in gnotobiotic animals and the tumor response to various carcinogenic treatments. Data from these studies indicate that the development of some neoplasms is influenced by the microbial environment, while that of others is not.

In gnotobiotes as in CONV animals, the most frequently occurring neoplasms have been the most studied. Thus, hemopoietic neoplasms (e.g., lymphomas and leukemia) in mice have received the greatest attention. Spontaneous development of thymic lymphoma has been studied in AKR, CFW, RFM, and ICR mice. Thymic lymphoma, which affects almost all CONV AKR mice, also is the cause of death in most GF AKR mice (6). When large numbers of mice are studied, however, the mortality rate from the disease appears to be slightly greater in the GF mice (7). In untreated RFM and ICR mice, thymic lymphoma occurs in lower incidence than in AKR mice and with a slightly greater incidence in GF as compared with CONV mice. These differences, however, are not statistically significant. A population of CFW mice with an unusually high incidence of lymphoblastic leukemia in the conventional environment were derived and studied as gnotobiotes. The GF mice had a greatly reduced incidence of this form of leukemia (9), an incidence comparable to that seen in other sublines of this strain reared in conventional environments by other investigators. Since GF newborns foster-nursed on CONV females from the "high leukemia colony" developed a high incidence of leukemia, and CONV newborns from that colony foster-nursed on GF females had a low incidence of leukemia, it seems likely that derivation of the gnotobiotic subline resulted in exclusion of some enhancing factor transmitted through the milk, possibly an oncogenic virus which is not present in other sublines of this strain of mice. In all other cases, however, thymic lymphoma appears spontaneously in GF mice at a somewhat higher incidence and somewhat earlier than in their CONV counterparts.

Reticulum cell sarcoma is also a common spontaneous hemopoietic neoplasm of mice, and the incidence of this disease has been determined in untreated GF ICR and RFM mice. In both strains the incidence of reticulum cell sarcoma is higher in CONV than in GF mice although in the case of ICR mice the sample size is not large and the difference is not statistically significant (8). The difference in time of onset and incidence of reticulum cell sarcoma in RFM mice, however, is statistically significant (see Table I). Recent unpublished data from our laboratory indicate that this difference is due principally to an

TABLE I. Summary of Cumulative Mortality Curves, i.e., Mean Age at Death (MAD) of GF and CONV RFM and C3H Mice for Different Causes of Death (see ref 38 for statistical techniques used)

Neoplasm	Strain	Sex	GF MAD $\pm$ SE	CONV MAD $\pm$ SE	P Values
Reticulum cell sarcoma	RFM	male + female	808 $\pm$ 19	703 $\pm$ 10	P⟨0.001
Mammary tumors	C3H	female	901 $\pm$ 32	870 $\pm$ 27	P⟩0.20
Liver tumors	C3H	male	823 $\pm$ 26	900 $\pm$ 19	P⟩0.20
Liver tumors	C3H	female	977 $\pm$ 29	907 $\pm$ 31	0.02⟩P⟩0.01
Nonendocrine + lung tumors	RFM	male + female	746 $\pm$ 51	649 $\pm$ 44	P⟩0.20
Malignant tumors	RFM	male + female	776 $\pm$ 35	677 $\pm$ 39	P⟩0.20

earlier onset of the disease in CONV mice.

Neoplasms developing in endocrine tissues of mice have also been studied extensively, especially breast tumors. In a small sample of ICR mice, there was no difference in the final incidence of mammary neoplasms (8). Casual observation of a C3H breeding colony suggested that the incidence of mammary neoplasms was lower than expected from data on CONV mice (10), but a careful analysis of retired female breeders from GF and CONV colonies showed no significant difference in risk of developing mammary tumors (11). Likewise, recent data from our laboratory show no difference in mortality rate due to breast tumors between GF and CONV virgin C3H females (Table I). Spontaneous ovarian tumors have also been studied in RFM and C3H mice. Although the yield of tumors in RFM female mice is small, there is no significant difference between GF and CONV mice (Table II). The incidence of spon-

TABLE II. Incidence of Different Neoplasms Seen at Necropsy in GF and CONV Mice (see ref 38 for statistical techniques used)

Neoplasm	Strain	Sex	Incidence % in GF at			Incidence % in CONV at			P values
			500 days	750 days	1000 days	500 days	750 days	1000 days	
Ovarian	RFM	female	0	0	67	0	0	7	P)0.20
Ovarian	C3H	female	0	47	50	0	27	59	P)0.20
Endocrine	RFM	female	0	0	83	0	20	26	P)0.20
Lung	RFM	male	0	67	83	22	27	67	0.20)P)0.10
Lung	RFM	female	18	36	48	17	43	100	P)0.20
Nonendocrine + lung	RFM	male+ female	8	8	40	6	14	23	P)0.20

taneous ovarian tumors in the C3H strain is considerably higher than in the RFM strain. There is also no difference in incidence of ovarian tumors in C3H virgin females (see Table II). There is no difference between GF and CONV RFM mice in the development of endocrine tumors when the various types (e.g., breast, ovarian, adrenal, thyroid) are pooled (Table II).

Other types of nonhemopoietic tumors have also been studied. The incidence of hepatoma in untreated male 40-week-old C3H mice has been reported by Grant and Roe (12) to be less in GF mice than in mice from their "minimal disease" colony. On the other hand, data from our laboratory suggest that the development of hepatomas in C3H male mice is not different throughout most of the life span although CONV males have an increased mortality rate from the tumor in the last third of life. The overall differences, however, are not sifnificant (see Table I). In female C3H mice there is a difference in mortality from liver tumors but in this case the GF mice have an

117

earlier mortality than their CONV counterparts (Table I). This apparent inconsistency suggests that further work will be necessary to clarify whether or not the microbial environment influences the development of hepatoma. Lung tumors in RFM mice have also been extensively studied. These tumors are generally small, papillary adenomas which only rarely appear to contribute to the death of the animal. The incidence of these tumors in germfree RFM male and female mice is not significantly different from that of their conventional counterparts (see Table II). For RFM mice, the incidence of all tumors other than endocrine and lung tumors is not significantly different either for those causing death (Table I) or for those occurring as incidental findings at death (Table II). Further, the incidence of malignant tumors in RFM mice is not significantly affected by the microbial environment (see Table I).

Thus, in summary, it appears that some spontaneous murine hemopoietic neoplasms are seriously affected by the absence of a conventional microbial environment whereas most, if not all, spontaneously occurring nonhemopoietic tumors are unaffected by the same alteration in microbial environment.

The induction of neoplasms in gnotobiotic animals has also been studied but with conflicting results. As in the case of spontaneous neoplasms, the microbial environment has its greatest effect on the expression of induced hemopoietic tumors. The incidence of radiation-induced myelogenous leukemia in RFM mice is greatly reduced in the absence of a microbial environment, but the incidence of thymic lymphoma is slightly (but not significantly) elevated (13). On the other hand, the induction of solid tumors by chemicals and by radiation has shown variable results. Grant and Roe (12) demonstrated that the incidence of DMBA-induced hepatomas in C3H mice is reduced in the absence of microbial environment, and others (14) have shown that urethane-induced lung tumors are likewise reduced in incidence in several mouse strains when the conventional microbial environment is absent. Intraperitoneal injection of mineral oil or its active components into CONV BALB/c mice results in the formation of abdominal plasma-cell tumors in a large number of cases. McIntire and Princler (15) failed to induce plasma-cell tumors in GF BALB/c mice so treated, but instead induced reticulum cell sarcoma. However, when the injection of mineral oil is accompanied by antigenic stimulation of the Peyer's patches, GF BALB/c mice do develop such tumors (16). Pollard and Salomon (17) have demonstrated that subcutaneous injection of methycholanthrene results in a similar incidence of lung tumors in GF and CONV mice. However, radiation-induced ovarian tumors and Harderian-gland tumors do not appear to be influenced by the microbial environment (18). Whether the differences observed with chemical carcinogens are the result of differences in location and metabolism of the chemical or the result of differences in promoting effects associated with microbial environment is not clear at this time.

Another species which has been extensively studied in the absence of a

TABLE III. Proportion of Tumors that are Malignant in GF and CONV Wistar Rats

Experiment reported by:	Ref. no.	Proportion (all tumors)	95% conf. interval	Proportion (breast tumors)	95% conf. interval
Conventional					
Paget & Lemon	21	.386	.326 – .448	–	–
Crain	22	.335	.270 – .405	.016	.001 – .083
Bullock & Curtis	23	.593	.550 – .636	.074	.035 – .146
Koletsky & Gustafson	24	.083	.018 – .225	–	–
Walpole et al.	25	.533	.266 – .787	–	–
Hueper	26	.469	.325 – .617	.000	.000 – .250
Ratcliffe (females)	27	.171	.125 – .225	.068	.039 – .111
Ratcliffe (males)	27	.432	.283 – .590	.000	.000 – .206
Kim et al.	28	.151	.068 – .276	.000	.000 – .166
Reinke et al.	29	.182	.082 – .327	.000	.000 – .236
MEAN		.334	.207 – .461	.053	.033 – .077
Germfree					
Pollard et al. '63	20	.077	.004 – .327	.167	.009 – .598
Pollard & Kajima '70	20	.000	.000 – .500	.000	.000 – .776
MEAN		.056	.000 – .242	.125	.006 – .500

microbial environment is the rat. Although at least three strains of rats have been examined for development of spontaneous neoplasms for many years, the data are as yet only qualitative. On the basis of limited data, Pollard (19) concluded that GF rats remain free of malignant tumors, suggesting some modification of the aging process. The published data are very few and are not matched by control CONV populations. An analysis of the difference between the ratio of malignant tumors to tumors of all types for GF Wistar rats (20) and CONV Wistar rats (21-29) suggests that the GF rats have a lower proportion of malignancy than the CONV. However, since the upper 95% confidence limit for the pooled GF data lies within the 95% confidence interval of the mean for the pooled CONV data and, since the GF data are compatible with the data from at least 4 of the 10 reported CONV populations, a more positive statement is not warranted. Further, it is clear that there is no significant difference in ratio of malignant breast tumors to total breast tumors (the most common tumor observed in aged female rats of this strain) between GF and CONV Wistar rats. Thus, while it is clear that GF rats also develop spontaneous neoplasms, both benign and malignant, attempts to quantitatively compare the incidences must await additional data.

Discussion

The microbial environment alters the expression of neoplasia of the hemopoietic system and in some cases influences the expression of tumors induced by chemical carcinogens. The relationship of these data to the principal theories of pathogenesis of neoplasia is important. The relation of viral infection to induction of neoplasms, particularly of hemopoietic neoplasms is well known. However, it has been clearly shown that there are no differences in susceptibility to oncogenic virus between gnotobiotic and CONV mice and rats (see ref 30). All GF mouse strains show evidence of oncogenic virus in their tissues but no such virus has been observed in germfree rats (30). These observations are consistent with the data from conventional animals of the same species. Thus, it does not appear that the differences in incidence of hemopoietic neoplasms in GF and CONV animals can be explained by a difference in the presence of, or susceptibility to, oncogenic virus. While the relation of somatic mutations to the induction of neoplasms has been repeatedly suggested, no studies have been made on the accumulation of somatic mutations in gnotobiotic rodents.

It is well known that host factors are important to the ultimate expression of neoplastic growths. Such promoting factors as nutritional state, immune competence, and rate of DNA synthesis may well affect the final incidence of neoplasms of different organs. Thus the microbial environment may, by altering such host factors, alter the incidence of neoplasms. The immune competence, both humoral and cellular, of gnotobiotic animals has been extensively studied. These studies demonstrate that GF animals have a slightly but consistently greater immune competence than their CONV counterparts (see ref 18). Such an increase in immune competence might explain a general reduction in the total numbers of neoplasms in GF animals but not the selective pattern which is seen. If the difference between incidences of hemopoietic neoplasms in GF and CONV mice are to be explained on the basis of immune competence, it is necessary to postulate an enhanced antigenicity of these types of tumors as compared to tumors of other organs. Enahnced antigenicity of virus-induced tumors has been clearly demonstrated (31). While this hypothesis would predict the observed decrease in incidence of myelogenous leukemia nd reticulum cell sarcoma, a decreased incidence of thymic lymphoma in GF mice would also be expected. Thymic lymphoma is not decreased, however, in GF mice.

It has been demonstrated that nutritional deficiencies can result in a reduction in the incidence of neoplasms (32). The effect does not appear to be selective but seems to affect neoplasms of all tissues. Thus it would be difficult to explain the selective effect reported here on the basis of nutritional deficiencies. The lact of a consistent response in the development of spontaneous hepatomas of C3H mice may, however, be related to nutrition since these tumors are particularly sensitive to dietary alteration (33). Another factor of significance to the development of neoplasia is increase in cellular proliferation. Rapidly proliferating tissues are more sensitive to carcinogenic treatment than are their more slowly proliferating counterparts, and treatments which induce cell proliferation frequently increase the incidence of neoplasms in tissues treated with carcinogens (see ref 34). The microbial environment influences the amount of DNA synthesis in some, but not all, cellular compartments, principally those producing granulocytes (18), lymphocytes (35), and intestinal epithelial cells (36). Thus the effect of the microbial environment on the induction of myelogenous leukemia by radiation has been explained on the basis of a reduced proliferation of the granulocytic compartment (37). Differences in incidence of reticulum cell sarcoma in RFM mice may also be related to antigenic stimulation of the reticulum cells in lymphatic tissues. Thus, while the relative importance of various host factors in influencing the ultimate expression of neoplasia is not clear, studies on the role of the microbial environment in the pathogenesis of spontaneous and induced neoplasms may help to clarify the mechanisms of carcinogenesis.

Acknowledgements

Research sponsored by the United States Atomic Energy Commission under contract with the Union Carbide Corporation.

References

1. Pollard, M., *Perspectives in Virology IV,* M. Pollard ed.), Academic Press, New York, New York, p. 257, (1964).
2. Ward, T. G., *Fed. Proc. 20:* 150 (1961).
3. Salomon, J. C., "The Germfree Animal in Research," (M. E. Coates, ed), Academic Press, New York, New York, p. 227, (1968).
4. Pollard, M., and Kajima, M., *Proc. Int. Conf. Radiat. Biol. and Cancer, Kyoto,* p. 175, (1966).
5. Walburg, H. E. Jr., Upton, A. C., Tyndall, R. L., Harris, W. W., and Cosgrove, G. E.., *Proc. Soc. Exp. Biol. Med. 118:* 11 (1965)..
6. Pollard, M., Kajima, M., and Teah, B. A., *Proc. Soc. Exp. Biol. Med. 120:* 72 (1965).
7. Walburg, H. E. Jr., and Cosgrove, G. E., *Advances in Experimental Medicine and Biology, Vol. 3,* "Germ-free Biology: Experimental and Chemical Aspects," (E. A. Mirand and N. Back, eds), Plenum Press, New York, New York, p. 135, (1969).
8. Walburg, H. E. Jr., and Cosgrove, G. E., *Exp. Gerontol. 2:* 143 (1967).
9. Nielsen, A. H., Amelunxen, R. E., Kornhaus, J., Sheek, M., and Werder, A. A., in "Germfree Research: Biological Effect of Gnotobiotic Environments," (J. B. Heneghan, ed.), Academic Press, New York, p. 137, (1973).
10. Kajima, M., and Pollard, M., *J. Bacteriol. 90:* 1448 (1965).
11. Pilgrim, H. I., and Lebrecque, A. D., *Cancer Res. 27 (1):* 584 (1967).
12. Grant, G. A., and Roe, F. J. C., *Nature 222:* 1282 (1969).
13. Walburg, H. E. Jr., and Cosgrove, G. E., *Proc. 1st Europ. Symp. on Late Effects of Radiation,* (P. Metalli, ed.), Comitato Nazionalle Energia Nucleare, Rome, p. 50, (1970).
14. Burstein, N. A., McIntire, K. R., and Allison, A. C., *J. Nat. Cancer Inst. 44: 212 (1970).*
15. McIntire, K. R., and Princler, G. L., *Immunology 17:* 481 (1969).
16. Hanna, M. G., Yang, W. K., and Walburg, H. E. Jr., (In preparation).
17. Pollard, M., and Salomon, J. C., *Proc. Soc. Exp. Biol. Med. 112:* 256 (1963).

121

18. Walburg, H. E. Jr., *Proc. IVth Int. Cong. Radiat. Res.,* Evian, France, (In press).
19. Pollard, M., *Proc. Nat. Conf. on Research Animals in Medicine,* (L. T. Harmison, ed.), (In press).
20. Pollard, M., and Kajima, M., *Amer. J. Pathol. 61:* 25 (1970).
21. Paget, G. E., and Lemon, P. G., "The Pathology of Laboratory Animals," (W. E. Ribelin and J. R. McCoy, eds.), C. C. Thomas, Springfield, Illinois, p. 382, (1963).
22. Crain, R. C., *Amer. J. Pathol. 34:* 311 (1958).
23. Bullock, F. D., and Curtis, M. R., *J. Cancer Res. 14:* 1 (1930).
24. Koletsky, S., and Gustafson, G. E., *Cancer Res. 15:* 100 (1955).
25. Walpole, A. L., Roberts, D. C., Rose, F. L., Hendry, J. A., and Homer, R. F., *Brit. J. Pharmacol. 9:* 306 (1954).
26. Hueper, W. C., *J. Nat. Cancer Inst. 16:* 447 (1955).
27. Ratcliffe, H. L., *Amer. J. Pathol. 16:* 237 (1940).
28. Kim, U., Clifton, K. H., and Furth, J., *J. Nat. Cancer Inst. 24:* 103 (1960).
29. Reincke, U., Stutz, E., and Wegner, G., *Z. Krebsforsch. 66:* 165 (1964).
30. Pollard, M., *Perspectives in Virology. V.,* "Virus-Directed Host Response," (M. Pollard, ed.), Academic Press, New York, New York, p. 267, (1967).
31. Severi, L., "Immunity and Tolerance in Oncogenesis," 2 vols., (L. Severi, ed.), Division of Cancer Research, Perugia, Italy, (1970).
32. Ross, M. H., and Bras, G., *J. Nutr. 87:* 245 (1965).
33. Tannenbaum, A., and Silverstone, H., *Cancer Res. 9:* 162 (1949).
34. United Nations Scientific Committee on the Effects of Atomic Radiation, Annex G, Experimental Induction of Neoplasms by Radiation, United Nations, N.Y., (In press).
35. Olson, G. B., and Wostmann, B. S., *J. Immunol. 97:* 267 (1966).
36. Lesher, S., Walburg, H. E. Jr., and Sacher, G. A. Jr., *Nature 202:* 884 (1964).
37. Walburg, H. E. Jr., Cosgrove, G. E., and Upton, A. C., *Int. J. Cancer 3:* 150 (1968).
38. Hoel, D. G., and Walburg, H. E. Jr., *J. Nat. Cancer Inst.,* (In press).

SPONTANEOUS TUMORS IN JAPAN-BORN GERMFREE RATS

Masasumi Miyakawa
Laboratory of Germfree Life Research, Kawashima, Japan

and

Yukiko Sumi and *Yutaka Uno*
Institute of Germfree Life Research,
Nagoya University School of Medicine, Nagoya, Japan

Introduction

A colony of Japanese-born rats was established in 1963 at Nagoya University School of Medicine after a long series of experiments, which had been started in 1954. This paper reports the spontaneous tumors that were observed in these germfree rats which were propagated up to the 12th generation during the period from 1963 to 1967.

Four strains of rats (Gifu hybrid, Fisher, Donryu and Wistar strains) employed for this experiment were propagated at the Nagoya University School of Medicine. The Gifu hybrid was the offspring of the rats originally derived from Gifu Prefecture, Japan. The Donryu strain was produced by H. Sato by repeating brother-sister matings for more than twenty generations. The Fisher strain was originally imported from the United States. The Wistar strain was obtained from the Takeda Chemical Co., Japan. Germfree rats which were derived from mothers by Cesarean operation were reared by forced hand-feeding using a gastric catheter. Although the rats of all 4 strains reached maturity, only the Wistar strain was propagated in germfree state to the 12th generation. When spontaneous tumors were observed in these rats, the rats were killed and subjected to histopathological examinations on tumor tissues, regional lymph nodes and endocrine organs. Tissues were fixed in formol-Zenker solution, sectioned and stained with hematoxylin-eosin, periodic acid-Schiff reaction, silver impregnation for reticulum, Mallory's aniline blue, Masson's trichome, Van Gieson's picrofuchsin and pyronin-methylgreen for plasma cells. The immuno-fluorescent technique was also employed to confirm the identity of antibody producing cells.

123

Results

Of 634 germfree adult rats (351 females), 7 had spontaneous neoplasms: 5 mammary fibroadenomas, 1 cortical adenoma of the adrenal and 1 thymoma (Table I).

TABLE I. Frequency of Spontaneous Tumor in Germfree Adult Rats of Wistar Strain (On and After Second Generation)

Kind of Tumor	No. Tumor / Total Females	No. Tumor / Total Males
Fibroadenoma	5/351	
Cortical Adenoma	1/351	
Thymoma		1/283

Rats of the first generation which grew to adulthood through forced hand-feeding, consisted of 7 Gifu hybrid (5 females), 2 Fisher strain rats (1 female), 4 Donryu strain rats (1 female), and 20 Wistar strain rats (12 females). However, none of them had spontaneous tumors during their lifetime. It is noteworthy that no mammary tumors were found in germfree female rats of the first generation which were hand-fed and did not experience lactation.

TABLE II. Generation and Age of Rats Bearing Fibroadenoma and Size of Each Tumor

	Generation	Age (days)	Size of Tumor (cm)
No. 1	2nd	522	5.9 x 5.5 x 4.8
No. 2	3rd	604	6.4 x 5.1 x 6.3
No. 3	4th	519	1.5 x 1.2 x 0.8
No. 4	5th	292	1.0 x 0.8 x 0.7
No. 5	10th	852	4.7 x 4.0 x 3.6
Average		502	

As shown in Table II, 5 fibroadenomas were found in rats of the Wistar strain at ages ranging from 292 days to 852 days. A tumor was found in each group of the 2nd, 3rd, 4th, 5th and 10th generation. The tumors varied in size from a small nodule 1.0 x 0.8 x 0.7 cm in dimension to a large firm lobulated mass measuring 6.4 x 5.1 x 6.3 cm. They were located in the subcutaneous tissue, and were well defined and easily separated from adjacent muscular tissues. The cut surface of the tumors for the most part showed nodules of various sizes. Microscopic examination revealed that the tumor consisted of the epithelial and connective tissue components. The relative distribution of each component varied in case and portion. In some cases the connective tissue exceeded the epithelial component; the connective tissue which varied in amount, density and maturity, proliferated and circumscribed the epithelial cells of the glands and ducts (Fig. 1). Fusiform fibroblasts proliferated in small

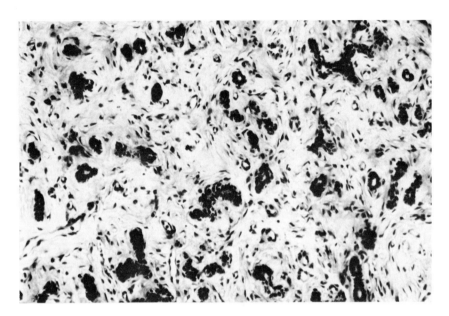

FIG. 1. H & E x 100. Fibroadenoma with overgrowth of the connective tissue which embraced the gland- and duct-like structures.

nodules, showing cellular stroma. In the older ones, excess fibrosis apparently induced glandular components to atrophy by pressure and resulted in hyalinization of the connective tissues. When the epithelial tissue was prominent, the epithelial elements formed gland- or duct-like structures lined with a single layer of columnar or cuboidal cells. In occasional cases the epithelial component increased at the expense of the connective tissue, and the histologic appearance was more like that of an adenoma (Fig. 2). In germfree rats, cellular components involving infiltrating cells were scanty, in general, in the contact zone between the normal host tissue and the tumor tissue. Table III notes the weights of the regional lymphnodes (axillary or abdomino-inguinal). The lymphnodes taken from the tumor side of the body were larger than those of the opposite side. The numbers of pyroninophilic plasma cells in the medullary cords of the lymph nodes of the tumor side were few in number, compared to those lymph nodes taken from the opposite side. These pyroninophilic cells contained gammaglobulins, according to the fluorescent antibody technique. The pituitary and adrenal glands of germfree rats with fibroadenomas were examined. The

125

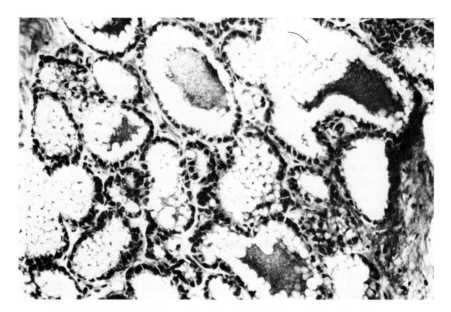

FIG. 2. H & E x 100. Preponderating epithelial elements in a fibroadenoma.

TABLE III. Wet Weight of Regional Lymphnodes of Rats Bearing Fibroadenomas (mg)

	Tumor Side (mg)	Tumor Free Side (mg)
No. 1	12.0	8.5
No. 2	14.0	9.0
No. 3	36.5	14.5
No. 4	7.5	6.2
No. 5	19.5	10.5
Average	17.9	9.7

relative weights of the pituitary and adrenal glands per gram body weight of germfree rats showed no remarkable difference between the tumor bearing group and the tumor-free group (Table IV). By microscopic examination, a cortical adenoma was found in the adrenal gland of one rat which carried a breast fibroadenoma. It was difficult to determine whether there was a relationship between the cortical adenoma and the mammary fibroadenoma.

One thymoma was found in a germfree Wistar rat, which had been hand-fed. This tumor was observed in a male germfree rat of the 5th generation group at 830 days of age. The tumor was extended from the position of the thymus to the heart which was forced to move to the left side. Further, it

TABLE IV. Weight of the Pituitary and Adrenal Glands of Rats Bearing Fibroadenoma
(mg per 100 gm body weight)

	Tumor Bearing Cases 292-852 Days of Age	Tumor Free Cases 314-720 Days of Age
Pituitary	4.57 ± 0.57* (5)**	4.65 ± 0.67 (10)
Adrenal (both sides)	17.34 ± 3.13 (5)	18.38 ± 2.91 (10)

*Standard deviation.
**The number of rats is indicated in parentheses.

extended into the right pleural cavity and compressed the hilar region to cause the atelectasis of the right lung. It invaded ventrally into the pericardium at the apex of the heart and the diaphragm. It infiltrated anteriorly destroying the sternum and upwards to the atrium and auricle of the heart, destroying cardial musculature, and around the trachea and the aorta (Fig. 3). By microscopic examination, it was revealed that the tumor consisted of epithelial reticular tissue admixed with lymphocytes. The epithelial reticular cells were polymorphic and occasionally spindle shaped. Occasionally, these epithelial cells formed small whorles, resembling Hassall's corpuscles (Fig. 4). However, they showed no evidence of cornification. The infiltrating lymphocytes mingled with the epithelial cells in varying proportion were present in different parts of the tumor. The tumor was designated a malignant thymoma on the basis of its

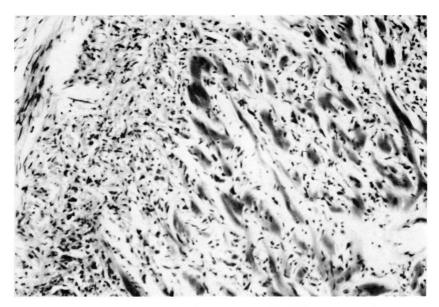

FIG. 3. H & E x 100. The auricular muscle infiltrated by thymoma cells.

127

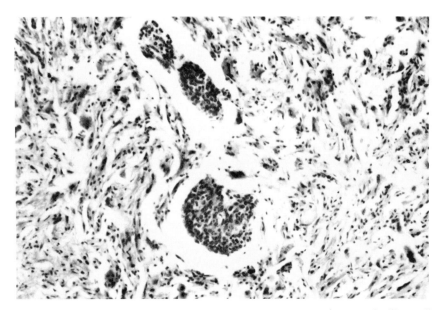

FIG. 4. H & E x 100. Thymoma with epithelial cells forming Hassall's corpuscles-like small whorles.

characteristic lympho-epithelial properties and its autonomous behavior. Muscular atrophy, red cell aplasia and lymphopenia which were reported to be found in conventional rats bearing thymomas were not observed in the germfree rat bearing this thymoma. The marked plasma cell response which was observed in the contact zone between a methylcholanthrene-induced fibro-sarcoma (particularly at the early stage of development) and the host tissue, was not observed in the germfree rat bearing the spontaneous malignant thymoma.

Conclusions

1) In 634 germfree adult rats (351 females) subjected to observation, 7 had spontaneous neoplasms: mammary fibroadenomas in 5 females, a cortical adenoma of the adrenal gland in 1 female, and a thymoma in 1 male.

2) Fibroadenomas were found at average age of 502 days.

3) One rat bearing a mammary fibroadenoma had a small cortical adenoma in the adrenal gland. No abnormality, however, was found in the pituitary glands of these rats.

4) A malignant thymoma was observed in a male germfree rat at the age of 830 days.

5) A plasma cell response in the germfree host with the spontaneous malignant thymoma was not observed, compared with that of the germfree host

against tumors induced by methylcholanthrene.

References

1. Crain, R. C., *Am. J. Path. 34:* 311 (1958).
2. Ratcliffe, H. L., *Am. J. Path. 16:* 237 (1940).
3. Heiman, J., *Am. J. Cancer 22:* 497 (1934).
4. Pollard, M., and Teah, B. A., *J. Nat. Cancer Inst. 31:* 457 (1963).

STUDY ON TRANS-SPECIES INDUCTION OF RETICULAR TISSUE NEOPLASMS IN GERMFREE CFW$_W$ MICE

Alvar A. Werder, Anne H. Nielsen, Remi E. Amelunxen,
O. J. Mira, and *Martha Sheek*
Department of Microbiology, University of Kansas School of
Medicine, Kansas City, Kansas 66103, U.S.A.

Introduction

It has been postulated (1) that: a) the genetic information for C-type viruses responsible for the development of reticular tissue neoplasms may be present in all vertebrates as repressed viral genomes and, b) the expression of oncogenic effects of these viruses may be influenced by environmental factors such as exposure to radiation and carcinogens, as well as by aging. Recently, evidence for the oncogenic expression of previously undetected genetic information apparently occurred by the formation of pseudotype viruses consisting of components derived from the viral genomes of two mammalian species (2, 3). Thus, it appears that so-called trans-species induction of viral oncogenesis by *in vivo* rescue of C-type viruses from species in which such viruses had not been demonstrated previously has been accomplished.

In the present study we have attempted to determine if trans-species induction of oncogenesis to mice has occurred. Therefore, utilizing a colony of germfree CFW$_W$ (4) mice, comparisons were made between: a) the oncogenic expressions of endogenous oncogenes involving reticular tissues and, b) the oncogenic effects which resulted from inoculations of cellular or of cell free preparations of lymphoreticular neoplasms from three foreign species (avian, canine and human). The former group (a) will be referred to as endogenous neoplasms and the latter group (b) as exogenous neoplasms.

Results

Endogenous lymphoreticular neoplasms. The endogenous lymphoreticular neoplasms have all been of the lymphocytic cell type. This is demonstrated by these results which are included in the data presented in Table I: a) During a ten year study 5,085 germfree and exgermfree mice have been observed until they reached the age of 6 to 24 months. To facilitate experimental procedures at times mice were removed from the germfree to an exgermfree environment which consisted of sterilized cages, food, and bedding. The mice raised in both the germfree and exgermfree environments have been designated as CFW_W (4) mice. A total of 13 of these mice developed lymphomas of lymphocytic cell type. b) The inoculation of cells from a cell culture of tissue from germfree embryos into suckling CFW_W mice resulted in lymphocytic leukemia in all of 23 mice inoculated. c) By exposing exgermfree young adult mice to radiation as previously described by Pollard and Matsuzawa (5), 43 of 106 mice developed lymphocytic lymphomas.

Though the neoplasms resulting from aging and x-radiation were lymphomas, in serial passages leukemia-lymphoma complexes were invariably produced. By the term lymphoma we refer to the development of enlarged lymph nodes and/or extranodal tumor masses. When malignant tissues were implanted subcutaneously, progressively growing tumors developed. When only leukemia developed (for example, as a result of the inoculation of the cell culture mentioned above), large numbers of malignant cells were observed in peripheral blood and these leukemic cells did not grow locally following subcutaneous implantation. When leukemia-lymphoma complexes were serially passaged, either by subcutaneous or intraperitoneal routes, lymphomas and leukemia developed in the recipients.

C-type particles have been observed in the mice with lymphomas and leukemias (6) and these neoplasms can be transmitted with inoculations of cell free preparations of malignant tissue (7). To assure effective transmission the neoplasms usually were serially passaged with homogenized tissue. The type of neoplasm, that is the leukemia-lymphoma complex or only leukemia, and the cell type were consistently maintained in all serial passages. As can be seen from the results in Table I, these characteristics have been maintained for many consecutive passages.

Comparisons of endogenous and exogenous lymphoreticular neoplasms. In

TABLE I. Endogenous Lymphoreticular Neoplasms in Germfree
and Exgermfree CFW_W Mice.

Type of induction	No. neoplasms total no. mice	Lymphocytic neoplasms	Last continuous passage*
Aging	13/5085	100%	77th
Inoculation of murine cell culture	23/23	100%	35th
Whole body radiation	43/106	100%	25th

*Cell type remained lymphocytic in all the passages.

132

order to attempt trans-species induction to the mice we inoculated specimens prepared from avian, canine and human lymphoreticular neoplasms. The preparations, usually obtained from the donors less than 4 hours before inoculation into the mice, consisted of whole blood, whole bone marrow, homogenized tumor tissue, or filtered cell free specimens (7). In one instance a cell culture of canine tumor tissue was used (8). The one specimen of avian source was a histiocytic lymphoma with numerous C-type viral particles. The recipients of this avian neoplasm also developed histiocytic lymphomas. Eight specimens were obtained from each of the other two species. Four of the donors, two from each species, had lymphocytic neoplasms. The murine recipients developed reticular neoplasms of the same cell type. The other donors had reticular neoplasms of reticulum, plasmacytic and undifferentiated cell types. Again, the recipients had similar cell types. The recipients of the canine cell culture developed reticulum cell leukemia; the donor also was diagnosed as having reticulum cell leukemia. A total of 52 mice developed lymphoreticular neoplasms following the inoculation of avian, canine and human specimens. In Table II we compare the incidences of endogenous and exogenous lymphocytic neoplasms. It can be seen that all 79 of the endogenous neoplasms were lymphocytic whereas only 12 of 52 exogenous neoplasms were lymphocytic.

TABLE II. Incidence of Reticular Tissue Neoplasms of Lymphocytic Cell Type.

Types of neoplasms*	No. with lymphocytic cell type total no. neoplasms
Endogenous	79/79
Exogenous	12/52

*See text for definition of terms.

Immunologic studies have been started for further comparison of the two groups of neoplasms, i.e., endogenous and exogenous. An example, which is typical of the results obtained with immunoprotection tests, will be presented. In these experiments, mice approximately 6 weeks of age, were implanted subcutaneously with approximately 10 million tumor cells. One to two weeks later a similar dose of a second tumor was implanted subcutaneously at a second site. The first tumor usually was implanted in the neck region and the second in the left or right groin. Only lymphomas could be used since the leukemias did not develop locally when inoculated subcutaneously. The results obtained with the immunoprotection tests are presented in Table III. Two tumors were used as second, or challenging tumors: the endogenous tumor had developed as a spontaneous tumor in a germfree mouse and had been passaged 43 consecutive times and the exogenous tumor had developed in a mouse following the

TABLE III. Effects of Active Immunization on Transplantable Tumors.

Immunizing tumors	Challenging tumors	Persistent tumors	
		no./no. mice	%
None (3x)	Endogenous	17/30	56
Homologous, Endogenous (2x)	Endogenous	1/20	5
Heterologous, Endogenous (5x)	Endogenous	4/50	8
Exogenous (4x)	Endogenous	17/40	42
None (3x)	Exogenous	14/30	47
Homologous, Exogenous (2x)	Exogenous	0/20	0
Heterologous, Exogenous (4x)	Exogenous	18/40	45
Endogenous (3x)	Exogenous	13/28	46

*Numbers in (x) indicate number of attempts with 8 to 10 mice per group.
Homologous indicates same tumor was used for immunization and challenge.
Heterologous indicates different tumors were used for immunization and challenge.

inoculation of human tissues and had been passaged 66 consecutive times. Both of the challenging tumors were lymphocytic leukemia-lymphoma complexes. In non-immunized mice, 56% of the endogenous and 47% of the exogenous tumors grew progressively. It can be observed from the data that evidently the two challenging tumors contained tumor specific antigens (TSA), since homologous (see Table III for definition) combinations of immunizing and challenging tumors resulted in the highest proportion of rejections. The heterologous endogenous tumors appeared to share the TSA of the challenging endogenous tumor whereas the four exogenous tumors used for immunization did not share the TSA with the endogenous tumor. On the basis of the results presented, the TSA of the challenging exogenous tumor was not shared by any of the ɔ endogenous and 2 heterologous exogenous tumors used to immunize the mice. In other experiments of this type we have shown similar results when 4 exogenous and 5 endogenous tumors were studied, i.e. all the endogenous tumors shared TSA and each exogenous tumor had a differentiating TSA.

Conclusions

It appears from the data presented that there are two distinct groups of lymphoreticular neoplasms in the mice of this study. One group consists of endogenous neoplasms. Apparently on the basis of cell type and TSA there is a consistency to these markers which suggests that a single oncogene is being expressed.

The other group consists of reticular neoplasms which developed following the inoculation of tissues from avian, canine and human species. The differences in cell types and the apparent specificity of the TSA for each of these exogenous tumors indicate the presence of other than endogenous oncogenes being expressed. Based upon these data and the present state of knowledge, it appears that the exogenous neoplasms are at least in part under the influence of genetic information supplied by the inoculated tissues.

Acknowledgement

Supported in part by Flossie E. West Memorial Fund.

References

1. Huebner, R. J., and Todaro, G. J., *Proc. Nat. Acad. Sci. U.S.A. 64:* 1087 (1969).
2. Aaronson, S. A., *Virology 44:* 29 (1971).
3. Gilden, R. V., Ororszlan, S., and Heubner, R. J., *Virology 43:* 722 (1971).
4. Nielsen, A. H., Amelunxen, R. E., Kornhaus, J., Sheek, M., and Werder, A. A., in "Germfree Research: Biological Effect of Gnotobiotic Environments," (J. B. Heneghan, ed.), Academic Press, New York, p. 137, (1973).
5. Pollard, M., and Matsuzawa, T., *Proc. Soc. Exp. Biol. Med. 116:* 1967 (1964).
6. Chapman, A. L., Nielsen, A., Cohen, H., Larsen, W. E., and Werder, A., *Proc. Soc. Exp. Biol. Med. 122:* 1022 (1966).
7. Nielsen, A. H., "Viral oncogenic studies in conventional CFW and germfree CFW_W mice," Ph.D. Thesis, University of Kansas School of Medicine, (1969).
8. Chapman, A. L., Bopp, W. J., Brightwell, A. S., Cohen, H., Nielsen, A. H., Gravelle, C. R., and Werder, A. A., *Cancer Res. 27:* 18 (1967).

135

NATURAL TRANSMISSION OF LEUKEMIA AND MAMMARY TUMORS IN CONVENTIONAL AND GERMFREE CFW$_W$ MICE

Anne H. Nielsen, Remi E. Amelunxen, James Kornhaus,
Martha Sheek and *Alvar A. Werder*
Department of Microbiology, University of Kansas School
of Medicine, Kansas City, Kansas 66103, U.S.A.

Introduction

The occurrence of leukemia and mammary tumors in successive generations of mice has been studied in many laboratories. Usually the mode of natural transmission for both malignancies has been reported as being "vertical" rather than "horizontal" (1, 2). For mammary tumors, variation for type of "vertical" transmission appears to depend upon the strain of virus being studied. For leukemias there appear to be differences dependent upon whether the disease was spontaneous or laboratory induced. In the former situation the mode of transmission has been reported as having a chromosomal pattern whereas in the latter it usually was postnatal, mainly through milk (3).

In the present study comparisons were made on the incidence and natural transmission of leukemias and mammary tumors to successive generations in CFW$_W$ (4) mice. The following viral-host systems were compared: spontaneous mammary tumors and leukemias in germfree and conventional mice, and serially passaged spontaneous and laboratory induced leukemias.

Results

Incidence of malignancies. Conventional CFW mice, originally purchased from Carworth Farms, New City, New York, had been randomly bred in our laboratories for nearly 10 years before we developed a germfree colony derived by Cesarean section in 1962. When the conventional mice were used for short term studies no malignancies were observed. However, when experimental procedures required observation periods of six months or longer, a moderately high incidence of leukemias and mammary tumors developed in the mice. Consistently, the incidence of leukemias has been approximately 30% in breeders of both sexes by the time the mice have attained the age of two years. Breeding females had a similar incidence for mammary tumors by this age. In

TABLE I. Incidence of Naturally Occurring Leukemia and Mammary Tumors in Conventional CFW Mice.

No. mice	Mice with leukemia No.	%	Mean time of death (mo.)	Mice with mammary tumors No.	%	Mean time of death (mo.)
			Breeders			
213 males	62	29	10.7	0		
168 females	45	27	9.1	39	23	12.1
			Nonbreeders			
99 males	27	27	10.8	0		
98 females	33	33	10.8	0		

Table I we present results obtained from an experiment when breeders and non-breeders were observed for the development of leukemias and mammary tumors. There was a striking consistency for the incidence and mean time of death of leukemia in the four groups of mice, i.e. both sexes in breeders and non-breeders. Mammary tumors developed only in breeding females with the mean time of death at a slightly later age than that observed for the leukemias.

The germfree colony, started with 24 mice, 10 males and 14 females, has produced approximately 7,000 mice in 22 successive generations. The techniques for maintaining a germfree environment were similar to those described previously (4, 6). To facilitate experimental procedures at times mice were removed from the germfree to an exgermfree environment consisting of sterilized cages, food and bedding. The mice raised in both the germfree and exgermfree environments have been designated as CFW_W (7) mice. The markedly reduced incidences of leukemias and mammary tumors observed in breeding germfree and exgermfree mice are depicted in Table II. Only leukemias of the lymphocytic cell type were observed in conventional, germfree and exgermfree mice.

Natural transmission of malignancies. The natural transmission of spontaneous leukemias and mammary tumors in the conventional mice was

TABLE II. Incidence of Naturally Occurring Leukemia and Mammary Tumors in Germfree and Exgermfree CFW_W Mice from 1962 to 1971.

No. mice	% leukemias	Mean time of death (mo.)	% mammary tumors	Mean time of death (mo.)
		Germfree		
1030 males	⟨0.5	15.2	0.0	—
1546 females	⟨0.5	13.1	⟨1.5	13.4
		Exgermfree		
1274 males	0.0	—	0.0	—
1235 females	⟨0.5	10.6	⟨0.5	12.0

mainly by postnatal means. This was demonstrated by two experiments: a. Cesarean derived infants from leukemic conventional females did not develop either malignancy when foster nursed by exgermfree females. b. Leukemic conventional females transmitted both malignancies to suckling natural offspring as well as to foster nursed exgermfree infants. Both groups of infants had similar incidences of the two neoplasms. By comparison, spontaneous leukemias and mammary tumors of the germfree and exgermfree mice were not transmitted to any of more than 500 infants of female parents with either of these malignancies.

Leukemias developing in the germfree mice following the influence of three different environmental factors have been serially passaged with the inoculation of homogenized tissue. Periodically, infants of inoculated females which survived for a sufficient length of time to bear young were observed for malignancies. The environmental situations which resulted in the development of leukemia were: a. aging, b. exposure of embryonic tissue to cell culture techniques (unpublished data) and c. exposure of young adult mice to whole body irradiation (4). As may be observed from the data in Table III, less than two percent of the offspring of the leukemic female parents developed leukemia.

TABLE III. Transmission of Leukemia to Offspring of Leukemic Mice; Parents were Inoculated with Leukemias Endogenous to Germfree or Exgermfree CFW$_W$ Mice.

Leukemic strains due to these environmental factors	No. of offspring	No. with leukemia	Age* at time of death (mo.)
Aging	100	1	8
Murine cell culture	35	0	–
Radiation	44	2	14,17
Totals	179	3 (1.6%)	

*Offspring were observed until the age of 2 years.

One strain of leukemia associated with mammary tumors of conventional mice and one strain of leukemia of exgermfree mice have been transmitted with consistency to offspring by a postnatal route. In female progeny of the conventional leukemic mice both leukemias and mammary tumors developed with relatively high frequency, 58% and 36%, respectively. It is of interest that 64% of the leukemic female offspring also developed mammary tumors. The male offspring had only a 24% incidence of leukemia and no mammary tumors. The leukemia from the exgermfree mice developed following the inoculation of a cell culture derived from canine leukemic tissue (8). This leukemia has been transmitted with high efficiency via milk to infants for 21 successive generations. Though the incidence in the infants was relatively high (approximately 70%), none of the females developed mammary tumors. The incidence of leukemia was similar in both sexes. The data on natural transmission obtained with these two leukemias are presented in Table IV.

TABLE IV. Comparison of Postnatal Transmission of Two Serially Transmitted Leukemias to Progeny of Leukemic Mice.

Source of neoplasms*	No. mice	% leukemia	Mean time of death (mo.)	% mammary tumors	Mean time of death (mo).
		Females			
Conventional mice	370	58**	9.5	36	10.0
Exgermfree mice	218	72	8.5	0	—
		Males			
Conventional mice	384	24	9.4	0	—
Exgermfree mice	246	65	7.4	0	—

*See text for description.
**65% of females with leukemia also had mammary tumors.

Conclusions

There were marked differences in the modes of transmission of naturally occurring leukemias and mammary tumors. Both malignancies were transmitted mainly by postnatal routes in conventional mice. By contrast, both malignancies were transmitted sporadically and, apparently, only by prenatal routes in germfree and exgermfree mice.

It appeared that laboratory induced leukemias endogenous to the germfree and exgermfree mice, i.e. induced by exposure of embryonic tissue to cell culture techniques or exposure of mice to whole body irradiation, were not transmitted to infants of leukemic females.

Only one strain of leukemia in exgermfree mice was transmitted consistently and with high efficiency to infants by postnatal means. There were striking differences between this leukemia and the leukemia of the conventional mice which was also transmitted postnatally. The former leukemia developed with similar incidence in both sexes and was not associated with mammary tumors. The leukemia in the conventional mice, on the other hand, was associated with mammary tumors in females in a majority of instances. The incidence of leukemia in the females was twice that of the males.

Perhaps the oncongenic viruses associated with these different neoplasms are genetic variants which might be identifiable by physico-chemical techniques.

Acknowledgement

Supported in part by the Flossie E. West Memorial Fund.

References

1. Bentvelzen, P., Daams, J. H., Hageman, P., and Calafat, J., *Proc. Nat. Acad. Sci. U.S.A. 67:* 377 (1970).
2. Huebner, R. J., and Todaro, G. C., *Proc. Nat. Acad. Sci. U.S.A. 64:* 1087 (1969).
3. Law, L. W., and Moloney, J. B., *Proc. Soc. Exp. Biol. and Med. 108:* 715 (1961).
4. Nielsen, A. H., *Viral oncogenic studies in conventional CFW and germfree CFW$_W$ mice.* Ph.D. Thesis, University of Kansas School of Medicine (1969).
5. Reyniers, J. A., *Ann. N.Y. Acad. Sci. 78:* 47 (1959).
6. Wagner, M., *Ann. N.Y. Acad. Sci. 78:* 89 (1959).
7. Chapman, A. L., Nielsen, A., Cohen, H., Larsen, W. E., and Werder, A., *Proc. Soc. Exp. Biol. and Med. 122:* 1022 (1966).
8. Chapman, A. L., Bopp, W. J., Brightwell, A. S., Cohen, H., Nielsen, A. H., Gravelle, C. R., and Werder, A. A., *Cancer Res. 27:* 18 (1967).

CHEMOTHERAPY OF SPONTANEOUS LEUKEMIA IN GERMFREE AND CONVENTIONAL AKR MICE

Morris Pollard and *Nehama Sharon*
Lobund Laboratory, University of Notre Dame
Notre Dame, Indiana 46556, U.S.A.

Introduction

Most immunosuppressive (IS) and cytotoxic antineoplastic drugs render the patient susceptible to endogenous and exogenous infections (1, 2). Under such circumstances, many patients die of infections rather than the diseases for which they were being treated. This therapeutic limitation leaves the impression that potentially useful drugs are not being assessed adequately.

In attempts to correct this problem, hospital patients have been subjected to protective measures such as antibiotic decontamination and maintenance in protected, insulated germfree rooms, prior to IS therapy (3, 4). In spite of these environmental (ecological) improvements, patients are still suffering from activated viral, mycotic, and antibiotic-resistant bacterial infections.

In an attempt to secure more complete assessments of chemotherapeutic measures, we have resorted to the use of germfree AKR mice which develop virus-related lymphatic leukemia spontaneously (5) in high incidence and in predictable pattern. Secondary bacterial infections pose no problem in them. The AKR mouse, originally developed by Furth and associates (6), is now in the 24th generation under germfree (GF) status. Their manifestations and patterns of lymphatic leukemia are the same as in the stock from which they had been derived. At average age 8 months (range 3 to 13 months), they appear rough, kyphotic, and dyspneic. The lymphoreticular tissues are swollen and infiltrated with anaplastic cells, many of which are in mitosis. In advanced stages, the visceral organs are heavily infiltrated and distorted by accumulations of neoplastic cells. Mice usually die within 10 days after appearance of symptoms. Diagnosis of the disease on the basis of symptomatology is remarkably accurate.

Materials and Methods

As preliminary to chemotherapeutic trials, GF and conventional CFW mice and Fischer rats were compared for relative sensitivities to cyclophosphamide

(CPA, *Cytoxan*, provided by Mead-Johnson Co., Evansville, Indiana). Groups of animals were inoculated intraperitoneally (IP) with a series of increasing doses/Kg body weight of freshly dissolved CPA, and they were observed for effect. Then infralethal doses of CPA were administered at weekly intervals, in order to compare survival rates between GF and conventional animals; and those that died were examined for gross and microscopic evidence of disease.

Results

GF rats and mice tolerated larger doses of CPA than conventional counterpart animals; also they survived longer under IP administrations of the drug than conventional animals (7). All doses are recorded in mg/Kg body weight. Five of 8 GF Fischer rats survived 8 daily injections of 25 mg CPA, while only 1 of 6 conventional rats survived a similar sequence of 20 mg of CPA. Larger doses of CPA were lethal to GF rats (Table I). Also, 2 of 4 GF Sprague-Dawley rats survived 8 inoculations of 50 mg CPA, and all of 4 survived treatments with 25 mg.

TABLE I. Effect of 8 Daily Intraperitoneal Inoculations of Cyclophosphamide In Germfree and Conventional Fischer Rats

Mg/Kg body weight	Germfree Dead (days)*	Conventional Dead (days)
75	8/8 (10)	6/6 (7)
50	8/8 (12)	6/6 (7)
25	3/8 (13)	6/6 (9)
20		5/5 (9)
15		2/6 (14)
10		0/6

*Number dead/number on test (days after onset of treatment)

GF and conventional CFW mice were administered CPA at weekly intervals for 5 weeks; and they were observed for a total of 8 weeks for effect. At a dose level of 5 x 125 mg, all GF mice survived for at least 8 weeks, but all of the conventional mice were dead. At a dose level of 5 x 250 mg, 2 of 10 GF mice died, and 10 of 10 conventional mice were dead by the 8th week. The lymphoreticular tissues in all treated mice were depleted, and the conventional mice had pneumonia.

Among 21 conventional AKR mice (age 5 months) which were administered 100 mg CPA per week continuously, half of them were dead at 17 weeks after onset of treatments. There were 4 survivors at 33 weeks, 3 of which were leukemic. All of 18 germfree counterpart AKR mice, with the same schedule of CPA treatments, survived for 33 weeks. The treated conventional AKR mice showed lesions of pneumonia and cystitis, in addition to the depletion of the lymphoreticular system.

Most of our untreated GF AKR mice develop lymphatic leukemia at average age 8 months (range 3 to 13 months) (8). Saline-treated GF AKR mice were dead of leukemia at average age 8 months, and they died within 10 days after onset of symptoms. However, the CPA-treated GF AKR mice survived up to age 13 months without evidence of leukemia. When the CPA treatment was discontinued, leukemic lesions appeared in them.

Forty GF AKR mice with clinical signs and symptoms of leukemia were subjected to a schedule of CPA treatments, as follows: each was administered one dose of approximately 1000 mg, and then 100 mg at weekly intervals thereafter. All of the mice survived beyond the expected expiration period of 10 days and 65% (26 mice) survived longer than 50 days. Twenty five percent (11 mice) survived over 100 days after onset of treatments. Five mice survived over 150 days (8). We do not have data on the ultimate survival time of all mice under treatment because the schedule was terminated after 150 days. At autopsy, the lymphoreticular tissues in all of the survivors were depleted, but we noted small foci of anaplastic cells in the depleted thymus glands which represented, presumably, evidence of continued leukemogenesis.

There are advantages in the use of GF mice for chemotherapy of virus-induced proliferative lesions. This has been clearly defined in therapy trials with GF Haas strain mice (9) which have congenitally acquired, persistent infection with lymphocytic choriomeningitis (LCM) virus. Administrations of CPA in schedules similar to those described in this report were effective in preventing and reversing the lesions associated with this syndrome (10, 11). The lesions were for the most part reflective of an over-active immunogenic system: swollen lymphoreticular tissues, elevated serum globulins, infiltrations of visceral organs with reticulum and plasma cells, glomerulonephritis, and reticulum cell sarcomas. The treated mice remained viremic, and lesions reappeared on cessation of treatment within the period of the original incubation period of 5 months (11).

Administrations of CPA prevented the development of leukemia in GF AKR mice, but it was necessary that the treatment schedules be continuous. CPA therapy of leukemic mice prolonged their longevity significantly, but they were not cured. As with the LCM in Haas strain mice, the disease was only suppressed by treatment.

GF mice with spontaneously-elicited neoplastic diseases provides an excellent controlled test system for assessment of cytotoxic therapeutic agents. Such studies should serve to clarify the pathogenic processes, and to determine if "cures" might be possible under optimum conditions.

Conclusions

Since germfree animals are free of bacterial flora, they tolerate more intensive therapeutic regimes with immunosuppressive drugs than conventional counterpart animals which often die of secondary infections. This thesis was applied with benefits to germfree AKR mice which otherwise developed leukemia spontaneously. Administrations of cyclophosphamide prevented the development of leukemic lesions, and reversed temporarily the lesions that had already developed. The treatment was directed at the lesions, not at the virus responsible for them.

Acknowledgements

Supported in part by funds from the St. Joseph County and Elkhart County (Indiana) Cancer Societies, and U.S.P.H.S. RR 00294.

References

1. Schwartz, S. A., and Perry, S. Jr., *Amer. Med. Assoc. 197:* 105 (1966).
2. Hughes, W. T., *Am. Jr. Dis. Children 122:* 283 (1971).
3. Perry, S., *Cancer Res. 29:* 2319 (1969).
4. Bodey, G. P., Gehan, E. A., Freireich, E. J., and Frei, E. III, *Am. Jr. Med. Sci. 262:* 138 (1971).
5. Pollard, M., Kajima, M., and Teah, B. A., *Proc. Soc. Exp. Biol. and Med. 120:* 72 (1965).
6. Furth, J., Sibold, H. R., and Rathbone, R. R., *Am. Jr. Cancer 19:* 521 (1933).
7. Pollard, M., and Sharon, N., *Jr. Nat. Cancer Inst. 45:* 677 (1970).
8. Pollard, M., and Sharon, N., *Proc. Soc. Exp. Biol. and Med. 137:* 1494 (1971).
9. Pollard, M., Sharon, N., and Kajima, M., *Proc. Soc. Exp. Biol. and Med. 127:* 755 (1968).
10. Sharon, N., and Pollard, M., *Nature (London) 224:* 707 (1969).
11. Sharon, N., and Pollard, M., *Arch. fur die Gesamte Virusforschung 34:* 278 (1971).

ANTITHROMBIN ACTIVITY IN DECONTAMINATED AND CONVENTIONAL RATS WITH ACUTE LEUKEMIA

H. Rasche, D. Hoelzer, M. Dietrich and *A. Keller*
Center for Internal Medicine and Pediatrics
and Center for Basic Clinical Research
University of Ulm, Ulm, Germany

Introduction

The use of gnotobiotic techniques is very well established today in the management of acute leukemia. Besides the danger of infection, these patients exhibit a high risk of bleeding complications due to thrombocytopenia. Nonetheless the lack of hemorrhage in patients with severe thrombocytopenia is not an uncommon clinical finding. Bleeding occurs very often by some precipitating factors as fever, bacterial and viral infection, and septicemia (1-3). There is some clinical evidence that reverse isolation and microbial decontamination of patients with acute leukemia during cytostatic therapy can reduce the number of hemorrhagic complications by a yet unknown mechanism (4). It is the aim of the present study to investigate the influence of decontamination and reverse isolation on the hemostatic defect of rats with a transplanted acute leukemia.

Materials and Methods

Animals. Male rats of the inbred strain BD IX were used in all experiments. Four groups of animals were examined: Group 1 — 10 conventional rats as controls; Group 2 — 10 animals after a decontamination period of 10 days; Group 3 — 8 animals with transplanted acute leukemia and peripheral white blood cell count between 250,000 — 400,000 cells/cmm; Group 4 — 8 decontaminated animals with transplanted acute leukemia and peripheral white blood cell count between 250,000 — 400,000 /cmm.

Performance of decontamination. The decontamination of the microbial flora was achieved by non-absorbable antibiotics: Bacitracin, Neomycin and Pimaricin (fungistatic agent). The antibiotics have been given in the sterile drinking water after the animals have been thirsty for 24 hours. Microbiological tests showed no microbial growth in the fecal samples after 3 days.

147

Induction of leukemia. The rat leukemia which we have used was first induced by Ivankovic in a rat of the BD IX strain by injection of ethyl-nitroso-urea. The leukemia is transferable by intravenous and intra-peritoneal injection of peripheral blood cells. There is no evidence for viral etiology. It is an acute leukemia which from its cytochemical properties can best be classified in medicine with the monocytic or myelo-monocytic leukemias. For the present experiments we have used a standard injection of 10^7 cells given intravenously through a tail vein.

Blood collection and clotting tests. Blood was obtained from ether-anesthetized animals by aortic puncture after laparotomy. Four ml of blood were drawn into a plastic syringe containing 1 ml of 0.1 m Na-citrate solution, transferred to a siliconized glass tube and centrifuged for 10 min at 3000 g. The plasma was kept deep frozen until tested.

Laboratory investigations on the hemostatic mechanism (thrombela-stography, fibrinogen, partial thromboplastin time, thromboplastin time, thrombin time, factor XIII) were determined as described elsewhere (5). Progressive antithrombin activity was determined according to a method patterned after the thrombin generation test of Pitney and Dacie (6) and exactly described by Hensen and Loeliger (7). The volume of the incubation mixture was 1.5 ml (0.75 ml distilled water, 0.5 ml thrombin solution 15 μ/ml, 0.25 ml heat-defibrinated plasma). Incubation was at 37°C in glass. At the designated intervals over a seven minute period 0.1 ml of this incubation mixture was transferred to a substrate mixture consisting of 0.2 ml Michaelis' buffer pH 6.7 and 0.2 ml pooled normal plasma. Clotting time was determined at 37°C in glass. A straight line (clotting time − incubation time) is obtained by plotting the increasing clotting times (sec) against the tested incubation time (min).

Results

Rats of the inbred strain BD IX without leukemia. After a decontamination period of 10 days there were no differences in the hematocrit, the platelet count and in the total leucocyte count between the gnotobiotic rats and the conventional control group.

The examination of thrombelastographic parameters fibrinogen, partial thromboplastin time, thromboplastin time, thrombin time, and factor XIII-activity gave similar results in the conventional and decontaminated rats (Table I).

Decontaminated rats exhibited an enhanced thrombin inhibiting capacity in heat-defibrinated plasma samples compared with their conventional counter-parts. As demonstrated in Figure 1, the remaining thrombin activity at all incubation times tested was lower in the decontaminated group, indicating a higher progressive antithrombin level. The differences were tested by Student's

**TABLE I. Results of Various Blood Clotting Tests In Decontaminated and Conventional
Rats of the Inbred Strain BD IX**

Clotting test	Decontaminated rats		Conventional rats		Significance of differences in Student's t-test
	Range	Mean	Range	Mean	
Thrombelastography r (min)	1.5 − 4.0	2	1.2 − 3.9	2.2	p ⟨ 0.5
k (min)	1.0 − 2.5	1.8	1.0 − 2.8	2.0	p ⟨ 0.5
max_e	214 − 128	142	210 − 134	136	p ⟨ 0.2
Fibrinogen (mg %)	150 − 380	270	210 − 360	240	p ⟨ 0.3
Partial thromboplastin time (sec)	49 − 68	53	52 − 67	55	p ⟨ 0.5
Thromboplastin time (sec)	15.2 − 21.3	19.5	16.3 − 20.5	18.9	p ⟨ 0.5
Thrombin time (sec)	29.1 − 36.5	32.1	28.3 − 37.2	33.0	p ⟨ 0.3
Factor XIII (% of a pooled normal rat plasma)	75 − 125	105	70 − 125	100	p ⟨ 0.5

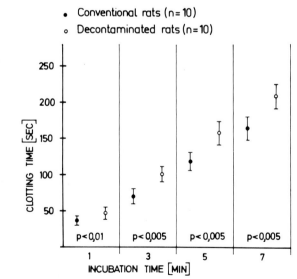

FIG. 1. Antithrombin III-activity in conventional and decontaminated rats of the inbred strain BD IX.

t-test and found to be statistically significant.

Rats of the inbred strain BD IX bearing an acute myelo-monocytic leukemia. The platelet and leukocyte count remains constant up to the third day after transplantation of 10^7 leukemic cells to the animals. During the next three days there is a significant increase of leukemic blood cells and values between $250,000 - 400,000$ cells/cmm are reached at the fifth or sixth day. During the same period a marked fall of the thrombocytes can be observed which is in agreement with a fall of the megakaryocytes in the bone marrow. It is important to emphasize that in the present study we only used animals in this final stage of the experimental acute leukemia. There were no obvious differences between the decontaminated and the conventional group in the development of the leukemia and in the behavior of peripheral thrombocyte and total leukocyte count.

In thrombelastographic examinations there was evidence of marked disturbances of the coagulation system in the leukemic animals, though they only exhibited a slight but inconstant prolongation of the partial thromboplastin time, thromboplastin time and the thrombin time. There was a significant increase of fibrinogen and a reduction of factor XIII-activity. No characteristic differences between the decontaminated and the conventional group could be observed.

The most important change of the clotting factors induced by the transferable leukemia in the rats was the marked increase of progressive antithrombin activity in the blood as it is demonstrated in Figure 2. It was remarkable that this increase was less pronounced in decontaminated animals indicated by the shorter clotting times at the different incubation times. It was not possible to give mean values of these examinations in this group because several clotting times became indefinitely long ($\rangle$ 700 sec) at the incubation times tested. The points in the figure therefore represent the single values for each animal under investigation.

Discussion

Our results concerning the coagulation system of conventional and decontaminated rats were in agreement with previously published data of Waaler *et al.* (8) and Mandel and Travnicek (9) who compared germfree and conventional animals except the small but statistically significant difference in progressive antithrombin activity between the conventional and decontaminated group in our study. As to our knowledge, comparable data have never been published before. Yet we were not able to differentiate whether this finding was caused by the lack of the microbial flora, indicating a specific host-microbial interaction, or by the use of the nonabsorbable antibiotics of which Neomycin has been shown to be very active in the recipient, even though less than 1% is absorbed.

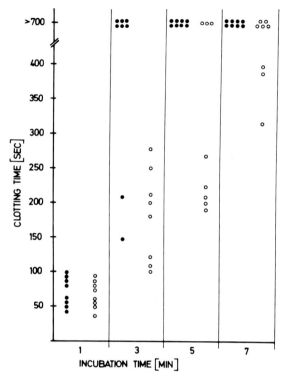

FIG. 2. Antithrombin III-activity in conventional and decontaminated rats of the inbred strain BD IX after transplantation of acute leukemia, (L5222).

The remarkable result in the leukemic animals was the significant increase of progressive antithrombin activity in defibrinated plasma samples compared with non-leukemic control rats. This activity was less pronounced in the gnotobiotic group than in the conventional control group.

There are two inhibitors of thrombin which can be identified in human plasma; alpha$_2$-macroglobulin and antithrombin III which is a substantial protein with the electrophoretical mobility of an alpha-globulin. There are indications in the literature that rats differ from most mammals in that the normal range of concentration of the alpha$_2$-macroglobulins in the serum includes or comes very close to zero (10); while these animals show the appearance of a slow alpha$_2$-globulin fraction in a number of pathological conditions including neoplastic growth (11, 12, 13). This peculiar protein is absent from the serum of the normal adult rat (11, 14) and is chemically, immunologically and probably functionally similar to the alpha$_2$-globulin of humans (10). Also there may be

151

relationships to the findings of Zacharia and Pollard (15) who observed elevated levels of alpha-globulins in sera from germfree tumor-bearing rats.

In further studies it must be clarified if the described protein alterations in rats are responsible for the enhanced antithrombin activity in leukemic animals and why this activity is obviously reduced in a gnotobiotic state.

Summary

Rats of the inbred strain BD IX, both conventional and gnotobiotic, with a transplanted acute myelo-monocytic leukemia showed a disturbance of blood coagulation within 6 days after the graft. The analysis of various clotting factors showed a marked increase of the activity of progressive antithrombin in defibrinated plasma samples which could explain partially the hemostatic defect. The increase of antithrombin was significantly less pronounced in rats in a gnotobiotic state – induced by antibiotic decontamination in a laminar air-flow bench – compared with the conventional controls.

Acknowledgements

The authors wish to thank Frl. R. Hieber and Fr. U. Ertl for competent technical assistance.

The work was supported in part by the Deutsche Forschungsgemeinschaft and Fraunhofer Gesellschaft.

References

1. Gaydos, L, A., Freireich, E. J., and Mantel, N., New Engl. J. Med. 266: 905 (1962).
2. Corrigan, J. J., Walker, L. R., and May, N., New Engl. J. Med. 279: 851 (1968).
3. Cohen, P., and Gardener, F. H., Arch. Intern. Med. 117: 113 (1966).
4. Rasche, H., Dietrich, M., Widmer, K., and Hiemeyer, V., in "Leukaemie," (R. Gross, ed.), Springer Heidelberg-Berlin-New York (In Press).
5. Hiemeyer, V., Rasche, H., and Diehl, K., Haemorrhagische Diathesen, G. Thieme-Verlag, Stuttgart, (1972).
6. Pitney, W. R., and Dacie, J. V., J. Clin. Path. 6: 9 (1953).
7. Hensen, A., and Loeliger, E. A., Thrombos. Diathes. Haemorrh. 9, Suppl. 1: (1963).
8. Waaler, B. A., Gustafsson, B. E., Hauge, A., Nilsson, D., and Amundsen, E., Proc. Soc. Exp. Biol. Med. 117: 444 (1964).
9. Mandel, L., and Travnicek, J., in "Advances in Germfree Research and Gnotobiology," (M. Miyakawa and T. D. Luckey, eds.), Iliffe Book Ltd., London, p. 89, (1968).
10. Heim, W. G., Nature 217: 1057 (1968).
11. Beaton, G. H., Selby, A. E., Veen, M. J., and Wright, A. M., J. Biol. Chem. 236: 2005 (1961).
12. Bogden, A. E., Cancer Res. 21: 1258 (1961).
13. Weimer, H. E., and Benjamin, D. C., Amer. J. Physiol. 209: 736 (1965).
14. Heim, W. G., Nature 193: 491 (1962).
15. Zacharia, T. P., and Pollard, M., J. Nat. Cancer Inst. 42: 35 (1969).

CELL TRANSFORMATIONS IN GERMFREE FISCHER RATS

Miriam R. Sacksteder, Louis Kasza,
Jerry L. Palmer and *Joel Warren*
Germfree Life Research Center
Fort Lauderdale, Florida 33314, U.S.A.

Introduction

Inasmuch as the rat is relatively free of indigenous viruses when compared with other rodents, it is not surprising that studies of rat leukemia have been relatively neglected. However, for those of us who still have some reservations about a universal virogenic basis for all neoplasms, the spontaneous rat tumors offer an intriguing field of study.

The ideal system for such investigation would be: 1) a highly inbred host of uniform and defined genetic composition; 2) it should have a reasonably well characterized incidence of spontaneous tumors; 3) the animal should be free of infection and of morphologically detectable virions; and 4) it should be maintained in a gnotobiotic state for obvious reasons of reducing horizontal contamination. The germfree Fischer 344 rat generally meets these requirements. In the following, we shall describe preliminary studies of a spontaneous, transplantable lymphatic leukemia, the "Nova rat leukemia," which appeared in an aged germfree rat. We shall also discuss the malignant transformation *in vitro* of embryonic cells derived from normal, germfree Fischer rats in this colony.

Results

Experimental. Our line of germfree Fischer rats was originally established at the National Cancer Institute in 1965 by Cesarean section. We received this colony in 1968 and have maintained it by brother-sister matings. It was screened serologically for indigenous viruses in 1969, and tumors were examined by electron microscopy at 6 month intervals since then. All have been free of virions (we are indebted to Dr. H. Chopra of the National Cancer Institute for the performance of these examinations). Rats of this colony are uniformly responsive to the injection of methyl-cholanthrene (MCA) with the development of fibrosarcomata within 90-120 days. In this respect they do not differ from conventional members of this line.

Table I. Occurrence of Spontaneous Tumors in Germfree Fischer Rats

GLRC* Generation	Sex	Age (days)	Date Observed	Approx. Population	Tumor
1 Gen No. 5	M	632	7-22-70	50	Auricular Carcinoma
1 Gen No. 6	F	585	6-12-70	44	Renal Tumor
1 Gen No. 6	F	763	12-9-70	50	Mammary Fibrosarcoma
1 Gen No. 6	M	890	4-14-71	50	Mammary Fibrosarcoma
2 Gen No. 12	F	506	1-8-71	60	Leukemia
1 Gen No. 5	F	833	2-9-71	38	Mammary Adenocarcinoma
1 Gen No. 10	M	668	4-5-71	45	Mammary Fibrosarcoma
1 Gen No. 5	F	833	2-9-71	50	Mammary Fibrosarcoma
2 Gen No. 12	M	885	1-23-72	45	Leukemia
2 Gen No. 14	F	398	10-18-70	55	Lung Carcinoma
3 Gen No. 12	M	474	11-5-71	32	Leukemia

*Germfree Life Research Center

Beginning in 1970, 11 tumors appeared when the animals had reached 1½ to 3 years of age (Table I). Because the isolator population of rats was reduced periodically by the removal of aged animals, the incidence of tumors can only be approximated at 2 − 5%. This probably represents only a minimal percentage. Leukemia appeared in 3 rats at 474, 506 and 885 days, respectively.

Nova Rat Leukemia (NRL) − Animal Studies. On January 8, 1971, a moribund rat was found to have massive splenomegaly, lymphoid hyperplasia, and only moderate liver enlargement in spite of marked sinusoidal infiltration by leukemic cells. Depending on the route of injection, suspensions of splenic tissues or of leukocytes produced leukemia or solid tumors in Fischer rats in approximately three weeks; and on successive passages, the incubation period has stabilized at 10-12 days. Less than 20 cells are invariably lethal, and we suspect that a single leukemic cell will colonize Fischer rats. There has been no pattern of age-related susceptibility with this line. The NRL is less pathogenic in Sprague-Dawley rats, and approximately 30% of animals recover from clinical neoplasia, or remain free of tumors.

The disease resembles the acute mononuclear leukemia of conventional Fischer rats. In animals infected with 1,000 − 10,000 cells by the i.p. or s.c. routes, the white blood count rises very slowly until the 10th − 12th day when a precipitous terminal leukocytosis appears. The large, elongated nuclei and polar accumulation of microsomes are characteristic of the Nova rat leukemic cell. The NRL cell does not contain the chloroleukemia granules present in the established tumors described by Shay and Jones. The latter were DMBA and radiation induced, respectively (1, 2).

Attempted Virus Isolation from the Nova Rat Leukemia. Cell-free extracts of tumor have failed to induce disease in newborn or weanling rats which were observed for long periods. Repeated examinations of NRL tumors and of leukocytes by electron microscopy have failed to reveal any evidence of virions.

We came to the conclusions from the above evidence, that no viral agent is present in the Nova rat leukemia.

Immunological Studies of Nova Rat Leukemia. We have expended considerable effort in an attempt to detect various types of antibody in the sera of Fischer and of Sprague-Dawley rats bearing the Nova rat leukemia, and of animals vaccinated with formaldehyde-killed suspensions of leukemic cells. Sera from rats of all ages have been tested for cytotoxic antibody by metabolic inhibition, by the trypan blue procedure, and for complement fixation antibody. All have been negative with the exception of a single Fischer rat which recovered from NRL while receiving 2% DMSO by mouth. The serum of this animal was repeatedly toxic for NRL cells *in vitro* to a titer of 1:6. Whether this suggests that low doses of antigen may be more effective is under investigation.

Cell Culture of Spontaneous and Induced Rat Tumors of Germfree Rodents. We have established monolayer cultures of the Nova, Shay, and Jones leukemias. Cells from all propagate equally well in Medium 199 with 30% calf serum for initial plating, after which the serum level can be reduced to $3 - 5\%$. The cultures are uniform fibroblasts, and resemble normal rat fibroblasts. Morphological differences among these cell lines are slight.

Various passage levels of each of these lines have been examined for their ability to induce tumors in either newborn or weanling Fischer or Sprague-Dawley rats. It was found that primary cultures rapidly lost oncogenicity between the 4th and 10th days after initiation in tissue culture. Periodic testing of successive transfers of cell cultures remained incapable of inducing tumors even though the generation time of the cultures shortened, and the cells flourished *in vitro*. However, 10 months from the initial establishment of the NRL in tissue culture, pooled cells of the 7th, 11th, 27th and 28th passages were exposed to 5-iodo deoxyuridine (IUDR) at a concentration of 20 μg for five successive transfers. At the end of this period, these cultures were trypsinized and the cells were inoculated into newborn Fischer rats. Tumors resembling lymphosarcomata developed in each of 7 animals. Virions were not observed in the cells by electron microscopy. Unfortunately, untreated NRL cells were not available as controls for this experiment, and when the entire study was repeated, it was found that the cell cultures, without IUDR, also produced tumors. We conclude that this represents a spontaneous re-acquisition of tumorigenicity. We are now investigating whether the "reactivated" line of NRL will induce leukemia, as well as solid tumors.

Malignant Transformation of Embryonic Rat Fibroblasts Derived from Germfree Animals. In 1970, we established a culture of fibroblasts from the embryonic tissues of a healthy germfree Fischer rat. Subcutaneous inoculations of the 6th, 10th and 23rd sub-cultures failed to induce tumors in weanling

155

Table II. Malignant Transformation of Rat Embryo Fibroblasts
On Prolonged Passage *in vitro*

Date	Days	Cell Passage	Treatment	Amount/Duration (µg) (days)		Rat Age (weeks)	Tumor	Time to Tumor (days)
12/21/70		1						
2/2/71	42	6*	None	−		4	0/5	−
3/10/71	80	10	None	−		4	0/5	−
7/8/71	198	23	None	−		8	0/4	−
2/10/72	408	50*	None	−		4	1/3	45
3/1/72	427	54	None	−		4	8/10	26
3/10/72	437	56	None	−		4	4/7	16
9/3/71	253	30	Tobacco Tar No. 38	10 mcg.	5 days	4	5/5	124 − 151
12/8/71	348	36	Tobacco Tar No. 38	1 mcg.	20 days	1	2/4	91 − 109
2/10/72	408	50	Tobacco Tar No. 38	10 mcg.	5 days	4	2/5	38
2/10/72	408	50	Tobacco Tar IRI	10 mcg.	5 days	4	2/5	38
3/1/72	427	54	Tobacco Tar No. 38	10 mcg.	5 days	4	5/10	28
3/1/72	427	54	Tobacco Tar IRI	10 mcg.	5 days	4	7/10	28
3/1/72	427	54	Tobacco Tar No. 11	10 mcg.	5 days	4	3/10	28
3/1/72	427	54	Tobacco Tar No. 13	10 mcg.	5 days	4	3/10	27
3/1/72	427	54	Tobacco Tar No. 17	10 mcg.	5 days	4	3/10	
3/1/72	427	54	Tobacco Tar No. 23	10 mcg.	5 days	4	5/10	28
3/1/72	427	54	Tobacco Tar No. 25	10 mcg.	5 days	4	0/10	
3/1/72	427	54	Tobacco Tar No. 26	10 mcg.	5 days	4	3/10	
3/10/72	437	56	MCA	10 mcg.	8 days	4	4/18	16

*Negative for virus by electron microscopy (Dr. Chopra).

Fischer rats (Table II). In contrast, the 30th and 36th passages, exposed to 10 µg of tobacco tar condensates, were found to be malignant when injected into weanling rats, and they induced highly metastatic fibrosarcomata which involved almost every organ of the animal. These findings led us to examine this line more extensively. Cell cultures of the 50th, 54th, and 56th passages were also injected subcutaneously into weanling Fischer rats. Tumors developed from the cells of each of these passage levels, and the incubation times decreased from 45 to 16 days, as shown in Table II. These tumors are readily transmissable by homogenates to normal Fischer rats in series. The same passages, when exposed to 10 different tar condensates (10 µg) also induced identical neoplasms in all animals, with incubation times essentially identical with those of control, untreated cultures. In our opinion, tars do not play a transforming role in the system, but "spontaneous" transformation to malignancy, as observed in this cell line, probably accounts for all of these observations.

Conclusions

Our older conception that leukemia in rats, and particularly gnotobiotic animals, was infrequent has now been revised, largely due to the efforts of Moloney and his associates (3). With the exception of a single report of Weinstein and Moloney (4), these tumors appear to be free of particles suggestive of virions. In our laboratory we have been unable to isolate any infectious agent from cell-free extracts of several tumors and a leukemia which were inoculated into newborn or weanling syngeneic rats.

Rapid loss of oncogenic potential in serially cultured leukemic cells within a few weeks was unexpected. The regaining of tumorigenicity with continued sub-culture could provide a very useful system for study of "switch-on" mechanisms.

Beginning with the early reports of Gey (5) it is established that serial propagation of rat fibroblasts, derived from conventional animals, would eventually become malignant after 30-100 transfers. In his work with rat liver cultures, Sato noted that this change was not always related to a loss of diploidy or a change in morphology (6). Sharon and Pollard observed transformation of Wistar germfree rat embryo cell cultures as early as the 14th passage (7); the resulting tumors grew rapidly but could not be transferred. The fact that transformation of our fibroblast lines occurred in roughly the same chronological period (one year) as is needed for spontaneous tumors to appear in the germfree Fischer parent rat, suggests that the latter may arise from predetermined genetic loci whether the cell remains in its parent or is cultured *in vitro*. We hope to observe the spontaneous tumors of this germfree colony for a period of years as this represents a model of human neoplasia in which evidence of a viral etiology remains unresolved.

Acknowledgements

This research was supported by Contract PH43-65-95 with the National Cancer Institute, National Institutes of Health, Bethesda, Maryland; and a grant from the Damon Runyon Memorial Foundation.

References

1. Shay, H., Gruenstein, M., and Marx, H. E., *Cancer Res. 11:* 29 (1951).
2. Jones, R., cited in D. S. Rosenthal and W. C. Moloney, *Proc. Soc. Exp. Biol. Med. 126:* 682 (1967).
3. Moloney, W. C., Boschetti, A. E., and King, V. P., *Cancer Res. 30:* 41 (1970).
4. Weinstein, R. S., and Moloney, W. C., *Proc. Soc. Exp. Biol. Med. 118:* 459 (1965).
5. Gey, G., *Cancer Res. 1:* 737 (1941).
6. Sato, J., in "Cancer Cells in Culture," (H. Katsuta, ed.), Univ. of Tokyo Press, Tokyo, (1968).
7. Sharon, N., and Pollard, M., *Cancer Res. 29:* 1523 (1969).

BIOSYNTHESIS OF HEPATOTOXINS IN GERMFREE AND CONVENTIONAL MICE

Nehama Sharon, C. Fred Chang and *Morris Pollard*
Lobund Laboratory, University of Notre Dame
Notre Dame, Indiana 46556, U.S.A.

Introduction

Nitrosamines (NA) induce an extensive array of neoplasms in experimental animals (1, 2), and are likely to be causally related to human cancer. They have been found in tobacco, grains, alcoholic beverages and fish meal (3-6). Nitrosamines can be synthesized in the stomach and in gastric contents of animals after oral feeding with combined non-toxic doses of nitrites and secondary amines (7-11). While the *in vitro* synthesis of nitrosamines from nitrites and secondary amines occurred in the presence of enteric bacteria, the role of microbial flora in the *in vivo* synthesis of nitrosamines was not known. This paper describes experiments performed with germfree and conventional mice in an effort to clarify the role of microbial flora in the *in vivo* synthesis of NA from nitrites and secondary amines.

Materials and Methods

Sodium nitrite ($NaNO_2$) (certified A.C.S. grade) and dimethylamine hydrochloride (DMA) (Matheson, Cole and Bell) were employed in all of the experiments. Solutions of the chemical compounds were freshly prepared in sterile distilled water. For use in GF animals, the solutions were sterilized by passing through a Millipore filter (0.45μ) into sterile glass ampules. The ampules were heat sealed and sprayed with 2% peracetic acid before being introduced into the sterile plastic isolator. The solutions were administered individually by gavage to groups of mice after 6 hours of starvation. They were given water 2 hours and food 16 hours after drug feeding.

Three strains of mice (C3H, Swiss-Webster and CFW), germfree and conventionals, weighing between 15-25 g were used. Sodium nitrite and DMA were administered alone or in combinations. The mice were observed up to 3 days, at which time the survivors were killed by ether anesthesia. Post mortem examinations were carried out on all of the animals. Livers were fixed in Bouin's solution, and tissue sections thereof were stained with hematoxylin and eosin.

Results

All doses of drugs are expressed in mg/Kg body weight. The highest nontoxic dose of $NaNO_2$ for conventional CFW mice, 100 mg, was used throughout the experiments. It was used separately or combined with 2500 or 3500 mg of DMA. Table I summarizes the results: administration of 100 mg

TABLE I. Liver Necrosis In Conventional CFW Mice Following Oral Administration
of Dimethylamine and Sodium Nitrite

Dose (mg/Kg)		Mortality at 24 hours/		Mice with necrosis/	
DMA	$NaNO_2$	Total No. of mice		Total survivors	
0	100	0/14	0%	0/14	0%
2500	0	0/25	0%	0/25	0%
3500	0	3/23	13%	0/20	0%
2500	100	3/17	17%	9/14	66%
3500	100	17/26	65%	8/9	89%

$NaNO_2$ combined with 2500 mg of DMA caused death in 3 of 17 mice (17%) within 24 hours after the feeding. Lesions of liver necrosis were observed in 9 of 14 survivors (66%) on the third day after treatment. When 3500 mg of DMA and 100 mg $NaNO_2$ were administered, 65% died within 24 hours; and 89% of the survivors developed liver necrosis. Mice treated with either $NaNO_2$ or DMA did not develop liver lesions on the third day. Mice which died within 24 hours after combination of the drug were free of liver necrosis. The severity of the lesions appeared to be dose-dependent.

Germfree (GF) CFW mice were more susceptible to the toxic effect of $NaNO_2$ than conventional CFW mice: 100 mg killed all of the mice, and 3500 mg of DMA killed 40% of the treated mice. Therefore, 75 mg of $NaNO_2$ was used in the GF Mice, instead of the 100 mg which was used in the conventional mice. Seventy-five mg of $NaNO_2$ was used individually or combined with 2500 mg and 3500 mg of DMA. Liver necrosis was not observed in mice treated with either DMA or $NaNO_2$, as was described with conventional CFW mice. However, in contrast to the results with conventional mice, liver necrosis was not observed in the survivors of the combined treatment regime, when they were examined on the 3rd day (Table II). GF CFW mice were susceptible to the higher dose of DMA: 40% of the mice died after they were fed with 3500 mg of DMA alone; and all of the mice died when this dose was combined with 75 mg of $NaNO_2$.

Conventional and GF Swiss-Webster mice each tolerated 100 mg of $NaNO_2$; and when this dose was combined with 2500 mg or 3500 mg of DMA, many of them died within 24 hours, and necrotic lesions were observed in the livers of the 3 day survivors (Table III). The liver lesions were dose-dependent

160

TABLE II. Liver Necrosis in GF CFW Mice Following Oral Administration of
Dimethylamine and Sodium Nitrite

Dose (mg/Kg)		Mortality at 24 hours/		Mice with necrosis/	
DMA	NaNO$_2$	Total No. of mice		Total survivors	
0	75	0/6	0%	0/6	0%
2500	0	1/24	4%	0/23	0%
3500	0	8/20	40%	0/12	0%
2500	75	2/5	40%	0/3	0%
3500	75	5/5	100%	—	—

and ranged from small local foci to large diffuse areas (Fig. 1). Each drug, alone, did not cause liver necrosis in the mice which survived the acute toxic effect. Conventional and GF C3H mice tolerated the 100 mg of NaNO$_2$ as was observed with the Swiss-Webster mice. After they were fed with combinations of NaNO$_2$ and DMA, they developed liver lesions (Table IV).

The GF mice were free of microbial flora during the entire course of the experiments; and the conventional mice were free of pathogenic microorganisms.

Conclusions

The results of the experiments with CFW mice suggested that the microbial flora might be required for *in vivo* synthesis of hepatotoxic compounds from mixture of NaNO$_2$ and DMA. However, the data received from the experiments with Swiss-Webster and C3H mice indicated that the microbiological flora was not required for the *in vivo* synthesis of the hepatotoxic agents. The three strains of conventional mice and the GF C3H and SW mice showed 2 distinct responses following the administration of combinations of NaNO$_2$ and DMA: a) an acute toxic response which killed mice within 24 hours and b) liver necrosis which was observed in the survivors after 3 days. The second response was not observed in the GF CFW mice. The development of liver necrosis was probably dependent on the dose of DMA and NaNO$_2$

TABLE III. Liver Necrosis In GF and Conventional SW Mice Following Oral
Administration of Dimethylamine and Sodium Nitrite

Dose (mg/Kg)		Mortality at 24 hours/ Total No. of mice		Mice with necrosis/ Total survivors	
DMA	NaNO$_2$	GF	Convent.	GF	Convent.
0	100	0/11-0%	0/11-0%	0/11-0%	0/11-0%
2500	0	0/10-0%	0/10-0%	0/10-0%	0/10-0%
3500	0	3/11-27%	0/10-0%	0/8-0%	0/10-0%
2500	100	6/20-30%	4/17-24%	2/14-14%	4/13-31%
3500	100	9/15-60%	7/18-39%	4/6-66%	8/11-73%

161

TABLE IV. Liver Necrosis in GF and Conventional C3H Mice Following Oral
Administration of Dimethylamine and Sodium Nitrite

| Dose (mg/Kg) | | Mortality at 24 hours/ Total No. of mice | | Mice with necrosis/ Total survivors | |
DMA	NaNO$_2$	GF	Convent.	GF	Convent.
0	100	0/6-0%	0/13-0%	0/6-0%	0/13-0%
2500	0	0/5-0%	0/13-0%	0/5-0%	0/13-0%
3500	0	0/5-0%	0/13-0%	0/5-0%	0/13-0%
2500	100	2/7-28%	1/22-5%	3/5-60%	3/21-14%
3500	100	3/7-43%	15/23-65%	1/4-25%	1/7-14%

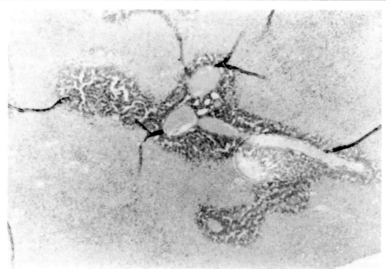

FIG. 1. Section of liver from germfree Swiss-Webster mouse at 3 days following oral administration of NaNO$_2$ and dimethylamine. Note the extensive necrosis in the liver parenchyma. Hematoxylin and eosin stain x 4.

administered to the mice. The high susceptibility of the GF CFW mice to the toxic effect of NaNO$_2$ interfered with the administration of the minimal dose of NaNO$_2$ required for that effect to be manifested.

We assume that the appearance of hepatic necrosis after 3 days was a result of *in vivo* synthesis of nitrosamines from the NaNO$_2$ and DMA (11). The differences between the strains of mice could be a result of a unique susceptibility to the toxic effects of NaNO$_2$, a pharmacogenetic effect.

Acknowledgements

Supported in part by funds from U.S.P.H.S. Grant R01 OH 00342 and the Marion County Cancer Society, Indiana.

References

1. Magee, P. N., and Barnes, J. M., *Advances in Cancer Res. 10:* 163 (1967).
2. Lijinsky, W., and Epstein, S. S., *Nature 225:* 21 (1970).
3. Druckery, H., Steinhoff, D., Beuthner, H., Schneider, H., and Kdorner, P., *Arzneimittel -Forsch. 13:* 320 (1963).
4. Sakshange, V. J., Sognen, E., Hansen, M. A., and Koppang, N., *Nature 206:* 1261 (1965).
5. Neurath, G., *Experientia 23:* 400 (1967).
6. McGlashan, N. D., Walters, C. L., and McLean, A. E. M., *Lancet 2:* 1017 (1968).
7. Sanders, J., and Burkle, G., *Z. Krebsforch. 73:* 54 (1969).
8. Sen, N. P., Smith, D. C., and Schwinghamer, L., *Food Cosmet. Toxicol. 7:* 301 (1969).
9. Sanders, J., *Arzneimittel-Forsch. 20:* 418 (1970).
10. Asahina, S., Friedman, M. A., Arnold, E., Miller, G. N., Mishkin, M., Bishop, Y., and Epstein, S. S., *Cancer Res. 31:* 1201 (1971).
11. Klubes, P., and Jondorf, W. R., *Res. Comm. Chem. Path. Pharmacol. 2:* 24 (1971).

163

THE ENHANCEMENT OF BONE MARROW COLONY-STIMULATING FACTOR PRODUCED BY FRIEND VIRUS (FV-P) INFECTION IN GERMFREE MICE

Edwin A. Mirand and *Joseph G. Hoffman*
Roswell Park Memorial Institute
New York State Department of Health, and
State University of New York at Buffalo,
Buffalo, New York 14203, U.S.A.

Introduction

The colony-stimulating factor (CSF) is found in elevated titers in sera and urines of humans and mice with leukemia or in various hematopoietic and certain infectious diseases (1-5). CSF stimulates the growth of granulocytic and mononuclear cell colonies of bone marrow in semisolid agar medium (5). The number and proliferation of colonies *in vitro* depends on the continued presence of CSF (6), suggesting that it may be a specific leukopoietin.

The exact role CSF plays *in vivo,* particularly on leukopoiesis, remains obscure, primarily because of its short lifetime *in vivo* and lack of large pools of a purified preparation of CSF. Attempts to isolate large amounts of CSF led to our finding (7) that unilateral or bilateral ureteral ligation elevates serum CSF in non-infected germfree mice for several days. Current data reported in this communication reveal further marked enhancement of serum CSF with ureteral ligation of germfree mice infected with polycythemic strain of Friend Virus (FV-P).

FV-P was discovered by Mirand *et al.* in 1961 (8-12) and has been a most useful tool in studying fundamental problems in hematology. FV-P produces a disease resembling polycythemia vera in man and the germfree mouse is much more susceptible to FV-P than the conventional or the conventionalized mice. Other reasons why germfree mice were used in this study are as follows: a) the uniformity of peripheral blood leukocyte counts and lower variability in number of bone marrow colony-forming cells (13); b) the serum concentrations of the CSF are known to be uniformly low in germfree mice (14); c) the effect of FV-P had to be studied in the absence of extraneous PPLO and bacterial infections; and d) it appeared to us to be a desirable biological test animal to observe viral induced granulopoiesis and its relationship to an endocrine regulatory mechanism.

Materials and Methods

Mice. Twelve-week-old germfree female Hauschka-Mirand ICR Swiss mice were obtained from the Charles River Breeding Laboratories (North Wilmington, Massachusetts) and were maintained in Trexler-type plastic germfree isolators (15). Inbred 8-week-old conventional DBA/1 males were obtained from the Roswell Park Memorial Institute West Seneca Breeding Colony. Infection by FV-P was accomplished by injection, i.p., of 0.2 cc of spleen filtrate at 10^{-1} titer. At 9 days post-infection unilateral ureteral ligation was carried out.

Germfree isolation technique. Strict germfree isolation was maintained throughout the course of the study, with routine cultures of food and feces to detect any inadvertent break in technique (15). The surgical procedures were performed in the germfree isolators. Animals were removed from the germfree isolators immediately before collection of blood and bone marrows for analysis.

Bleeding. White blood counts, differential counts, and hematocrits were performed with blood obtained from the tail vein of an unanesthetized mouse. The mouse was anesthetized with ether and killed by bleeding from the axillary vessels, using Pasteur pipettes for blood collection. Clots were allowed to contract for 1 to 2 hr at room temperature, and the sera was stored at $-20°C$.

Bone marrow collection. Using a hypodermic syringe and needle, the entire plug of bone marrow from a single femur was expressed into 2 ml of bone marrow collecting fluid (modified Eagle's medium with 10% fetal calf serum and 10% trypticase soy broth). A single cell suspension was prepared by repeated pipetting, and was counted in a hemocytometer chamber.

Assay for bone marrow *in vitro* colony-forming cells. Mouse bone marrow cultures were established, using a technique described extensively elsewhere (4, 16). In brief, double-strength modified Eagle's medium containing 20% fetal calf serum and 20% trypticase soy broth was mixed with an equal volume of 0.6% agar in distilled water. Sufficient bone marrow cells were added to aliquots of the mixture to give final cell concentrations of 5×10^4, 2.5×10^4, and 1.25×10^4 nucleated cells/ml of culture medium. Then 1 ml of each cell suspension was pipetted in a separate 35 mm plastic petri dish containing 0.02 ml of mouse serum from a pool of known colony-stimulating activity (4). Triplicate plates were prepared for each cell concentration.

Plates were allowed to gel at room temperature for 20 min, and were incubated without change of medium in a humidified incubator at 37°C with a continuous flow of 5% CO_2 in air. Plates were scored after 7 days of incubation, using an X 30 dissecting microscope. The criteria for colony scoring have been described previously (1, 2). At these cell dosages, there was a linear relationship between the number of cells cultured and the number of colonies developing for a specified bone marrow. Accordingly, colony counts in plates containing different numbers of bone marrow cells were adjusted, and each count was expressed as the mean number of colonies per 10^6 cultured cells. This latter value was used in determining the number of *in vitro* colony-forming cells per femur.

Assay of serum colony-stimulating factor. Each serum of germfree mice to be tested was pipetted into 35 mm plastic petri dishes at doses of 0.0125, 0.025, and 0.05 ml. A single cell suspension of pooled DBA/1 bone marrow cells from one femur each of three mice was added to the bone marrow culture medium to give a final cell concentration of 50,000 nucleated cells/ml, and the mixture was held at 37°C. A 1 ml aliquot was pipetted into each petri dish and mixed thoroughly with the serum. Incubation and scoring were done as described for the colony-forming cell assay. As in previously reported work, there was found to be, in general, a linear relationship between serum dose and the number of colonies forming on each plate (1, 2). The data to be described refer only to colony stimulation by 0.025 ml dose levels, since this dose has allowed good discrimination between inactive and active sera, and is not subject to technical problems of surface drying frequently encountered with higher doses of mouse serum (2).

Operations. All operations were performed in the germfree isolator. Operative and sham-operative groups were anesthetized with 0.2 ml of pentobarbital injected intraperitoneally. The abdomen was opened through a midline incision, and the left ureter was securely ligated with a 4-0 silk ligature. The incision was closed with clips. The technique for the sham-operative animals was similar, except that instead of ureteral ligation, a small area of the lumbar abdominal wall was suture-ligated. The ureteral ligation and sham-operation were performed on alternate mice, using a single set of instruments. At the completion of the study, all animals were autopsied and all of the mice with ureteral ligations had developed hydronephrosis.

Results

Colony formation. Upon stimulation by active serum CSF, loose globular cell clusters developed in the agar. Between the colonies were scattered single cells and micro-colonies containing 2 to 10 cells. Colonies, as scored at 7 days, usually contained 20 to 500 cells. When assayed 6 days after surgery, animals with unilateral ureteral ligation had serum CSF activities that were, on the average, four times as high as those of nonoperative controls. Sham-operative animals had levels of serum CSF equivalent to those in normal animals. The difference between the operative groups and the normal and sham groups was significant, p being less than 0.01 (Fig. 1). In FV-P infected animals the unilateral ureteral ligature increased serum levels of CSF to 6 times that in the non-operated controls. The levels of CSF in infected mice were at least double that found in non-infected but non-operated, sham-operated, and unilateral

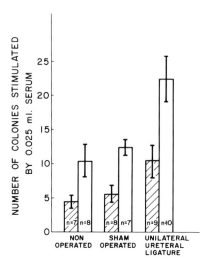

FIG. 1. Number of *in vitro* granulocytic-mononuclear colonies developing 7 days after stimulation by 0.025 ml serum collected from non-infected and infected FV-P germfree mice 6 days after unilateral ureteral ligation, sham operation, or non-operative, zero time. Standard deviations are indicated. Ligation at 9 days after virus infection. Diagonal shading denotes non-infected mice. Number of animals in each experiment denoted by "n".

ureteral ligatured mice.

Peripheral blood determinations. There was no significant difference among the hematocrits of the non-infected mice although these had heightened total leukocyte counts in the ureteral ligation group. The lymphocyte count was not altered by the infection (Fig. 2). The FV-P had its most pronounced effect on the polymorphonuclear cells of ligatured mice where the cell count was 50,650 per cmm as compared with 1,372 per cmm in the non-operated, uninfected mice (Fig. 2). In all cases FV-P infected animals showed a greatly increased (at least 10 times) polymorphonuclear count over the non-infected. To a much lesser extent this increased count shows in the eosinophilic and mononuclear cell count of FV-P infected mice (Fig. 2).

Bone marrow colony-forming cells. There was no detectable difference in the number of colony-forming cells per femur in each of the 3 non-infected groups of mice (Fig. 3). The absolute number of colonies developing from a specified bone marrow appears to depend upon the strength of the stimulating serum. Hence, the values for colony-forming units per femur are relative, and represent only a portion of the number of colonies that might develop after maximum stimulation. In the infected group the non-operated and sham-operated animals show an increased but not significant number of colony forming cells per femur (Fig. 3). The unilateral ureteral ligatured group shows a slight increase in colony forming cells over the non-infected mice.

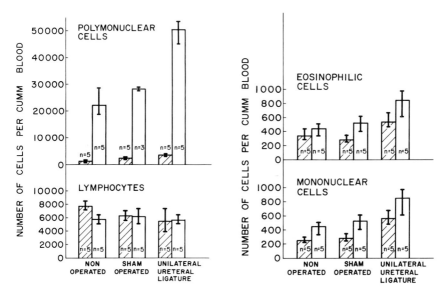

FIG. 2. Number of polymorphonuclear, lymphocytic, mononuclear and eosinophilic cells in peripheral blood at 6 days after unilateral ureteral ligation, sham operation, and non-operative, mice. Ranges of values of counts are indicated. Ligation at 9 days after virus infection in germfree mice. Diagonal shading denotes non-infected mice. Number of animals in each experiment denoted by "n."

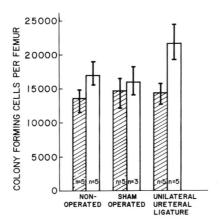

FIG. 3. Number of *in vitro* colony forming cells in femoral bone marrow of germfree mice 6 days after unilateral ureteral ligation, sham operation, or non-operative, zero time. Ligation 9 days after virus infection. Range of values are indicated. Diagonal shading denotes non-infected mice. Number of animals in each experiment denoted by "n."

Discussion

The marked enhancement of CSF levels in serum by the unilateral ureteral ligation in germfree mice reveals the granulocytic function of CSF in the presence of the massive polycythemia (erythrocytopoiesis and granulocytopoiesis) induced by FV-P. The enhancement had been found and elucidated in the previous study (7) on the effect of ligation in germfree animals without infection and without a polycythemia. The results of that work are fully corroborated here with additional findings showing that the erythropoietic and granulocytic stimulation induced by FV-P appear to be independent of one another. This is borne out further by Mirand (10) who showed that viral induced erythropoiesis is not erythropoietin (ESF) related since no detectable ESF was found in the plasma or urine of infected FV-P animals and anti-ESF had no effect on preventing viral-induced erythrocytopoiesis (11).

While other studies with leukemia (1, 2) and following viral infection (4) have not shown a consistent relationship between peripheral blood granulocytes and the level of CSF, they have not excluded the possibility of an existence of such a relationship. The effects on leukopoiesis of infection and of leukemia have not been amenable to analysis. However, the present data show a strong correlation between the polymorphonuclear cell count and the amounts of CSF in circulation. There is the possibility that this correlation comes about by the virus altering some endocrine regulatory mechanism that causes a marked granulocytosis to occur. The marked levels of CSF found point to its being the *in vivo* stimulating factor for polymorphonucleocytes; it may properly be called a specific leukopoietin, granulopoietin.

The fact that we see high levels of CSF in the serum of both non-infected and infected germfree mice brings up the question whether the metabolism of this serum factor in the germfree mouse resembles what we observe for erythropoietin (ESF). We have previously reported (16, 17) that an augmented response to ESF occurs in germfree mice. Several possible mechanisms for this enhanced response were proposed: a) increased numbers of ESF-committed stem cells are present or that an increased sensitivity of these elements to ESF exists in the germfree animal; b) the internal environment of the germfree animal favors an augmented activity of the ESF; this could conceivably occur if the level of a circulating erythropoiesis inhibitory factor was reduced in the germfree animal; or c) a diminution in the rate of destruction of the ESF characterizes the germfree animal. In the latter connection, the liver has been suggested as a site of inactivation of ESF (18, 19) and this could be the same case for CSF. The fact that the liver is less developed in the germfree than in the conventional animal (20, 21) might be interpreted as favoring this possibility. Mirand *et al.* (22) recently have shown that, in the germfree animal, disappearance of exogenous ESF from the blood of germfree mice is much longer than conventional mice.

Stating again, the possible mechanisms for these findings might include a reduced ability of the liver to destroy ESF in the germfree animal and, even perhaps, a decreased capacity of blood-forming organs in germfree mice to utilize ESF at the same rate as conventional mice. What we find for ESF will have to await further clarification for CSF since the state of findings for this factor, CSF, is still being defined.

Summary

Six days after unilateral ureteral ligation the serum levels of colony-stimulating factor (CSF) are four times as high as in non-operative germfree mice. In germfree mice infected with polycythemic Friend Virus (FV-P), the unilateral ureteral ligation raises serum CSF to marked levels that are six times those in non-operated, non-infected controls. In mice subjected to unilateral ureteral ligature, the polymorphonuclear cell count in the peripheral blood is increased by a factor of 36 by FV-P infection. The data support the hypothesis that CSF functions *in vivo* as a specific leukopoietin and FV-P may be responsible for altering some endocrine regulatory mechanism involving leuko-poietin leading to a marked granulocytopoiesis.

Acknowledgements

This study was supported in part by grants from the American Cancer Society (VC-82), the U. S. Public Health Service (CA-07745), and the John A. Hartford Foundation, Inc.

References

1. Robinson, W. K., Metcalf, D., and Bradley, T. R., *J. Cell. Physiol. 69:* 83 (1967).
2. Metcalf, D., and Foster, R. S. Jr., *J. Nat. Cancer Inst. 39:* 1235 (1967).
3. Foster, R. Jr., Metcalf, D., Robinson, W. K., and Bradley, T. R., *Brit. J. Haematol. 15:* 147 (1967).
4. Foster, R. S. Jr., Metcalf, D., and Kirchmyer, R., *J. Exp. Med. 127:* 853 (1968).
5. Metcalf, D., *Med.J. Aust. 2:* 739 (1971).
6. Metcalf, D., and Foster, R. Jr., *Proc. Soc. Exp. Biol. Med. 126:* 758 (1968).
7. Foster, R. S. Jr., and Mirand, E. A., *Proc. Soc. Exp. Biol. Med. 133:* 1223 (1970).
8. Mirand, E. A., Hoffman, J. G., Grace, J. T. Jr., and Trudel, P. J., *Proc. Soc. Exp. Biol. Med. 107:* 824 (1961).
9. Mirand, E. A., Prentice, T. C., Hoffman, J. G., and Grace, J. T. Jr., *Proc. Soc. Exp. Biol. Med. 106:* 423 (1961).
10. Mirand, E. A., *Science 156:* 832 (1967).
11. Mirand, E. A., Steeves, R. A., Lange, R. D., and Grace, J. T. Jr., *Proc. Soc. Exp. Biol. Med. 128:* 844 (1968).
12. Steeves, R. A., Fjelde, A., and Mirand, E. A., *Proc. Nat. Acad. Sci. U.S.A. 68:* 2391 (1971).
13. Metcalf, D., and Foster, R. S. Jr., in "Germfree Biology: Experimental and Clinical

Aspects," (E. A. Mirand and N. Back, eds.), Vol. 3, Plenum Press, New York, p. 383, (1969).

14. Metcalf, D., Foster, R. S. Jr., and Pollard, M., *J. Cell Physiol. 70:* 131 (1967).
15. Mirand, E. A., and Grace, J. T. Jr., *Nature (London) 200:* 92 (1963).
16. Mirand, E. A., and Gordon, A. S., *Experientia 24:* 492 (1968).
17. Mirand, E. A., Gordon, A. S., and Murphy, G. P., in "Germfree Biology: Experimental and Clinical Aspects," (E. A. Mirand and N. Back, eds.), Vol. 3, Plenum Press, New York, p. 111, (1969).
18. Jacobsen, E. M., Davis, A. K., and Alpen, E. L., *Blood 11:* 937 (1956).
19. Prentice, T. C., and Mirand, E. A., *Proc. Soc. Exp. Biol. Med. 95:* 231 (1957).
20. Miyakawa, M., Uno, Y., and Asai, J., "The Reticuloendothelial System, Morphology, Immunology and Regulation," (Kyoto), Nissha, Kyoto, Japan, p. 132, (1965).
21. Thorbecke, G. J. and Benacerraf, B., *Ann. N. Y. Acad. Sci. 78:* 247 (1959).
22. Mirand, E. A., Gordon, A. S., Zanjani, E. D., Bennett, T. E., and Murphy, G. P., *Proc. Soc. Exp. Biol. Med. 139:* 161 (1972).

SECTION V

GNOTOBIOTIC ENVIRONMENTS IN DENTISTRY

THE PERIODONTIUM OF OLD GERMFREE AND CONVENTIONAL RATS

S. Rovin, W. Sabes and *L. R. Eversole*
Department of Oral Pathology, University of Kentucky College of Dentistry

and

H. A. Gordon
Department of Pharmacology, University of Kentucky College of Medicine
Lexington, Kentucky 40506, U.S.A.

Introduction

There are conflicting reports of the occurrence of periodontal disease in germfree rodents, as characterized by apical migration of the gingival epithelial attachment and periodontal bone loss. Non-inflammatory, naturally occurring periodontal disease was reported in Sprague-Dawley rats, but only a few animals were studied (1). Another study showed apical proliferation of the epithelial attachment with increasing age in germfree Cobb strain rats, but only one animal was as old as 9 months (2). Other workers reported the absence of epithelial proliferation in the gingiva of germfree Wistar rats (3) and in our own laboratory, peridontal disease did not occur in Fischer rats even in the face of silk ligatures placed subgingivally around their mandibular first molars (4). The present study was done to either corroborate or negate the other reports of naturally occurring periodontal disease in germfree rats.

Materials and Methods

Twenty-four germfree and 24 conventional Sprague-Dawley rats were used. The rats were retired breeders obtained at age 16 months and sacrificed at 24 months, which is considered to be senescence. All of the rats were fed the same steam sterilized diet, 5010-C and maintained in our laboratory as reported previously (4).

The rats were given pentobarbital and decapitated, the mandibles were removed, bisected, fixed in 10% neutral buffered formalin and decalcified in 5% buffered formic acid. After paraffin embedding, the mandibles were cut at 8 microns mesio-distally, stained with hematoxylin and eosin and examined microscopically.

175

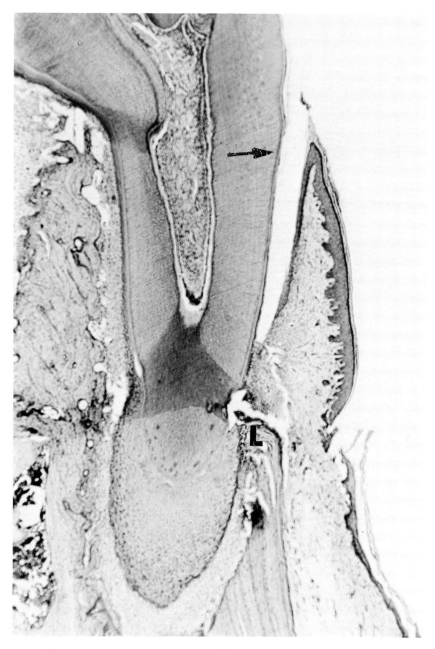

FIG. 1. Mesial root of first molar showing bone loss (L) and apical proliferation appreciably past the cemento-enamel junction (arrow). H&E X76.

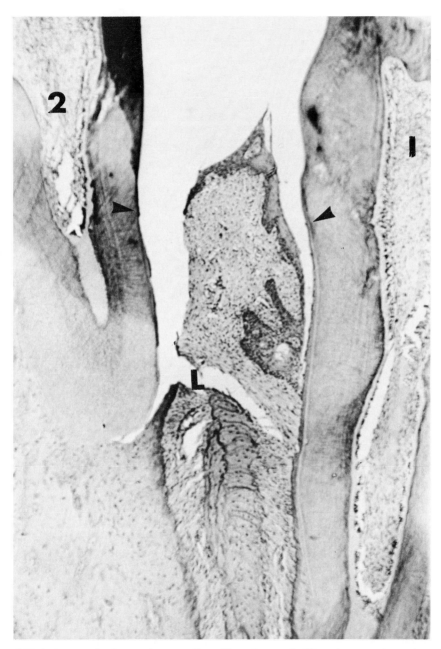

FIG. 2. Interproximal area between first (1) and second (2) molars showing apical proliferation at the distal of the first molar and to a lesser extent at the mesial area of the second molar. Arrows show the cemento-enamel junction, and the bone level (L) is normal. Separation of tissue from the second molar is artifactual. H&E X76.

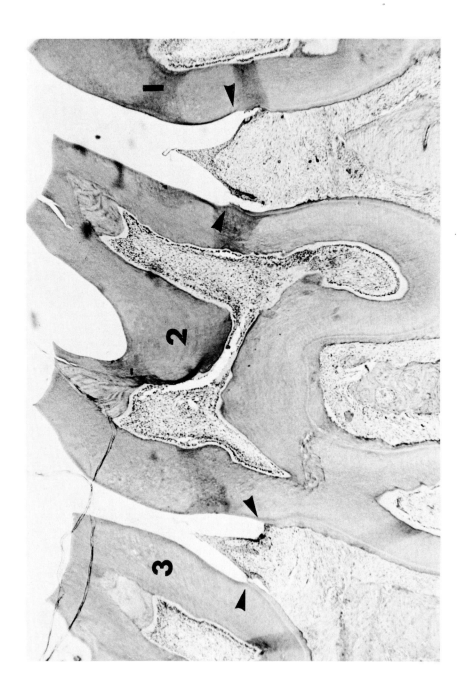

Results

All of the animals, germfree and conventional, had identical findings. There was apical proliferation of the epithelial attachment and histologic evidence of bone loss on the mesial area of the first molars (Fig. 1). There was slight apical proliferation of the epithelial attachment, but no evidence of bone loss in the interproximal area between the first and second molars (Fig. 2). There was slight to no apical proliferation of the epithelial attachment in the interproximal area between the second and third molars (Fig. 3) and none on the distal area of the third molar. Also, in the latter sites, there was no evidence of bone loss.

In all instances of apical proliferation and bone loss there was no evidence of associated inflammation. An inflammatory response was seen only in conjunction with the impaction of hair and this occurred to the same extent as reported in our earlier studies (4).

Discussion

Since the findings were identical with or without the presence of microbes, their explication rests with other factors, namely age, genetics and chewing pattern of the animals. Evidence against epithelial attachment proliferation and bone loss being a concinnitant of aging is the variation in the extent of apical proliferation and bone loss from the first to the third molar. By itself, aging would not be expected to produce differences in destruction in the same tissue. Aging combined with some genetic influence might account for the findings, but this is only speculation. One can conceive of an animal being genetically programmed to show varying patterns of loss in the same tissue with aging. A third factor that must be considered is the effect of the occlusal forces generated by chewing. Although there is no supporting experimental evidence, it is very likely that the greatest forces applied during chewing were on the first molars of these animals, which coincides very well with the greatest loss of periodontal tissue occurring around these teeth.

The results of this study coupled with earlier studies indicate that although apical proliferation of the epithelial attachment occurred and is by definition periodontal disease, the absence of inflammation rules against it being equated to that in humans.

FIG. 3. Mesial-distal section showing both interproximal areas with levels of epithelial attachment and underlying alveolar bone. Molars are numbered and arrows show the cemento-enamel junction. H&E X40.

Summary

Histologic specimens from the periodontium of 24 germfree and 24 conventional senescent Sprague-Dawley rats revealed bone loss on the mesial area of the mandibular first molars, decreasing degrees of apical proliferation of the gingival attachment from the gingiva of the first molar to the third molar, but no evidence of inflammatory periodontal disease. The findings were explained as being the combined result of aging, genetics and pattern of chewing.

Acknowledgements

This investigation was supported by U.S.P.H.S. Research Grant DE-02351 from the National Institute of Dental Research, National Institutes of Health, Bethesda, Md.

References

1.   Baer, P. N., and Fitzgerald, R. J., *J. Dent. Res. 45:* 406 (1966).
2.   Hodess, H., Goldman, H. M., and Ruben, M. P., *J. Dent. Res. 43:* 833 (1964).
3.   Fitzgerald, R. J., Jordan, H. V., and Stanley, H. R., *J. Dent. Res. 39:* 923 (1960).
4.   Rovin, S., Costich, E. R., and Gordon, H. A., *J. Perio. Res. 1:* 193 (1966).

PERIODONTAL DISEASE IN GNOTOBIOTIC AND CONVENTIONAL RICE RATS

Sam Rosen, Fred Meyer and *Steven P. Pakes*
The Ohio State University
Columbus, Ohio 43210, U.S.A.

Introduction

The rice rat, *Oryzomys palustris*, has proven to be an animal that is uniformly and consistently susceptible to periodontal disease (1-3). Although this animal is an excellent tool for the study of periodontal disease, the etiologic microbial spectrum is not as well established for this disease as it is in dental caries. Microbial studies on conventional rice rats have shown that high counts of enterococci and actinobacilli are associated with periodontal disease (4). *Odontomyces viscosus* was able to cause the disease in hamsters (5). In gnotobiotic albino rats, *Streptococcus mutans*, an organism capable of forming dextran from sucrose, induced periodontal disease in addition to dental caries (6). Certain levan as well as dextran forming streptococci can induce this disease in germfree albino rats provided that a high concentration of sucrose is in the diet (7). Periodontal disease was also induced in gnotobiotic rats by *Actinomyces naeslundii* (8). In evaluating 31 strains of Gram positive rods it was found that *A. naeslundii, O. viscosus,* certain bacilli and diphtheroids caused marked subgingival plaque formation, root caries, and alveolar bone loss in gnotobiotic rats and/or hamsters (9).

The germfree albino rat has served a useful purpose in distinguishing etiologic microorganisms in dental caries. Therefore, it follows that the germfree rice rat could be used for the same purpose for periodontal disease. The value of using germfree rather than conventional animals inoculated with specific microorganisms is that the guesswork of interaction with resident flora is eliminated.

Results

After establishing that cross-suckling between newborn rice rats and albino rats was possible in the conventional environment, attempts were made to derive germfree rice rats. Unborn rice rats were delivered by hysterorectomy into

181

isolators in which germfree albino rats had given birth within 48 hours. The albino mother refused to accept these animals until the young were saturated with a fecal slurry made with fecal pellets obtained from cages housing germfree albino rats. A litter of four rice rats was successfully weaned. At this point, a sterility check revealed that a mold, *Aspergillus niger,* contaminated the isolator. The weaned rice rats were maintained in this environment. Other than making a mat in the drinking water, the mold was without deleterious effect to the animals. Charles River 7RF (Agway) diet was used to maintain these animals. A rice rat was removed at 82 days of age and at 94 days of age, sacrificed, and examined for the periodontal syndrome. The two remaining rats, a male and a female, were kept in the isolator for 23 weeks. These rats did not produce any young, and they also were examined for the periodontal syndrome. Comparisons of the syndrome were made with conventional rice rats of comparable age and diet. Twenty-three week old rice rats in conventional environment exhibited marked food and hair impaction at the gingival margin, destruction of the gingival tissue and severe resorption of alveolar bone (Fig. 1). Rice rats of the same age reared under our gnotobiotic conditions exhibited slight food and hair impaction, but no gelatinous plaque was observed on the tooth surface or gingival margin. Gingival tissue was healthy and the alveolar bone was resorbed slightly only in a small area of the anterior root of the first mandibular molar

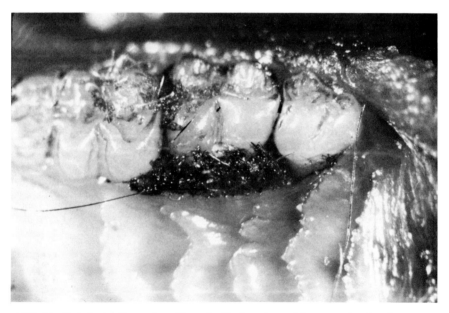

FIG. 1A. Periodontal disease in a 23 week old rice rat reared in conventional environment. Hair and debris packed into gingival sulcus in maxilla.

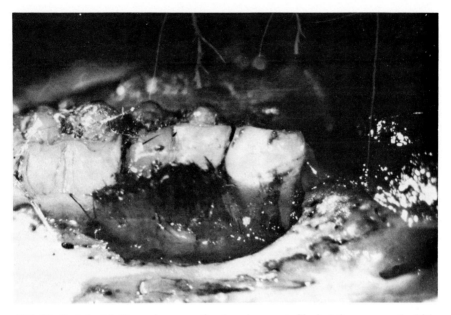

FIG. 1B. Periodontal disease in conventional environment. Gingival tissue removed which revealed depth of accumulation of hair and debris.

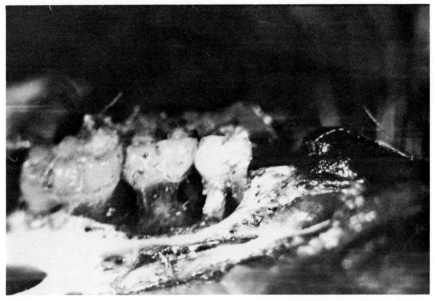

FIG. 1C. Periodontal disease in conventional environment. Debris removed which revealed alveolar bone loss.

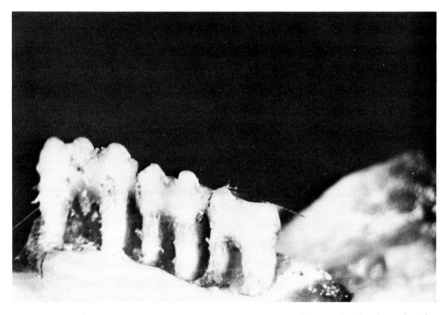

FIG. 1D. Periodontal disease in conventional environment. Severe alveolar bone loss in mandible.

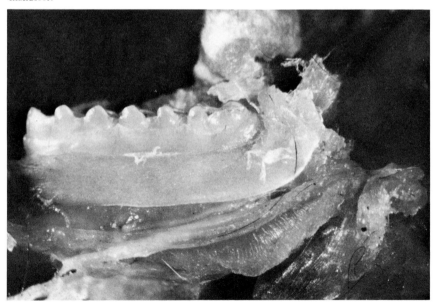

FIG. 2A. Periodontal disease in a 23 week old rice rat reared in gnotobiotic environment. The only cultivable organism was *Aspergillus niger*. Intact mandible.

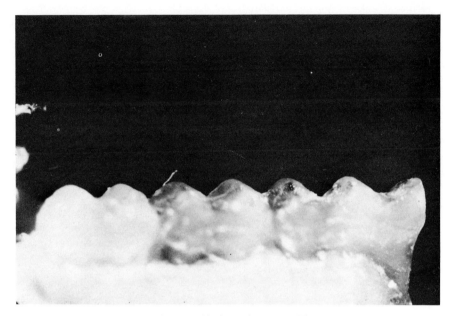

FIG. 2B. Periodontal disease in gnotobiotic environment. Tissue removed and revealed slight alveolar bone loss at anterior of first molar.

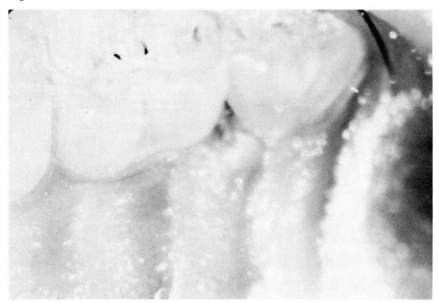

FIG. 2C. Periodontal disease in gnotobiotic environment. Debris accumulation between second and third molar.

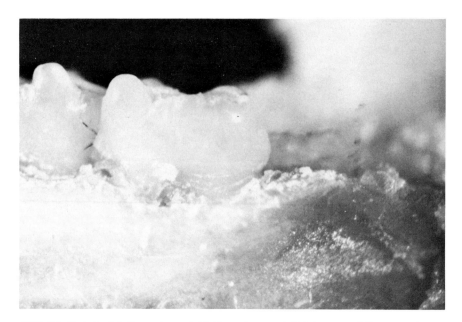

FIG. 2D. Periodontal disease in gnotobiotic environment. Debris removed from area shown in Fig. 2C and revealed slight alveolar bone loss.

and in areas of the third molar where there was a slight accumulation of debris (Fig. 2).

The teeth, cecum, liver, heart and stomach from the two rats that remained in the isolators for 23 weeks were cultured on Sabouraud's and blood agars. No growth was observed on blood agar and the mold could be recovered only from the teeth and cecum of one of the animals. The ceca of both of these rats were noticeably enlarged.

Conclusions

The rice rat may be derived by relatively simple procedures and reared by a foster albino rat. Rice rats reared in a gnotobiotic environment in which the mold, *A. niger,* was the only cultivable microorganism present developed periodontal disease only slightly when compared to conventional rice rats of comparable age on a comparable diet.

References

1. Gupta, O. P., and Shaw, J. H., *Oral Surg. 9:* 592 (1956).
2. Gupta, O. P., and Shaw, J. H., *Oral Surg. 9:* 727 (1956).
3. Mulvihill, J. E., Susi, F. R., Shaw, J. H., and Goldhaber, P., *Arch. Oral Biol. 12:* 733 (1967).

4. Socransky, S. S., MacDonald, J. B., Sawyer, S. J., and Auskaps, A. M, *Arch. Oral Biol.* *2:* 104 (1960).
5. Jordan, H. V., and Keyes, P. H., *Arch. Oral Biol. 9:* 401 (1964).
6. Gibbons, R. J., Berman, K. S., Knoettner, P., and Kapsimalis, B., *Arch. Oral Biol. 11:* 549 (1966).
7. Gibbons, R. J., and Banghart, S., *Arch. Oral Biol. 13:* 297 (1968).
8. Socransky, S. S., Hubersak, C., and Propas, D., *Arch. Oral Biol. 15:* 993 (1970).
9. Socransky, S. S., Hubersak, C., Propas, D., and Rozanis, J., I.A.D.R. abstracts (1970).

THE PERIODONTIUM OF GERMFREE DOGS

Max A. Listgarten
Center for Oral Health Research, University of Pennsylvania
Philadelphia, Pennsylvania 19104

and

James B. Heneghan
Department of Physiology, Louisiana State University School of Dentistry
New Orleans, Louisiana 70119, U.S.A.

In germfree beagles, approximately 9 months of age, the gingival connective tissue contained accumulations of plasma cells and lymphocytes in close proximity to the junctional and sulcular epithelium. The localization of the cells probably reflected a response to foreign substances diffusing from the gingival sulcus, rather than a response to mechanical injury. Although conventional beagles are naturally susceptible to periodontal disease, no tissue breakdown was noticeable in these animals, as well as those of an older group of beagles ranging in age from 20 months to 3½ years. The older animals demonstrated varying degrees of polymorphonuclear leukocytic infiltration of the junctional epithelium, and chronic inflammatory cells in the adjacent connective tissue. However, this was not accompanied by any apical migration of the junctional epithelium, or any detectable alveolar bone loss. Dental plaque, which consists to a large extent of microorganisms, was obviously not present in these animals. However, a stained, markedly thickened acquired pellicle was noted on a number of posterior teeth. This material consisted of an amorphous, bacteria-free organic matrix, up to 0.4 mm in thickness, which demonstrated a layered pattern typical of appositional growth. It was most probably derived from salivary components.

The details of these experiments have been published elsewhere: Listgarten, M. A., and Heneghan, J. B.: "Chronic Inflammation in the Gingival Tissue of Germfree Dogs," *Arch. Oral. Biol. 16:* 1207 (1971); and Listgarten, M. A., and Heneghan, J. B.: "Observations on the Peridontium and Acquired Pellicle of Adult Germfree Dogs," *J. Periodont.* (In Press).

INFLAMMATION AFTER PULP EXPOSURE OF TEETH IN GERMFREE, DEFINED FLORA AND ISOLATOR CONVENTIONAL MICE

Edward White, D. P. Riley, Linda Wiles and *Jeanne Joyce*
Department of Microbiology and Immunology, School of Dentistry
University of Southern California, Los Angeles, California 90007, U.S.A.

Introduction

The microbial contribution to inflammatory reactions and its effect on healing is of general concern and interest. Surgical trauma to teeth and other oral tissues has been used to study the relationship between bacterial flora and healing (1-3). A model of exposed dental pulps and microbial infection offers a unique opportunity to observe microbe-host and inflammation-healing inter-relationships because of the nature of the pulp-environment interface. The exposed dental pulp may serve as a continuous avenue for environmental stimuli to deeper connective tissues and bone or become walled off either by calcific deposits or mucosa. With walling off, sequestered foreign material may become trapped within the root canal. This model offers stimulus-response possibilities not found elsewhere in the body.

There is disagreement in the literature about the effect of the microbial flora on healing of surgical wounds. Recently, host-microbial relationships have been reviewed (4). Some studies have found that there are no differences in inflammatory reaction and healing following oral surgical trauma in germfree and conventional mice (1, 2). However, other studies of oral trauma in rats (3) and assorted other trauma in mice (5) and guinea pigs (6) have shown disparate inflammatory responses between germfree and conventional animals. The results of this investigation support the latter observations.

Beyond the microbial effects on inflammation and healing is the clinical concern of the bacterial etiology of pulpal disease. An understanding of the etiological parameters of pulpal necrosis, pulpitis, and periapical inflammation is obscured by a lack of definition of the contribution of traumatic and microbial influences. Clearly, bacteria must play a role in some instances of pulpal pathology, but the specific offending organisms have not been elucidated. Alternatively, it is proposed that pulpal pathology may develop in an apparent absence of microbial involvement. This empirical observation lends support to the endodontic dogma that dental pulps may become irreversibly necrotic from trauma alone. Necrosis would be the result of physical insult, e.g., a blow to a tooth, cavity preparation, temperature extremes, et cetera. Within the pulp spaces of the tooth, the inflammatory response would be perpetuated and intensified by noxious substances liberated from damaged tissue. This stagnated material may then induce a destructive inflammatory reaction in the periapical spaces; all in the absence of any microbial contribution. Although the experimental protocol followed in this investigation does not duplicate trauma on intact teeth, it does offer the possibility of comparing responses to oral trauma and differing microbial infections of germfree, defined flora and conventional mice.

Materials and Methods

Eighty young adult CD-1 Swiss Webster albino female mice were received from Charles River Farms. They were divided into approximately equal groups and entered into five isolators. The mice were maintained on a diet of L-356 (General Biochemical Co.) and water *ad libitum.* Twenty young adult Specific Pathogen Free CD-1 Swiss Webster albino female mice were maintained in a non-sterile isolator and served as isolator conventional animals. The mice were individually anesthetized with Metophane (Pitman Moore, Inc.). The maxillary left molars of all mice were cut off at or near the gingival margin with curved iris scissors.

Four isolators were monoinfected with pure cultures of one of the following organisms: alpha streptococci, *Candida albicans, Staphylococcus aureus,* or *Staphylococcus epidermidis.* The alpha strep. was an indigenous strain isolated from the oral cavity of mice. Oral inoculations of each mouse were made with cotton-tipped applicators at the time of surgery, 24, 48, 72 hours, and 4 days, post-surgery. One group of germfree mice was not inoculated. The experimental mice were identified by groups designations and are defined in Table I. Usually two mice in each group were sacrificed at 4, 8, 15, 22 days, and 4, 8, and 12 weeks post-surgery. Maxillae were fixed, decalcified, serially sectioned and stained with hematoxylin and eoisin. The lungs of germfree and monocontaminated mice were prepared for histological evaluation for all

TABLE I. Summary of Microbial Exposure of Mice Following Surgical Trauma

Group		Inoculum
I	Germfree	None
II	Defined flora	alpha streptococci
III	Defined flora	*Candida albicans*
IV	Defined flora	*Staphylococcus aureus*
V	Defined flora	*Staphylococcus epidermidis*
VI	Isolator conventional	None

192

specimens subsequent to the 4 day sacrifice period.

Samples for bacteriological monitoring were obtained from the cecum and reported as positive or negative for growth. Oral swabs of sacrificed mice were cultured beginning with the 15 day specimens.

Results

Microscopic examinations of normal and operated maxillae were directed toward evaluation and scoring of intensity of inflammatory and healing responses in applicable samples. For this paper, inflammatory responses were graded primarily by the intensity of inflammatory cellular infiltration. The scores were recorded as zero (0) for those specimens with no definable inflammatory cell infiltrate. Plus one (+) denoted minimal, plus two (++) moderate, and plus three (+++) dense inflammatory cell inflitration. Figure 1 shows the frequency of inflammatory response scores for all groups and is a composite of samples for all time periods after surgical trauma. A more comprehensive description of the histological observations of these samples will be included in a future publication.

In the germfree mice that were not infected (Group I), the 4 day samples showed some focal necrosis and intrapulpal hemorrhage. Specimens from subsequent sacrifice periods consistently revealed overall patterns of repair.

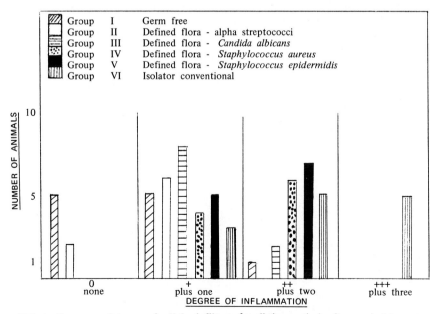

FIG. 1. Summary of degree of cellular infiltrate for all time periods after surgical trauma.

Reactive cellular stroma characterized earliest samples and irritation-tertiary-dentin-characterized the latter. The inflammatory cellular infiltration was either within normal limits or minimal with equal frequency for Group I (one exception) (Fig. 1). Rarely was any definitive alteration from normal noted in the periapical tissues of this group.

Group II mice inoculated with alpha streptococci had a slightly greater incidence of minimal cellular infiltration than Group I. No instance of moderate or dense cellular infiltration was noted for this group. Interpretation of the results from this group is difficult because of the inability to culture streptococci from the oral cavity of these mice throughout the experimental period. Cecum cultures were positive for bacterial growth after 21 days. The microorganisms were not identified, however. Results from histological evaluation of lung samples would be consistent with bacterial infection for this group (see below).

C. albicans inoculated mice (Group III) demonstrated predominantly minimal to moderate inflammatory responses only (Fig. 1). Surprisingly, Groups IV and V, *S. aureus* and *S. epidermidis* inoculated respectively, had responses quite similar to each other and more intense than Groups II and III. Moderate, rather than minimal, cellular infiltrates were slightly more common for these groups. No samples were scored as dense (Fig. 1). Nonetheless, Groups IV and V, *Staphylococcus sp.* infected, had vigorous inflammatory reactions.

Almost half of the isolated conventional animals (Group VI) had dense infiltrations, an equal number with moderate, and a few with minimal infiltration. This group clearly had a greater intensity of inflammatory responses than the other groups.

Individual variation of inflammation and/or repair was noted for any time period within all groups. Generally, inflammatory responses persisted throughout this study for *Staphylococcus sp.* infected and isolator controls (Groups IV, V, VI). Inflammation occurred early, either persisted at a minimal level, or disappeared completely in samples beyond 15 days for *Candida sp.* and streptococci inoculated Groups II and III.

Lung samples from germfree mice (Group I) were free of inflammation and were similar to normal non-traumatized germfree mice. Interestingly, all samples of lungs from mice subjected to trauma and infected with bacteria and fungi showed varing degrees of chronic focal inflammation, particularly in the upper half of the lungs of the left and right upper lobes. These areas were characterized by collections of large macrophages in the alveolar spaces and associated thickening of the alveolar walls (7).

Conclusions

These data indicate that microbial infection was essential to initiate and sustain a vigorous inflammatory response in the surgically exposed dental pulps and associated tissues of mice. Conversely, germfree mice had none to minimal inflammation after cutting off the crowns of molar teeth. Similar observations have been made in experiments designed to characterize inflammatory reactions of the periodontium. Our results and conclusions are quite consistent with the findings that bacteria are required to induce gingival inflammation in defined-flora animals (8, 9). In general, healing as measured by a return to normal, deposition of tertiary dentin, and subsiding inflammation was delayed or prevented within 12 weeks for isolator conventional and *Staphylococcus sp.* infected mice.

Realizing that there were exceptions within every group, one can generalize about the spectrum of inflammatory potential for differing microbial flora: flora of isolator conventional mice seemed to have the highest inflammatory potential; *Staphylococcus sp.* next in a lower order of magnitude; followed by *Candida sp.*; with streptococcus being the least offensive of all organisms introduced. A definite gradient appeared between the various groups and would probably exist for any other organisms tested.

Another interesting facet of this study was the apparent diminution of inflammatory infiltration noted in the groups infected with *Streptococci sp.* and *Candida sp.* Interestingly, a mild to moderate response was evident for the first 15 days and subsided for the remainder of the experimental period. This could mean that the host was able to resist any further microbial insult after the initial deleterious effects associated with trauma. In effect, these animals could accommodate the microorganisms, and their pulps be predominantly healed. However, no such accommodation was consistent for *Staphylococcus sp.* infected or isolator conventional groups. These findings for isolator conventional animals were in agreement with earlier studies (10).

As a model for evaluating the interrelationships between microbial effects and inflammation, dental pulps have great potential. Closed or open wounds can be created and noxious material introduced into pulp canals, thereby acting with a "depot" effect for sustained action.

Finally, for speculation, I would propose that trauma, within the bounds of reason, does not cause irreversible pulpal death. For that matter, I would additionally propose that trauma alone does not induce intensive inflammatory reactions in any tissues or organs. I would further suggest that microbial input or some other suitable antigenic stimulus is essential for induction and sustenance of inflammation beyond initial necrotic and vascular changes. Pulpal death in humans would then be the result of an interplay between trauma and microbial infection. Whether pulpal death ultimately occurs or not would depend upon host resistance and virulence of organisms (bacteria, fungi, viruses?). Bacterial may be "seeded" into the systemic circulation at a far greater frequency than is presently supposed. If so, this would provide ample opportunity for bacteria to get into irritated pulps by anachoresis (11). The result of this infection, subsequent to trauma, could lead to necrosis. The observations of this study, in a small measure, support the hypothesis that trauma and bacteria in concert contribute to chronic inflammation.

Acknowledgements

This investigation was supported in part by Grant 5-PO6-RR00407-03 from Animal Resources Branch, Division of Research Resources, N.I.H., to the School of Medicine, University of Southern California.

We wish to thank Robert Dorfman, Drs. R. D. Buckley and C. G. Loosli for their advice and assistance.

References

1. Rovin, S., Costich, E. R., Fleming, J. E., and Gordon, H. A., *J. Oral Surg. 24:* 239 (1966).
2. Rovin, S., Costich, E. R., Fleming, J. E., and Gordon, H. A., *Arch. Pathol. 79:* 641 (1965).
3. Kakehashi, S., Stanley, H. R., and Fitzgerald, R. J., *Oral Surg. Oral. Med. Oral Path. 20:* 340 (1965).
4. Gordon, H. A., and Pesti, L., *Bacteriol. Rev. 35:* 390 (1971).
5. Perkins, E. H., Nettesheim, P., Morita, T., and Walburg, H. E., Jr., in "The Reticuloendothelial System and Atherosclerosis," (N. R. Di Luzio and R. Paoletti, eds.), Plenum Press, New York, p. 175, (1967).
6. Miyakawa, M., in "Recent Progress in Microbiology," (G. Tunevall, ed.), Almquist and Wiksell, Stockholm, p. 299, (1959).
7. Loosli, C. G. (unpublished results).
8. Rovin, S., Costich, E. R., and Gordon, H. A., *J. Periodont. Res. 1:* 193 (1966).
9. Gibbons, R. J., Berman, K. S., Knoettner, P., and Kapsimalis, B., *Arch. Oral Biol. 11:* 549 (1966).
10. Glickman, I., Pruzansky, S., and Ostrach, M., *Am. J. Orthodont. Oral Surg. 30:* 263 (1947).
11. Gier, R. E., and Mitchell, D. F., *J. Dent. Res. 47:* 564 (1968).

COMPARISON OF ANTICARIES EFFECTS OF DIFFERENT POLYGLUCANASES IN LIMITED-FLORA HAMSTERS INFECTED WITH *STREPTOCOCCUS MUTANS*

R. J. Fitzgerald
Veterans Administration Hospital
Miami, Florida 33125

D. B. Fitzgerald
Institute of Oral Biology, Univ. of Miami
Miami, Florida 33136

and

T. H. Stoudt
Merck Sharp and Dohme Research Laboratories
Rahway, New Jersey 07065, U.S.A.

Introduction

The limited flora hamster, like the specific pathogen free animal, may be considered a type of gnotobiote if the definition of that term is extended to its broadest sense. In animals of these categories the knowledge of the associated microbiota encompasses not so much the identity of the members of the microflora that is present but rather the types of microbial elements which are absent (1). Specifically, in the case of the hamsters used in the experiments to be described, the animals were demonstrably free from microorganisms which could induce coronal caries or root surface caries when high sucrose diets were fed. These animals have been reared under "clean colony" conditions and the breeding stock has been monitored periodically by challenge with a cariogenic diet to insure the absence of a caries conducive flora.

Animals of this type have been employed to demonstrate the etiological role of *Streptococcus mutans* in the production of dental caries (2) and in establishing the importance of the sucrose mediated production of extracellular polysaccharides by these organisms in the formation of adherent plaque deposits of cariogenic microorganisms on the surfaces of the teeth (3, 4, 5).

In the case of *S. mutans* the major portion of the extracellular polysaccharide material produced from sucrose consists of polyglucans with a smaller proportion of polyfructans. The polyglucan fraction consists of dextrans (alpha 1-6 linked glucan) with varying amounts of 1-2, 1-3, and 1-4 linked glucans depending on the strain of *S. mutans* employed (6, 7). Fitzgerald et al (5) have shown that administration of an enzyme from *Penicillium funiculosum* NRRL No. 1768 could inhibit plaque formation and caries development in hamsters infected with *S. mutans* and receiving a high sucrose diet. It has already been reported that this enzyme which is an exoenzyme specific for $\alpha,1$-6 linked polyglucans varied in its ability to attack artificial plaques *in vitro* depending on the strain of *S. mutans* used to grow the plaques (8). It was therefore of interest to determine the effects of different polyglucanases on plaque formation and caries in hamsters infected with strains of *S. mutans* which produced plaque deposits *in vitro* that were relatively resistant to the $\alpha,1$-6 polyglucanase.

Materials and Methods

Enzyme preparations. The polyglucanase preparations were experimental products produced by Merck, Sharp and Dohme Research Laboratories. They differed in the nature of the organism which produced them, degree of purity, and substrate specificity. The *P. funiculosum* enzyme was an exoenzyme which attacked only $\alpha,1$-6 linkages. The *Penicillium sp.* enzyme was an endoenzyme which possessed activity against both $\alpha,1$-6 and $\alpha,1$-2 linkages. The streptomyces enzyme has not been fully characterized as yet but none of the enzyme preparation showed activity against $\alpha,1$-3 or $\alpha,1$-4 linkages. Unit activity of the enzymes was expressed according to Tsuchiya et al (9) using a linear $\alpha,1$-6 linked dextran as the standard substrate. The enzymes were dissolved in the distilled water provided as drinking water to the animals and the solutions were freshly prepared every two days.

Animal Test System. Weanling hamsters of the Institute of Oral Biology stock were distributed in groups of 3 in screen bottom cages at 21 days of age and provided with cariogenic Diet 2000 which contained 56 percent sucrose (10). The animals were infected orally with 24 hour Todd-Hewitt Broth cultures of the appropriate test organism. One week later, after plaque formation had started, the administration of the enzyme solutions was begun. Both food and drinking solutions were continuously available. The animals were sacrificed and the molar dentition scored for plaque and caries (11, 12) 42 days after they were infected; which meant that the enzymes had been administered for the last 35 days of this period.

Test Microorganisms. *S. mutans* strains SL-1R and K1-R (6715) which were known to form *in vitro* plaques that were relatively resistant to *P. funiculosum* dextranase (8) were employed in these tests. These organisms had been induced to streptomycin resistance to facilitate their isolation and identification from oral swab samples. They were abundantly present in the

198

mouths of the infected animals during the course of the tests and were not recovered from uninfected control animals.

Results

Table I presents the effects of a crude and a highly purified dextranase from *P. funiculosum* on the development of dental caries in hamsters infected with *S. mutans* strains SL-1R and K1-R (6715). Although the organisms differ in their odontopathic activity both enzyme preparations were comparably effective as inhibitors of caries development, indicating that the crude enzyme preparation did not contain other types of enzyme activity which might affect the caries experience of the animals.

TABLE I. Effect of Dextranase on Caries in Hamsters Receiving Sucrose Diet No. 2000.

S. mutans Strain	Enzyme Purity	Number Animals	Caries Score
SL-1R	8%	6	5.3
	90%	6	4.4
	Controls	6	19.5
K1-R (6715)	8%	6	8.3
	90%	6	3.1
	Controls	6	61.4

Dextranase administered in drinking water (500 units/ml)
Duration of test: 42 days

When polyglucanases of different types were administered to hamsters infected with strain SL-1R at levels which were comparable with respect to their activity on a linear dextran (α,1-6 polyglucan), both the antiplaque effects and the anticaries effects were essentially similar for the different enzymes (Table II).

Discussion

Caries induction in our strain of limited flora hamsters through infection with *S. mutans* and the use of a high sucrose diet closely simulates the conditions of a classical monoinfection experiment in gnotobiotes for these hamsters do not possess an indigenous cariogenic flora of significant consequence. This factor has made these animals extremely useful for the assessment of the cariogenic potential of various microorganisms without the necessity of employing the more exacting techniques required for the usual type of gnotobiotic test system. The presence in these animals of an indigenous but non-cariogenic microflora approximates more closely the normal oral ecologic

TABLE II. Effect of Polyglucanases on Plaque and Caries in Hamsters Infected with *S. mutans* **(SL-1R).**

Source	Type	Enzyme Conc.	Number Animals	Plaque Score	Caries Score
Penicillium funiculosum	Exo	500 u/ml	9	5.3	3.9
Penicillium sp.	Endo	500 u/ml	9	6.4	6.6
Streptomyces sp.	?	500 u/ml	9	7.1	1.3
Infected controls	—		9	21.4	45.3
Uninfected controls	—		9	6.2	3.8

Duration of test: 42 days

situation involving a mixed microbiota and, in contrast to the monoinfected gnotobiote, permits inferences to be made regarding the ability of potential cariogenic microorganisms to become established in the oral ecosystem as well as to induce disease. The problem of measuring the implantation of test organisms in the oral environment of the hamster has been simplified by the employment of mutants "labelled" by the induction of antibiotic resistance, a technique which permits their simultaneous recovery and identification from oral samples on culture media rendered selective by the incorporation of the antibiotic to which they are resistant (2).

Suggestions that the cariogenic potential of *S. mutans* is associated with the ability to produce adherent plaque deposits by the elaboration of extracellular polyglucans from sucrose (13, 14) have been substantiated by the demonstration that plaque formation and caries may be inhibited by dextranase administration to hamsters infected with this organism. The demonstration that *S. mutans* can produce several types of insoluble polyglucans which may be resistant to degradation by dextranases which specifically attack $\alpha,1$-6 linkages (6, 7, 8) has engendered the idea that enzymes or mixtures of enzymes with broader specificity could be more effective in the control of plaque formation and caries.

In the present studies however, an exo-dextranase from *P. funiculosum* which attacked only $\alpha,1$-6 linked polyglucans effectively suppressed plaque deposition and caries development in hamsters infected with two strains of *S. mutans* which *in vitro* also produced other polyglucans from sucrose that were

200

not attacked by this enzyme (8). The polyglucans produced by *S. mutans* strain SL-1R from sucrose *in vitro* contained a mixture of alpha 1-6, 1-2 and 1-3 linked glucans and were degradable by an endoenzyme preparation from a penicillium species which produced α,1-6 and α,1-2 glucan hydrolases (7). Nevertheless we have observed that microbial plaque formation and caries development in hamsters infected with strain SL-1R were inhibited to the same extent by the *P. funiculosum* exo-dextranase, the *Penicillium sp.* endoenzyme preparation and an incompletely characterized α,1-6 polyglucanase containing preparation from a *Streptomyces* when these enzyme preparations were administered on the basis of comparable α,1-6 glucan hydrolase activity.

Although it is not specifically known that the same spectrum of polyglucans is produced *in vivo* in hamsters as is produced *in vitro* by this organism, dextranase resistant polyglucans have been found in well established human dental plaques (7, 16) and we have noted (unpublished experiments) that direct application of the *P. funiculosum* dextranase to 3 week old plaque deposits of hamsters infected with *S. mutans* K1-R or SL-1R has frequently resulted in the deposits becoming loosened in their entirety or breaking up into smaller enzyme resistant fragments which no longer adhered to the teeth. In contrast hamster plaques formed *in vivo* by *S. mutans* E-49, which *in vitro* formed dextranase susceptible polyglucans, were almost completely dissolved by this enzyme.

It should be noted that in the *in vitro* plaque tests only 10 units/ml of dextranase were used at pH 7.1 (8) whereas the animals received 500 units per ml of drinking water. Also the pH of the plaques *in vivo* must have been closer to the optimum for dextranase activity (ca. pH 5.0), since it has been shown that plaque pH can fall to below this level in hamsters within minutes after contact with sucrose (15) and the animals usually followed each period of food consumption with a short period of drinking the enzyme solution. However, while these differences may affect quantitatively the susceptibility of α,1-6 polyglucans to dextranase (α,1-6 glucan hydrolase), they should have no bearing on other polyglucans in hamster plaques which are not attacked by this enzyme.

We interpret these results to indicate that, *in vivo,* α,1-6 polyglucans may exist at the interface between the bulk of the plaque and the outer tooth surface forming, at least in part, the adhesive substance which anchors the plaque. Once this is attacked by dextranase the cariogenic plaque, even though it may contain other polyglucans, can easily be dislodged. New plaque formation would be largely prevented by continuous availability of dextranase in the drinking water.

Some independent support for this aspect of plaque control is available from *in vitro* studies of Walker (17) on the regulatory mechanisms of polyglucan synthesis in oral streptococci. She has suggested that α,1-6 glucans are the initial extracellular polyglucans formed from sucrose and that the synthesis of other linkages is a secondary phenomenon. If this mechanism also applies intraorally to the *S. mutans* hamster caries model system it appears plausible that the effectiveness of the various enzyme preparations was due principally to their content of α,1-6 glucanhydrolase activity. The enzyme continuously available in the drinking water apparently broke down the extracellular α,1-6 polyglucans soon after they were elaborated and before other more resistant polymers were formed in significant amounts. Under these circumstances the application of polyglucanases with specificities for other types of glucan linkages would not be expected to contribute appreciably to plaque and caries inhibition.

On the other hand, it is conceivable that enzyme preparations with multiple substrate specificities would prove more useful as potential plaque control agents in humans where there would be less likelihood that enzyme therapy could be conducted on a continuous basis and more opportunity that the mixed oral flora could produce a variety of extracellular polysaccharides in the plaque deposits.

Summary

In a caries test system using limited flora hamsters three different enzyme preparations were equally effective when compared on the basis of their α,1-6 glucanhydrolase activity in preventing plaque formation and caries induction by *S. mutans* strains capable of forming, *in vitro,* polyglucans which were substantially resistant to attack by *P. funiculosum* dextranase, an exoenzyme which attacks only α,1-6 polyglucans. Since these enzymes were administered continually in the drinking water it is suggested that these results were due to the prompt destruction of the α,1-6 polyglucans produced by these organisms from sucrose before they could be further modified by the formation of other linkages and before they could contribute to the buildup of plaque deposits of cariogenic organisms on the teeth of the animals.

Acknowledgements

Supported in part by N.I.H. Grant DEO-2552-04S1.

References

1. Fitzgerald, R. J., *J. Dent. Res. 42:* 549 (1963).
2. Fitzgerald, R. J., and Keyes, P. H., *J. Amer. Dent. Assn. 61:* 9 (1960).
3. Krasse, B., *Archs. Oral Biol. 10:* 233 (1965).
4. Frostell, G., Keyes, P. H., and Larson, R. H., *J. Nutrit. 93:* 65 (1967).
5. Fitzgerald, R. J., Keyes, P. H., Stoudt, T. H., and Spinell, D. M., *J. Amer. Dent. Assn. 76:* 301 (1968).
6. Guggenheim, B., and Schroeder, H. E., *Helv. Odont. Act. 11:* 131 (1967).
7. Stoudt, T. H., Unpublished results, (1971).
8. Fitzgerald, R. J., Spinell, D. M., and Stoudt, T. H., *Archs. Oral Biol. 13:*75 (1968).
9. Tsuchiya, H. M., Jeanes, A., Bricker, H. M., and Wilham, C. A., *J. Bact. 65:* 513 (1952).

10. Keyes, P. H., and Jordan, H. V., *Archs. Oral Biol. 9:* 377 (1964).
11. Fitzgerald, D. B., and Fitzgerald, R. J., *Archs. Oral Biol. 17:* 215 (1972).
12. Keyes, P. H., *J. Dent. Res. 28:* 523 (1959).
13. Gibbons, R. J., *Caries Res. 2:* 164 (1968).
14. Fitzgerald, R. J., and Jordan, H. V., in *Art and Science of Dental Caries Research,* pp. 79-86, (Edited by R. S. Harris), (1968).
15. Charlton, G., Fitzgerald, D. B., and Keyes, P. H., *Archs. Oral Biol. 16:* 655 (1971).
16. Minah, G. E., Loesche, W. J., and Dziewiatkowski, D. D., *Archs. Oral Biol. 17:* 35 (1972).
17. Walker, G. J., *J. Dent. Res. 51:* 409 (1972).

OBSERVATIONS ON THE CARIOGENIC ASSESSMENT OF STREPTOCOCCI IN GNOTOBIOTIC RATS, WITH REFERENCE TO THE TAXONOMY OF *STREPTOCOCCUS MUTANS*

D. K. Blackmore
Medical Research Council Laboratory Animals Centre

D. B. Drucker
Manchester University Department of Bacteriology & Virology

and

R. M. Green
University of Wales Dental School, United Kingdom

Introduction

A rapid method for the evaluation of the cariogenicity of streptococci in gnotobiotic rats has been previously described (1). Although this initial contribution only described the effect of one strain of organisms (OMZ 61) it was suggested that the system might provide a reproducible method for the rapid evaluation of potentially cariogenic streptococci. Using these techniques other strains of streptococci were successfully investigated (2).

Materials and Methods

In the present study, 21 different strains of streptococci were investigated using similar techniques. Nine of these strains were tested at intervals ranging from 6 – 20 months. The strains of organisms investigated included those previously described by other workers as *Streptococcus mutans* and of known cariogenicity, organisms not previously studied in animals, and those previously considered as non-cariogens. Table I summarizes the materials and methods employed during this study. The majority of the organisms studied *in vivo* were also subjected to extensive *in vitro* investigations, which allowed them to be classified by numerical taxonomic methods as described by Drucker and Melville (3).

Results

The strains of streptococci and the incidence of fissure caries induced in

205

TABLE I. Summary of Materials and Methods

Strain of rat . . . . Gnotobiotic inbred AGUS
Number of rats used 290
Number of litters 80
Age of rats at beginning of experiment . . . . 21 − 24 days
Duration of experiment . . . . 21 days
Method of caries assessment . . . . Lower molar sections
Number of strains of streptococci investigated 22
Number of strains tested more than once 9
Interval between retesting . . . . 6 − 20 months

the lower molars of the gnotobiotic rats are shown in Table II. The results of repeating the tests at varying intervals are given in Table III. A dendrogram, based on the *in vitro* characteristics of various streptococci, studied by the present authors and other workers in animal models, is shown in Fig. 1. This dendrogram also includes other streptococci which have not been studied in relation to their possible cariogenicity. It should be noted that streptococci strains 2M2, JR8LG and 112 exhibited rather different cariogenic properties when re-tested in gnotobiotic rats. 2M2 is a strain of streptococcus known to produce a mutant capable of producing plaque (4). In the first experiment the organism apparently failed to produce extracellular polysaccharide and was of low cariogenicity. In the subsequent experiment, the extracellular poly-saccharide producing mutant spontaneously occurred and was associated with much higher cariogenic properties. In the case of JR8LG, it was noted that in the second experiment the organism underwent some form of change which resulted in a different colonial morphology. It is assumed that this change was linked with slight changes in its cariogenic potential.

Strain 112 was classified as of intermediate cariogenicity when first tested. A second series of experiments was then designed whereby the organism was inoculated orally into one group of rats, and then three weeks later direct oral swabs of these rats were used to contaminate a further series of three week old germfree rats. Oral swabs from this second group were used to contaminate a third group three weeks later. On the first passage in the second experiment no fissure caries were produced, but on second and third passages, strain 112 again produced sufficient fissure lesions (a mean of between 4 and 5) to be classified as of intermediate cariogenicity. These findings lead one to suggest that the *in vitro* culture of a potential cariogen may reduce its cariogenicity, but once this capability has been restored, relatively reproducible results can be obtained.

Strain D282 exhibited a slightly lower cariogenicity on each subsequent test, but each time it could be unequivocally classified as highly cariogenic. When D282 was initially tested in both gnotobiotic and specific pathogen free (S.P.F.) AGUS rats of the same inbred strain, there was a similar effect in relation to the introduction of fissure caries. Although proximal lesions also

206

TABLE II. Comparative Cariogenicity

Cariogenicity	Strain of Streptococcus and previous specific terminology	Total number of fissure lesions lower molars
High	D282 (*S. mutans*)	11.3
	BHT (*S. mutans*)	9.0
	2M2	8.9*
	OMZ 61 (*S. mutans*)	8.1
Intermediate	P1	6.5
	112	5.0
Low	2F2 (*S. pyogenes*)	3.75
	S69 (*S. faecium*)	3.6
	PK1	3.5
	JC2	3.25
	D65	2.9
	D182	2.5
	167	2.5
	JR8LG	2.0
	SBEL	1.75
	2M2	1.75
	S39 (*S. liquefaciens*)	0.9
Negative	15 (*Pneumococcus*)	NIL
	207 (*S. equi*)	NIL
	S61 (*S. durans*)	NIL
	S68 (*S. liquefaciens*)	NIL
	S70 (*S. faecium*)	NIL
	112	NIL*
	JR8LG	NIL*

*Results of second test

occurred in both groups, the S.P.F. animals were less affected. Only the gnotobiotic animals developed buccal and lingual lesions. Subsequent experiments with gnotobiotic rats failed to reproduce these smooth surface lesions.

AGUS inbred strains of rats have been used for all the gnotobiotic experiments described in this paper. More recently, an inbred strain of hooded rats has also been employed. When both strains of rats were orally inoculated with strain OMZ 61, fissure caries only were induced in the AGUS rats, while both proximal and fissure lesions occurred in the hooded rats.

Drucker and Melville (3) discussed the classification of oral streptococci of human and rat origin, and pointed out that frequently the term *S. mutans* had been applied to any cariogenic streptococcus. In their study they defined a Phenon G, which included five known cariogenic strains: BHT, FA-1, AHT,

TABLE III. Repetition of Experiments

Strain of Streptococcus	1st Experiment				2nd Experiment				3rd Experiment				Interval between experiments
	No. of rats	T	B	C	No. of rats	T	B	C	No. of rats	T	B	C	
D.282	12	11.3	10.1	5.8	11	10.8	8.9	5.9	8	8.8	5.4	2.0	14 and 12 mo.
JC.2	4	3.25	0.5	0	8	2.3	0	0	7	5.2	2.7	1.4	14 mo. and 3 weeks*
112	4	5.0	2.5	0	8	0	0	0	6	4.3	1.5	0.5	20 mo. and 3 weeks*
2F2	4	3.75	1.5	0	3	2.0	0.3	0	–	–	–	–	15 months
PK.1	4	3.5	1.25	0	3	3.7	0.7	0	–	–	–	–	6 months
167	4	2.5	0.25	0	4	1.25	0.25	0	–	–	–	–	6 months
JR8Lg	4	2.0	0	0	12	0	0	0	–	–	–	–	20 months
SBEL	4	1.75	0	0	2	2.5	0.5	0	–	–	–	–	4 months
2M2	4	1.75	0.5	0	12	8.9	3.4	1.1	–	–	–	–	20 months

T = Mean total number of fissure lesions
B = Mean number of advanced lesions
C = Mean number of very advanced lesions
* = 2nd and 3rd experiments carried out at 3-weekly intervals by direct transmission from experimentally infected rats.

OMZ 61 and E 49. They suggested that only this group of streptococci warranted the specific terminology of *S. mutans*, and that it should not be applied to many other cariogenic strains including SL-1 and K1R. This suggestion was in keeping with the findings of Orland *et al.* (5), and implies that although all strains of *S. mutans* are cariogenic, not all cariogenic streptococci are necessarily *S. mutans*. *In vitro* studies on strain D 282 also suggest that it is a true strain of *S. mutans*.

It will be noted (see Table III) that with the exception of the mutant form of 2M2 all other strains of highly cariogenic streptococci investigated in this study were *S. mutans*, while all others, although the majority showed some degree of cariogenicity, could not be classified taxonomically within this specific group.

Conclusions

Of the twenty-one strains of streptococci investigated, seventeen showed

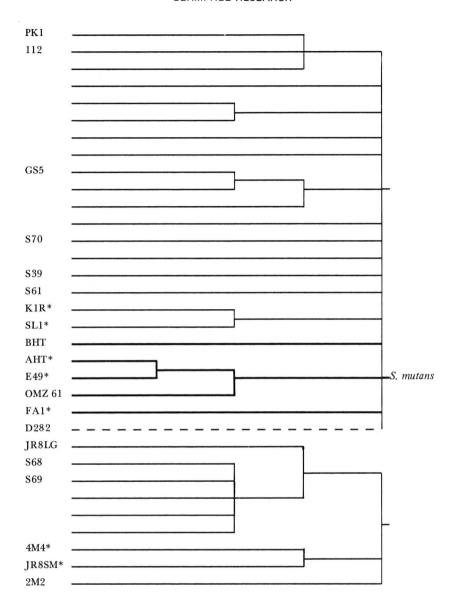

*Not investigated for cariogenicity in present study.

FIG. 1. Dendrogram of Streptococci based on their *in-vitro* characteristics

some degree of cariogenicity, but only four strains were classified as highly cariogenic. Further investigations suggested that *in vivo* cariogenicity tests using gnotobiotic inbred rats resulted in a high degree of reproducibility, provided that there were no obvious changes in other characteristics of the organisms being tested. These results also suggest that strains of streptococci which are classified as *S. mutans* by extensive taxonomic studies are more highly cariogenic than other strains. This test system allowed organisms previously incorrectly termed *S. mutans* to be differentiated from those strains which justified such specific terminology on the basis of the taxonomic scheme of Drucker and Melville (3).

References

1. Blackmore, D. K., and Green, R. M., *Archs. Oral Biol. 15:* 1149 (1970).
2. Blackmore, D. K., Drucker, D. B., and Green, R. M., *Archs. Oral Biol. 15:* 1377 (1970).
3. Drucker, D. B., and Melville, T. H., *Archs. Oral Biol. 16:* 845 (1971).
4. Tanzer, J. M., and McCabe, R. M., *Archs. Oral Biol. 13:* 139 (1968).
5. Orland, F. J., Blayney, J. R., Harrison, R. W., Reyniers, J. A., Trexler, P. C., Ervin, R. F., Gordon, H. A., and Wagner, M., *J. Am. Dent. Ass. 50:* 259 (1955).

RELATIONSHIP OF SPECIFIC ANTIBACTERIAL AGGLUTININS IN SALIVA TO DENTAL CARIES IN GNOTOBIOTIC RATS

Morris Wagner
Department of Microbiology, University of Notre Dame
Notre Dame, Indiana 46556, USA

Introduction

Attempts to immunize man and experimental animals against dental caries date back to the 1930's (1, 2). A review of this area of research by Wagner (3) and work done since that time indicate that immunization experiments in man, conventionally-reared animals or animals in "relative states of gnotobiosis" have been unsuccessful, inconclusive or have given opposing results in the hands of different investigators. For example, at the 1970 Annual Meeting of the International Association for Dental Resarch, Gaffar *et al.* (4) reported significant reduction of caries in immunized hamsters while Tanzer *et al.* (5) were unable to immunologically protect rats from smooth surface caries.

A test of the hypothesis that specific immunization can prevent or significantly reduce the incidence and severity of dental caries depends on at least two assumptions: (a) All the potential viable cariogenic agents present in the oral cavity should be known to the investigator so that homology between cariogenic and immunogenic agents can be attained; (b) immunological protection will depend on the ability of the host to secrete protective antibody to the oral cavity.

With regard to point (a) above, it is well known that dental caries have a multiple etiology. The following cariogenic organisms have been described: *Streptococcus faecalis* (3, 6, 7), *S. faecalis* var. *liquefaciens* (3), *S. mutans* (8), *S. mitis* (9), *S. salivarius* (9), *S. sanguis* (10, 11), *Lactobacillus casei* (7, 12), *L. acidophilus* (13). In addition, *Odontomyces viscosus* (14), *Actinomyces naeslundii,* a diptheroid rod and a bacillus species have been reported to have cariogenic activity of the root caries type (15). Perhaps other yet unknown cariogenic microorganisms exist. It is therefore not too surprising that earlier attempts to immunize man and conventionally-reared animals were largely unsuccessful because of the investigator's inability to know and control the oral flora and an inability to match the cariogenic agents present with their homologous immunogens.

211

With regard to point (b) preceding, many investigators attempting anticaries immunization have failed to measure the immune response, or have measured antibody in serum but not in saliva. It is known that salivary antibody levels are not necessarily related to serum levels, that serum IgA and locally synthesized (salivary gland) IgA are selectively secreted via the salivary glands to the oral cavity and that the ability to secrete may be genetically controlled independently of the serum levels of antibody.

The use of the gnotobiotic animal in testing the hypothesis that specific immunization can decrease or prevent dental caries offers a number of advantages that circumvent the above mentioned problems. Susceptible gnotobiotic rats can be inoculated orally with a single specific cariogenic culture. Half of the animals can then be immunized with a homologous bacterin, leaving the nonimmunized animals as controls. Thus, the serum and salivary antibody produced is directed against only a single type of microorganism.

Materials and Methods

In the present study, germfree Lobund-Wistar rats were used unless otherwise indicated. Weanling rats were inoculated orally with a pure culture of the cariogenic bacterial strain and the immunized groups of animals were started on the immunization protocol on the same day that the oral inoculation with the viable agents was given. The immunogen was a formalin-killed washed whole-cell bacterin made from the homologous cariogenic agent and was given subcutaneously in a dose of 1×10^9 cells in saline on days 0, 3, 6 post oral association with the viable agent. At day 9 and at approximately 30 day intervals thereafter, a similar dose of bacterin in Freund's Complete Adjuvant was given over a total experimental period of 150 days. Serum and salivary titers of agglutinating antibody were determined during the course of the experiment and terminally. Terminal titers and gross caries scores are reported here.

Results and Discussion

Earlier studies (7) had indicated that some rats gnotobiotically mono-associated with a homofermentative strain of lactobacillus developed caries while others did not. Furthermore, animals with the higher salivary antibody titers had little or no caries while rats with low or no titers developed lesions. Since the inverse relationship between salivary agglutinins and cariogenesis had been observed in animals that had not received any parenteral antigenic treatment, a number of experiments were performed to test the anticaries immunization hypothesis further.

A summary of three immunization experiments in gnotobiotic rats harboring S. faecalis (ND 547) as cariogenic agent is shown in Table I. Specific immunization virtually eliminated caries incidence. All animals in the non-

212

TABLE I. Caries Scores and Salivary Agglutinin Titers in Nonimmunized and Specifically Immunized Gnotobiotic Rats Monoassociated with *Streptococcus faecalis.*

	Immunized	Nonimmunized
Total number of rats	18	23
Rats with caries	3	23
Rats caries-free	15	0
Mean caries score	0.17	8.26
Maximum score	1	30
Minimum score	0	3
Mean salivary titer*	60	6.5
Titer range**	32-128	0-32

*reciprocal of geometric mean of 2 fold dilution titer.
**reciprocal of dilution titer.

immunized groups developed caries while only 3 of 18 rats (1 rat in each of the three immunized groups) developed caries among the immunized animals. Each of these three caries-positive rats had a minimal observable lesion, score = 1. It was noted that rats with salivary titers above 1:32 were all caries-negative, rats with titers below 1:32 were caries-positive and rats showing titers of 1:32 were pivotal, some being positive and some negative.

A series of other immunization experiments was done using other known cariogenic agents. Results are shown in Table II. Again, specific immunization

TABLE II. Caries Scores and Salivary Antibody Titers in Immunized and Nonimmunized Gnotobiotic Rats Monoassociated with Various Cariogenic Bacteria

	Nonimmunized			Immunized		
	No.	Titer	Score	No.	Titer	Score
Streptococcus mutans (GS-5)	6	7.1	18.8	6	71.8	0
Streptococcus (Exp. 1) *sanguis*-like No. 167	4	53.8	0.5	5	84.4	0
Streptococcus (Exp. 2) *sanguis*-like No. 167	7	5.9	11.6	9	69.1	0
Lactobacillus casei(ND 465)	4	6.7	2.3	4	53.8	0

Titers are expressed as the reciprocal of the geometric mean for the group while caries scores are expressed as the arithmetic mean.

prevented cariogenesis by *S. mutans, S. sanguis* and *L. casei.* It should be noted that the first *S. sanguis* experiment resulted in high salivary titers and virtually no caries in the nonimmunized controls. The nonimmunized animals in the second experiment had low titers, active caries and the immunized animals were protected. The reason for the discrepancy between nonimmunized controls in the two experiments is not known but the data still support the earlier observations that there is an inverse relationship between salivary titer and caries activity. Rosen (16) has reported that caries experience in *L. casei* mono-associated gnotobiotic rats varied considerably from experiment to experiment. Results ranged from appreciable caries in one experiment to zero caries in the next, despite the use of the same rat strain, the same type of diet and the same bacterial strain. Unfortunately, he presented no salivary antibody data for his groups of animals.

Additional experiments were designed to test the hypothesis that the difference in caries susceptibility between genetically derived Harvard caries-resistant (CR) and caries-susceptible (CS) rats may have an immunologic basis (17-19). Germfree Harvard weanling CR and CS rats were inoculated orally with viable *S. faecalis* (ND 547) and maintained monoassociated for five months. The CR rats responded to the monoassociation alone (without parenteral injection) with high serum and salivary titers and with little or no caries. In contrast, CS rats developed serum and salivary antibody more slowly, never attained the salivary titers reached by CR rats and they developed extensive caries.

Under parenteral immunization, the CR monoassociated rats maintained high serum and salivary antibody levels and remained caries-free. The immunized CS rats also developed high serum levels of antibody but their salivary antibody level remained low and no anticaries protection was observed in that both immunized and nonimmunized rats developed extensive caries. Thus, CR and CS rats both responded well to parenteral immunization in terms of circulating serum antibody but differed markedly in their ability to deliver protective levels of antibody to the oral environment. These findings suggest that there is an immunologic basis for genetic difference in caries susceptibility for the two rat strains.

Some of the CR rats, monoassociated with *S. faecalis* were bred within the isolator unit. Second generation animals displayed salivary antibody titers and caries experience intermediate between results reported for the first generation CR and CS animals. Since the first generation animals were exposed to *S. faecalis* only after 3 weeks of germfree life while second generation animals were exposed at birth or possibly even prenatally, the data suggest that prenatal or neonatal exposure to the specific antigenic stimulus may result in a suboptimal immune response and thus an increase in caries incidence and intensity. More work is needed to verify whether a state of partial tolerance brought about by early exposure to antigenic stimulation by the cariogenic organism can indeed reverse the "genetic" resistance of CR rats. The present preliminary observations suggest that this may be the case.

Conclusions

1. Gnotobiotic rats monoassociated with specific cariogenic bacteria and fed a high carbohydrate diet develop caries.
2. Dental caries incidence can be reduced to virtual elimination by specific immunization against a known cariogenic organism in the gnotobiotic rat.
3. Caries incidence appears to be inversely related to the specific agglutinating antibody levels attained in saliva.
4. The early exposure of a host animal to cariogenic bacteria may lead to a decrease in the homologous antibody levels in saliva and allow an increase in caries incidence and severity.
5. An immunologic basis for genetic resistance to dental caries is implied.

Acknowledgements

This work was supported in part by NIH Grant DE-01887, the B-0 Scientific Research Foundation and the University of Notre Dame.

References

1. Jay, P., Crowley, M., and Bunting, R. W., *J. Am. Dent. Ass. 19:* 265 (1932).
2. Jay, P., Crowley, M., Hadley, F. P., and Bunting, R. W., *J. Am. Dent. Ass. 20:* 2130 (1933).
3. Wagner, M., Doctoral Thesis, Purdue University, West Lafayette, Ind. (1966). *Dissert. Abstr. 27 (2),* (1966).
4. Gaffar, A., Marcussen, H. W., Huffner, J., and Kestenbaum, R. C., Proc. 48 Gen. Meet. I.A.D.R., p. 124, (1970).
5. Tanzer, J. M., Hageage, G. J., and Larson, R. H., Proc. 48 Gen. Meet. I.A.D.R., p. 165, (1970).
6. Orland, F. J., Blayney, J. P., Harrison, R. W., Reyniers, J. A., Trexler, P. C., Ervin, R. F., Gordon, H. A., and Wagner, M., *J. Am. Dent. Ass. 50:* 259 (1955).
7. Wagner, M., and Orland, F. J., *Proc. Ind. Acad. Sci. 73:* 75 (1967).
8. Fitzgerald, R. J., Jordan, H. V., and Stanley, H. R., *J. Dent. Res. 39:* 923 (1960).
9. Gibbons, R. J., and Banghart, S., *Archs. Oral Biol. 13:* 297, 697 (1968).
10. Shklair, I. L., Coykendall, A. L., Carroll, P. B., and Tow, H. D., Proc. 45 Gen. Meet. I.A.D.R., p. 69, (1967).
11. Shklair, I. L., and Rosen, S., *J. Dent Res. 48:* 1313 (1969).
12. Rosen, S., Lenney, W. S., and O'Malley, J. E., *J. Dent. Res. 47:* 358 (1968).
13. Fitzgerald, R. J., Jordan, H. V., and Archard, H. O., *Archs. Oral Biol. 11:* 473 (1966).
14. Keyes, P. H., and Jordan, H. V., *Archs. Oral Biol. 9:* 377 (1964).
15. Socransky, S. S., Hubersak, C., Propas, D., and Rozanis, J., Proc. 48 Gen. Meet. I.A.D.R., p. 86, (1970).
16. Rosen, S., *Archs. Oral Biol. 14:* 445 (1969).
17. Peri, B. and Wagner, M., *Bact. Proc. 71:* 107 (1971).

18. Peri, B., and Wagner, M., (1973) to be published in detail elsewhere.
19. Peri, B., Doctoral Thesis, University of Notre Dame, Notre Dame, Indiana (1970).

EFFECTIVENESS OF HIGH SPEED DENTAL DRILLS AS NEBULIZERS AND CONTROL OF THE GENERATED AEROSOLS

Gerard McGarrity and *Lewis Coriell*
Institute for Medical Research
Camden, New Jersey 08103

and

Don Trachtenberg and *Victor Long*
School of Dental Medicine, University of Pennsylvania
Philadelphia, Pennsylvania 19104, U.S.A.

Introduction

Several studies have demonstrated increased bacterial aerosols during use of the high-speed dental handpiece (1-3). However, the extent and properties of these aerosols has varied, and one report stated airborne bacteria to be greater with use of the conventional handpiece than with the high-speed instrument (4). There are many variables that can account for this, especially the air pressure and water flow rates, and Litsky *et al.* have mentioned the need for proper sampling technique (5). The variables in environmental sampling during high-speed drilling demonstrates the need for an *in vitro* assay system in which an accurate appraisal could be made of the handpiece as an aerosol generator.

The purpose of these studies was to minimize the number of environmental variables so that an accurate appraisal could be made of the high-speed dental handpiece as an aerosol generator. On the basis of these studies control measures are suggested to minimize risk to dental operatory personnel.

Methods

Initial studies were performed in a 3x4x3 ft. plastic germfree isolator. A Starflite portable dental handpiece was operated inside the unit through glove ports; the pump for the handpiece was outside the isolator. The two basic types of experiments performed in this unit were: 1) drilling of extracted human teeth mounted on a dental arch and measuring the number of airborne dust particles with a Dynac Model M 101 electronic dust counter (6); and 2) immersing the drill into a beaker containing 50 ml of a suspension of T3 bacteriophage of

Escherichia coli for 30 sec. Samples of T3 aerosols were obtained 6 in. from the site of nebulization with 50 ml plastic syringes containing 10 ml of broth. The phage was assayed by standard bacteriophage techniques (7). T3 phage was used as a tracer aerosol since it can be grown in large numbers; is innocuous to personnel; easy to assay; and is stable in aerosol. It has been nebulized in our laboratories several hundred times to test the efficiencies of various filters and to determine the effectiveness of air curtains (8, 9). Phage aerosols were also sampled with an Andersen sampler (6) with methods already described (8). Air pressure in the handpiece was 30 psi; relative humidity in the isolator was 65 ± 2% R.H.

Results

T3 phage was nebulized inside the enclosure a total of 17 times. Air samples obtained immediately after drilling averaged 5.8×10^7 PFU/ft^3 air, ranging from 7.3×10^6 to 2.8×10^8 PFU/ft^3. Samples obtained 5 and 10 minutes after nebulization averaged 8.4×10^6 and 6×10^6 PFU/ft^3 air respectively. The relatively long life of the phage aerosol suggested small, nonsedimenting particles.

To determine particle size, samples of the nebulized phage were obtained by Andersen samplers. Immediately after nebulization, the majority of particles were 1 to 5 microns in size. Fewer phage particles were recovered 5 and 10 min later, but the majority were still between 1 and 5 microns.

Long-lived aerosols were also obtained when human teeth mounted on a dental arch were drilled inside the isolator. The sampling probe of an electronic particle counter was positioned 6 in. from the site of drilling. There was an average of 10,000 particles/ft^3 before drilling. After 30 sec of drilling, counts increased to several hundred thousand per cubic ft. In a test representative of 25 experiments, counts increased from a background of 9,000/ft^3 to 243,000/ft^3 when the handpiece was operated without making contact with the teeth. These were mainly water droplets. Counts remained elevated until sampling was discontinued 60 min later. There was a great variation observed in these counts in individual tests. When counts returned to baseline levels, the handpiece contacted the tooth for 30 sec. Counts increased from an average of 9250/ft^3 to 475,000/ft^3 minutes after drilling. Counts averaged 304,000 and 242,000 30 and 60 min after drilling respectively.

Nebulization of phage and tooth particles was performed in a 6 x 10 x 7 ft room to compare results obtained in the closed environment of the plastic isolator with those obtained in a larger room of a size similar to a small dental operatory. Samples of phage and dust particles were obtained 6 in. from the point of release to approximate the distance between patient and dental personnel. Only the technician performing the sampling was in the room during these tests. Air is introduced into this room through a bank of HEPA filters which comprise the entire ceiling. Vertical air velocity in the room with the blowers in operation can be varied from 10 to 100 fpm, the latter speed constituting what is commonly known as laminar airflow.

With the blowers not in operation, phage tests showed an average of 2.3 x 10^5 PFU/ft^3 air in the stagnant atmosphere of this room 1 min after nebulization; the same average was detected at the same sampling site 10 min later. These averages were calculated from 6 tests.

Phage studies performed at an air velocity of 10 fpm showed an average of 3.1 x 10^2 PFU/ft^3, approximately a three log decrease from control values. Samples obtained 5 min later showed essentially no phage. When the air velocity was increased to 25 fpm, no phage was detected in 6 tests immediately after nebulization or 5 min later.

When extracted human teeth mounted in a dental arch were drilled in this room without ventilation, dust counts increased from an average of 20,900/ft^3 to 277,750 (averages of 4 tests). Ten min after drilling counts averaged 198,600 and remained higher than 100,000 until 30 min when sampling was discontinued.

When these studies were repeated with an air velocity of 10 fpm, an average of 5,695 particles were detected in the 1 min period immediately after drilling and this decreased to an average of 120 two min later.

These studies were performed with 1 technician in the room and a minimum of activity. To determine the effect of activity on the minimum air velocity to eliminate airborne contamination, a subject was seated in the center of the room while the operator held the handpiece inside the subject's mouth, for 1 min. No tooth contact was made. A third person held an Andersen bacterial air sampler 6 in. from the mouth. The variables in this series of investigations were no ventilation in the room, and ventilation at velocities of 10 and 25 fpm.

Results showed an average of 109 CFU/ft^3 detected when the system was not in operation; there was no significant difference with an air velocity of 10 fpm. This was based on observations of 47 experiments performed with no ventilation and 41 with velocity at 10 fpm. With a velocity of 25 fpm, an average of 3.3 CFU/ft^3 were detected.

Discussion and Conclusions

Dense aerosols of viable and nonviable particulates were generated by the high-speed dental handpiece and persisted for long periods, indicating the presence of many small sized particles. This was confirmed by Andersen samplers, which demonstrated that immediately after nebulization, the majority of the particles had an equivalent diameter of 1 to 5 microns. Five and 10 min later, a less concentrated aerosol was evidenced, but the majority of particles were still 1 and 5 microns. Particles in this size range have the potential to penetrate human alveoli (6).

The aerosol generated in the isolator by actual drilling of extracted teeth had a slower decay rate since biological inactivation was not a factor and was influenced solely by the sedimentation rate and minimal air currents inside the isolator. This aerosol consisted of water droplets and tooth particles.

Vertical flow air of 25 fpm velocity can maintain viable and nonviable airborne particles near zero levels during use of the high-speed handpiece. These results demonstrate that the 100 fpm employed in conventional laminar airflow systems is not needed to control aerosols generated in the dental operatory, and more economical flow rates can be employed (10).

It is difficult to make definite recommendations in the absence of demonstrable hazards to dental personnel and patients. Litsky *et al.* have referred to some potential infections that can occur (5). Grundy has reported cause and effect relationships between use of the air turbine and appearance of respiratory, alimentary, ocular and skin symptoms (11). Baunoe reported possible transmission of infectious hepatitis to dentists (12). These two studies however, were based on responses to questionnaires rather than on prospective clinical studies. More studies are needed to quantitate the infectious hazard of high-speed drilling to dental personnel, patients, and visitors to the dental operatory, especially in light of evidence indicating possible airborne spread of serum hepatitis (13).

Less is known about the fate of tooth particulates and amalgam. The present studies demonstrate that dense aerosols containing mostly small sized particles are generated during high-speed dental drilling, and these remain in the atmosphere for prolonged periods. Atmospheric particles, both viable and nonviable, will remain airborne until they sediment onto flat surfaces, are breathed or vented. The small sized particles in aerosols from dental equipment will not sediment under normal conditions. Ventilation and filtration systems normally encountered in dental operatories are not sufficient to purge the area of these aerosols. This means that the occupants of these rooms are constantly inhaling air heavily contaminated with viable and nonviable particles. We recommend studies be made on the possible effects these aerosols may have on personnel, and increased ventilation rates be employed in operatories to minimize exposure. Cost effectiveness studies would have to determine the optimum ventilation rate, but it is obvious from published reports that the usual ventilation systems in operatories are not capable of removing generated contamination.

Acknowledgements

The authors wish to thank Vicky Ammen, Judi Sarama and Mary Federico for technical assistance.

This work was supported by grants from the John Hatford Foundation, the State of New Jersey and by N.I.H. General Research Support Grant Nos. FR5582 to the Institute for Medical Research and RR05337-11 to the University of Pennsylvania.

References

1. Madden, R. M., and Hausler, W. J., *J. Dent. Res. 42:* 1146 (1963).
2. Pistocco, L. R., and Bowers, G. M., *U.S. Navy Newsletter 40:* 24 (1962).
3. Brown, R. V., *J. Dent. Children 32:* 112 (1965).
4. Kazantizis, M. G., *Proc. Roy. Soc. Med. 54:* 242 (1961).
5. Litsky, B. Y., Mascis, J. D., and Litsky, W., *Oral Surg. 29:* 25 (1970).
6. Mazzarella, M. A., and Flynn, D. D., "Introduction to Experimental Aerobiology," Wiley-Interscience, p. 437, (1969).
7. Adams, M. H., "Bacteriophages," Interscience Publishers Inc., (1959).
8. Coriell, L. L., and McGarrity, G. J., *Appl. Microbiol. 16:* 1895 (1968).
9. Coriell, L. L., and McGarrity, G. J., *J. Amer. Assoc. Contam. Control 1:* 16 (1969).
10. Coriell, L. L., McGarrity, G. J. and Blakemore, W. S., in "Germfree Research: Biological Effect of Gnotobiotic Environments," (J. B. Heneghan, ed.), Academic Press, New York, p. 43, (1973).
11. Grundy, J. R., *Dent. Practit. 17:* 17 (1966).
12. Baunoe, J. H., *Tandlaegebl. 63:* 407 (1959).
13. Almeida, J. D., Kulatilake, A. E., Mackay, D. H., Shackman, R., Chisholm, G. D., MacGregor, A. B., O'Donoghue, E. P. N., and Waterson, A. P., *Lancet 2:* 849 (1971).

SECTION VI

NUTRITION AND METABOLISM

THE BREAKDOWN OF STARCH AT DIFFERENT LEVELS IN THE DIGESTIVE TRACT OF THE AXENIC, GNOTOXENIC AND HOLOXENIC CHICKEN

O. Ivorec-Szylit
Laboratoire de Recherches sur la Conservation
et l'Efficacite des Aliments

P. Raibaud
Station Centrale de Recherches Laitieres et de
Technologie des Produits Animaux
C.N.R.Z. — 78 — Jouy-en-Josas

and

P. Schellenberg
Station de Pathologie Aviaire
C.R.V.Z. — 37 — Tours, France

Introduction

It is generally recognized in the domestic fowl, as in a monogastric, that the digestion of starch takes place mainly in the duodenum for cereal starch and in the ceca for raw tuberous root starch. The crop is usually considered as reservoir for the digesta in the chick, but it has a large microflora (1) and can play a role in digestion (2). This role of the crop is marked by the formation of the products of hydrolysis (oligosaccharides) and of fermentation (D and L lactic acids and volatile fatty acids) (3). Starch digestion is practically completed when the digesta reach the duodenum.

In order to separate the effects of the microflora, we have compared the extent and nature of the breakdown of starch at different levels in the digestive tract of axenic (germfree) gnotoxenic and holoxenic (conventional) chickens.

Results

The major emphasis of this investigation has been upon determination of soluble carbohydrates, glucose, D and L lactic acid by methods already described (4).

The crop. In the holoxenic animal, as in the axenic animal, amylase

225

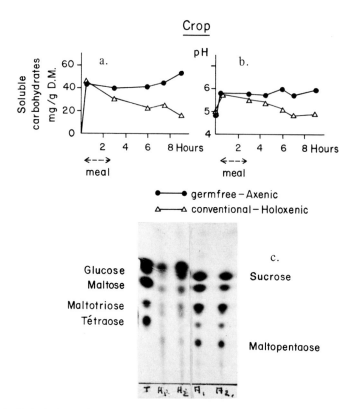

FIG. 1. Carbohydrate digestion in the crop during the 9 postfeeding hours. a) Quantitative evolution of the soluble carbohydrates. b) Evolution of the pH. c) Qualitative composition of the digesta, A. Axenic – H. Holoxenic.

activity can be found in the crop; however, it is much weaker in the axenic. In addition, both quantitative and qualitative differences can be observed (Figs. 1a and 1c) in the abilities of axenic and holoxenic chicks to use the diet starch. In the former, the carbohydrate concentration does not decrease during the post-feeding hours and the absence of glucose and the presence of tetraose characterizes breakdown due to the saliva. By contrast, in the latter, the presence of glucose which constitutes 50 to 90 per cent of the glucide fraction shows the influence of bacterial amylases.

In the crop of the holoxenic chicken, two enantiomorphes of lactic acid are formed, in similar and quite important quantities (3 per cent) accompanied by a fall in pH from 6 to 4.

In the absence of a microflora, there are only small quantities of L lactic acid (0.06 per cent) of endogenous origin. The change in concentration which is observed during the course of digestion in the holoxenic animal does not occur in the axenic and there is no change in the pH (Fig. 1b).

The crop contains a substantial microbial population, in particular *Lactobacillus sp.* homofermenters (7×10^9 per g of D.M.), heterofermenters (10^9 per g of D.M.) and a facultative anaerobic *Streptococcus sp.* (6×10^4 per g of D.M.); we have also noted bifidobacteria (10^9 per g of D.M.) in some cases.

Two strains of bacteria, a *Lactobacillus sp.* and a *Streptococcus sp.* isolated from the crop of a holoxenic cock, both of which produced D and L lactic acid *in vitro*, were used to inoculate the axenic chickens. The results obtained *in vivo* showed apparent important differences, first from the results obtained *in vitro*, and secondly between the two strains which had been implanted in equal numbers in the digestive tract (Table I).

TABLE I. Implantation of Monoflora at Different Levels of the Digestive Tract

	Lactobacillus (log 10)	*Streptococcus* (log 10)
Crop	7.5	7.7
Duodenum	6.2	5.5
Ceca	9.4	9.4

In the chicken having a monoflora of *Streptococcus sp.* as in the axenic chick, the sucrose present in the diet is not degraded and there is no formation of glucose and of lactic acid.

In the chicken having a monoflora of *Lactobacillus sp.* as in the holoxenic, the pH falls but the appearance of glucose was mostly due to the degradation of the shortest chain carbohydrates (sucrose − maltose). Maltopentaose always remained. Furthermore, the *Lactobacillus sp.* only produces L lactate from these sugars whereas *in vitro*, as already said, it also produces the D isomer (Table II).

The duodenum. The amount of short-chain carbohydrates (Fig. 2a) present in the duodenum, like the pH (Fig. 2b), is greater in the absence of microflora and is represented mainly by glucose and by traces of maltotriose and maltopentaose (Fig. 2c). At this level of digestion, the absence of a qualitative difference between axenic and holoxenic chickens shows that the main digestive activity is due to enzymes of animal origin.

The ceca. As in the crop, the quantitative (Fig. 3a) and the qualitative (Fig. 3c) composition of the carbohydrates contained in the ceca differs between holoxenic and axenic birds. In the holoxenic, there is only a low quantity of carbohydrate (2 per cent); this practically does not change during the digestive

TABLE II. Influence of Monoflora in the Starch Breakdown in the Crop

	pH		Evolution of soluble carbohydrates			Lactic acids (mg/g D.M.)	
			quantitative (mg/g D.M.)		qualitative		
	3H	6H				L +	D −
			3H	6H			
Axenic	5.80	6.02	38.5	42.9	Sucrose++ Maltose+ Triose++ Tetraose Penta+	0.6	−
Streptococcus sp.	5.80	5.87	28.3	25.4	Sucrose++ Maltose+ Triose++ Penta	0.6	−
Lactobacillus sp.	5.66	5.00	29.6	9.0	Glucose+ Triose Penta+	31.0	−

process and is made up exculsively of glucose. In contrast, in the axenic animal there is a considerable accumulation of carbohydrate, which is maximal 7 hours after the start of the meal and contains practically all the products of starch breakdown. The pH is always higher in the absence of flora but we note similar evolution for both with a minimum between the 4th and 6th post-feeding hours (Fig. 3b). Implantation of bacteria in the axenic bird modifies the plan of carbohydrate breakdown. Furthermore, marked differences are observed between the ability of the *Lactobacillus sp.* and *Streptococcus sp.* to utilize these carbohydrates (Table III).

Finally, in the holoxenic chicks, nearly no starch is left at the duodenum level (2 per cent); on the contrary, in the axenic chicks, appreciable concentration (15 per cent) of starch is found in the feces.

Discussion and Conclusions

In the absence of microflora, the process of starch breakdown is modified throughout the digestive tract. Post-feeding change of pH in the crop, the duodenum and the ceca already account for differences in the glycolysis of the different metabolites.

It has been shown in the crop itself that the first stages of starch digestion

Duodenum

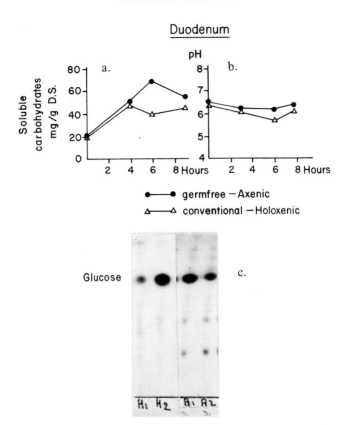

FIG. 2. Carbohydrate digestion in the duodenum during the 9 postfeeding hours. a) Quantitative evolution of the soluble carbohydrates. b) Evolution of the pH. c) Qualitative composition of the digesta, A. Axenic – H. Holoxenic.

depend on the bacteria, and that the lactic acid in the two isomers is produced by the bacteria and not by the crop epithelium.

The observations made on holoxenic subjects are in agreement with our results in the monoxenic (*Lactobacillus sp.*). The crop of these two types of animals is the first important site of proliferation of the *Lactobacillus sp.* which is responsible for the production of lactic acid and the fall of the pH. However, we have seen that this production is, in fact, different because the type of lactic acid formed by the monoxenic is not the same as in the holoxenic. It is possible that an association of two or more strains of bacteria are necessary to remove the differences between the holo and monoxenic birds. It seems that the function of bacterial associations can have a very important effect on the metabolism of the host.

We notice that results concerning lactic acid formation *in vitro* and *in vivo*

229

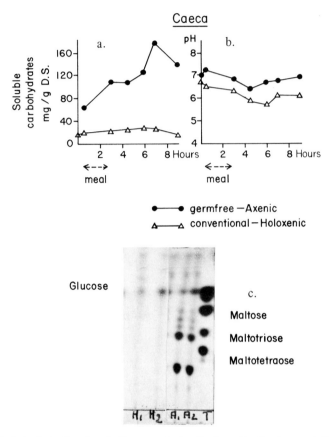

FIG. 3. Carbohydrate digestion in the caeca during the 9 postfeeding hours. a) Quantitative evolution of the soluble carbohydrates. b) Evolution of the pH. c) Qualitative composition of the digesta, A. Axenic — H. Holoxenic.

are not related either to *Lactobacillus sp.* or to *Streptococcus sp.* We have reconfirmed previous observations on the function and/or formation of bacterial enzymes which develop differently *in vitro* than in the digestive tract.

The work of Lepkovsky (5) showed that the amylase activity in the digestive tract of the chicken is greatly elevated in the ceca and cloaca in the absence of intestinal microflora; pancreatic amylase is usually destroyed by the bacterial proteases in the holoxenic bird. This could explain the presence of the products of starch breakdown and starch itself beyond the level of the duodenum in the axenic chicken. However, the animal does not seem to benefit from the presence of these pancreatic enzymes because it lacks essential bacteria.

These results lead us to reconsider the function of pancreatic amylase which is classically considered to be the only enzyme hydrolyzing starch in the

TABLE III. Influence of Monoflora on the Starch Breakdown in the Ceca

	pH		Evolution of short-chain carbohydrates		
			quantitative (mg/g D.M.)		qualitative
	3 H	6 H	3 H	6 H	
Axenic	6.8	6.7	110	130	Glucose+ Triose++ Penta++
Streptococcus sp. . .	6.8	6.8	91	91	Hexa+ Penta+++ Tetra+
Lactobacillus sp. . .	5.70	5.50	38	50	Hexa+ Penta+++

digestive tract of the chicken. It appears from the results of our investigation of digestion in the crop and the ceca that salivary amylase plays a part and that bacterial enzymes have a function which cannot be ignored. This could explain in part why the digestion of starch only declines by 26% (72% compared with 98%) after pancreatectomy of the chicken (6).

We do not know to what extent this unusual digestion of starch in the axenic chicken influences its energy metabolism but pertinent studies are in progress in our laboratory. We are also endeavoring to determine which bacterium or association of bacteria are able to hydrolyze starch *in vivo* in the digestive tract of the gnotoxenic chicken.

References

1. Lev, M., Briggs, C. A. E., *J. Appl. Bact. 19:* 224 (1956).
2. Bolton, W. *Proc. Nutr. Soc. 21:* 24 (1962).
3. Ivorec-Szylit, O., Mercier, Ch., Delesque, M., and Calet, C., 13e Congres d'Agriculture, Kiev (U.S.S.R.), p. 234, (1966).
4. Ivorec-Szylit, O., and Szylit, M., *Ann. Biol. Anim. Bioch. Biophys. 3:* 353 (1965).
5. Lepkovsky, S., Wagner, M., Furuta, F., Ozone, K., and Koike, T., *Poultry Sc. 43:* 722 (1964).
6. Ariyoski, S., Koike, T., Furuta, F., Ozone, K., Matsumura, Y., Dimick, M. K., Hunter, W. L., Wang, W., and Lepkovsky, S., *Poultry Sc. 43:* 232 (1964).

INTERRELATIONSHIPS BETWEEN THE GUT MICROFLORA AND THE RESPONSE OF CHICKS TO UNIDENTIFIED GROWTH FACTORS

Gordon F. Harrison and *Roy Fuller*
National Institute for Research in Dairying,
Shinfield, Reading, England

Introduction

The presence of unidentified growth factors in fish solubles has been accepted for many years. Harrison and Coates (1) showed that this growth promoting activity was dependent on the microflora. Conventional chicks did not grow as well as their germfree counterparts and the growth depression was overcome by a dietary supplement of fish solubles.

Harrison and Coates (2) showed that when a bacteria-free filtrate of an aqueous extract of excreta from conventional chicks was given to germfree chicks growth was not depressed, thus confirming that the presence of the bacterial moiety was necessary. However, the filtrate did increase the thickness of the wall of the small intestine.

Monoassociation of chicks with *Streptococcus faecalis* var. *liquefaciens* caused a small non-significant growth depression, but when given with the filtrate growth was markedly depressed. This growth depression was entirely overcome by fish solubles.

It seemed likely that the filtrates contained a viable agent since only a small quantity (0.2 ml) resulted in a thickening of the gut that persisted for 4 weeks, and an attempt was made to verify this.

Results

Germfree chicks were given the filtrate of conventional origin and 2 weeks later an extract of their excreta was administered to germfree birds. The gut weight was significantly increased by the extract (Table I). Thus the gut thickening effect of the original filtrate survived the passage and gave further evidence of the presence of a viable organism in the filtrate. Confirmation was provided by immunoelectrophoretic analysis of sera from chicks dosed with the filtrate and from those not dosed. In dosed birds the intensity of the IgG arc was more pronounced indicating an antibody response to the filtrate (Fig. 1). Thus it

TABLE 1. Effect on Gut Weight of Filtrates Prepared from Excreta of Germfree Chicks or of Chicks Dosed with the Conventionally Derived Filtrate

| | Treatment | |
Without filtrate	With germfree filtrate	With passaged filtrate
26.8	25.2	31.7

Mean gut weights (mg/g) at 4 weeks

is certain that the filtrate contains a viable agent probably of viral nature.

During experiments to evaluate the effect of fish solubles on the *Streptococcus sp.* and the filtrate, it was observed that the growth depressing effect lessened and eventually disappeared. The growth of dosed chicks improved and became as good as that of those not dosed (Fig. 2). At first it was assumed that either the streptococcus or the agent in the filtrate had become less potent. To see if this was so, new cultures of the organism were made from the original freeze-dried material, a new streptococcus was isolated and a filtrate was prepared from excreta obtained from another Institute. In no case could a

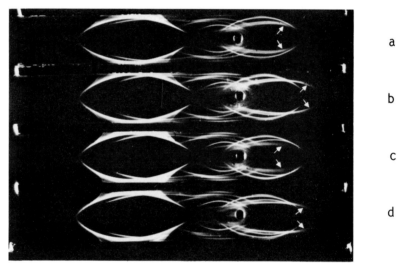

Chicks receiving a. basal diet
b. basal diet + filtrate
c. fish solubles diet
d. fish solubles diet + filtrate

FIG. 1. Immunoelectrophoretic analysis of chick sera.

234

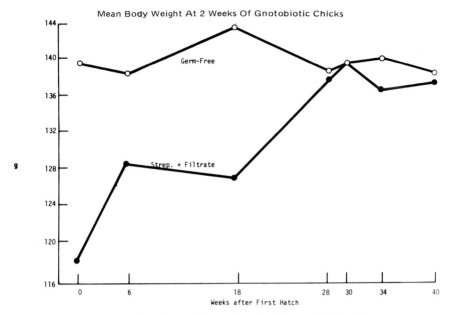

FIG. 2. **Elimination of growth depressing effect in gnotobiotic chickens.**

growth depression be obtained when chicks were dosed with the bacteria and the filtrate.

In these experiments chicks were obtained over a period of 40 weeks from one breeding flock maintained at this Institute. This suggested that the gradual lessening of the growth depressing effect was due to increasing resistance to the activity of the streptococcus-filtrate mixture. When chicks from another source were dosed with the streptococcus-filtrate mixture that was previously ineffectual, their growth was depressed. Thus chicks of different origin may differ in their susceptibility to the growth depressing agents.

Fig. 3 illustrates the difference between growth of chicks derived from the early stages of the hen's laying cycle and from the later stages. It is clear that when dosed with *S. faecalis* plus filtrate, birds derived from younger hens grew less well than those derived from older hens. Those that were not dosed grew equally well.

If this reflects an increasing resistance to a growth depression reversible by dietary fish solubles, a similar trend should be detectable in conventional birds. We therefore examined results of experiments with conventional chicks hatched every other week for 4 years and involving a different flock of hens each year. The mean weights of birds with and without dietary fish solubles, from the first 6 and last 6 hatches from all flocks is shown in Fig. 4. Although the difference between the two lots of chicks is not quite as large, there is no doubt that it is

235

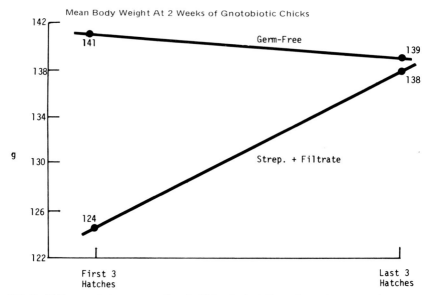

FIG. 3. **Difference between growth of chicks derived from the early stages of the hens laying cycle and from the later stages.**

similar to that obtained with chickens given the streptococcus-filtrate mixture.

If the difference in growth between the 'early' and 'late' chicks involves the filterable agent, a corresponding difference in the effect of the filtrate alone on the gut weight might be expected. The gut weights of 'early' and 'late' chicks from 2 flocks of hens are shown in Fig. 5, where it can be seen that the effect of the filtrate is equally great in both groups. Thus it is unlikely that the filterable agent responsible for gut thickening is involved in the diminishing growth depression.

Unpublished work by G. C. Cheeseman and R. Fuller in this Institute showed that the 7S content of chicken serum increases with the age of the chicken up to at least 77 weeks. This is shown in Fig. 6. If the level of 7S material is taken as an index of the immunological response of the chicken the striking increase in response persists during the laying period. Since antibody levels in egg yolk are directly proportional to those in the serum of the dam (3), the older the dam is, the higher will be the serum antibody level in the yolk and hence in the chick. This increase in antibody may thus account for the diminishing effect of the growth depressing agents on these birds. Such an explanation may also account for the widely reported variability in the growth response to dietary fish solubles that has frustrated attempts to elucidate the mode of action of fish solubles in improving the growth of chicks.

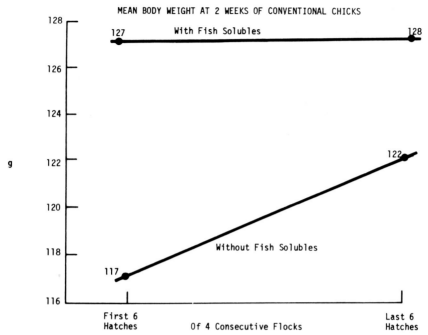

FIG. 4. Growth of conventional chicks over a 4 year period with a different flock of hens each year. The mean weights of birds with and without dietary fish solubles, from the first 6 and last 6 hatches from all flocks.

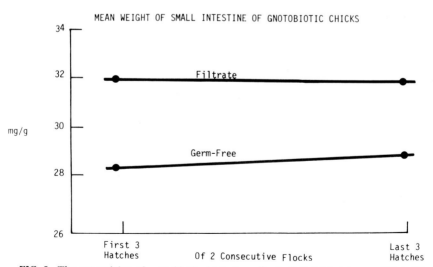

FIG. 5. The gut weights of gnotobiotic chicks from "early," first 3 hatches, and "late," last 3 hatches from 2 flocks of hens.

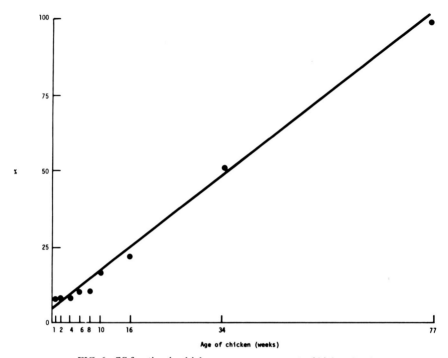

FIG. 6. 7S fraction in chicken serum as a percent of highest level.

Conclusions

Dietary fish solubles can overcome the growth depression caused by administering a streptococcus plus a filterable agent which probably contains a virus. The resistance of chicks to the growth depression depends, at least in part, on the age of the dam, which, as it increases, may confer increasing immunity on the progeny. This may explain the great variability in growth response to fish solubles.

References

1. Harrison, G. F., and Coates, M. E., *Proc. Nutr. Soc. 28:* 70A (1969).
2. Harrison, G. F., and Coates, M. E., *Br. J. Nutr. 28:* 213 (1972).
3. Brierley, J., and Hemmings, W. A., *J. Embryol. exp. Morph. 4:* 34 (1956).

THE INFLUENCE OF THE ANTIBIOTICS AUREOMYCIN AND MOENOMYCIN (FLAVOMYCIN) ON GERMFREE CHICKS UNDER STRESS CONDITIONS

G. Riedel
Vorstand: Prof. DDr. DDr. h.c. J. Bruggemann
Institut fur Tierphysiologie der Tierarztlichen
Fakultat Munchen, Germany

Introduction

Until now a positive effect of nutritive doses of antibiotics in the diet on growth was observed only in conventionally but not in germfree reared chicks (1-3). Therefore it was suggested that increased body weight gain registered in conventional chicks fed diets with nutritive levels of antibiotics is attributable to changes in the intestinal flora.

Our studies were based on the fact that compared to conventional control chicks, growth rate of germfree chicks is about 10 – 20% higher. In Figure 1 such results obtained in our department (4) are shown, which are in agreement with findings of others (1, 2). It was assumed that the retarded growth of the conventinoal chicks might be due to a stress exerted by the intestinal flora which can be reduced by nutritive doses of antibiotics. Provided this assumption holds, growth retardation of germfree chicks caused by an artificial stress should be also alleviated by nutritive levels of antibiotics (5).

Materials and Methods

Broiler chicks, (Nichols/Lohmann) were used for all experiments. The animals hatched and were raised in plastic isolators. A semi-synthetic diet and water was offered *ad libitum.* For sterility control once a week samples of feces, diet and water were obtained from the isolators. At the end of the experiments one animal per unit was checked for mycoplasmas and viruses.

To test the hypothesis previously mentioned, the following experimental design was applied: In all experiments the animals kept in each isolator were divided in four groups. The experimental groups used are characterized in Table I. Unlike groups 1 and 2 the experimental diets of groups 3 and 4 contained either 10 mg/kg Aureomycin (CTC) or 10 mg/kg Flavomycin (Moenomycin).

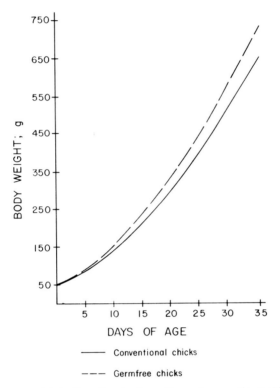

FIG. 1. Growth rate of germfree and conventional chicks.

As stressors either sterilized milk or *Salmonella pullorum* toxin were injected i.m. in groups 2 and 4.

Results and Conclusions

The injection of sterilized milk (Fig. 2) in the CTC-experiment resulted in a marked growth depression in group 2 compared to group 1. Between groups 3 and 4 there was no difference in weight gain. Injection of *S. pullorum* toxin (Fig.

TABLE I. Experimental Plan

group	antibiotics (10 mg/kg diet)	stress
1	−	−
2	−	+
3	+	−
4	+	+

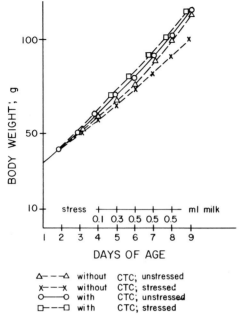

FIG. 2. Action of Aureomycin (CTC) on germfree chicks.

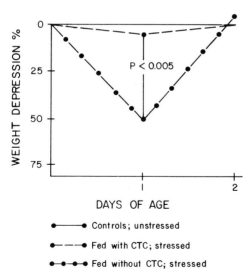

FIG. 3. Reduced weight gains of germfree chicks fed with or without aureomycin (CTC) after stress with *Salmonella pullorum* toxin.

3) also caused a decrease of weight gain in group 2, compared to group 1. In addition growth in group 4 was reduced slightly compared to group 3 in this experiment. However, the difference between groups 1 and 2 was significantly ($P\langle0.005$) larger than between groups 3 and 4.

Similar results were obtained (Fig. 4) when the diets contained 10 mg/kg Flavomycin (Moenomycin) (6). In this experiment sterilized milk was

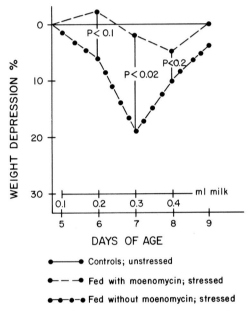

FIG. 4. Action of Moenomycin after stress on germfree chicks.

injected as stressor.

This finding was unexpected since only traces of Moenomycin are absorbed from the intestine. Maybe this small amount of Moenomycin absorbed is sufficient to cause the effect observed.

These findings indicate that nutritive levels of antibiotics stimulate growth in germfree chicks under certain conditions. Hence the effect of nutritive doses of antibiotics on growth of conventional chicks might be due not only to influences on the intestinal flora but also to changes in metabolism.

References

1.   Coates, M. E., Fuller, R., Harrison, G. F., Lev, M., Suffolk, S. F., *Brit. J. Nutr. 17:* 141 (1963).
2.   Forbes, M., Park, J. T., *J. Nutr. 67:* 69 (1959).
3.   Lev, M., Forbes, M., *Brit. J. Nutr. 13:* 78 (1959).

242

4. Merkenschlager, M., Merkenschlager, M., Losch, U., Riedel, G., *Tierarztl. Umschau 22:* 132 (1967).
5. Bruggemann, J., Merkenschlager, M., Schmidt, H., Riedel, G., Schole, J., *Z. Tierphysiol., Tierernahrg. u. Futtermittelkde. 25:* 321 (1969).
6. Riedel, G., Reiter, H., Losch, U., (In Preparation).

IMPROVED LACTATION IN GERMFREE MICE FOLLOWING CHANGES IN THE AMINO ACID AND FAT COMPONENTS OF A CHEMICALLY DEFINED DIET

Julian R. Pleasants, Bernard S. Wostmann and *Bandaru S. Reddy*
Lobund Laboratory, University of Notre Dame,
Notre Dame, Indiana 46556, U.S.A.

Introduction

The value of a chemically-defined (CD) water-soluble diet for germfree (GF) animals needs little elaboration. The combination of the germfree state with feeding of CD diet means that we can know for the first time exactly what an animal must be provided from outside itself in order to function normally. This provides a baseline from which to determine the influence of the resident microbial flora on nutritional requirements. Sterilization of water-soluble, low molecular weight diet by filtration preserves the chemical definition of the diet and at the same time provides the opportunity for elimination of antigens. Ultrafilters with a cutoff point of 5,000 or 10,000 molecular weight can be used to eliminate impurities likely to be antigenic. As had been hoped, the elimination of antigens in the diet of GF mice eliminates the residual gamma globulins detected by immunoelectrophoresis in the serum of GF mice fed natural or semi-synthetic diets (1-3). The combination of GF animals and CD diet thus provides an immunological baseline for determining the primary effects of externally derived antigens on the immune system.

Development at Lobund Laboratory of a CD diet adequate for reproducing colonies of GF rodents has progressed steadily (4-6), integrating results of our own experiments with new developments in the science of nutrition and in the understanding of the physiology of the GF animal. At the last international meeting in Louvain in 1969, we reported our results to date with a chemically defined diet consisting of a water solution of amino acids, glucose, B vitamins, and minerals, and an ethyl linoleate solution of vitamins A, D, E and K. A colony of GF CFW mice had reproduced into the 5th generation on this diet, indicating its qualitative adequacy, but the rate of reproduction was too low to provide animals for general experimental use. A colony of inbred GF C3H mice could not continue reproduction on this type of diet until we had made drastic quantitative changes, reported in Louvain, in the amino acid and mineral levels

245

of the diet. Since that time the GF C3H colony also reproduced into the 5th generation, but again with too low a reproductive efficiency to permit much experimental use of the animals. Only half of the litters were weaned, the number per litter weaned was 3, and the young averaged 5 g at 21 days against an expected weaning weight of 9 g for this strain fed natural-type diet. Further clues to nutritional deficiency were the matted fur of the young animals in the first weeks after weaning, and the symmetrical loss of fur by some adult animals, especially reproducing females. Some individual young mice also refused to consume the fat supplement, which was fed separately from the diet, and these mice had to be discarded. Observations on the feeding schedule of reproducing female mice led to the hypothesis that their primary deficiency was one of total diet intake, since they only slightly increased their level of intake during pregnancy and lactation in comparison with mice fed natural-type diets. Experiments were therefore set up to determine if diet intake was limited by very high concentrations of some nutrient(s) in the blood plasma after consumption of CD diet. Coincidentally, the changes of amino acids involved in these experiments were also accompanied by a change from defined fat to corn oil, dictated by a drastic cut in funding. This change also required an increase in total fat intake, since corn oil is only 50 to 60% linoleate. Thus the daily fat supplement was increased from 0.15 ml to 0.25 ml per mouse. When greatly

TABLE I. G/100 g Water-soluble Nutrients In Diet 487WS-15

Solution 1: To 156 ml glass-distilled water at 70°C add:

Leucine	1.44	Asparagine	0.84
Phenylalanine	0.60	Arginine HCl	0.66
Isoleucine	0.78	Threonine	0.60
Methionine	0.78	Lysine HCl	1.44
Tryptophan	0.30	Histidine HCl·H_2O	0.60
Valine	0.60		

Cool solution to room temperature and add:

Glycine	0.24	Ca fructose $(PO_4)_2$	4.7
Proline	1.20	$CaCl_2 \cdot 2H_2O$	0.6
Serine	1.08	$MgCl_2 \cdot 6H_2O$	1.5
Alanine	0.48	NaCl+KI*	0.07
Na Glutamate	2.76	Bmix 111E3	0.066
Ethyl Tyrosine HCl	0.60	Choline Cl	0.25
Ferrous gluconate	0.04	$K(CH_3COO)$	1.06
Salt mix 35	0.062	Final volume	167 ml

*NaCl containing 0.55 mg KI

Solution 2: Dissolve 76.65 g anhydrous α-D-glucose in glass-distilled water at 70°C, and make up to 167 ml.

Filter and store the 2 solutions separately in the isolator. Mix 1:1 daily for feeding.

improved reproduction followed these changes, it then became necessary to institute other experiments to demonstrate the relative roles played in this improvement by the amino acid change and by the lipid change, and also by a later trace element change. The results of these experiments form the basis of this progress report. The basal diet 487WS-15 and the 3 different lipid supplements are shown in Tables I and II.

Materials and Methods

The amino acids were L form, NRC grade, and were obtained either from General Biochemicals, Inc. or the Vivonex Corp. The B vitamins, vitamins D, E and K, ferrous gluconate and monocalcium fructose diphosphate were also obtained from GBI. Other minerals were Fisher Certified reagents or equivalent. Vitamin A palmitate was supplied by Hoffman-LaRoche. The purified lipids were made on special order by Nu Chek Prep, Elysian, Minn. In the experiment testing the effect of vanadium, this was added in the form of sodium orthovanadate (Na_3VO_4, K&K Laboratories) to provide 25 μg V per 100 g solids, as recommended by Schwarz and Milne (7). Plasma free amino acids were determined in a Technicon Automatic Amino Analyzer, Model TSM, as described by Reddy et al. (8).

TABLE II. Supplements To Diet 487WS-15

0.062 g salt mix 35 contains, in mg:			
Mn(acetate)$_2$·4H$_2$O	45	(NH$_4$)$_6$Mo$_7$O$_{24}$·4H$_2$O	0.3
ZnSO$_4$·H$_2$O	11	Na$_2$SeO$_3$	0.018
Cu(acetate)$_2$·H$_2$O	3	Co(acetate)$_2$·4H$_2$O	0.09
Cr(acetate)$_3$·H$_2$O	2	NaF	0.5

0.066 g Bmix 111E3 contains, in mg:			
Thiamin HCl	0.5	Riboflavin	0.75
Pyridoxine HCl	0.63	Niacin	3.75
Biotin	0.1	i-Inositol	25.0
Folic acid	0.15	Ca pantothenate	5.0
Vitamin B$_{12}$(pure)	0.06	p-aminobenzoic acid	30.0

Lipid supplement: each mouse received daily in a dish 0.25 ml (0.225 g) of one of the following:

	E3	E4	E5
Ethyl linoleate, g		0.11	
Trilinolein, g			0.11
Triolein, g		0.11	0.11
Corn oil, g	0.22		

Each mixture provided the following vitamins: 4.3 μg vitamin A palmitate (7.8 I.U.); 48 μg vitamin K$_1$; 4.4 mg DL-α-tocopheryl acetate, 2.2 mg DL-α-tocopherol, and 0.0192 μg vitamin D$_3$ (0.77 I.U.).

The mice were maintained in Trexler type plastic isolators and tested by routine procedures (9). Pairs were housed in stainless steel wire cages 5" x 6" (3). Females were given ash-free filter paper for nesting material before parturition. The diet solutions, water, and lipid supplements were filtered into the isolator through a Millipore GS filter (0.22 μ pore size). The filter holder was mounted in a Tygon pipe sealed to the top of the isolator and sprayed with peracetic acid before insertion of the autoclaved holder (3, 5). The water-soluble diet was offered in overhead brown bottles having holes 1/16" in diameter drilled in the plastic lid. Water was available in similar bottles. The lipid supplement was measured daily into a 1" diameter stainless steel planchette welded to a heavy disk of stainless steel.

Results

The levels of plasma free amino acids 30 minutes after a feeding of our previous diet 487WS-5 (24% total amino acids) were compared to levels reported (11) for conventional (CV) mice fed natural type diets, and to the levels in our GF C3H mice fed natural type diet L-485 (10). Isoleucine and leucine levels were 3 times control levels, an important difference for amino acids which are only slowly metabolized. When the level of total amino acids was reduced from 24% of solids to 14% of solids (diet 487WS-15), while maintaining the same relative proportion of amino acids, there was a drastic reduction, to nearly normal levels, of the plasma concentrations of threonine, lysine, leucine, and isoleucine, which had previously been 2.5 to 10 times the levels seen in the CV and GF controls. Thus the change in dietary amino acid levels from 24% to 14% appeared to bring about a normalization of plasma free amino acid levels.

Concomitant with the change in dietary amino acid levels, corn oil had replaced ethyl linoleate as the source of essential fatty acid. Following these 2 simultaneous changes, there was a dramatic improvement in the growth of suckling young. It could already be seen in the first several days of nursing, when growth and skin pigmentation were obviously superior to those of earlier litters. The first 6 litters weaned after the amino acid and lipid changes averaged 10 g at weaning, in contrast to 5 g in mice whose mothers were consuming 487WS-5 plus ethyl linoleate. Furthermore, the corn oil was accepted by all weanlings. There was no incidence of shaggy fur in the weeks following weaning. However, there was no reduction in the number of litters lost at birth. This was 8/14 lost on the new diet, similar to 35/71 litters lost on the previous diet.

In order to determine if the amino acid reduction or the change from ethyl linoleate to corn oil, or the increase in total lipid was responsible for improved lactation, the amino acid level was held constant, and the available females were divided into 2 groups, one continuing on 0.25 Ladek E3 with corn oil, the other receiving daily 0.25 ml of a mixture of equal parts ethyl linoleate and highly purified triolein, with the usual fat-soluble vitamins (Ladek E4, Table II). When this mixture proved unacceptable to some young at weaning, a comparison was made of the acceptability of purified trilinolein and ethyl linoleate. When the former proved much more acceptable, it was substituted for ethyl linoleate in Ladek E4, producing Ladek E5, which was fed thereafter.

TABLE III. Effects of Dietary Changes on Reproduction and Development.
Basal Diet 487WS-15 for All Groups.

	Lipid	E3	E4	E5	E5
	Vanadium	–	–	–	+
Litters born		15	12	24	7
Litters weaned		9	6	8	6
% litters weaned		60	50	33	86
Young born		47+	30+	71+	26
Young weaned		32	17	21	21
% young weaned		⟨68	⟨57	⟨30	81
No. weaned/litter weaned		3.6	2.8	2.6	3.5
Aver. wgt. at 21 days		8.8	9.6	7.8	8.1
Acceptability of lipid		Good	Poor	Good	Good
Incidence of shaggy fur		None	Freq.	Occas.	Occas.
Fur loss in adults		Occasional on all lipids			

Comparative results are shown in Table III. Normal weaning weights were obtained on all 3 types of lipid supplement, but the litters with 5 or more young were underweight at weaning. Fur was shaggy after weaning in groups on purified fat but not in groups fed corn oil. At this point in the experiment, Schwarz and Milne (7) reported the essentiality of vanadium for maximum growth of conventional rats fed a highly purified CD diet and maintained in plastic rather than stainless steel cages. Vanadium did not, however, prevent the shaggy fur also seen by Schwarz and Milne in their experiments. Although our mice are maintained in stainless steel cages, the amount of vanadium available to the mice from this source could be quite variable. One part of the group fed purified fat was therefore given a supplement of vanadium added to the water-soluble portion of the diet. Preliminary results with this new diet indicate that it dramatically increased the percentage of litters weaned, without eliminating the shaggy fur syndrome, or the loss of fur in some adult females.

Conclusions

Increased weight of the young at weaning was due to the decrease in total amino acid content from 24% to 14% of solids. Further improvement may be possible by adjusting the level of individual amino acids. The effect of corn oil in increasing the percentage of litters weaned can be duplicated by adding vanadium to the diet of mice fed defined lipid. Trilinolein is much more acceptable to weanling mice than ethyl linoleate and almost as acceptable as corn oil. Neither defined lipid prevented shaggy fur in the immediate post-weaning period. This symptom, and the occasional loss of fur by adults in all groups will first be investigated by addition of other trace elements, such as tin (12). It is concluded that reproduction at the level achieved on defined lipid plus vanadium can support extensive experimental use of the GF animal-defined diet system.

Acknowledgements

Supported by N.I.H. grant HD00855, by Biomedical Sciences Support Grant RR-07033-06 from the General Research Resources, Bureau of Health Professions and Manpower Training, N.I.H., and by the University of Notre Dame.

References

1. Wostmann, B. S., Pleasants, J. R., and Bealmear, Patricia, *Federation Proc. 30:* 1779 (1971).
2. Wostmann, B. S., Pleasants, J. R., Bealmear, Patricia, and Kincade, P. W., *Immunol. 19:* 443 (1970).
3. Wostmann, B. S., Pleasants, J. R., and Reddy, B. S., in "Husbandry of Laboratory Animals," (M. L. Conalty, ed.), Academic Press, London, p. 187, (1967).
4. Pleasants, J. R., Wostmann, B. S., and Zimmerman, D. R., *Lab. Anim. Care 14:* 37 (1964).
5. Pleasants, J. R., in "The Germfree Animal in Research," (M. E. Coates, ed.), Academic Press, London, p. 47, (1968).
6. Pleasants, J. R., Reddy, B. S., and Wostmann, B. S., *J. Nutr. 100:* 498 (1970).
7. Schwarz, K., and Milne, D. B., *Science 174:* 426 (1971).
8. Reddy, B. S., Pleasants, J. R., and Wostmann, B. S., *Proc. Soc. Exp. Biol. Med. 136:* 949 (1971).
9. Institute of Laboratory Animal Resources, National Research Council, *Gnotobiotes,* National Academy of Sciences, Washington, D.C. (1970).
10. Kellogg, T. F., and Wostmann, B. S., *Lab. Anim. Care 19:* 812 (1969).
11. Drewes, Patricia A., and McKee, R. W., *Nature 213:* 411 (1967).
12. Schwarz, K., and Milne, D. B., *Biochem. Biophys. Res. Comm. 40:* 22 (1970).

DIGESTIBILITY AND BALANCE STUDIES OF GNOTOBIOTIC PIGS

R. Kenworthy
Unilever Research Laboratory
Colworth House, Sharnbrook,
Bedford, United Kingdom

Introduction

Information is accumulating on the effects of the intestinal microflora on intestinal mucosal morphology and epithelial cell turnover (1-6), but there is a marked lack of information regarding the significance of these effects on gut function. It was decided therefore to examine the influence of *Escherichia coli* on digestibility of dietary nutrients in gnotobiotic pigs, during the time phase when morphological changes were known to occur (3).

Materials and Methods

The experiments have been carried out with germfree and infected gnotobiotic pigs on a liquid milk diet (3). They were maintained in metabolism crates inside plastic isolators and feces and urine collections were made daily. Analyses of excreta included estimations of protein, oil and nitrogen free extract (NFE).

Results

Fecal water and NFE output from germfree animals increased as they aged. Protein excretion remained reasonably constant, but oil output decreased towards the end of the observation periods.

Infection resulted in increased output of water and protein and, in some pigs, there was a disturbance in excretion of oil and NFE; this soon stabilized however (see Fig. 1).

Conclusions

The pattern of NFE excretion in the germfree pig indicates a progressive inability to utilize the carbohydrate fraction of the diet, i.e. lactose; a conclusion consistent with the observations of Bailey, Kitts and Wood (7) that there is

251

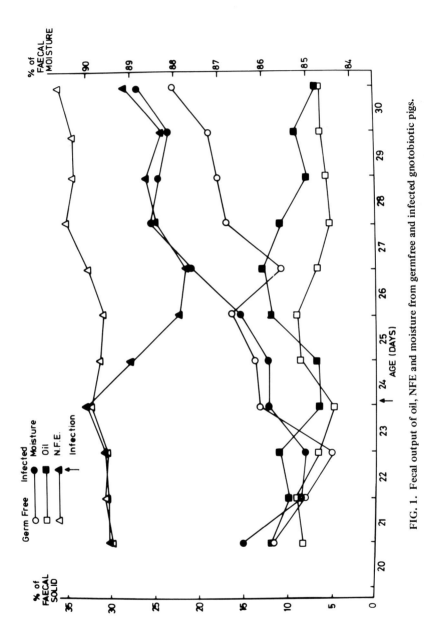

FIG. 1. Fecal output of oil, NFE and moisture from germfree and infected gnotobiotic pigs.

reduced lactase activity in the small intestine of piglets about 2 weeks after birth.

Although no attempt was made in these experiments to compare intestinal lactase activity in young germfree and conventional pigs, it is interesting that an apparent deficiency occurs in both these animals since observations on germfree rats (8) have shown distinctly higher dissaccharidase levels (including lactase) than in conventional controls. The salient factor here is probably the age of the animals under study, since the pigs were only a few weeks old and the observations of Reddy and Wostman (8) related to adult rats. It is possible that the germfree pigs did not have time to adapt from an established pattern.

The increased excretion of protein after infection is likely to be due primarily to the inflammatory response and epithelial cell desquamation, and the disturbances in oil and NFE outputs probably reflect an effect of microbial metabolism on the intestinal epithelial cells.

References

1. Abrams, G. D., Bauer, H., and Sprinz, H., *Lab. Invest. 12:* 355 (1963).
2. Gordon, H. A., and Bruckner-Kardoss, E., *Am. J. Physiol. 201:* 175 (1961).
3. Kenworthy, R., *J. Comp. Path. 80:* 53 (1970).
4. Kenworthy, R., *J. Clin. Path. 24:* suppl. (Roy. Coll. Path.), *5:* 138 (1971).
5. Kenworthy, R., and Allen, W. D., *J. Comp. Path. 76:* 291 (1966).
6. Sprinz, H., Kundel, D. W., Dammin, G. J., Horowitz, R. E., Schneider, H., and Formal, S. E., *Amer. J. Path. 39:* 681 (1961).
7. Bailey, C. B., Kitts, W. D., and Wood, A. J., *Canad. J. Agric. Sci. 36:* 51 (1956).
8. Reddy, B. S., and Wostmann, B. S., *Archs. Biochem. Biophys. 113:* 609 (1966).

THE SIGNIFICANCE OF THE INTESTINAL MICROFLORA ON THE GROWTH OF JAPANESE QUAIL FED DIETS CONTAINING NAVY BEANS

D. J. Jayne-Williams and *D. Hewitt*
National Institute for Research in Dairying
University of Reading, England

Introduction

It is well recognized, for example see Liener (1), that the inclusion of raw legumes in animal diets frequently gives rise to poor growth and sometimes death. Kakade & Evans (2) reported that raw navy beans (*Phaseolus vulgaris*) caused severe growth depression and death of rats within 28 days; rats given a similar diet containing mildly autoclaved beans gained weight. Similar effects with chicks of the domestic fowl were observed by Hewitt & Coates (3) who also noted that the growth of germfree chicks fed diet containing raw beans was only slightly depressed. Jayne-Williams & Hewitt (4) studied the growth depressing and lethal effects of raw navy bean diets on Japanese quail. Some of the results and fresh data are outlined in the following contribution.

Methods

The diets used contained either raw (R) or autoclaved (A) navy bean meal. Meal A was autoclaved at 121°C for a nominal 5 minutes. The meal was mixed with an equal weight of basal diet containing casein, maize starch, vitamins, salts, maize oil and small amounts of methionine, arginine and glycine. A navy bean-free rearing diet (S) was also used. For gnotobiotic work the diets were sterilized by irradiation with 5 Mrads from a ^{60}Co source.

Results

All of 16 conventional (CV) day old quail provided with diet R died within 8 days, whereas all of the same number of birds given diet A survived (mean body weight at 8 days, 16.2 $\pm$ 0.7g). There were no deaths among 23 germfree (GF) day-old birds given diet R, but the mean body weight at 8 days was lower (14.1 $\pm$ 0.4g) than that of similar birds given diet A (17.0 $\pm$ 0.4g). CV and GF quail which had been reared for 14 days on diets before being given the experimental diets showed similar trends except that mortality on diet R was reduced. Irrespective of the microbiological state of the environment, all birds given diet R showed significant enlargement of the pancreas. It is clear from the foregoing that raw navy beans only exhibit a lethal effect in the presence of the intestinal microflora. Experiments were therefore undertaken to determine which, if any, particular component of the intestinal microflora was responsible for death. Various techniques, including the use of an anaerobic isolator similar to that described by Aranki (5), were used to isolate pure cultures of bacteria from the intestinal contents of sickly CV quail on diet R. The total of 149 isolates caused death when administered to GF birds on diet R. On the basis of the results of a number of tests (including sensitivity or resistance to penicillin and neomycin) the collection was subdivided into 6 groups, each of which was then separately tested by administering to GF birds on diet R.

Only one group, comprising 6 Gram negative rods and 1 Gram positive coccus, caused high mortality. The coccus tested on its own proved innocuous, whereas one representative of the 6 rods was lethal. All these 6 organisms were shown to be coliforms. Removal of all coliforms from the collection of 149 isolates left a residue which, though causing growth depression, was non-lethal.

The possibility that a heat-labile constituent(s) of the raw beans was altering the quantitative or qualitative aspects of the intestinal microflora was then investigated.

Counts of coliform bacteria (Difco MacConkey's agar: 2 d at 37°C) were made on the pooled contents of 6 segments of the gastrointestinal (g.i.) tracts of 4 CV quail fed either diet R, diet A, or diet S. The segments examined were: the crop; the first, third, fifth and last sevenths of the small intestine; and the ceca. In addition, lactobacilli (medium of Rogosa, Mitchell & Wiseman (6): 2 days anaerobically at 37°C), streptococci (medium of Barnes (7): 1 day aerobically at 37°C) and total anaerobes (ETSA medium of Aranki (5): 2 days at 37°C) were enumerated.

There was close agreement between the coliform counts obtained on the first 4 sites with birds given diets R and S; the counts with birds given diet A were consistently lower, however, but in no instance by more than 1.6 log cycles. The cecal counts were highest with diet R (4.3×10^9/g) and lowest with A (1.3×10^7/g); diet S was intermediate (1.1×10^8/g). Pseudomonads were also cultivated on the MacConkey's agar and occurred in all sites of birds fed diets R and A in the range $10^5 - 10^6$/g; they were only present in the crop samples of birds given diet S and at a count of 10^5/g. Counts of lactobacilli in the crop and small intestine of birds fed diet R were consistently lower (between 1 and 2 log cycles) than those in birds fed the other diets; but cecal counts were similar. Total counts and those of streptococci were generally similar (within 1 log cycle) in all birds.

It thus appeared that, apart from the occasional differences recorded above − the importance of which it is difficult to assess − the feeding of diets containing raw beans had no influence on the numbers of certain broad groups including coliforms, present in different segments of the quail g.i. tract. Examination by the IMViC and other tests recommended in Report (8) of representative colonies of coliforms picked from count plates showed the following distribution of types: diet R − 22 strains of *Escherichia coli* I; diet A − 12 strains of *E. coli* I, 1 of *Klebsiella aerogenes*; diet S − 5 of *E. coli* I, 1 of *E. coli* III, 3 of *K. aerogenes.* Thus no gross alteration in the qualitative picture resulted from feeding the raw beans.

Confirmation of the observations that raw beans had no marked influence on the quantitative and qualitative aspects of the coliform population of the quail intestine was obtained with gnotobiotic birds. A group of 3 week-old GF quail in the same isolator was subdivided into 3 cages and provided with diets R, A and S, respectively. After a period of 5 days on these diets, all birds were given drinking water containing a culture of *E. coli,* previously shown to cause the death of young gnotobiotic quail on diet R. A week later 4 birds from each group were killed by ether and the contents of each of 4 segments of the g.i. tract pooled. Coliform counts were determined on well mixed samples on MacConkey's and nutrient agar. The counts for each segment (crop, upper and lower small intestine and ceca) proved to be similar (all within 0.8 log cycles and two-thirds within 0.2 log cycles) irrespective of the diet.

Further gnotobiotic experiments were then conducted to determine whether the coliforms derived from birds fed the raw bean diet were peculiar to such birds or indeed peculiar to quail fed any of the diets. Pure cultures of coliforms were, therefore, isolated from quail on different diets, and from the feces of healthy chickens (2 isolates), goat, mouse, guinea pig, calf and rabbit (1 isolate from each). These cultures were introduced separately into isolators containing two groups of 10-13 GF quail chicks on diets R and A, respectively. In all instances high mortalities (mostly 100%) were recorded for quail fed diet R and low or no mortalities for birds fed diet A.

Body temperatures, determined *per anum* with an electronic thermometer, showed that CV quail on the raw bean diet exhibited hypothermia when compared with birds on diets A and S. Fig. 1 shows the body temperatures and mean weights of quail that had been reared for 21 days on diet S before being switched to diets R or A. When a group of the birds surviving on diet R for 6 days was switched to diet A no further deaths occurred, and body temperatures and growth rates soon returned to normal. Body temperatures of GF quail fed the two diets remained similar over a test period of 14 days.

Conclusions

It is clear that the death of CV quail fed diet containing raw navy beans depends on the combined effects of heat-labile principles in the beans and the

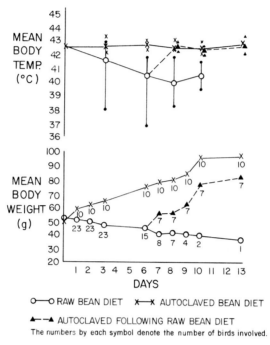

O—O RAW BEAN DIET   x—x AUTOCLAVED BEAN DIET

▲--▲ AUTOCLAVED FOLLOWING RAW BEAN DIET

The numbers by each symbol denote the number of birds involved.

FIG. 1. Effect of diet on body weight and temperature.

coliform components of the intestinal microflora. Furthermore, no indications were obtained of the raw bean diet having elected abnormal numbers or types of coliform bacteria, or of the lethal strains being peculiar to the quail g.i. tract. Hypothermia has been observed in mice injected with the lipopolysaccharide endotoxins of Gram negative bacteria (9, 10) and it seems likely that the reduced body temperature observed in quail fed raw bean diet is a manifestation of coliform endotoxemia. In addition to other heat-labile toxic factors (such as trypsin inhibitors), navy beans and other legumes are known to contain phytohemagglutinins, PHA (1). It has been shown (11) that the injection of *P. vulgaris* PHA into mice leads to depression of the phagocytic activity of the reticuloendothelial system (RES). Were ingested PHA to act in a similar way, the animal would be unable to contain intestinal bacteria which, as Fuller & Jayne-Williams (12, 13) have shown with young chicks, are able to translocate from the lumen of the gut into the lymph, blood, liver, etc. Endotoxemia and death could therefore rapidly ensue. Work is at present in progress to assess the effects of raw bean diets on the ability of the quail RES to clear injected carbon and bacterial cells, and on the lethal effects of incorporating purified PHA (concanavalin A from jackbeans) into quail diets. The results are to be published elsewhere.

Acknowledgements

The authors are indebted to Mrs. D. J. Bathe, Miss M. A. Cook, Mrs. E. Nechutna, Miss S. Lewington and Messrs. C. D. Burgess, J. P. Fordham, and D. A. F. Miles for invaluable assistance.

References

1. Liener, I. E., *Toxic Constituents of Plant Foodstuffs,* Academic Press, New York, (1969).
2. Kakade, M. L., and Evans, R. J., *Br. J. Nutr. 19:* 269 (1965).
3. Hewitt, D., and Coates, M. E., *Proc. Nutr. Soc. 28:* 47A (1969).
4. Jayne-Williams, D. J., and Hewitt, D., *J. Appl. Bact. 35:* 331 (1972).
5. Aranki, A., Syed, S. A., Kenney, E. B., and Freter, R., *Appl. Microbiol. 17:* 568 (1969).
6. Rogosa, M., Mitchell, J. A., and Wiseman, R. F., *J. Bact. 62:* 132 (1951).
7. Barnes, E. M., *J. Appl. Bact. 19:* 193 (1956).
8. Report, *J. Appl. Bact. 19:* 108 (1956).
9. Zahl, P. H., and Hutner, S. H., *Proc. Soc. Exp. Biol. Med. 56:* 156 (1944).
10. Anderson, W. H., and Broderson, R., *Proc. Soc. Exp. Biol. Med. 70:* 322 (1949).
11. Lozzio, B. B., Machado, E., and Lozzio, M. L., *J. Reticuloendo. Soc. 6:* 466 (1969).
12. Fuller, R., and Jayne-Williams, D. J., *Br. Poult. Sci. 9:* 159 (1968).
13. Fuller, R., and Jayne-Williams, D. J., *Res. Vet. Sci. 11:* 368 (1970).

259

CAUSES AND POSSIBLE CONSEQUENCES OF CECAL ENLARGEMENT IN GERMFREE RATS

Bernard S. Wostmann, Bandaru S. Reddy and *Edith Bruckner-Kardoss*
Lobund Laboratory, Department of Microbiology, University of Notre Dame
Notre Dame, Indiana 46556

and

Helmut A. Gordon and *Bhagwan Singh*
Department of Pharmacology, College of Medicine, University of Kentucky
Lexington, Kentucky 40506, U.S.A.

Introduction

Germfree rodents accumulate high molecular weight mucopolysaccharide material in their enlarged cecum (1). High speed centrifugation of cecal contents yields a supernatant containing 5 to 10 mg of such material per ml. Upon chromatography of the supernatant via Bio-Rex 70 (weak cationic resin, hydrogen form (2)) much of the polysaccharide material appears in the first eluate, indicating its strong negative charge. In conventional cecal contents this material is essentially absent (1).

Further purification via Sephadex G 200 gel filtration reveals several molecular weight fractions ranging from approx. 200,000 to 50,000. Preliminary analytical data of the highest molecular weight fraction indicate a protein content less than 5%, and the presence of hexosamine, hexuronic acid and sialic acid in molar ratios of approximately 5:3:1. They suggest that in the absence of microbial enzymes material derived both from intestinal mucosa (acidic mucopolysaccharides containing sulfated equimolar hexosamine-hexuronic acid complexes), and mucuous secretions (hexosamine-sialic acid complexes) accumulate in the cecum (3).

Hexosamine was determined after hydrolysis of samples in 2 N HCl at 100°C for 3 hours and purification via Dowex-50 W columns as described by Boas (4). Eluates were neutralized and hexosamine content determined spectrophotometrically using the Boas modification of the Elson and Morgan method (5). Hexuronic acid was determined after treatment of the sample with concentrated sulfuric acid, using the color reaction with carbazol as described by Dische (6). Sialic acid was determined after hydrolysis in 0.05 N sulfuric acid at

261

80°C for 1 hour. The hydrolyzates were used for the thiobarbituric acid assay of sialic acids according to Warren (7).

Upon continuous antibiotic treatment of conventional mice (300 ppm Penicillin G with drinking water) a similar carbohydrate material starts to accumulate in the cecum. In this model a direct relationship was found between the influx of water into the enlarging cecum (as depicted by dry matter content), and the appearance of high molecular weight, hexosamine and hexuronic acid containing materials during the establishment of a transient

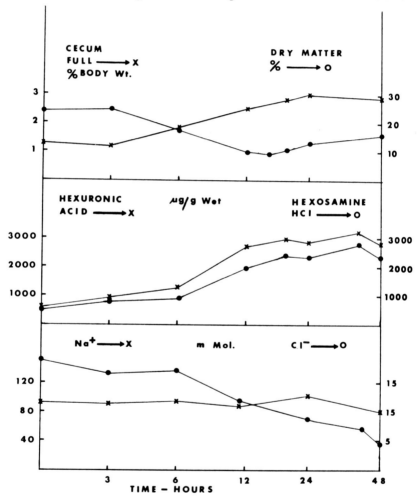

FIG. 1. Change in cecal size, cecal dry matter, Na⁺ and Cl⁻ concentration with the appearance of hexuronic-hexosamine containing material in the cecum of conventional mice fed 300 ppm Penicillin with the drinking water.

"germfree" state in the cecum between 15 and 48 hours after the start of the experiment. During this time Cl⁻ concentration in the cecal supernatant dropped to approximately 25% of its original value, while Na^+ concentrations remained at the level found in the untreated conventional (and similarly in the germfree) mouse cecum (Fig. 1). In studies with germfree rats the high molecular weight, negatively charged material was found capable of attracting water from the blood into the cecal fluid, while apparently inhibiting adequate functioning of the Na^+ transport dependent water outflow because of the resulting inadequate supply of absorbable negatively charged ions (1). Under germfree steady state conditions chloride ion concentration in the cecum may reach almost nonexisting levels, while only $4 - 7$ mEq/l HCO_3^- are maintained via diffusion of CO_2. Similar data have been reported by Asano (8, 9). In addition, our observations suggest a loss of intestinal muscle tone resulting from the elimination of direct or indirect flora effects (10). This last factor presumably is a major cause for the permanent cecal enlargement found in non-germfree rodents continuously treated with combinations of oral antibiotics which allow reestablishment of a modified intestinal microflora after an initial "germfree" period (11).

The cecum of the germfree rodent thus reaches a size determined by the accumulation of water-attracting macromolecules, the ensuing limitation set upon water efflux, and the reduced muscular tonus. The cecal enlargement appears to have a profound influence on function and metabolism (Table I). On the one hand our recent data, and those reported by Combe at this conference (12) again indicate that food consumption and growth of the germfree rat are similar to that of its conventional counterpart. On the other hand oxygen uptake, cardiac output and blood volume are consistently reduced in the intact germfree rat (13, 14). When, however, the enlarged cecum is removed surgically, leaving a passage between small and large intestine intact (15), then cardiac output and O_2 uptake are restored to normal, respectively near normal range (16). This last observation clearly links the phenomenon of cecal enlargement to various metabolic deviations found in the germfree rat.

A number of liver functions appear to be affected in a way consistent with the lower metabolic rate in the germfree state (Table I). Arterial blood flow was found to be approximately 60% of normal, and thiamine levels 2/3 of conventional values (17), suggesting a reduced or incomplete catabolism particularly of carbohydrates for the production of chemical energy. Reduction in activity of both glucose-6-phosphate dehydrogenase (60%) and 6-phosphogluconate dehydrogenase (80%) were found, suggesting de-emphasis of the hexosemonophosphate shunt and reduced availability of NADPH via this mechanism. No significant compensatory activation of malic enzyme (NADP-specific malate dehydrogenase) is indicated by the data. The lower level of succinic acid dehydrogenase activity (68%) suggests reduced energy yielding catabolism via the tricarboxylic acid (TCA) cycle, and a link to a possible

TABLE I. Metabolic Data in Adult Male Germfree and Conventional Wistar Rats[1]
(Means ± SE)

	GF	Conv	GF/Conv
Cardiac output[2] (ml/min/kg)	137 ± 7	203 ± 11	(.80)
O_2 consumption[2] (ml/min/kg)	11.5 ± 0.4	15.2 ± 0.4	(.76)
Liver			
Regional arterial blood flow[3] (ml/min/g)	0.27 ± 0.04	0.53 ± 0.04	(.51)
Thiamine[3] (μg/g)	6.8 ± 0.1	9.1 ± 0.3	(.75)
Glucose 6-P dehydrogenase[4] (units/g protein)	17.8 ± 0.7	29.6 ± 2.6	(.60)
6-P gluconate dehydrogenase[4] (units/g protein)	36.4 ± 1.4	45.3 ± 2.7	(.80)
Succinic dehydrogenase[4] (units/mg prot.)	179 ± 2	264 ± 10	(.68)
Malic enzyme[4] (units/g prot.)	19.4 ± 1.1	17.0 ± 1.7	(1.14)
Cytochrome oxidase[4] (units/mg prot.)	758 ± 37	628 ± 35	(1.21)
ATP-citrate lyase[4] (units/g prot.)	12.1 ± 1.0	7.2 ± 0.5	(1.68)
FA-synthetase complex[4] (units/g prot.)	21.4 ± 1.0	14.4 ± 1.7	(1.49)

[1]Age: 3-4 months. 6 or more animals per observation.
[2]Wostmann et al. (16)
[3]Wostmann et al. (17)
[4]Reddy et al. (19)

thyroid hypofunction (18) implied by the reduced O_2 intake. On the other hand both the citrate cleaving enzyme and the fatty acid synthetase complex demonstrated increased activity (168% resp. 149%), while mitochondrial cytochrome oxydase activity was increased to 121%. A detailed report on metabolic enzymes in the germfree rat liver is in preparation (19).

Glucose 6-phosphate dehydrogenase and 6-phosphogluconate dehydrogenase activities in liver and kidneys were assayed by the method of Glock and McLean (20), and NADP-specific malate dehydrogenase activity was assayed by the method of Ochoa (21). ATP-citrate lyase and fatty acid synthetase activities in liver were measured by the procedures based on the method of Srere (22) and Smith *et al.* (23) respectively. Succinic dehydrogenase and cytochrome oxidase activities in liver were determined by methods described by Potter (24) using a differential respirometer.

The presently available data (Table I) seem to agree with the supposition that in the germfree rat liver, reduced activity of the TCA cycle leads to an increased transfer of accumulating citrate from the mitochondrion to the cytoplasm. Here the enzyme systems involved in formation of acetyl-CoA, and its conversion to fatty acids appear to be activated, presumably by the increase in citrate concentration (25). However this system may lack NADPH necessary for chain elongation, since the hexosemonophosphate shunt evidently operates at low level, and malate production via the TCA cycle must be low. This would leave only mitochondrion derived isocitrate as a potential reductant for cytoplasmic NADP. As a result the germfree rat forms less rather than more body fat than its conventional counterpart (13). Citrate apparently escapes via the circulation and into the urine of the germfree rat, where it was found in five fold excess by Gustafsson (26).

At this point the question arises whether the above is the cause of, or the result from, the reduced oxygen demand. To obtain further information we measured oxygen uptake by liver slices with a Clark-type oxygen electrode, and found no difference between germfree and conventional rodents (Table II).

This observation seems to suggest an "external" limitation rather than a primary reduction in potential requirement of a strongly metabolically active tissue like the liver. Desplaces *et al.* (29), who were the first to draw attention to the reduced oxygen use of the germfree rat, also reported a decreased uptake of $131I^-$ by the germfree rat thyroid. The reduced activity of the succinic acid dehydrogenase (Table I) could conceivably point in the same direction since

TABLE II. O_2 Uptake by Rat Liver Slices[1] (Means $\pm$ SE)

	mμmol/min/g wet tissue
Germfree (6)	728 ± 41
Conventional (6)	705 ± 40
Conventional	480^2

[1]Approx. 150 mg, in 3 ml Krebs-Henseleit solution at 30°C. Rat: Fisher C344 (male). Diet: L-462 (27).
[2]Estabrook *et al.* (28)

265

TABLE III. Thyroid Function Tests in Germfree and Conventional Male Rats
(Means ± SE)

Strain (age) Location Diet	T-3 Units[1]		T-4 I/100 ml[2]		
	GF	Conv	GF		Conv
Fischer C344 U.K.[3] L 462[6]	53.4 ± 1.5 *s*[8]	66.1 ± 2.0	3.3 ± 0.2	*s*	4.6 ± 0.2
(3-4 m)	(13)	(8)	(14)		(9)
Wistar, N.D.[4] L 474E$_{29}$[7]	42.8 ± 2.3 *s*	50.7 ± 1.8	4.4 ± 0.2	*ns*	4.2 ± 0.1
Lobund (3.4 m)	(12)	(11)	(9)		(7)
Fischer C344 U.K.[5] L462	55.7 ± 1.2 *s?*	60.2 ± 1.8	2.7 ± 0.2	*ns*	2.6 ± 0.2
(5 m)	(10)	(6)	(10)		(13)

[1]Thyroxine-binding protein; percentage ^{125} thyroxine retained in test after exposure to 200 μl serum. Miles Laboratories, Elkhart, Ind. U.S.A.
[2]·Bound and free thyroxine iodine. Miles Laboratories, Elkhart, Ind. U.S.A.
[3]Univ. of Kentucky Sept. 1971
[4]Univ. of Notre Dame Dec. 1971
[5]Univ. of Kentucky March 1972
[6]Practical type diet, 24% protein (27)
[7]Semi-synthetic diet. Basis: rice, starch + 24% protein (30)
[8]*s* means P<0.05; *s?* P = 0.06; *ns* = non significant

Rivlin (18) has pointed out that hypothyroidism may lead to reduced activity of flavo protein dependent dehydrogenases. However, our recent studies of thyroid function by means of commercially available tests (Table III), combined with morphological (Table IV) and histological data thus far have failed to reveal a clear cut functional deficit in the germfree rat. Levenson (13) reported finding no appreciable difference between serum PBI and serum thyroxine iodine concentrations of germfree and conventional rats. At best the present data indicate some lag in development of the endocrine system of the germfree rodent. Nomura (31) has obtained data on testosterone production in gnotobiotic mice which seem to point in the same direction. Such a phenomenon could, on the other hand, also be construed as a **result** of the generally lower metabolic rate of the germfree rodent.

As indicated earlier, fractionation procedures for the cecal supernatant call for chromatographic separation via the hydrogen form of Bio-Rex 70, a weak cationic exchange resin. Late in the elution with $0.01 - 0.25$ N NaOH as described by Gordon and Kokas (2), dark Fe containing pigments appear. On furthur chromatography via AG 1-X$_4$ (quarternary ammonium resin) these yield a well defined pigment fraction designated by these authors as α-pigment. This substance has been held responsible for the refractoriness of various tissues of the germfree rodent to endogenous or exogenous epinephrine. This is suggested by studies that demonstrate: a) stimulatory effect of germfree cecal supernatant

TABLE IV. Endocrine Morphology of Germfree and Conventional Male Rat[1]

Strain (age)	Location	Diet	Status	Body wt.	Adrenal	Thyroid	Pituitary	Testes
				g	mg%	mg%	mg%	mg%
Fischer C344 (1½ m)	U.K.	L 462	GF	100	18.3	5.9	—	1157
			Conv	96	20.9[s]	7.1[s]	—	1355[s]
Wistar, Lobund (3-4 m)	N.D.	L 474E29	GF	300	13.6	5.4	2.4	780
			Conv	329	12.7	6.5[s]	2.9[s]	800
Fischer C344 (5 m)	U.K.	L 462	GF	278	13.4	5.4	3.0	978
			Conv	314	12.4	4.8	2.8	946

Explanation of symbols: See Table III. Only significant differences indicated.

[1] 10 or more experimental animals per experimental group.

on the rhythmic villus contraction of dogs (2); b) epinephrine-inhibitory effect imparted to mesenteric microvessels of conventional rats on topical application of germfree cecal supernatant (32); and c) observations which indicate that the microvessels of the mesocecum of germfree rats are refractory to epinephrine (33, 34). α-pigment was further purified by gel filtration on Sephadex G 50. Results indicate (Fig. 2) that the pigment obtained from germfree rat cecal content consists almost exclusively of a peptide-like material with molecular weight approximately 4800. When these materials were tested on the dog villus preparation (2), where enhancement of villus contraction indicates an epinephrine inhibitory effect, we found that almost all activity residing in the terminal eluate of the cationic resin can be recovered as α-pigment. A comparable pigment fraction of approximately 10% of the amount in the germfree cecum was found in conventional rat cecal content. However, less than half of this material has a molecular weight of 4800, the balance consists of several apparently inactive fractions with molecular weight between 4000 and 1800. Conventional rats treated via the drinking water with a mixture of bacitracin, streptomycin, and mycostatin (35), showed a substantial amount of the 4800 molecular weight, pharmacologically active material although other distinct fractions with molecular weight between 3000 to 10,000 were obviously present (Fig. 2).

Gordon and Kokas (2) have pointed to the analogy between the action of α-pigment and the previously established epinephrine antagonistic action of ferritin. Since ferritin is desquamated with the intestinal mucosa and thus enters the lumen of the gut with its proteases, we have digested ferritin with a mixture of trypsin and chymotrypsin. Reddy (30) had shown that especially in the

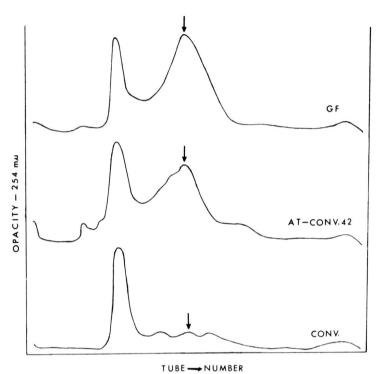

FIG. 2. Sephadex G 50 purification of α-pigment preparations from germfree (GF), 42 days antibiotic treated (AT-Conv. 42) and Conventional (CONV) rats. Indicator at left: cytochrome C; indicator at right: bromophenolblue. Arrow indicates α-pigment.

germfree cecum, the concentration of these enzymes is approximately 4 times as high as under conventional conditions. Upon Sephadex G 50 filtration of the resulting material there appeared, besides unchanged ferritin, a number of distinct low molecular weight entities ranging from 3,000 and 7,000. The activities of these fractions are presently under investigation. Thus far one fraction, with a molecular weight slightly lower than α-pigment (approximately 4,000) was found to have an activity similar to that of α-pigment.

Germfree rodents show reduced intestinal propulsion, especially in the cecum (36). The prolonged residence time in the enlarged germfree cecum with its relatively high levels of proteases would not only result in an ideal milieu for proteolytic digestion, but would allow at least partial absorption of molecular weight entities of 4800 or thereabouts. At present the physiological activity of α-pigment is studied in relation to the earlier established epinephrine insensitivity of the precapillaries of the germfree rat and its potential effect on the circulatory system, and to possibly related functional and/or metabolic

268

characteristics of the germfree rat.

Summary

In the absence of degrading enzymes of microbial origin germfree rodents accumulate high molecular weight, negatively charged mucopolysaccharide material in the cecum causing colloid osmotic water attraction coupled to a paucity of diffusible negative ions necessary for solute coupled water transport. The resulting cecal enlargement leads in germfree rats to an approximately 25% reduction in metabolic rate. These rats demonstrate extensive shifts in function and intermediary metabolism, the latter leading to a loss of high energy metabolites such as citrate in the urine. Other data suggest some delay in maturation of the endocrine system. The enlarged cecum harbors higher than normal concentrations of proteolytic enzymes. This leads to enhanced formation and to accumulation of pharmacologically active materials such as α-pigment, which under conventional conditions would be subject to further microbial degradation. α-pigment is a polypeptide with molecular weight of approximately 4800 and 0.2% Fe, which demonstrates strong catecholamine inhibitory properties and is considered a possible breakdown product of ferritin. Present studies seek to relate the occurrence of α-pigment to functional and metabolic deviations found in the germfree rat.

Acknowledgements

The authors gratefully acknowledge the technical assistance of Mr. Barrett F. Schwartz, and Mr. Roger W. Valentine, students at the University of Kentucky. This research was supported by U.S.P.H.S. Grants HD-00855 and AM-14621.

References

1. Gordon, H. A., and Wostmann, B. S., in "Germfree Research: Biological Effect of Gnotobiotic Environments," (J. B. Heneghan, ed.), Academic Press, New York, p. 593, (1973).
2. Gordon, H. A., and Kokas, E., *Biochem. Pharmac. 17:* 2333 (1968).
3. Spiro, R. G., *Ann. Rev. Biochem. 39:* 599 (1970).
4. Boas, N. F., *J. Biol. Chem. 204:* 544 (1953).
5. Elson, L. A., and Morgan, W. T. J., *Biochem. J. 27:* 1824 (1933).
6. Dische, Z., *J. Biol. Chem. 167:* 189 (1947).
7. Warren, L., *J. Biol. Chem. 234:* 1971 (1959).
8. Asano, T., *Proc. Soc. Exp. Biol. Med. 124:* 424 (1967).
9. Asano, T., *Proc. Soc. Exp. Biol. Med. 131:* 1201 (1969).
10. Gordon, H. A., Bruckner-Kardoss, E., Staley, T. E., Wagner, M., and Wostmann, B. S., *Acta. Anat. 64:* 367 (1966).
11. Savage, D. C., and Dubos, R., *J. Exp. Med. 128:* 97 (1968).
12. Combe, E., in "Germfree Research: Biological Effect of Gnotobiotic Environments,"

269

(J. B. Heneghan, ed.), Academic Press, New York, p. 305, (1973).

13. Levenson, S. M., *Ann. N. Y. Acad. Sci. 176:* 273 (1971).
14. Gordon, H. A., Wostmann, B. S., and Bruckner-Kardoss, E., *Proc. Soc. Exp. Biol. Med. 114:* 301 (1963).
15. Bruckner-Kardoss, E., and Wostmann, B. S., *Lab. Anim. Care 17:* 542 (1967).
16. Wostmann, B. S., Bruckner-Kardoss, E., and Knight, P. L., *Proc. Soc. Exp. Biol. Med. 128:* 137 (1968).
17. Wostmann, B. S., Knight, P. L., Keeley, L. L., and Kan, D. F., *Fed. Proc. 22:* 120 (1963).
18. Rivlin, R. S., *Adv. Enzyme Regulation 8:* 239 (1970).
19. Reddy, B. S., Wostmann, B. S., and Pleasants, J. R., (Submitted for publication).
20. Glock, G. E., and McLean, P. *Biochem. J. 55:* 400 (1953).
21. Ochoa, S., in "Methods of Enzymology, Vol. 1," (S. P. Colowick and N. O. Kaplan, eds.), Academic Press, New York, p. 739, (1955).
22. Srere, P. A., *J. Biol. Chem. 234:* 2544 (1959).
23. Smith, S., Gagne, H. T., Pitelka, D. R., and Abraham, S., *Biochem J. 115:* 807 (1969).
24. Potter, V. R., in "Manometric Techniques," (W. W. Umbreit, R. H. Burris and J. F. Stauffer, eds.), Burgess Publishing Co., Minneapolis, Minn., p. 162, (1964).
25. Lane, M. D., Moss, J., Ryder, E., and Stoll, E. *Adv. Enzyme Regulation 9:* 237 (1971).
26. Gustafsson, B. E., and Norman, A., *J. Exp. Med. 116:* 273 (1962).
27. Wostmann, B. S., *Ann. N. Y. Acad. Sci. 78:* 175 (1959).
28. Estabrook, R. W., Shigematsu, A., and Schenkman, J. B., *Adv. Enzyme Regulation 8:* 121 (1970).
29. Desplaces, A., Zagury, D., and Sacquet, E., *C. R. Acad. Sci. Paris 257:* 756 (1963).
30. Reddy, B. S., Pleasants, J. R., and Wostmann, B. S., *J. Nutr. 97:* 327 (1969).
31. Nomura, T., Ohsawa, N., and Kageyama, K., Saito, M., and Tajima, Y., in "Germfree Research: Biological Effect of Gnotobiotic Environments," (J. B. Heneghan, ed.), Academic Press, New York, p. 515, (1973).
32. Bruckner, G., in "Germfree Research: Biological Effect of Gnotobiotic Environments," (J. B. Heneghan, ed.), Academic Press, New York, p. 535, (1973).
33. Baez, S., and Gordon, H. A., *J. Exp. Med. 134:* 846 (1971).
34. Baez, S., Bruckner, G., and Gordon, H. A., in "Germfree Research: Biological Effect of Gnotobiotic Environments," (J. B. Henegan, ed.), Academic Press, New York, p. 527, (1973).
35. Wiseman, R. F., in "Germfree Research: Biological Effect of Gnotobiotic Environments," (J. B. Heneghan, ed.), Academic Press, New York, p. 441, (1973).
36. Abrams, G. D., and Bishop, J. E., *Proc. Soc. Exp. Biol. Med. 126:* 301 (1967).

THE BILE ACIDS OF THE MOUSE: EFFECT OF MICROFLORA, AGE AND SEX

H. Eyssen, G. Parmentier, J. Mertens and *P. De Somer*
The Rega Institute, University of Leuven,
Leuven, Belgium

Introduction

Although the mouse has been extensively used as an experimental animal in nutritional research, basic knowledge of the bile acid metabolism of this species is sparse. Cholic acid is considered to be the predominating bile acid of the mouse (1-3), in addition to smaller amounts of muricholic acids and microbially formed bile acid metabolites (2, 3).

Germfree animals are well suited for studying the metabolism of the primary bile acids. In the present investigations, we studied the effect of microflora, age and sex, on the bile acids of the mouse.

Materials and Methods

All animals were inbred C3H mice fed a semi-synthetic diet for at least 2 weeks prior to the experimental period. The composition of L-356R diet has been described previously (4). The food of both the germfree and the conventional animals was steam-sterilized for 25 min at 121℃. The germfree animals were kept in Trexler-type flexible film isolators.

Bile acids were determined by gas-liquid chromatography of the methyl ester acetates or the trimethylsilyl ethers on a column of 1% OV-1 or 3% QF-1 at 252℃, using a flame-ionization detection system. The analytical procedure is described in more detail elsewhere (5).

Results and Discussion

Figure 1 shows gas-liquid chromatograms of the methyl ester acetates of the bile acids in bladder bile of 5 month old male mice. The bile of conventional mice contained approximately 75% of cholic acid; smaller peaks corresponded to the muricholic acids and to several unidentified substances. In contrast, the bile acid pattern in germfree mouse bile was dominated by β-muricholic acid which accounted for 60% of the total bile acid; cholic acid accounted for 30% and

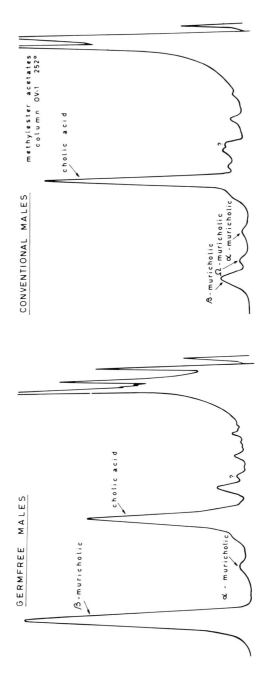

FIG. 1. Bile acids in the bladder bile of 150-day old germfree and conventional male mice fed a purified L-356R diet. Gas-liquid chromatography of the methyl ester acetates on a column of 1% OV-1 at 252° C.

minor components for approximately 10%.

The cause of the low concentration of β-muricholic acid in conventional bile — apparently in the absence of microbially formed conversion products — remains to be established. One could speculate that intestinal microorganisms decompose β-muricholic acid. Transformation of β-muricholic acid into an unabsorbable derivative is an alternative hypothesis. Finally, it cannot be excluded that intestinal bacteria or their metabolites directly affect the bile acid synthetizing systems in the liver cells.

Subsequent experiments showed that, in germfree mice, the relative amounts of β-muricholic and cholic acid depend upon the age and sex of the animal. The bile acids of 10 day old mice consisted almost exclusively of cholic acid, with only trace amounts of α- and β-muricholic acid. Significant amounts of β-muricholic acid were found in bile of 15 day old mice, and the relative concentrations of this bile acid progressively increased with age (Fig. 2). In 8 month old germfree male mice, for instance, β-muricholic acid accounted for more than 75% of the bile acids in bladder bile. In the females, however, the increase of the ratio of β-muricholic to cholic acid progressed more slowly and stabilized at a value of approximately 1 to 1 at the age of 5 months.

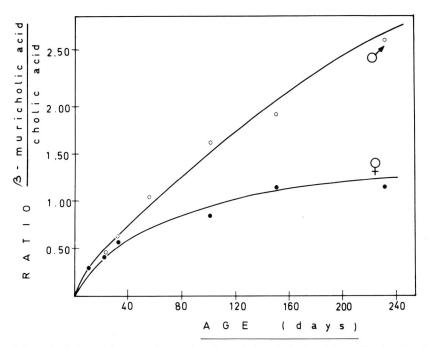

FIG. 2. Evolution of the ratio of β-muricholic to cholic acid in the bladder bile of male and female germfree mice between the age of 10 days and 8 months.

These experiments raised the question whether female mice produced less β-muricholic acid, or more cholic acid. This was studied by measuring the daily output of fecal bile acids in 3 month old animals. If we assume a steady state in the adult mouse, the daily fecal excretion of bile acids should correspond to the daily production. As shown in Table I, males and females excreted approximately the same amount of β-muricholic acid. Males, however, eliminated only one fourth of the amount of cholic acid excreted by the females. This indicates that the lower β-muricholic to cholic acid ratio in female mice is mainly due to the synthesis of more cholic acid, not to less production of β-muricholic acid.

TABLE I. Fecal Bile Acids of 3 Month Old Germfree Mice

	Fecal excretion mg/animal/24 hr*	
	Males	Females
Cholic acid	0.07	0.29
β-Muricholic acid	0.60	0.62
Minor components**	+0.10	+0.10
Unidentified compound***	+0.66	+0.40
TOTAL	1.43	1.41
Body weight (g)	30	24.5

*Determined by gas-liquid chromatography.
**Mainly α- and Ω-muricholic acids, plus traces of a compound eluting at the location of hyodeoxycholic acid.
***Presumably a dihydroxy bile acid with a double bond in the nucleus.

The data in Table I reveal another feature of bile acid metabolism in germfree mice. Feces of both males and females contained significant amounts of an unidentified compound. Assuming that the detector response to the unidentified compound was the same as the response to the other bile acids, it could be calculated that the unidentified peak accounted for 46% and 28% of the fecal bile acids in males and in females, respectively. On thin-layer and gas-liquid chromatography, the unidentified compound had the characteristics of a bile acid. The results of the mass spectrometry suggested that the substance was a dihydroxy bile acid, differing from the normal bile acid series by the presence of a double bond in the steroid nucleus. The respective positions of the hydroxyl groups and the double bond have not yet been determined.

The relative retention time of one of the smaller unidentified peaks in chromatograms of bladder bile corresponded to the retention time of the unidentified substance in feces. This suggested that the unidentified compound was secreted with the bile, but accumulated in the feces because it was poorly absorbed from the small intestine. More evidence for this hypothesis was obtained from an experiment in which the bile acid pattern was determined separately in different segments of the intestine. As shown in Table II, the unidentified compound accounted for less than 2% of the bile acids in the bile and in the small intestine, for 51% in the cecum plus colon, and for 46% in the feces.

TABLE II. Relative Amounts of Bile Acids in Various Sections of the Intestine of Germfree 3 Month Old Male Mice

	Bile acids (percent of total)			
	Bile	Small intestine	Cecum + colon	Feces
Cholic acid	23.0	20.9	5.9	4.9
β-Muricholic acid	68.0	68.7	34.9	42.0
Minor components	7.5	8.5	8.3	7.0
Unidentified compound	1.5	1.9	50.9	46.1

The efficiency of absorption of the individual bile acids has not yet been studied in detail. From the data in Table II it could be calculated, however, that the ratio of β-muricholic to cholic acid increased from a value of 2.9 in the bile to 3.3 in the small intestine, to 5.9 in the cecum plus colon, and to 8.9 in the feces. These results suggest that conjugated β-muricholic acid is significantly less efficiently reabsorbed than conjugated cholic acid.

Although the body weights of female mice were 20% lower than those of the males, the daily output of fecal bile acids was almost identical in both groups. This indicates that female mice produced 20% more bile acids per unit of body weight. Similar results were obtained from an experiment in which the total bile acid pools were determined in the gall bladder plus the gastro-intestinal

TABLE III. Bile Acid Pools in the Gall Bladder Plus the Intestine of 3 Month Old Germfree Mice Fed A Semi-synthetic L-356R diet

	Bile acid pool mg per mouse	
	Males	Females
Cholic acid	1.8	4.6
β-Muricholic acid	7.7	5.0
Minor components	±1.9	±1.9
TOTAL	11.4	11.5
Body weight (g)	30	24.5

tract. The data in Table III show that, despite the lower body weights, the bile acid pools of females were as high as those of males. Hence, when calculated on a body weight basis, female mice had a 20% larger pool of bile acids than the males.

Summary and Conclusions

The present investigations confirm that cholic acid is the predominating bile acid in adult conventional mice. Cholic acid and β-muricholic acid are the major bile acids in the bile of adult germfree mice.

Synthesis of β-muricholic acid does not start until 2 weeks after birth. From that time on, the ratio of β-muricholic to cholic acid progressively increases with age, to reach a value of 2.5 in 8 month old germfree males. In females, this ratio increases more slowly and becomes stabilized around a value of 1 at the age of 5 months. The results of our experiments seem to indicate that this difference between males and females could be explained by the fact that female mice produce 4 times as much cholic acid as the males.

An unidentified compound accounts for 46% and 28% of the fecal bile acids in male and female germfree mice, respectively. According to the mass spectrometric data, this substance could be a dihydroxy bile acid with a double bond in the steroid nucleus. Preliminary results indicate that only small amounts of the unidentified bile acid are secreted in the bile, but that the relative concentration increases in the distal segments of the intestine because the substance is poorly reabsorbed.

Acknowledgements

This work was supported by a grant from the "Fonds voor Collectief Fundamenteel Onderzoek" — Contract No. 43 of the "Onderling Overlegde Acties." The skillful technical assistance of R. Massonet is gratefully acknowledged.

References

1. Haslewood, G. A. D., and Wootton, V., *Biochem. J. 47:* 584 (1950).
2. Danielsson, H., and Kazuno, T., *Acta Chem. Scand. 13:* 1141 (1959).
3. Beher, W. T., Baker, G. D., Anthony, W. L., and Penney, D. G., *Proc. Soc. Exptl. Biol. Med. 116:* 442 (1964).
4. Eyssen, H., Van den Bosch, J. F., Janssen, G. A., and Vanderhaeghe, H., *Atherosclerosis 14:* 181 (1971).
5. Eyssen, H., Parmentier, G., Compernolle, F., Boon, J., and Eggermont, E., *Biochem. Biophys. Acta. 273:* 212 (1972).

276

BIOHYDROGENATION OF LONG-CHAIN FATTY ACIDS BY INTESTINAL MICROORGANISMS

H. Eyssen, G. De Pauw and *P. De Somer**
The Rega Institute, University of Leuven
Leuven, Belgium

Introduction

Intestinal bacteria transform lipids, neutrol sterols, steroid hormones and bile acids into a variety of metabolites, some of which might have important pharmacological activities. Previous investigations demonstrated that intestinal microorganisms profoundly modify the fecal fatty acid pattern of the rat (1). These experiments also suggested that intestinal bacteria hydrogenated unsaturated C_{18} fatty acids to yield stearic acid. However, although linoleic acid-reducing bacteria were isolated from rumen contents (2-4), the isolation of fatty acid-hydrogenating bacteria from the intestine of mammals has not yet been reported.

The present investigations demonstrate that hydrogenation of oleic and linoleic acid can be carried out *in vitro* with mixed cultures of anaerobic fecal microorganisms from the rat. In addition, a microorganism was isolated which, under certain conditions, hydrogenates linoleic acid.

Results and Discussion

Figure 1 shows gas-liquid chromatograms of fecal long-chain fatty acids of germfree and conventional rats fed a 9% corn oil diet. In the germfree animals, the fecal fatty acid pattern is simple and reflects the composition of the dietary corn oil and the tissue lipids. Conversely, conventional rats excrete a number of unidentified "bacterial" fatty acids, mainly eluted ahead of palmitic acid. Although these fatty acids have not yet been identified, they are of microbial origin, because they are not found in germfree feces. Attempts to isolate microorganisms producing these "bacterial" fatty acids were not yet successful.

There are also striking differences in the C_{18} fatty acid fraction. In germfree animals, the predominating C_{18} fatty acids, linoleic acid (18:2) and oleic acid (18:1), are unsaturated. The amount of stearic acid, a saturated

---

*Paper presented by P. De Somer

277

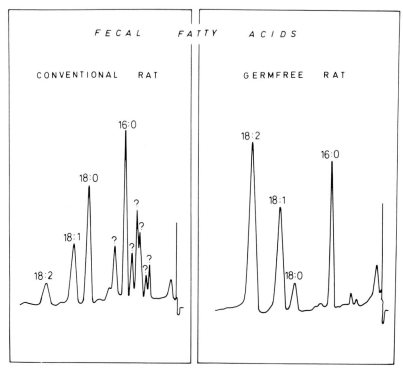

FIG. 1. Gas-liquid chromatography of the methyl esters of the fecal fatty acids of germfree and conventional rats fed a 9% corn oil diet. ? = unidentified "bacterial" fatty acids; 16:0 = palmitic acid; 18:0 = stearic acid; 18:1 = oleic acid; 18:2 = linoleic acid.

18-carbon fatty acid, is remarkably low. In conventional rats, the ratio of the unsaturated to the saturated C_{18} fatty acids is completely reversed. The amount of linoleic acid is significantly reduced, whereas stearic acid becomes the predominating C_{18} fatty acid.

Since the germfree and conventional animals excreted comparable amounts of C_{18} fatty acids, these data suggest that, in conventional rats, linoleic acid is converted into stearic acid by microbial enzymes. To obtain direct evidence that intestinal microorganisms are capable of hydrogenating unsaturated fatty acids, a culture medium was developed in which biohydrogenation of fatty acids could be demonstrated *in vitro*. This consisted of thioglycollate medium without added dextrose (BBL, No. 11,718), fortified with 1% yeast extract and 3% freeze-dried beef brain powder. Either sodium oleate or sodium linoleate were added to a final concentration of 4.5 or 3.5 mg/ml, respectively. When incubated in this medium under anaerobic conditions, suspensions of fecal microorganisms extensively hydrogenated the unsaturated fatty acids. The fatty acid hydrogenating activity could be maintained by subculturing in this medium

TABLE I. **Biohydrogenation of Linoleic Acid** *in vitro*

	Fatty acids (mg/ml)*	
	Culture medium	+ Feces from conventional rats
Bacterial fatty acids**	0	0.2
Palmitic acid (16:0)	1.1	1.1
Stearic acid (18:0)	1.1	2.6
Oleic acid (18:1)	2.3	1.9
Linoleic acid (18:2)	3.5	0.2
TOTAL	8.0 mg/ml	6.0 mg/ml

*Determined by gas-liquid chromatography of the methyl esters on a column of 18% DEGS.
**Unidentified fatty acids eluting before palmitic acid or between palmitic and stearic acid.

during at least 70 passages.

The results of a typical experiment are presented in Tables I and II. When incubated in a linoleic acid medium for 7 days, suspensions of fecal microorganisms did not produce "bacterial" fatty acids, and the amount of palmitic acid remained unaltered. There was, however, a 2.5-fold increase of the amount of stearic acid, whereas linoleic acid virtually disappeared from the culture medium. The concentration of oleic acid was slightly reduced. Similar results were obtained after incubation in an oleic acid medium. In that case, however, the most striking result was the increase of the stearic acid concentration at the expense of oleic acid. Under both conditions, significant amounts of C_{18} fatty acids were lost during incubation.

TABLE II. **Biohydrogenation of Oleic Acid** *in vitro*

	Fatty acids (mg/ml)*	
	Culture medium	+ Feces from conventional rats
Bacterial fatty acids**	0	0.2
Palmitic acid (16:0)	1.1	1.2
Stearic acid (18:0)	1.1	2.5
Oleic acid (18:1)	4.4	1.2
Linoleic acid (18:2)	0.6	0.2
TOTAL	7.2 mg/ml	5.3 mg/ml

*, ** — See footnotes to Table I.

To obtain direct evidence that stearic acid produced in these cultures arose from microbial hydrogenation of the unsaturated fatty acids – not from *de novo* synthesis – the cultures were incubated with ^{14}C-labeled oleic acid. In the unincubated culture medium, 100% of the radioactivity was found in the oleic acid fraction. Conversely, after 7 days incubation with fecal microorganisms, more than 93% of the radioactivity was found in the stearic acid fraction. Total recovery of radioactivity was about 85%.

In subsequent investigations, attempts were made to isolate the fatty acid-hydrogenating microorganisms from these mixed cultures on brain-oleate or brain-linoleate agar incubated under anaerobic conditions. It soon became clear, however, that biohydrogenation of unsaturated fatty acids is a complex phenomenon involving more than one microorganism.

From the original mixed culture, two subcultures were isolated. Subculture A was not pure and contained approximately 5 different species. Upon incubation with this culture *in vitro*, both oleic and linoleic acid were transformed into stearic acid. Gnotobiotic rats associated with subculture A exhibited a fecal C_{18} fatty acid spectrum comparable to that of conventional rats. However, "bacterial" fatty acids were not produced. So far, all attempts to isolate a pure culture of the stearic acid producing microorganism have failed.

Subculture B was a mixture of 3 species and transformed linoleic acid into an octadecenoic acid (presumably oleic acid) but failed to convert the latter into stearic acid. From this subculture a bacterium was isolated that, under certain conditions, hydrogenates linoleic acid to yield an octadecenoic acid with the retention time of oleic acid. The microorganism is a strictly anaerobic gram-positive rod. Although some cultures resisted heating to 56°C for 30 min, presence of spores was not observed and all strains were killed at 65° C. Branching was not observed. On the basis of these results, the microorganism has been tentatively classified into the genus eubacterium.

Neither the mechanism, nor the conditions for biohydrogenation of linoleic acid by this *Eubacterium sp.* have been completely elucidated. When grown in pure culture on the brain-thioglcyollate medium, the *Eubacterium sp.* transformed linoleic acid into another fatty acid which by gas chromatography and mass spectrometry was shown to be an isomer of linoleic acid (Fig. 2). Under these conditions, production of oleic acid could not be demonstrated. However, when the brain powder was omitted from the medium and the concentration of linoleic acid was reduced to one sixth of the usual amount added, 15 to 25% of the isomer was transformed into octadecenoic acid upon prolonged incubation in an atmosphere of pure hydrogen for 10 to 14 days.

In the presence of certain "helper" bacteria, the isomer was quickly and completely converted into octadecenoic acid. Several microorganisms, such as *Proteus sp., Escherichia coli* and several strains of *Clostridium sp.,* displayed "helper" activity. Strains of *Staphylococcus sp., Streptococcus faecalis* or

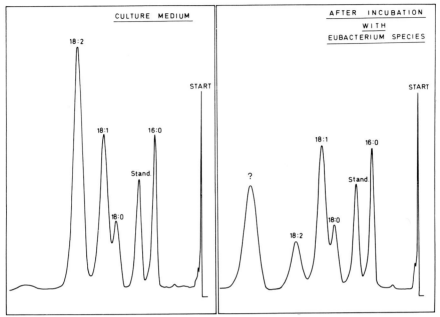

FIG. 2. Transformation of linoleic acid into a conjugated isomer by a pure culture of an unclassified *Eubacterium sp.* Gas-liquid chromatography of the methyl esters on a column of 18% DEGS. 16:0 = palmitic acid; Stand. = heptadecanoic acid internal standard; 18:0 = stearic acid; 18:1 = an octadecenoic acid with the retention time of oleic acid; 18:2 = linoleic acid; ? = isomer of linoleic acid with conjugated double bonds (see text). Brain-thioglycollate medium with linoleic acid added.

Lactobacillus sp., did not exert any "helper" function. It was also established that the "helper" bacteria by themselves did not hydrogenate linoleic acid or the isomer (Table III). When grown in pure culture on a linoleate medium, the *Eubacterium sp.* produced the isomer. A pure culture of *Proteus sp.* failed to transform linoleic acid. Association of both species resulted in production of octadecenoic acid. When the *Eubacterium sp.* was allowed to grow for 2 days as a pure culture, the resulting isomer was quickly hydrogenated upon addition of a suspension of *Proteus sp.* bacteria. However, when the *Eubacterium sp.* was killed by heating at 56°C prior to association with *Proteus sp.,* the isomer was not reduced. Upon incubation with a killed culture of *Proteus sp.* the *Eubacterium sp.* still produced the isomer, without further reduction. These investigations showed that, for quick and complete reduction of linoleic acid into octadecenoic acid to occur, both microorganisms must be actively developing.

The available evidence suggests that the two double bonds of the isomer are in the conjugated position. This would imply that the first step in the hydrogenation of linoleic acid is a shift of the double bonds to form a

TABLE III. "Helper" Activity of *Proteus sp.* in Biohydrogentaion of Linoleic Acid

Culture (+ linoleic acid)	End-product
1. *Eubacterium sp.* (5 days)	isomer
2. *Proteus sp.* (5 days)	no transformation
3. *Eubacterium sp.* plus *Proteus sp.* (5 days)	octadecenoic acid*
4. – *Eubacterium sp.* (2 days)	isomer
– plus *Proteus sp.* (5 days)	octadecenoic acid*
5. – *Eubacterium sp.* (2 days)	isomer
– killed at 56°C	
– plus *Proteus sp.* (5 days)	isomer
6. – *Proteus sp.* (2 days)	no transformation
– killed at 56°C	
– plus *Eubacterium sp.* (5 days)	isomer

*With the retention time of oleic acid on a column of 18% DEGS.

conjugated system. It should be noted that biohydrogenation of linoleic acid by *Butyrivibrio fibrisolvens* – a microorganisms isolated from the rumen of sheep – also could proceed via intermediate formation of a conjugated isomer (4).

The mechanism of the "helper" activity remains to be elucidated. One could imagine that, in spite of strict anaerobic techniques, the oxidation-reduction potential in a pure culture of *Eubacterium sp.* is not low enough to activate the hydrogenating enzyme systems. The observation that small amounts of octadecenoic acid were produced upon incubation of a pure culture in an atmosphere of pure hydrogen tends to support this view, but does not yet warrant the conclusion that the "helper" bacteria stimulate the production of oleic acid by creating an extremely low oxidation-reduction potential in the culture medium. Another possible explanation could be that the "helper" bacteria provide essential metabolites or suitable hydrogen donor systems. This, however, remains to be investigated.

Summary and Conclusions

The present investigations have shown that intestinal bacteria produce a number of unidentified "bacterial" fatty acids. The microorganisms producing "bacterial" fatty acids have not yet been isolated.

The intestinal microflora also hydrogenates unsaturated fatty acids. Biohydrogenation of linoleic or oleic acid into stearic acid was carried out by suspensions of fecal microorganisms *in vitro*. It was also shown that at least two microorganisms are involved in biohydrogenation of unsaturated fatty acids.

One of these microorganisms has been isolated. It is an unclassified *Eubacterium sp.* In pure culture it transforms linoleic acid into an isomer. Under certain conditions, e.g. prolonged incubation in an atmosphere of pure hydrogen, the pure culture transforms 15 to 25% of the isomer into oleic acid or a related octadecenoic acid. However, in presence of certain "helper" bacteria such as *Proteus sp., E. coli* or *Clostridium sp.,* the isomer is quantitatively transformed into octadecenoic acid in less than 72 hr. Although the mechanism of the "helper" function remains to be elucidated, it has been established that the "helper" bacteria by themselves do not hydrogenate linoleic acid or its isomer.

The second microorganism, responsible for reduction of oleic acid into stearic acid, has been grown in mixed cultures but has not yet been obtained in pure culture.

References

1. Evrard, E., Hoet, P. P., Eyssen, H., Charlier, H., and Sacquet, E., *Brit. J. Exp. Path. 45:* 409 (1964).
2. Polan, C. E., McNeill, J. J., and Tove, S. B., *J. Bacteriol. 88:* 1056 (1964).
3. Kemp, P., and White, R. W., *Biochem. J. 106:* 55 (1968).
4. Kepler, C. R., Hirons, K. P., McNeill, J. J., and Tove, S. B., *J. Biol. Chem. 241:* 1350 (1966).

URINARY CALCULI IN GERMFREE RATS: ALLEVIATED BY VARYING THE DIETARY MINERALS

J. Cecil Smith, Jr., E. G. McDaniel and *Floyd S. Doft*
Veterans Administration Hospital, Washington, D.C. 20422,
and National Institutes of Health, Bethesda, Maryland 20014, U.S.A.

Introduction

A significantly increased incidence of urolithiasis has been revealed in germfree rats fed a diet designed to produce zinc deficiency (1). Specifically, germfree rats fed a zinc deficient diet showed a 66 per cent incidence of urolithiasis compared to 9 per cent for conventional controls fed the same diet. Earlier, in 1962, Gustafsson and Norman reported 50 per cent of male germfree rats showed urinary calculi compared to none in conventional controls (2).

This report: 1) confirms the finding of increased incidence of urolithiasis in germfree rats fed a specific mineral mixture; 2) includes x-ray diffraction and infra-red spectrophotometric analyses of the calculi; 3) provides data showing the reduction of urinary calculi by altering the dietary minerals; 4) compares the chemical analysis of the calculogenic and less calculogenic mineral mixtures; and 5) advances a possible explanation for the increased urinary calculi in germfree animals fed the specific mineral mixture.

Materials and Methods

All experiments used 19-20 day old weanling germfree, ex-germfree and specific pathogen free (SPF) rats with initial weights of 40-45 grams. The rats were of the Sprague-Dawley strain with similar genetic origin. The experiments ranged from 40 to 124 days duration. Visual identification without magnification of calculi in either the bladder, ureters, and/or kidney constituted evidence of urolithiasis. Histological examination was made of selected kidneys and bladder showing urolithiasis. More complete details of experimental procedures previously have been published (1, 4). All diets used in these experiments were zinc deficient, 3.4 ppm zinc or less. The basal diet is shown in Table I.

Experiment I. This experiment compared the incidence of urolithiasis in animals fed the basal diet with rats fed a similar diet in which the Hubbell, Mendel and Wakeman (HMW) mineral mixture (3) was reduced from five to

TABLE I. Composition of Zinc Deficient Diet

		Percentage
Casein[1]		20
Corn starch		70
Corn oil		5

Vitamins per 100g diet		Minerals per 100g diet	
Vitamin A acetate	5500 USP units	$CaCO_3$	0.83
Vitamin D$_3$	1100 USP units	$CaHPO_4$	2.37
α-tocopherol acetate	75 mg	$MgSO_4$	0.25
Menadione	1 mg	KCl	0.58
Thiamine hydrocloride	6 mg	NaCl	0.33
Pyridoxine hydrocloride	2 mg	Na_2HPO_4	0.58
D-L calcium pantothenate	15 mg	$CuSO_4$ (anhydrous)	0.0006
Niacinamide	10 mg	$FeC_6H_5O_7 \cdot 5H_2O$	0.02
Ascorbic acid	100 mg	$MnSO_4 \cdot H_2O$	0.02
Biotin	1 mg	KIO_3	0.0008
Vitamin B$_{12}$	0.01 mg		
Choline chloride	100 mg		
p-aminobenzoic acid	5 mg		
Folic acid	1 mg		
Riboflavin	3 mg		

[1]Extracted with disodium ethylenediamine tetraacetate (Na_2EDTA) to lower the zinc content according to method described by Davis *et al., J. of Nutr. 78:* 445, 1962.

three per cent, with a phosphorus supplement added (0.50g of phosphorus/100 g of diet from 1.10g NaH_2PO_4 and 1.13g $NaHPO_4$). The casein was extracted with disodium ethylenediamonetetraacetate (Na_2EDTA) by a modification of Davis *et al.* (5) to lower the zinc concentration. The carbohydrate (cornstarch) was concomitantly increased from 70 to 72 per cent.

Experiment II. This experiment was designed to determine: 1) if changing the source of protein from extracted casein to egg white or 2) using a completely different mineral mixture, as described by Wesson (6), would decrease the incidence of urolithiasis. The diets were identical to the basal diet (Table I) except that 20 per cent egg white plus 1.2 per cent D-L threonine was substituted for the casein. In addition, in the second part of the experiment, 4 per cent Wesson mixture was substituted for the 5 per cent HMW.

Results

Experiment I. A comparison between the incidence of urolithiasis in germfree and conventional rats fed the basal diet with differing mineral mixtures is shown in Table II. As shown, alteration of the HMW mineral mixture (3) resulted in a marked reduction of urinary calculi in the germfree rats, with the

TABLE II. Incidence of Urolithiasis in Germfree and Conventional Rats Fed the Basal Diet with Original and Modified Mineral Mixture[1]

| Mineral Mixture | Urolithiasis | | | |
	Germfree		Conventional	
	Incidence (%)	No. of animals	Incidence (%)	No. of animals
5% HMW[2]	66	(31)	9	(22)
3% HMW + 0.5% phosphorus[3]	7	(28)	4	(26)

[1]Composition of basal diet in Table I.
[2]Hubbell, Mendel, and Wakeman (3).
[3]0.50g phosphorus per 100g of diet (The source of phosphorus was 1.10g NaH_2PO_4 plus 1.13g of Na_2HPO_4 per 100g of diet).

degree of involvement much less severe in comparable conventional rats.

Experiment II. The results of this experiment revealed that the incidence of urolithiasis was not decreased by substituting egg white for the extracted casein in the basal diet (Table III). The incidence of urinary calculi in germfree rats fed the egg white diet was identical, 66 per cent, to that in animals fed the basal casein diet (Table II). However when Wesson mineral mixture was used (4 per cent of the diet) instead of the HMW mixture (5 per cent of the diet) the incidence was decreased from 66 per cent to zero (Table III).

The calculi as analyzed by x-ray diffraction and infrared spectrophotometry were mainly composed of weddellite ($CaC_2O_4:2H_2O$) plus an organic phase which was not collagen or urea. Whewellite ($Ca_2O_4:H_2O$), newberyite ($MgHPO_4:3H_2O$), struvite ($NH_4MgPO_4:6H_2O$), apatite (Ca_3PO_4),

TABLE III. Incidence of Urolithiasis in Germfree and Conventional Rats Fed an Egg White Diet with Different Mineral Mixtures[1] (Experiment No. 2)

| Mineral Mixture | Urolithiasis | | | |
	Germfree		Conventional	
	Incidence (%)	No. of animals	Incidence (%)	No. of animals
5% HMW[2]	66	(6)	0	(6)
4% Wesson[3]	0	(7)	0	(8)

[1]The diet was similar to the basal diet (Table I) except egg white (20%) plus 1.2% D-L Threonine served as the protein source. The carbohydrate (corn starch) was changed to 68.8%. The percentages of vitamins and fat were identical to the basal diet in Table I.
[2]Hubbell, Mendel and Wakeman (3).
[3]Wesson (6).

brushite ($CaHPO_4:2H_2O$) or hydroxyl apatite [$3 Ca_3(PO_4)_2:Ca(OH)_2$] were not detected.

Discussion

The basal diet (Table I) used in these studies tends to be calculogenic since 9 percent of the conventional animals developed urolithiasis (1). The data demonstrate that the HMW mineral mixture was the main causative factor for the high incidence of urinary calculi (Tables II and III). This mineral mixture was also used by Gustafsson and Norman (2) who earlier reported increased urolithiasis in germfree rats. In addition, Van Reen *et al.* (7) reported conventional rats fed a diet with HMW mineral mixture showed a high incidence of calculi. Those investigators demonstrated that excess calcium was a causative factor. More recently, Schwarz (8) noted that conventional rats fed an amino acid diet containing the HMW mixture exhibited urolithiasis. Regarding the data in Table III, we are aware that calculogenic properties of the HMW and Wesson Mineral mixtures can not be accurately compared since the one diet contains 5 per cent HWM, whereas the other is composed of 4 per cent Wesson minerals. Since the data clearly demonstrate that the egg white diet containing 4 per cent Wesson minerals resulted in much lower incidence of urolithiasis compared to a similar diet with 5 per cent HMW mineral mixture, they again suggest 5 per cent HMW as a causative agent in germfree rats.

It is also recognized that the diets used in these studies were zinc deficient. However, we have no evidence to indicate that lack of zinc in our diets affected the development of calculi since both the calculogenic and less calculogenic diets were zinc deficient. King *et al.* (9) reported that zinc excretion was significantly greater in 22 patients with recurrent renal stone formation. However, they concluded that zinc excretion was probably a secondary phenomenon and suggested that zinc was not directly involved in renal stone formation.

A possible explanation for the increased incidence of calculi in the germfree rat fed our basal zinc deficient diet follows: First, the HMW mineral mixture (3) used in the basal diet favors calculi formation even in conventional rats. One reason for this is the abnormal calcium to phosphorus (Ca:P) ratio of 4.6:1 compared to 1.5:1 for the Wesson mixture as shown in Table IV.[1] In addition, the germfree rat reportedly absorbs and retains a higher percentage of dietary calcium compared to conventional controls, as well as excreting greater quantities of calcium via the urine, a condition favoring calculi formation (2, 10).

Urinary calculi confound nutritional experiments and are thus undesirable. However, because the calculi produced by the basal diet described here are

---

[1]For a critical review of dietary mineral mixtures see Greenfield, H., and Briggs, G. M., *Annual Review of Biochemistry 40:* 549 (1971).

TABLE IV. Chemical Analyses of Calculogenic and Less Calculogenic Mineral Mixtures[1]

	Grams/100g									
Mineral Mixture	CaO	P_2O_5	MgO	Na_2O	K_2O	MnO	Fe_2O_3	FeO	CO_2	Ca:P ratio
Calculogenic[2]	30.7	10.9	1.4	4.3	14.3	.02	.27	.12	22.6	4.6:1
Less Calculogenic[3]	19.7	22.0	1.5	5.8	22.4	.02	N.D.[4]	.26	2.6	1.5:1

[1]Methods used were those described by L. Shapiro and W. W. Brannock. U.S. Geological Survey Bulletin 1144-A, 1962, supplemented by atomic absorption spectrophotemetry.
[2]HMW Mineral Mixture (3).
[3]Wesson Mineral Mixture (6).
[4]Non-detectable.

calcium oxalates, similar in composition to the most common human urinary calculi (11), the germfree rat fed such a calculogenic diet could be a useful model for studying calcium oxlate formation.

Conclusion

An increased incidence of urolithiasis in germfree animals fed zinc deficient casein or egg white diets has been observed. Sixty-six per cent of the germfree rats fed the casein diet containing five per cent HMW mineral mixture exhibited urolithiasis. By lowering the HMW mineral mixture to 3 per cent of the diet and supplementing with 0.50% phosphorus the incidence of urinary calculi was reduced to 8 per cent in the germfree animals. Likewise, substituting Wesson mineral mixture (4 per cent of the diet) in place of the HMW Mineral mixture (5 per cent of the diet) resulted in fewer calculi. Thus the increased urolithiasis noted in germfree rats fed a basal zinc deficient diet could be nearly eliminated by varying the mineral mixtures resulting in a more favorable calcium to phosphorus ratio. There was no indication that the lack of zinc in the diets affected calculi formation since both the calculogenic and less calculogenic diets were zinc deficient.

Acknowledgements

The authors wish to express their appreciation to Dr. Mary Mrose and Frank Cuttitta, and other personnel of the Branch of Astrogeologic Studies, Chemistry of Cosmic and Related Materials Project, U.S. Geological Survey, Washington, D.C., for analyses of the calculi, mineral mixtures, and diets.

References

1. Smith, J. C. Jr., and McDaniel, E. G., *Invest. Urol. 9:* 518 (1972).
2. Gustafsson, B. E, and Norman, A., *J. Exp. Med. 116:* 273 (1962).

3. Hubbell, R. B., Mendel, L. B., and Wakeman, A. J., *J. Nutr. 14:* 273 (1937).
4. Smith, J. C., and Halsted, J. A., *J. Nutr. 100:* 973 (1970).
5. Davis, P. N., Norris, L. C., and Kratzer, F. H., *J. Nutr. 78:* 445 (1962).
6. Wesson, L. G., *Science 75:* 339 (1932).
7. Van Reen, R., Lyon, H. W., and Lossee, F. L., *J. Nutr. 69:* 302 (1959).
8. Schwarz, K., *J. Nutr. 100:* 1487 (1970).
9. King, L. R., Mulvaney, W. P., and Johnson, J. P., *Invest. Urol. 8:* 405 (1971).
10. Reddy, B. S., Pleasants, J. R., and Wostmann, B. S., *J. Nutr. 99:* 353 (1969).
11. Lonsdale, K., *Science 159:* 1199 (1968).

PROTEIN METABOLISM IN THE GERMFREE AND CONVENTIONAL CHICK

Marie E. Coates, D. Hewitt and *D. N. Salter*
National Institute for Research in Dairying
Shinfield, Reading, England

Introduction

In a previous investigation on protein digestion in the chick, Salter & Coates (1) obtained evidence that the gut microflora had a marked influence on the amount and type of nitrogenous material in the lower gut and excreta. Although this appeared to have little effect on the availability of dietary protein to the host, there were indications that bacterial activity altered the distribution of nitrogenous excretion products between the fecal and urinary components. This, if quantitatively significant, could give misleading results of protein quality evaluations done in a conventional environment. Nitrogen (N) balance studies with good and poor quality proteins have now been made on chicks to investigate further the effects of microbial activity on the utilization of dietary proteins.

The nutritional value of a protein may be low because it is deficient in one or more of the essential amino acids or because the availability of its component amino acids has been reduced by processing. Sesame meal, which contains little lysine, was chosen as representative of the first group and autoclaved cod fillet of the second; the corresponding good quality proteins were sesame meal supplemented with lysine and freeze-dried cod fillet.

Methods

Each experiment was conducted on germfree chicks kept in Gustafsson isolators and on their hatch mates reared in a conventional chick room. Groups of eight two-week-old chicks were used for each experimental treatment. They were housed in pairs in stainless steel cages with wire screen floors through which the excreta dropped into a tray of $0 \cdot 1$ N H_2SO_4. The food troughs were designed to prevent the birds from scattering diet into the excreta tray, and to allow the food intake of each pair to be accurately measured.

The composition of the diets is given in Table I. They were sterilized by γ-radiation at 5 Mrad, a procedure known to have little or no effect on the

TABLE I. Composition of the Experimental Diets

	N-free	Cod fillet	Sesame
Maize starch	86·95	70·95	32·90
Sesame meal[1]	—	—	55·0
Cod fillet[2]	—	16	—
Salt mixture[3]	6·0	6·0	6·0
Vitamin mixture[3]	0·8	0·8	0·8
Choline chloride	0·15	0·15	0·2
Inositol	0·10	0·10	0·10
Maize oil	5·0	5·0	5·0
Methyl cellulose	1·0	1·0	—

[1]For the lysine-supplemented diet 0.5% L-lysine was added at the expense of starch.
[2]Freeze-dried or autoclaved.
[3]The mineral and vitamin supplements were essentially similar to those of Salter & Coates (1).

nutritive value of proteins (2). Sterilized diets were fed to the birds in both environments.

The birds were given the N-free diet for one week. During the last three days food intake was measured and quantitative collections of excreta were made. The chicks were then given one of the test diets for a week, collections being made as before on the last three days. The procedure was repeated for a third week with the N-free diet. The N content of the excreta was determined and the mean excretion during the two periods on the N-free diet was used as a measure of the endogenous N loss. Uric acid was also determined in the excreta.

The net protein utilization (NPU) was calculated from the formula:

$$\text{NPU} = \frac{\text{Total N eaten} - (\text{Total N excreted} - \text{Endogenous N excreted})}{\text{Total N eaten}} \times 100$$

Results

The NPU values, with standard errors, for the four different diets in germfree and conventional environments are given in Table II.

There were very large differences in NPU values between the four diets,

TABLE II.

Diet tested	NPU value	
	Germfree	Conventional
Sesame	47 + 2·3	42 + 1·3
Sesame + lysine	60 + 0·2	63 + 1·8
Cod fillet	94 + 2·6	89 + 2·2
Autoclaved cod fillet	60 + 2·2	60 + 6·1

but no significant differences between the values found in the two environments. The total N excreted, with the amounts of N contributed by uric acid, are recorded in Table III.

TABLE III.

Diet tested	Type of chick	N in excreta (mg/g N intake)		Uric acid % of total N
		Total	Uric acid	
Sesame	GF	629	342	54·4
	CV	661	335	50·7
Sesame +	GF	487	215	44·1
lysine	CV	447	189	42·3
Cod fillet	GF	274	117	42·7
	CV	281	118	42·0
Autoclaved	GF	673	158	23·5
cod fillet	CV	629	189	29·6

During the periods on the test diet the total N excreted (mg/g N intake) was not significantly different in the two environments. However, during the periods when N-free diets were given the germfree birds excreted consistently more N than did their conventional counterparts. The mean values over the four experiments were, for germfree and conventional birds respectively, $9·6 \pm 0·4$ and $7·5 \pm 0·2$ mg/g food eaten, a difference that was statistically significant at P $\langle 0·05$. The percentage of N contributed by uric acid was 46·6 in the germfree and 54·7 in the conventional excreta.

Discussion

There are several ways in which the course of digestion of proteins might be influenced by the activity of the gut microorganisms, and the effects could be of benefit, detriment or indifference to the host. For instance, amino acids might be released from a poorly digestible protein through the action of microbial proteases. Conversely, free amino acids could be lost to the host if they were incorporated into microbial proteins. There are indications from our previous work (1) that amino acids and peptides reaching the lower gut undergo bacterial degradation with liberation and subsequent absorption of ammonia. This activity is unlikely to be of consequence to the host since much of the ammonia would be reexcreted in the urine after conversion to uric acid in the bird or urea in the mammal; only if it were used for the synthesis of tissue amino acids could it contribute towards the host's nutrition. More indirectly, the presence of a gut flora might, by modifying the morphology and perhaps the function of the gut, reduce the efficiency of uptake of amino acids from the intestine.

The nutritive value of a protein depends on the ease with which it is digested and on the efficiency with which the products of digestion are synthesized into tissue proteins. Animal tests for "true digestibility" and "biological value" of a protein attempt to assess these two properties. Both require measurement of fecal nitrogen excretion. When performed in a conventional environment the results are likely to be misleading if, as postulated above, bacterial action reduces the amount of N excreted in the feces without benefit to the host. The test for "net protein utilization" takes account of both digestibility and utilization, since it is a measure of the proportion of food N retained by the test animal. The retained N is calculated by subtracting the total N excreted in the urine and feces from the total N intake. Thus the distribution of N between two routes of excretion is irrelevant and the NPU value truly reflects the nutritive value of the protein to the test animal in either environment.

The germfree chick offers some advantage over the rat as a subject for N balance studies since it is not subject to cecal enlargement, a condition that might invalidate comparison with its conventional counterpart. It has the disadvantage, however, that fecal and urinary excretions are mixed in the cloaca before voiding and cannot be collected separately without surgical adaptation. Intact birds were used in the experiments reported here, hence the NPU value was the only measure of protein quality that could be calculated. There were very big differences, as expected, between the NPU values for the four diets tested, but little or none between values in the two environments. The small differences in favor of germfree birds given sesame or cod fillet were not statistically significant. Thus it can be concluded that, under the conditions of these experiments, microbial activity had no important effect on utilization of dietary proteins by the birds.

Uric acid is the chief end-product of protein catabolism in birds and forms the major nitrogenous constituent of the urine. The proportion of uric acid in the excreta therefore gave some idea of the distribution of N between urine and feces, even though separate collection of urine was not possible. The large differences in uric acid excretion reflect the differences in nutritive quality of the four test diets. The cod fillet was well digested and well retained, as judged by the relatively small amount of N either in the total excreta or in the uric acid portion. The autoclaving procedure had clearly reduced the digestibility of the cod fillet, since excretion of N was more than doubled on this diet. Uric acid excretion was also increased, indicating that some of the nitrogenous products absorbed from the diet had not been retained by the birds. The sesame diet was apparently well digested but poorly utilized, since the contribution of uric acid to the total N excreted was high. Supplementation with lysine markedly improved its retention by the bird.

The environmental differences in either the amounts of uric acid or the proportion it contributed to the total N excretion were small and statistically non-significant. Nevertheless they showed trends towards the kind of effects that might have been expected from microbial action on the types of protein tested. With unheated cod fillet, for example, results were identical in both environments. On this diet no effect of the microflora was to be expected, since little of the food protein reached the lower gut where the organisms are most numerous. On the diet containing autoclaved cod fillet, however, uric acid contributed a slightly higher proportion of the total N excretion in the conventional environment. Such a result could arise if nitrogenous material, possibly peptides or ammonia, released by microbial action had been absorbed but not retained by the host. On the sesame diets, with or without lysine, the proportion of uric acid N excreted was marginally higher in the germfree groups. This finding suggests a slightly better absorption of amino acids by the germfree birds, and is in accord with similar indications in our earlier work (1). In general, however, the absence of any marked difference in uric acid excretion in the two environments emphasizes the relative unimportance of the gut microflora in the digestion and utilization of dietary proteins by the chick.

The higher excretion of endogenous N in the germfree environment confirms an earlier observation by Miller (3). It may reflect a truly greater loss of N from the tissues of the germfree birds or, more likely, the N loss from conventional birds was only apparently smaller because the composition of endogenous N residues had been altered by the action of the microflora. The proportion of uric acid N to total N was higher in the conventional excreta, indicating that endogenous N is more subject to bacterial degradation than are the residues of dietary protein. Whether or not this leads to conservation of N for use by the host cannot be deduced from these experiments. The possibility remains to be investigated in a longer-term study.

References

1. Salter, D. N., and Coates, M. E. *Br. J. Nutr. 26:* 55 (1971).
2. Ley, F. J., Bleby, J., Coates, M. E., and Paterson, J. S., *Lab. Anim. 3:* 221 (1969).
3. Miller, W. S., *Proc. Nutr. Soc. 26:* X (1967).

ROLE OF CYSTEINE ETHYL ESTER AND INDIGENOUS MICROFLORA IN THE PATHOGENESIS OF AN EXPERIMENTAL HEMOLYTIC ANEMIA, AZOTEMIA, AND PANCREATIC ACINAR ATROPHY

Stanley M. Levenson, Dorinne Kan and *Charles Gruber*
Department of Surgery

and

Ernst Jaffe, Komei Nakao and *Eli Seifter*
Departments of Medicine, Pathology, and Surgery & Biochemistry
Albert Einstein College of Medicine
Bronx, New York 10461, U.S.A.

Introduction

Our laboratory has reported (1-3) a previously not reported syndrome of pancreatic acinar atrophy and fibrosis, azotemia and anemia which occured in conventional rats of the Sprague-Dawley and Fischer strains fed a chemically defined amino acid liquid diet (J_2, Table I) containing all compounds and ions known to be necessary for the growth and health of rats, and none in what appeared to be excessive levels. The abnormalities did not develop at all, or to a much less extent, in germfree (GF) rats fed this same liquid diet, or in conventional rats fed the ingredients of this liquid diet in solid form, or in rats fed other liquid diets of similar chemical composition. The severity of the abnormalities which develop is evident from Fig. 1, which contrasts the incidence of spontaneous death among IHO (conventional rats raised in isolators) and GF (germfree) rats. The abnormalities are as reproducible and predictable experimentally in conventional rats as is scurvy in conventional guinea pigs deprived of ascorbic acid.

We showed that the critical microbial factor(s) is present in the whole cecal contents (but not an ultrafiltrate of the cecal contents) of healthy conventional rats eating chow. This was evident when GF rats which were purposefully contaminated with the cecal contents of conventional rats eating a commercial rat chow "complete" diet, became anemic, azotemic and developed the pancreatic lesions when they were switched to the liquid amino acid diet J_2 while their GF littermates which were kept GF did not, despite their ingestion of the same liquid diet. We also have conducted experiments which indicated that it

297

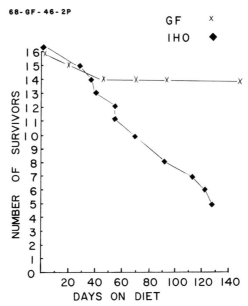

FIG. 1. Spontaneous deaths of germfree X and IHO ◆: Sprague-Dawley rats fed liquid diet J₂.

was the gut bacteria among the rat's microbial flora which were almost certainly the critical component. In particular, *Proteus sp.* and possibly staphylococci are involved.

The **pancreatic lesion** is characterized early by minimal inflammatory changes and beginning necrosis of acinar cells. The quiet acinar necrosis progresses, leading to pancreatic acinar atrophy, fibrosis, and fatty replacement. Fat absorption is markedly impaired (neither protein nor carbohydrate polymers have been tested). There is no glycosuria and the islets do not appear to be involved at least for many months. There are some metaplastic changes at the periphery of the islets after many months — the origin of the metaplastic cells has not been established yet (1).

The **livers** of the rats are normal grossly and microscopically. Despite the azotemia, the **kidneys** appear normal by gross and light microscopic examination.

The **erythrocytes** of the anemic rats were at first normochromic and normocytic and later slightly hypochromic and microcytic. Serum iron concentrations are similar in anemic and non-anemic rats; there is no blood loss. Our experiments showed that **the anemia is hemolytic** in nature (active bone marrow, reticulocytosis, increased ^{59}Fe uptake, decreased red blood cell survival time (by a factor of 2), splenomegaly, increased splenic iron) and that the "defect" is in red blood cells (established by cross-transfusion experiments) and includes a change in the absorption spectrum of hemoglobin. Splenectomy ameliorates but does not prevent the anemia. The anemia is neither prevented nor corrected by any of the known vitamins, singly or in combination, or by iron.

In contrast, feeding ultra-pure bovine serum albumin, ultra-pure α-lactalbumin, vitamin-free casein, or an acid hydrolysate of vitamin-free casein (to which tryptophan was added) prevented or cured the anemia and restored erythrocyte survival to normal and ameliorated the pancreatic lesion. However, feeding a supplement of amino acids in amounts and proportions similar to the composition of casein, or the ash of casein, had no prophylactic or therapeutic effects. Further, supplements of casein or casein hydrolysate ameliorate (though they do not prevent) the pancreatic lesion while a supplement of amino acids in amounts and properties similar to the casein does not affect the pancreatic lesion.

The role of the pancreas in hematopoiesis has not been well defined. The development of pancreatic acinar fibrosis because of anemia has not previously been reported. It is unlikely that the anemia is secondary to the pancreatic lesion

TABLE I. Composition of Liquid Amino Acid Diets

Amino Acids	116	J$_2$	L-479E
		g/liter Diet	
L-Cysteine ethyl ester HCl	0.55	2.42	
L-Tyrosine ethyl ester HCl	8.40	3.14	10.00
L-Asparagine		3.95	6.00
L-Serine	6.60	2.30	7.75
L-Proline	12.70	2.30	15.00
L-Aspartate	6.75	2.30	
L-Glutamate, mono-Na	25.60	27.95	30
L-Alanine	3.20	2.30	3.75
L-Arginine HCl	4.70	8.90	3.75
Glycine	2.05	13.94	2.50
L-Histidine HCl H$_2$O	2.85	3.38	2.75
L-Isoleucine	4.40	5.50	2.50
L-Leucine	7.00	7.30	4.00
L-Lysine HCl	6.50	11.80	6.25
L-Methionine	3.15	5.39	4.25
L-Phenylalanine	3.15	7.63	4.50
L-Threonine	4.40	5.00	2.50
L-Tryptophan	1.40	1.50	2.00
L-Valine	4.90	5.50	3.50
	108.30	122.50	111.00

*A table showing comparisons of the complete diets (including vitamins, minerals and fatty acids) is in *Federation Proceedings, 30:* 1785 (1971) (3).

since the anemia begins before there are substantial changes in the pancreas. The anemia observed here is different from that seen in patients with chronic pancreatic disease which is usually of a macrocytic type. Also, iron absorption is often increased in patients with pancreatic dysfunction; in our rats on the chemically defined diet iron absorption is normal. The anemia long precedes the azotemia, so a renal basis for the anemia is not likely.

Role of cysteine ethyl ester in the pathogenesis of the syndrome. In this report we will describe some of our studies conducted during the past year directed towards defining the pathogenesis of the syndrome, with particular emphasis on how the dietary chemical and host microbial factors interact to produce the hemolytic anemia, azotemia, and pancreatic acinar atrophy and fibrosis. Some of our other studies determining the nature of the red blood cell defect and hemoglobin abnormality in the anemic rats and determining the component(s) of the proteins and casein hydrolysate which is protective are to be described elsewhere.

The syndrome we have observed in rats in our experiments ingesting liquid diet J_2 differs substantially from the abnormalities so far described by other investigators studying: a) "chemically defined" amino acid diets; b) pancreatic acinar atrophy and fibrosis; c) nutritional or other hemolytic anemias; and d) amino acid imbalances, antagonisms and toxicities including those of methionine, homocysteine, cystine and cysteine(4). A review of this is in our published papers (2, 3) and in a detailed paper which is in preparation.

Materials and Methods

The formulations of three liquid diets, J_2, 116 (Greenstein, Winitz, and Otey (5)), and L-479E (Reddy, Pleasants, and Wostmann (6)), are listed in Table I. Diet J_2 leads to the pathologic syndrome of anemia, azotemia, and the pancreatic lesion while rats ingesting diet 116 do not become anemic or azotemic and either do not develop the pancreatic lesion, or develop it to a much less extent than rats ingesting diet J_2. When HCl was added to diet 116 to match the higher HCl content of diet J_2, no change in the "toxicity" of diet 116 was noted. Reddy, Pleasants and Wostmann (6) indicate that rats ingesting diet L-479E do not develop pancreatic abnormalities.

Among the differences in the composition of these diets are differences in the concentrations of certain amino acids. The higher concentration of cysteine ethyl ester in diet J_2 was suggested as critically involved first by E.S. of our group because: a) we (7) and Shapiro *et al.* (8) had previously found that it combined with menadione to form an adduct which interfered with prothrombin synthesis and led to vitamin K deficiency (this does not happen when vitamin K_1 is used as in diet J_2) and b) we could visualize it interacting with other ingredients in the diet and/or components in the rat's gut, including bacteria and their products, or metabolites resulting from the interaction of bacteria and other compounds. As a result, compounds may be formed which give rise to H_2S, acrylyl acid derivatives, effect the condensation of acrylyl or pyruvoyl derivatives to various amines, or compounds which are amino acid antagonists, e.g., a lysine analog (see references 2, 3 for further discussion of these points).

Results

To test the possibility that cysteine ethyl ester hydrochloride (C.E.E.HCl) is involved in the pathogenesis of the syndrome, diet J_2 was prepared with and without cysteine ethyl ester. In our normal preparation of diet J_2, C.E.E.HCl is the last of the solid ingredients added. Thus, a batch of diet was prepared and then halved; to one half, C.E.E.HCl in the normal concentration was added while none was added to the other half. We found that the rats drinking diet J_2 with C.E.E.HCl developed the full blown syndrome as usual, but none of the rats ingesting this diet without C.E.E.HCl did.

To extend this observation, an experiment was carried out in which diet J_2 was prepared up to the addition of C.E.E.HCl as noted above, but divided into thirds; to one third, C.E.E.HCl in the normal J_2 concentration (0.48% solid) was added, to another one third, C.E.E.HCl in the diet 116 concentration (0.11% solids) was added, and to the other one-third, no cysteine ethyl ester was added. At the same time, using the same batch of dietary ingredients, diet 116 was made up in a similar fashion so that one preparation contained no C.E.E.HCl, another the usual 116 C.E.E.HCl (0.11% solids), and the third the diet J_2 C.E.E.HCl concentration (0.48% solids).

As part of this same experiment, diet 116 was prepared with its usual composition but with added HCl in the amount normally present in diet J_2 and using the preparation techniques of diet J_2. The data are given in Table II.

TABLE II

C.E.E.HCl % Diet Solids		Anemia	Pancreatic Lesion
Diet J_2	0	0	0
	0.11	++	+++
	0.48	+++	+++
Diet 116	0	0	0
	0.11	0	+
	0.11*	0	0
	0.48	0	++

*Prepared by methods generally used to prepare diet J_2 and with added HCl to match the HCl content of diet J_2.

The data show that cysteine ethyl ester hydrochloride is critically involved, but that it is substantially more "toxic" when fed in diet J2 than in diet 116 and that this difference is not due to the modes of preparation or HCl contents of the diets.

We then conducted experiments to determine whether cysteine (hydrochloride) or cystine would induce the syndrome. It should be pointed out that the levels of cysteine ethyl ester used in these experiments is below that of other amino acids generally found to lead to imbalances or toxicities. The pathologic syndrome we have observed differs from those described for methionine, cystine and homocysteine. Some investigators have assumed that the ingestion of cystine and cysteine would lead to similar effects, but few studies with cysteine feeding have been reported. Cysteine ethyl ester was introduced into the formulation of amino acid liquid diets by Greenstein and his colleagues (9) because of its greater solubility than that of the free amino acid or the hydrochloride: " . . . relying upon the powerful tissue esterases to effect the hydrolysis of these compounds to the free amino acids." However, little is known about the metabolic fate of cysteine ethyl ester and it is possible that a significant proportion of it is absorbed unchanged and that it is "toxic" in this form since cysteine ethyl ester is apt to be a stronger nucleophilic agent than cysteine itself.

In parallel trials: a) **cysteine hydrochloride was substituted for cysteine ethyl ester hydrochloride** in liquid diet J2 and b) **cystine** was substituted for cysteine ethyl ester hydrochloride in diet J2 in the solid form.

The data indicate that cysteine ethyl ester and cysteine hydrochloride behave in dramatically different ways. Thus when cysteine hydrochloride was substituted in equimoler concentration for cysteine ethyl ester in liquid diet J2, neither anemia nor the pancreatic lesion developed (Table III).

In the experiments with solid diets we showed that when cystine was substituted for cysteine ethyl ester, no pancreatic lesion developed (solid diets were used because the relative insolubility of cystine prevents its being used in liquid diets) nor did any anemia develop.

The adverse effects of cysteine ethyl ester may be due to a direct effect of

TABLE III.

	Body wt.(g)	Hgb (g%)	Hct (%)	Pancreatic Lesion
Diet J2 Cysteine ethyl ester	191	9.0	30	3+
Modified Diet J2 Cysteine hydrochloride	240	17.3	49	0

*Sprague-Dawley rats, male, started on diets at 21-23 days of age; rats killed 61 days later.

302

this compound and/or to an effect after it has been converted to some other compound. Thus, we visualize the possible toxicity of cysteine ethyl ester as being due to either the reaction of cysteine ethyl ester with a body constituent because of the nucleophilic properties of this mercaptan, or the reaction of cysteine ethyl ester with certain other dietary or endogenous (e.g., of the rat's gut contents) constituents giving rise to either antimetabolites or a non-utilizable product thereby removing an essential metabolite from the diet. The indigenous flora may play a direct or indirect role in these processes.

Summary

We have presented data which show that the presence of cysteine ethyl ester (and **not** cysteine hydrochloride or cystine) is a necessary factor in the pathogenesis of this syndrome, but that its effects are conditioned by the physical state of the diet (liquid being much more "toxic" than solid), the composition of the diet, e.g., the other amino acids, and the presence of the indigenous flora in the rats. Studies exploring these aspects are described elsewhere. It is apparent that the esters of amino acids can not be assumed to be metabolically identical to the free base and that further investigation of various esters and tissue esterases is in order.

Acknowledgements

Supported in part by N.I.H. Grants AM-05664, 1 RO1 AM15144, 5-K5-GM-14,208 (Research Career Award, S.M.L.).

References

1. Geever, E. F., Seifter, E., and Levenson, S. M., *Brit. J. Exp. Path. 51:* 341 (1970).
2. Levenson, S. M., Kan, D., Gruber, C., Crowley, L., Jaffe, E. R., Nakao, K., Geever, E. F., and Seifter, E., *Ann. Surg. 174:* 469 (1971).
3. Levenson, S. M., Kan, D., Gruber, C., Crowley, L., Jaffe, E., Nakao, K., Geever, E., and Seifter, E., *Fed. Proc. 30:* 1785 (1971).
4. Harper, A. E., Benevenga, N. J., and Wohlhueter, R. M., *Physiol. Rev. 50:* 428 (1970).
5. Winitz, M., Birnbaum, S. M., Sugimura, T., and Otey, M. C., in "Amino Acids, Proteins and Cancer Biochemistry," (J. T. Edsall, ed.), Academic Press, New York, p. 9, (1960).
6. Reddy, B. S., Pleasants, J. R., and Wostmann, B. S., *J. Nutr. 97:* 327 (1969).
7. Seifter, E., Shapiro, R., Geever, E., Nagler, A., Rosenthal, M., and Levenson, S. M., in "Advances in Germfree Research and Gnotobiology," (M. Miyakawa and T. D. Luckey, eds.), The Chemical Rubber Co., Cleveland, Ohio, p. 96, (1968).
8. Shapiro, R., Rosenthal, N. A., and Gold, B. K., *J. Nutr. 97:* 389 (1969).
9. Greenstein, J. P., Birnbaum, S. M., Winitz, M., and Otey, M. C., *Arch. Biochem. Biophys. 72:* 396 (1957).

NITROGEN METABOLISM IN GERMFREE RATS

Etiennette Combe
Laboratoire des Metabolismes, INRA
Theix 63 — St. Genes Champanelle
France

Introduction

The purpose of this work was to investigate the nitrogen metabolism of rats as modified by the germfree environment. The use of germfree animals, in which no action of the intestinal microflora occurs, makes it possible to learn more of the digestive process which involves endogenous nitrogen secretion into the intestinal lumen.

It has been shown (1-4) that the daily fecal nitrogen excretion is higher in germfree than in conventional rats. In the present study, nitrogen balance and the amino acid composition of feces excreted by both groups of animals were investigated. The results were related to published (5) amino acid composition of cecal contents of germfree and conventional rats.

Methods

Eight germfree and 10 conventional, two month old male, rats were housed individually in stainless steel metabolism cages which allowed immediate separation of feces and urine. They received steam sterilized L 356 diet and water *ad libitum.* Food consumption, fecal and urinary excretion, as well as body weight, were recorded daily for two consecutive periods of six and five days (periods A and B).

Results

Table I shows the results of the second period (B), when it is reasonable to assume that the animals were accustomed to their new housing. Growth and food intake were similar in both germfree and conventional environments. However, differences occurred in fecal excretion; germfree rats excreted more material (dry matter and water) than conventional rats.

Samples of food, feces and urine of both groups were pooled for each period to allow determination of nitrogen (Kjeldhall) and total amino acids

TABLE I. Daily Growth, Food Intake, Fecal Excretion (g/day) in Germfree and
Conventional Rats, All Males, Fed L 356 *Ad Libitum*

Environment	Germfree	Conventional
No. of Animals	8	10
Body Weight	196 +6*	190 + 6
Growth	3.3 + 0.4	2.7 + 0.5
Food Intake	16.1 + 1.4	18.1 + 0.6
Fecal Excretion	2.64 + 0.21	2.04 + 0.15

*Mean + standard deviation.

(Moore and Stein, chromatography, after hydrolysis). Results given in Table II show that, when daily nitrogen ingestion was similar, fecal nitrogen excretion was higher in the germfree group. As a result, apparent digestibility of nitrogen was lower in germfree rats than in conventional rats. It is of interest to note that nitrogenous losses via urine were more important in the conventional than in the germfree group.

TABLE II. Nitrogen Metabolism in Germfree and Conventional Rats, All Males,
Fed L 356 *Ad Libitum* for Two Periods of 6 (A) and 5 (B) Days

Nitrogen mg/rat/day	Germfree		Conventional	
	A	B	A	B
Intake	617	581*	619	640
Fecal	120	159	92	94
Urinary	240	251	292	335
Apparent Digestibility (%)	80.5	72.6	85.1	85.3

*Germfree rats show an abnormal nutritional behavior in the B period. These results were not used to draw our general conclusions.

Apparent digestibility was calculated for each amino acid (Table III). Apparent digestibility of most amino acids appeared to be lower in the germfree environment; this was characteristic for tyrosine, serine, threonine and cystine. Conversely, the apparent digestibility of methionine was higher in the germfree than in the conventional gut. Some amino acids seem to have the same digestibility in both cases: these were valine, alanine, isoleucine and leucine, phenylalanine and lysine. The lower apparent digestibility of the amino acids in germfree rats may be relevant to the lack of reabsorption of nitrogenous compounds of digestive origin, such as pancreatic enzymes (6), mucoproteins (7), and desquamations.

In Table IV, the per cent amino acid composition of feces from germfree

306

TABLE III. Apparent Digestibility of Amino Acids (%) in Germfree and Conventional Rats, Fed L 356 *Ad Libitum*

Period	Germfree		Conventional	
	A	B*	A	B
Threonine	82.2	77.3	86.4	85.7
Serine	77.4	72.5	81.2	81.9
Alanine	86.9	84.6	84.6	84.7
Valine	90.3	87.7	89.3	88.9
Cystine	50.0	38.5	53.8	55.6
Methionine	90.7	89.6	87.9	86.7
Isoleucine	87.6	84.2	85.7	85.2
Leucine	92.6	90.6	90.9	90.9
Tyrosine	84.2	78.6	89.9	89.1
Phenylalanine	94.3	92.6	93.7	92.9
Lysine	90.6	85.8	90.8	91.1

*Germfree rats show an abnormal nutritional behavior in the B period. These results were not used to draw our general conclusions.

and conventional rats was compared to the per cent amino acid composition of insoluble materials from cecal contents. Amino acid composition differed only slightly in germfree and conventional feces. However, when a microflora — which is particularly poor in histidine — is present, the proportion of histidine in the feces was smaller. In the feces from germfree rats, the proportions of lysine, arginine and leucine were characteristic of amino acid composition of desquamations; the proportions of threonine and serine were similar to those of mucoproteins and pancreatic enzymes. These characteristics agree with those given previously for the amino acid composition of insoluble material from germfree cecal content.

TABLE IV. Amino Acid Composition (% of Total Measured Amino Acids) in Cecal Insoluble Material and in the Feces of Germfree and Conventional Rats Fed L 356 *Ad Libitum*

Amino Acids	Germfree			Conventional		
	Cecum*		Feces	Cecum*		Feces
	II	III	Total	II	III	Total
Threonine	8.2	5.6	5.3	3.9	5.0	4.4
Serine	12	7.0	8.9	14.1	6.0	8.0
Isoleucine	4.7	5.0	5.0	7.3	5.6	6.3
Leucine	4.2	8.7	5.3	3.1	8.4	6.9
Lysine	6.8	4.0	5.0	7.3	5.4	5.2
Histidine	2.2	2.2	1.9	1.9	2.2	1.8
Arginine	3.6	5.8	3.3	2.1	5.2	3.8

*Amino acids in cecum are calculated from Combe and Pion (5) in alcohol soluble — TCA insoluble material (fraction II) and alcohol — TCA insoluble material (fraction III).

Threonine, which is one of the essential amino acids, appeared to be less digestible in the germfree rat. It is a constituent of proteins and mucoproteins of endogenous origin, which were not attacked in the germfree rat, due to the lack of microbial degradation. Its proportion to the other amino acids was higher in the germfree than in the conventional feces and cecal contents.

Conclusions

Absence of a conventional microflora caused many modifications in the nitrogen metabolism of rats. It appeared that the pathways of excretion were modified. More nitrogen left the organism through the digestive tract than by other paths of excretion. It can be said also that the microflora plays an important part in the small intestine by degrading digestive enzymes, muco-proteins, and desquamations, and by utilizing the constituents for its own metabolic purpose. The similarity of the amino acid composition of feces as compared to that of cecal contents, however, does not completely exclude any digestive process (including absorption, etc.) along the large intestine.

References

1. Levenson, S. M., and Tennant, B., *Fed. Proc. 22:* 109 (1963).
2. Evrard, E., Hoet, P. P., Eyssen, H., Charlier, H., Sacquet, E., *Brit. J. Exp. Path. 45:* 409 (1964).
3. Luckey, T. D., *Ernahrungsforschung 10:* 191 (1965).
4. Hoskins, L. C., and Zamcheck, N., *Gastroenterology 54:* 210 (1968).
5. Combe, E., and Pion, R., *Ann. Biol. Anim., Bioch., Biophys. 6:* 255 (1966).
6. Corring, T., and Jung, J., *Nutr. Rep. Intern.* 6 (In Press).
7. Werner, J., *Acta Soc. Med. Upsala 58:* 1 (1953).

ELECTRON MICROSCOPIC STUDIES ON CARDIAC LESIONS IN GERMFREE AND CONVENTIONAL RATS FED DIET DEFICIENT IN VITAMIN B$_1$

Yukiko Sumi and *Junpei Asai*
Nagoya University School of Medicine, Nagoya

and

Masasumi Miyakawa, Masami Arakawa and *Masanori Kanzaki*
Laboratory of Germfree Life Research, Kawashima, Japan

Introduction

It has been generally accepted that flora-synthesized thiamine was not utilized by the host fed a complete diet but had some contribution to the host fed a thiamine-deficient diet through the secondary passage following coprophagy. This paper describes the influence of the flora-synthesized thiamine upon cardiac lesions of acute thiamine deficiency.

Materials and Methods

Three groups of male rats of Wistar origin were employed in this experiment. The first group consisted of germfree male rats established by hand-feeding at the Laboratory of Germfree Life Research, Kawashima, Japan. The second group consisted of conventional male rats with a tail cup designed to prevent coprophagy absolutely; these animals were called cupped rats. The third group consisted of conventional male rats without a tail cup, and were called non-cupped rats. The tail cup used in this experiment was made of glass in the shape of swellfish. It had a wide opening at the proximal end and a narrow one at the distal end. At the distal end the cup was attached on the tail with a needle. Each cupped rat was placed in a cage 10 x 20 x 15 cm with a rough meshed screen-bottom. At the time of necropsy, it was determined that the stomach of the cupped rats had no signs of coprophagy, whereas the stomach of the non-cupped conventional rats contained a considerable amount of feces. These three groups of rats were placed on a thiamine-deficient diet at the age of 35 days, and were reared for 23 or 28 days. The composition of the deficient-diet was shown in Table I. The experimental diet was steam-sterilized

TABLE I. Composition of Experimental Diet (100 gm)

Casein (vitamin-free)	23.0 gm
Corn starch	63.4 gm
Salts mix.	3.0 gm
Cellophane	3.0 gm
Corn oil (including fat soluble vitamin)	7.0 gm
Thiamine HCl (omitted)	6.0 mg
Riboflavin	3.0 mg
Nicotinamide	12.0 mg
Ca. pantothenate	30.0 mg
Choline HCl	250.0 mg
Pyridoxine HCl	4.0 mg
Biotin	1.0 mg
Folic acid	1.0 mg
Vitamin B12 (0.1%)	25.0 mg
PABA	2.5 mg
Inositol	100.0 mg
Ascorbic acid	200.0 mg

for 25 minutes at 121°C. The controls consisted of germfree and conventional rats fed a complete diet. All animals were weighed daily throughout the experimental period. On the 23rd or 28th day of thiamine-deficient period, some animals in each group were killed, and the hearts and the gastric and cecal contents were removed, weighed and the thiamine level was measured by thiochrome method modified by M. Fujiwara (6). The hearts were prepared for the light microscopic examination following a routine procedure. For the electron microscopic examination, auricular tissues were fixed in 4% glutaladehyde solution with sodium cacodylate buffer and post fixed in 2% osmium tetraoxide. The glycerol extraction treatment method was used to observe the pure actomyosin system. Following the ordinary electron microscopic procedure, the preparations were observed with an electron microscope Hitachi H58 apparatus. The remaining rats in all three experimental groups were observed until the death due to acute thiamine deficiency. Mitochondria of the heart were prepared by digestion of the heart muscle with Nagarse (bacterial proteolytic enzyme) by the method of Hatefi *et al.* (4) as modified by Ozawa (5). Electron micrographs of the samples were taken to test the mitochondrial population in the preparations. The uptake of oxygen was measured at 25°C with a Clark-type electrode (Beckman Co.). The experiments were carried out in a medium (5 ml) which contained 0.3 M mannitol, 10 mM KCl, 10 mM KH_2PO_4, 2.5 mM $MgCl_2$, 0.25 mM EDTA and 5 mM Tris-Cl. The pH was 7.4. Sodium succinate (10 mM) and ADP (0.2 mM) were added to the reaction mixture for oxidative phosphorylation. The rate of respiration in the presence of ADP divided by the rate in its absence was defined as the respiratory control index (RCI).

The control germfree and conventional male rats fed on a complete diet

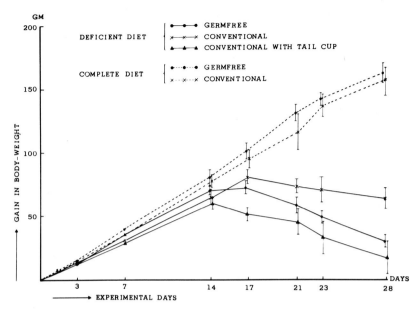

FIG. 1. Growth curves of germfree and conventional rats fed a thiamine-deficient diet and a complete diet.

were also subjected to the examinations described above.

Results

Growth. Figure 1 presents the growth curves of the three groups of rats on the thiamine-deficient diet and the two control groups on a complete diet. Although the body weight of the control germfree and conventional rats increased smoothly, all the rats on the thiamine-deficient diet lost weight after the 14th to 17th day. In these deficient rats, the weight loss was greater in the germfree and cupped conventional rats than in the non-cupped conventional rats with access to their feces. No significant difference was found in the weight loss between germfree and cupped conventional rats.

Survival days. After thiamine-deficient feeding had started, non-cupped conventional rats lived 48 to 59 days, germfree rats 32 to 38 days, and cupped rats 31 to 35 days. It was noteworthy that the non-cupped conventional rats, having access to their feces, lived longer than the rats of the other two groups.

Total thiamine in cecal and gastric contents. Total thiamine was measured in the contents of the cecum and the stomach of rats fed on a thiamine-deficient diet for 23 or 28 days. More thiamine was detected in the cecal contents of the cupped and non-cupped conventional rats with an intestinal flora than in the germfree rats (Table II). This suggested that thiamine was synthesized by the

TABLE II. Total Thiamine in Cecal and Stomach Contents of Germfree and Conventional Rats Fed A Thiamine-Deficient Diet

	Cecal Contents (μg/total cecal content/rat)		Stomach Contents (μg/total stomach content/rat)
	23 days	28 days	23 days
Germfree	0.47 + 0.02* (7)**	0.49 + 0.04 (10)	0.17 + 0.04 (5)
Cupped conventional	2.61 + 0.78 (7)	2.00 + 0.78 (10)	0.46 + 0.29 (5)
Non-cupped conventional	5.97 + 0.62 (7)	4.98 + 0.64 (10)	2.00 + 1.13 (7)

*Standard deviation
**Number of rats in sample

intestinal flora. It was also presumed that coprophagy had some influence on the flora-synthesized thiamine, since the total thiamine level was higher in the cecal contents of the non-cupped rats than in the cupped rats prevented from coprophagy. In the stomach contents of the thiamine-deficient rats, the germfree rats had an almost negligible amount of thiamine, the cupped conventional rats had a slightly higher value, while non-cupped conventional rats had a much higher value (Table II).

Total thiamine in the heart. The hearts of non-cupped conventional rats on a thiamine-deficient diet for 23 or 28 days had more thiamine than either germfree or cupped conventional thiamine-deficient rats (Table III). In the control animals on a complete diet, there was no significant difference between

TABLE III. Total Thiamine Levels in the Hearts of Germfree and Conventional Rats Fed A Thiamine-Deficient Diet for 23 and 28 Days and A Complete Diet (μg/total heart/rat).

	Thiamine-Deficient Diet		Complete Diet
	23 days	28 days	
Germfree	0.47 + 0.04* (7)**	0.31 + 0.03 (10)	8.71 + 0.44 (5)
Cupped conventional	0.41 + 0.07 (7)	0.32 + 0.05 (10)	
Non-cupped conventional	0.71 + 0.08 (7)	0.48 + 0.06 (10)	8.93 + 0.68 (5)

*Standard deviation
**Number of rats in sample

the total thiamine levels in the hearts of germfree and conventional rats.

Electron micrographs of the heart on a thiamine deficient diet for 23 days. Although muscular degeneration and interstitial fibrosis were observed by light microscopic examination of the heart of rats on a thiamine-deficient diet, it was difficult to find the difference in grade of cardiac lesions among the three experimental groups. Therefore, electron microscopic examination was performed. A small focal lesion of auricular muscle characterized by derrangement and destruction of myofilaments was observed by the electron micrograph of the heart of germfree rats fed on a thiamine-deficient diet for 23 days. Swelling and vacuolar degeneration of the mitochondria were found. The cupped thiamine-deficient rats had the same myofibrillar lesion characterized by derrangement and destruction of the myofilament. The mitochondria were also swollen and had partially disintegrated cristae. In the non-cupped thiamine-deficient conventional rats, the myofibrils appeared normal, although some mitochondria were swollen and had spotted clearing.

Electron micrographs of the heart on a thiamine-deficient diet for 28 days. Electron micrographs of auricular muscles of germfree thiamine-deficient rats revealed disruption and derrangement of the myofilaments accompanied with homogenized structureless masses. According to glycerol extraction treatment methods, the destruction of the actomyosin system became more evident.

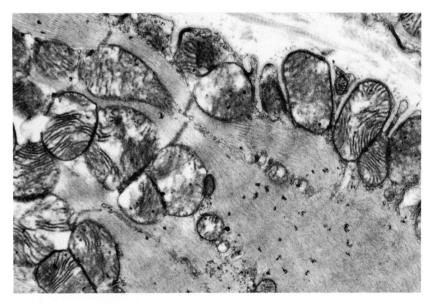

FIG. 2. Electron micrograph of the auricular muscle of a germfree rat fed a thiamine-deficient diet for 28 days. X 19,500. Note the disruption and derrangement of myofilament.

313

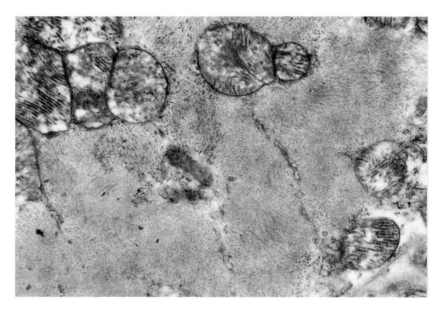

FIG. 3. Electron micrograph of the auricular muscle of a cupped rat fed a thiamine-deficient diet for 28 days. X 19,500. The cross section reveals the disappearance of myosin.

Mitochondria had disintegration of the cristae. These lesions of the myofibrils were widely distributed (Figure 2). Electron micrographs of the auricles of cupped, conventional thiamine-deficient rats had the same grade of myofibrillar disruption and a similar distribution of the cardiac lesions as in germfree rats. Myosin was not present in the cross section. Swelling, dissolution and disintegration of cristae were observed in mitochondria, some of which fell into cystic degeneration (Figure 3), whereas electron micrographs of the auricles of non-cupped thiamine-deficient conventional rats showed less myofibrillar lesions as compared to the germfree and cupped thiamine-deficient rats. The area of myofibrillar changes were not wide, and the sarcomeres appeared normal, although some of the mitochondria were slightly swollen and had partial dissociation of the cristae (Figure 4).

Oxygen uptake of mitochrondria. In the presence of succinate, no significant difference was found in the rate of oxygen uptake of the mitochondria prepared from rats under the various conditions. In the presence of both succinate and ADP, however, the mitochondria prepared from either thiamine-deficient germfree or cupped conventional rats had a lower rate of oxygen uptake than those of the controls and thiamine-deficient, non-cupped conventional rats. A low respiratory control index was noticed in the cases of thiamine-deficient, germfree and cupped conventional rats. From these results it might be considered that the mitochondria were loosely coupled in oxidative

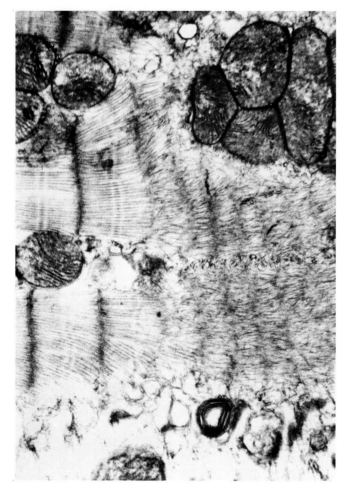

FIG. 4. Longitudinal section of the auricular muscle of a non-cupped rat fed a thiamine-deficient diet for 28 days. X 22,000. Myofibrillar changes are not as marked as compared to Figs. 2 and 3.

phosphorylation when germfree and cupped conventional rats were fed on a thiamine-deficient diet (Table IV).

Conclusions

1) The total thiamine content was higher in the hearts of non-cupped conventional rats fed a thiamine-deficient diet for 23 days or 28 days than in those of both germfree and cupped conventional rats fed a deficient diet for the

315

TABLE IV. Respiration of Heart Mitochondria In Rats Fed A Thiamine-Deficient Diet for 28 Days

Animals	Condition	$-\triangle 0$ mμ atoms/min/mg protein		RCI*
		Succinate	Succinate and ADP	
Germfree	Deficient	91	127	1.39
	Control	96	217	2.23
Conventional	Non-cupped deficient	97	184	1.90
	Cupped deficient	93	147	1.58
	Control	108	238	2.22

*Respiratory Control Index

same period.

2) Electron microscopic evaluation of the heart of rats fed a deficient diet for 23 or 28 days showed that non-cupped conventional rats had less destruction of myofilament than germfree rats and cupped conventional rats prevented from coprophagy.

3) The mitochondria of the heart might be loosely coupled in oxidative phosphorylation in germfree and cupped conventional rats fed a thiamine-deficient diet.

References

1. Wostmann, B. S., Knight, P. L., and Kan, D. F., *Ann. N.Y. Acad. Sci. 98:* 516 (1962).
2. Ashburn, L. L., and Lowry, J. V., *Arch. Path. 37:* 27 (1944).
3. Hackel, D. B., Goodale, W. T., and Kleinerman, J., *Am. Heart J. 46:* 883 (1953).
4. Hatefi, Y., Jurtshuk, P., and Haavik, A. G., *Arch. Biochem. Biophys. 94:* 148 (1961).
5. Ozawa, T., *Arch. Biochem. Biophys. 117:* 201 (1966).
6. Fujiwara, M., *Vitamin (Jap.) 9:* 148 (1955).

THE ROLE OF UREA IN THE HYPERAMMONEMIA OF ECK FISTULA DOGS

Francis C. Nance, Henry J. Kaufman and *David G. Kline*
Department of Surgery, Louisiana State University School of Medicine
New Orleans, Louisiana 70112, U.S.A.

Introduction

In a previous paper we reported that germfree dogs with Eck fistulas develop hepatic encephalopathy (1). These animals had histologic and bio-chemical evidence of hyperammonemia and exhibited the clinical symptoms of hepatic coma. In a subsequent paper we reported that after ingestion of a blood meal, germfree dogs with Eck fistulas had marked increases in blood ammonia as great as observed in conventional Eck fistula dogs (2). The present experiment was designed to assess the possible role of urea hydrolysis in the hyper-ammonemia of germfree Eck fistula dogs and to determine the presence or absence of a non-bacterial endogenous urease in the gastrointestinal tract of the dog.

Materials and Methods

Conventional dogs used in these experiments were mongrels of both sexes obtained from the L.S.U. Animal Care Facility. All had received a single injection of penicillin and streptomycin during a two-week period of quarantine prior to use but no antibiotics were administered subsequently.

Germfree dogs were purebred adult beagles of both sexes obtained from the L.S.U. Germfree Facility. The animals were Cesarean delivered into flexible film isolators and hand-fed with sterile synthetic bitchs' milk until weaning. Techniques of rearing germfree dogs have been previously published by Heneghan (3). All animals were fed chow containing 22% protein. The chow was heat-sterilized and supplemented with filter-sterilized vitamins.

Weekly cultures of fresh stool specimens were obtained to monitor the bacteriologic status of germfree animals. In addition, terminal cultures were obtained from all animals that died or were sacrificed prior to removal from the isolators.

End-to-side portacaval shunts were performed in 8 germfree and 10 conventional dogs under pentabarbital anesthesia. Conventional animals received from 250-500 ml of normal saline i.v. at the time of operation. Germfree animals were given 250 ml of low-molecular weight dextran during the operation to prevent clotting of the anastomosis.

All of the animals were allowed at least 2 weeks to recover from surgery before urea ingestion studies were performed.

Urea tolerance tests were carried out in a manner similar to that employed for blood ingestion. Fasting germfree and conventional dogs with and without Eck fistulas were sedated with propiopromazine 1 hour prior to study. After withdrawing a control venous blood sample for blood ammonia, an orogastric tube was passed into the stomach and 40 g of urea dissolved in 200 ml of sterile water was administered. At intervals of 3 and 6 hours following ingestion, venous blood samples were again obtained and analyzed for blood ammonia levels. Animals were given water *ad lib* following the ingestion of urea.

The Eck fistulas were inspected for patency in all animals at the time of sacrifice or necropsy. Six conventional dogs survived with patent shunts for 22 to 266 days. Six germfree dogs survived for 16 to 166 days. All dogs surviving the surgery developed signs of portasystemic encephalopathy and had hyperammonemia.

Blood ammonia levels were measured by the Hyland ion exchange resin technique.

Results

A total of 9 urea tolerance studies were performed in the 6 conventional animals with patent shunts. All developed massive rises in blood ammonia ranging from 125-681% of control values (Table I). Two conventional animals died in coma during the tests. A mean peak rise in blood ammonia of 416% over control levels was observed.

TABLE I. Changes In Blood Ammonia After Urea Ingestion Shunted Conventional Dogs

Animal No.	Control Ammonia $\mu g\%$	Peak Ammonia $\mu g\%$	Percent Change
727	40.5	300.0	+641.0
450	123.2	739.0	+500.0
904	300.0	675.0	+125.0
904	375.0	499.5	+033.0
148	330.0	1995.0*	+505.0
42	195.0	915.0	+369.0
42	225.0	1290.0	+473.0
42	189.0	720.0	+396.0
463	240.0	1875.0*	+681.0

*Died in Coma   Mean Change: 415.88%

TABLE II. Changes In Blood Ammonia After Urea Ingestion Shunted Germfree Dogs

Animal No.	Control Ammonia μg%	Peak Ammonia μg%	Percent Change μg%
1439	169.5	192.0	+13.0
1440	129.0	195.0	+51.0
1457	126.0	150.0	+19.0
1457	270.0	195.0	−28.0
1457	255.0	375.0	+47.0
1459	69.0	81.0	+17.0
1459	337.5	255.0	−24.0
1445	210.0	138.0	−34.0
1454	225.0	225.0	−00.0
1454	150.0	165.0	+10.0
1454	300.0	270.0	−10.0

Mean Change: 5.55%

Eleven urea tolerance tests were performed in the 6 germfree animals with patent Eck fistulas. Changes in blood ammonia ranged from −34% to +51% in the six hours after urea ingestion. The mean peak change observed in all tests was +5.6% (Table II).

Germfree animals experienced little or no increase in blood ammonia after urea ingestion. Conventional animals experienced a massive increase. Data from all urea tolerance studies are summarized in Figure 1.

Discussion

Our previous observations that hepatic encephalopathy could occur in the germfree Eck fistula dog have lead us to explore the possible sources of ammonia in the absence of a gastrointestinal flora. One obvious source is the kidney but this mechanism would seem inadequate to explain the marked hyperammonemia observed. The rises in blood ammonia we observed after ingestion of a blood meal indicated that there are sufficient endogenous non-bacterial enzymes within the gastrointestinal tract to hydrolyze dietary proteins to ammonia. That considerable ammonia production occurs in the gut is attested to by our unpublished observations of very high levels of ammonia (in excess of 1000 μg%) in the ileocolic vein of germfree animals. The present experiment was undertaken to evaluate yet another possible cause of hyperammonemia, i.e., hydrolysis of urea by mucosal ureases in the gut.

The presence of ureases in the gastric mucosa of a number of vertebrates was first reported by Luck (4). Since that time several investigators have explored the possibility that a mucosal urease was produced in the stomach or elsewhere in the gastrointestinal tract. It has long been recognized that fully half

319

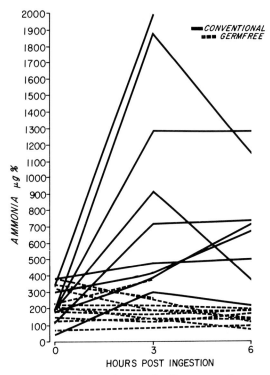

FIG. 1. Blood ammonia after urea meal.

of the bacterial species residing in the gastrointestinal tract are capable of hydrolyzing urea and this fact has greatly complicated efforts to prove the presence of endogenous non-bacterial urease. All investigators have agreed that the mucosal urease, if present, is located in the cells near the surface of the mucosa. The ubiquitous presence of urease producing bacteria has made all efforts at measuring urease activity suspect.

Kornberg and Davies (5) in their review and Dintzis and Hastings (6) in their experiments concluded, mainly on the basis of the effects of antibiotics on urease activity, that there were no mucosal ureases present in the animals they studied. Conway (7) has vigorously rejected these conclusions and reported significant urease activity in the surface epithelial cells of the mouse stomach. Fleshler and Gabuzda (8), in a careful clinical study, favored the concept that a non-bacterial urease was present in the stomach of patients. Belding and Kern (9) thought, on the basis of their studies in cats, that a mucosal urease must be present although they were unable to demonstrate urease activity in fetal gastric mucosa. Summerskill and co-workers (10, 11) in a number of clinical studies have concluded that there are probably significant mucosal ureases in humans but they were careful to point out the possibility of bacterial contamination.

In the only previous study in germfree animals Levenson (12) administered radioactively labelled urea to rats. The urea was given subcutaneously to 4 animals and intragastricly to one. The breakdown rate of urea in germfree animals was less than 1% that observed in conventional animals. Levenson concluded that no endogenous ureases were present in the rat.

On the basis of our experiments we conclude that there are no non-bacterial ureases in the dog. The evidence seems clear: little or no increase in blood ammonia was observed in our germfree Eck fistula animals after urea was given.

This conclusion does not invalidate present clinical approaches to the therapy of portasystemic encephalopathy. These measures are directed mainly towards bacterial ureases and it is clear that they play a large role in the hyperammonemia of conventional Eck fistula dogs and in humans with portasystemic shunts.

An important aspect of our observations is that there are considerable enzymatic pathways capable of producing large quantities of ammonia from ingested protein in the germfree animal. Efforts at treatment of hepatic coma must include something more than alteration of the bacterial flora since it is clear that the gastrointestinal tract is quite capable of making ammonia without the help of bacteria.

Summary

1) Previous observations that germfree dogs develop hyperammonemia and encephalopathy after portacaval shunts have been confirmed.

2) Conventional dogs with Eck fistulas developed massive rises in blood ammonia after ingesting 40 grams of urea.

3) Germfree dogs with Eck fistulas developed minimal changes in blood ammonia after ingesting 40 grams of urea.

4) The hyperammonemia of germfree Eck fistula dogs is **not** due to the presence of an endogenous non-bacterial urease.

Acknowledgements

Supported by U.S.P.H.S. Grant No. A1-10095-01 and by Grant No. RR-00272.

The considerable technical help of Mrs. Dianne P. Hines is gratefully acknowledged.

References

1. Nance, F. C., and Kline, D. G., *Ann. Surg. 174:* 856 (1971).

2. Nance, F. C., Batson, R. C., and Kline, D. G., *Surg. 70:* 169 (1971).
3. Heneghan, J. B., Floyd, C. F., and Cohn, I. Jr., *J. Surg. Res. 6:* 24 (1966).
4. Luck, J. M., *Biochem. J. 18:* 825 (1924).
5. Kornberg, H. L., and Davies, R. E., *Physiol. Events. 35:* 169 (1955).
6. Dintzis, R. Z., and Hastings, A. B., *Proc. Nat. Acad. Sc. 39:* 571 (1953).
7. Conway, E. J., Fitzgerald, O., McGeeney, K., and Geoghegan, F., *Gastroenterology 57:* 449 (1959).
8. Fleshler, B., and Gabuzda, G. J., *Gut. 6:* 349 (1965).
9. Belding, M. E., and Kern, F. Jr., *J. Lab. Clin. Med. 61:* 560 (1963).
10. Summerskill, W. H. J., and Wolpert, E., *Am. J. Clin. Nutr. 23:* 636 (1970).
11. Aoyagi, T., Engstrom, G. W., Evans, W. B., and Summerskill, W. H. J., *Gut. 7:* 631 (1966).
12. Levenson, S. M., Crowley, L. V., Horowitz, R. E., and Malm, O. J., *Science 234:* 2061 (1959).

SECTION VII

MICROBIOLOGY: INFECTIOUS DISEASES AND ANTIBIOTICS

HISTOPATHOLOGICAL AND BIOCHEMICAL RESPONSES OF GERMFREE AND CONVENTIONAL MICE WITH SALMONELLA INFECTION

Atsushi Ozawa and *Jinsaku Goto*
Department of Bacteriology
The Second Tokyo National Hospital

and

Yasushi Ito and *Hisao Shibata*
Department of Internal Medicine
The Second Tokyo National Hospital
Tokyo, Japan

Introduction

We have investigated, by sequential analysis, the histopathological changes which occur in the gut mucosa subsequent to the invasion by *Salmonella typhimurium* LT-2 in DKI mice, an inbred strain susceptible to *Salmonella enteritidis* infection. Furthermore, host responses to the superinfection of *Salmonella typhimurium* in antibiotic treated DKI mice repopulated by autochthonous *Escherichia coli* were investigated from the viewpoints of: bacterial multiplication, bacterial invasion, and histological findings in the intestinal epithelium by using bacteriological fluorescent antibody, and light microscopy techniques. Our investigations were also designed to study the role of enteric bacterial flora upon the host by comparing germfree mice with gnotobiotic mice monocontaminated with *E. coli* or *S. typhimurium* and conventional mice.

While the constancy of the "normal" enteric flora and its resistance to superinfection has been observed frequently, little is known about the underlying mechanisms.

Results

The sequential analysis of DKI mice challenged with *S. typhimurium LT-2.*
DKI mice challenged orally with 9×10^8 organisms of *S. typhimurium* usually succumbed within 7-9 days to a systemic infection with septicemia. The cecum

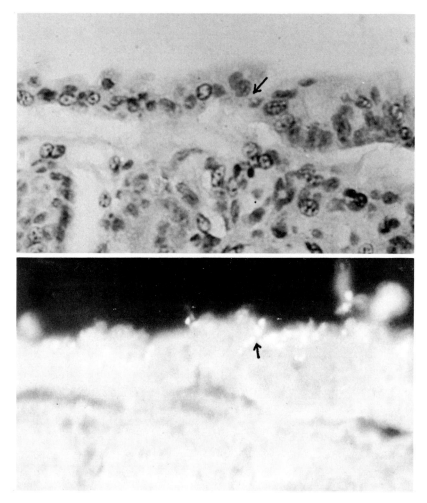

FIG. 1. A few fluorescing bacilli start to invade into the intestinal mucosa of the cecum by passing through or between epithelial cells at 6 hours after oral challenge with *S. typhimurium.* Arrows indicate fluorescing bacilli invading by passing between epithelial cells. Magnification: 400X

and large intestine were regarded as the primary sites of bacterial multiplication and bacterial invasion of orally administered *S. typhimurium* LT-2. This was determined by a sequential quantitative estimation of the number of bacteria recovered from the upper small intestine, lower small intestine, cecum, upper large intestine and lower large intestine.

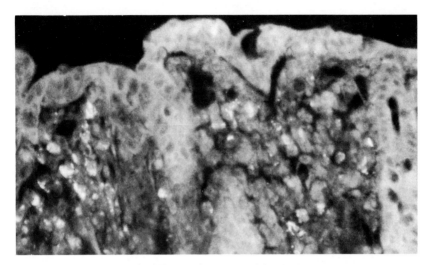

FIG. 2. Massive fluorescing bacilli were demonstrated in the lamina propria of the large intestine. Magnification: 300X

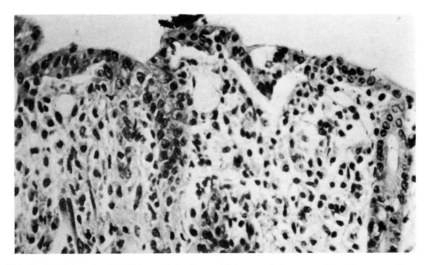

FIG. 3. Lamina propria of large intestine which revealed macrophage type reactions. Magnification: 300X

A few bacilli reached lamina propria by passing through or between epithelial cells at 6-24 hours after challenge and were engulfed by macrophages. This initiated the inflammatory responses with pyknosis, vacuolation and hyperplasia of epithelial cells (Fig. 1).

327

The marked invasion of fluorescing organisms into the lamina propria after 24 hours revealed the development of these histopathological changes: epithelial denudation which was characterized by macrophage accumulation, cellular infiltration which consisted of neutrophils in the intestinal mucosa, alterations of the crypt epithelium and edema in the submucosa (Figs. 2 and 3).

In general, bacterial multiplication, histological changes and the number of fluorescing bacilli in the epithelium of the small intestine were minor as compared with the inflammatory responses and number of invading fluorescing bacilli in the cecum and large intestine.

The sequential analysis of DKI mice superinfected with *S. typhimurium* **after introducing** *E. coli.* When 1.2×10^9 cells of *S. typhimurium* were administered orally to the DKI mice pretreated with 9×10^8 organisms of *E. coli,* the number of salmonella recovered from upper small intestine steadily fell for 48 hours following *S. typhimurium* inoculation. The multiplication of salmonella in cecum and large intestine of the mice inoculated with *E. coli* was partly suppressed by the presence of *E. coli,* as compared with the results obtained in the DKI mice monoinfected with *S. typhimurium.* These results suggest that bacterial persistence of *E. coli* in the gut lumen may be responsible for elimination of *S. typhimurium* from the gut.

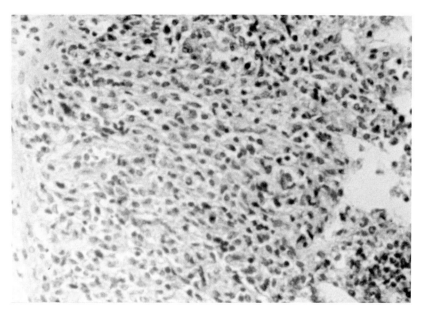

FIG. 4. Exudative inflammatory reactions which accompanied the infiltration of neutrophils were manifested in the large intestine 8 days after monocontamination of germfree mice with *S. typhimurium.* Magnification: 400X

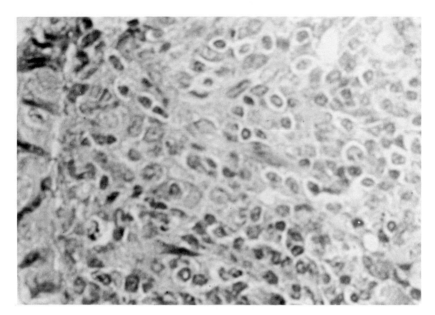

FIG. 5. Proliferative inflammatory lesions were demonstrated in the large intestine 12 days after monocontamination of germfree mice with *S. typhimurium*. Magnification: 400X

Ten to 72 hours after superinfection, a few fluorescing organisms of *S. typhimurium* characterized certain responses of the intestinal epithelium to the bacterial invasion. The inflammatroy reactions appeared 48 hours after infection. During the first 72 hours, numerous free organisms were seen in the gut lumen. At 72 — 96 hours after challenge, histological alterations in the mucosa of the cecum and large intestine were characterized by thickening of the lamina propria due to the accumulation of macrophage type of cells, lymphocytes, neutrophils and a mild epithelial desquamation.

The histological and biochemical studies on germfree mice, gnotobiotic mice monocontaminated with *E. coli* or *S. typhimurium*, and various conventional mice. Eight days after monocontamination of germfree mice with *S. typhimurium,* the histological changes in cecum and large intestine revealed exudative inflammatory reactions limited to the mucosa and submucosa rather than proliferative reaction. The proliferative reactions became evident at 12 days after monocontamination of germfree mice with *S. typhimurium* (Figs. 4 and 5).

Twelve days after monocontamination of germfree mice with *S. typhimurium,* no fluorescing bacilli were demonstrated in the epithelium and lumen of upper small intestine. At this stage a few fluorescing organisms which had invaded into the intestinal mucosa were demonstrated in the cecum and large intestine, despite massive numbers of fluorescing bacilli in the gut lumen.

The alkaline phosphatase activity, neutral fat and kunkel test on the sera obtained from conventional mice exhibited higher values than the germfree mice. Electrophoretic analyses on the sera derived from the mice sacrificed at 12 days after monocontamination of germfree mice with *S. typhimurium* demonstrated an increase of α_2 globulin and immunoglobulins as compared with those obtained in germfree mice and gnotobiotic mice monocontaminated with *E. coli*.

Conclusions

The present investigations have demonstrated that the primary sites of bacterial multiplication and bacterial invasion of *S. typhimurium* into the gut mucosa were the cecum and upper large intestine. Salmonella was capable of invading the mucosa by passing through or between epithelial cells. Epithelial desquamation of the mucosa may have been elicited by the disturbance of intestinal microcirculation subsequent to the proliferative reactions which accompanied macrophage accumulation in the lamina propria. The suppression of the development of histopathological lesions in the intestinal mucosa and bacterial invasion into the epithelial mucosa at earlier stages of *S. typhimurium* infection was ascribed to the presence of *E. coli* in its microflora. It would appear that the mechanisms in the development of histological lesions and bacterial invasion should be considered different from those of bacterial multiplication in the gut lumen. This emphasizes that studies on the role of the indigenous enteric flora in host reactions should be investigated in general aspects which include bacteriological, histological, histochemical and physiological evaluations.

STUDIES ON THE PATHOGENESIS OF *CANDIDA ALBICANS* BY THE USE OF GERMFREE MICE

Kazuo Iwata, Tatsuo Nagai and *Tatsuo Ikeda*
Department of Microbiology, Faculty of Medicine
University of Tokyo, Bunkyo-ku
Tokyo, Japan

and

Masahiko Okudaira
Department of Pathology
Kitasato University School of Medicine
Sagamiohno, Kanagawa-ken, Japan

Introduction

A few studies have been made on candida infections using germfree mice (1-3) and chicks (4, 5) and on diassociation with bacteria, *Escherichia coli* or *Streptococcus faecalis* (5, 6).

In view of the difficulties involved in the colonization of *Candida albicans* in the gastrointestinal tract of conventional animals by oral inoculation, a new line of germfree mice was used to examine the pathogenesis in relation to the morphogenesis and histopathology of the fungus. Another attempt, using germfree mice, was made to clarify the mechanism of opportunistic infections which are often caused by this fungus during treatment with antibacterial antibiotics in bacterial infections and by other factors such as steroids, in relation to diassociation with shigella.

Materials and Methods

Germfree mice of the CF No. 1/H strain of either sex, 5 weeks old, weighing 18 ± 1 g, which had been developed at the Hikari Plant, Takeda Chemical Industries, Ltd. (7), were employed during the present study. Rearing and experiments were carried out in plastic isolators under completely sterile conditions. *C. albicans* 6713 and *Shigella flexneri* 2a 5505 were selected as challenging organisms. For oral challenge of the former organism yeast form cells were used.

Results

PART I —Monoassociation with *C. albicans:* **Fluctuations of the number of** *C. albicans* **in the feces of germfree and conventional mice.** In conventional mice of the CF No. 1 strain which were inoculated orally with 10^7 and 10^8 viable cells of *C. albicans* per mouse, smaller numbers of organisms, $5 \times 10^3 - 5 \times 10^6/g$ (wet wt) were excreted in the feces after 24 hr. Within a few days fecal cultures from all individual animals became negative. Contrary to this, in the germfree mice which were inoculated with 10^3, 10^5 and 10^6 viable cells per mouse, a rapid increase in number of organisms was observed which reached a maximum number ($10^7 - 10^8$ cells/g) around the 10th day. The maximum plateau number was maintained up to the final day of observation, the 60th day. This result suggests that the entire intestinal canal of all animals had been colonized. The challenge, however, seemingly neither impaired the animal's health nor caused loss of body weight. Only the feces became softer.

A possible infection-enhancing effect of cortisone was investigated by using gnotobiotic mice whose tracts were colonized by challenge with *C. albicans.* Beginning 30 days after challenge with 10^3 or 10^5 viable cells of the pathogen, 0.1 mg of cortisone acetate was injected subcutaneously once a day for 25 successive days into each gnotobiotic animal. As a consequence, all animals gradually became moribund with considerable loss of body weight and diarrhea, and they succumbed approximately 8 weeks after challenge, although the number of organisms present was unchanged. This is suggestive that systemic infection developed in the hosts.

On the other hand, a possible chemotherapeutic effect of amphotericin B, an antifungal antibiotic, was tested on the course of colonization and/or infection in candida monoassociated mice. Beginning 30 days after challenge of 10^5 viable cells, 0.1 mg of the antibiotic was orally administered once a day for 25 days to each mouse. This treatment resulted in a dramatic reduction in the number of organisms in the feces, which ultimately became negative on culture. This displays evidence for an apparent healing of the infection.

Distribution of organisms in the gastrointestinal tract and various other organs of germfree mice. Every mouse in the above three experimental groups was examined for the distribution of the challenging organism in the contents obtained from different segments of the gastrointestinal canal and in the tissues of various other organs at autopsy.

The results obtained were found to be consistent with the above-mentioned data on the fluctuations of the number of organisms in the feces, as shown in Figure 1. In the group challenged with candida alone, the number of organisms in contents from every segment in the gastrointestinal canal existed at nearly the same level of $10^7 - 10^8$ cells/g (wet wt). From the upper part of the small intestine, however, a lesser number ($10^3 - 10^4$ cells/g) was noted, whereas the tissue homogenates of every other organ were negative on culture. The

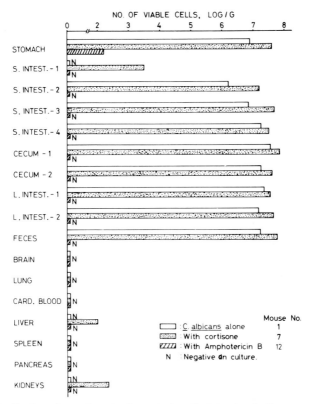

NO. OF VIABLE CELLS, LOG/G

STOMACH
S. INTEST. - 1
S. INTEST. - 2
S. INTEST. - 3
S. INTEST. - 4
CECUM - 1
CECUM - 2
L. INTEST. - 1
L. INTEST. - 2
FECES
BRAIN
LUNG
CARD. BLOOD
LIVER
SPLEEN
PANCREAS
KIDNEYS

Mouse No.
: C. albicans alone   1
: With cortisone   7
: With Amphotericin B   12
N : Negative on culture.

FIG. 1. Distribution of organisms in the gastrointestinal tract and other organs of germfree mice orally monoassociated with *C. albicans* alone, *C. albicans* with cortisone treatment, and *C. albicans* with amphotericin B administration. *C. albicans*: 6713 strain, 10^6 cells.

cortisone-treated group manifested similar results but the cultures of the spleen and kidney samples were positive upon culture with $10^2 - 10^3$ cells/g. This result indicates an apparent evidence for the development of systemic infection as described above. In contrast, the amphotericin B-administered group was found to be essentially different from the former two groups; no organisms were observed in all the specimens examined, with the exception of one mouse in whose stomach contents organisms were found in a small number (10^2 cells/g). This is also evidence for a healing process of infection.

Histopathological and morphological findings. At autopsy 8 weeks after challenge with *C. albicans*, the histopathological findings characteristic of germfree mice, particularly the digestive, hematopoietic and respiratory organs, were similar to previously reported results. Mice which were monoassociated with the pathogen alone manifested the following lesions: cell infiltration in the tissues of all the segments of the gastrointestinal tract, especially the stomach;

333

Experimental group	Results							
	Stomach		S. intest.		Cecum		L. intest.	
	L	M	L	M	L	M	L	M
Inoculation with								
C. albicans alone	++	++ / + / +	+	● / + / −	+	+ / − / −	+	++ / + / −
C. albicans plus Cortisone	##	## / + / ##	+	## / + / ##	+	## / + / +	+	## / + / ##
C. albicans plus Amphotericin B	±	+ / − / −	±	− / − / −	±	− / − / −	±	+ / − / −

L = Lesion. M = Morphogenesis; upper, yeast form; middle, germ tube form; lower, hyphal form. The grade of lesions; ###,very severe; ##,severe; #,moderate; +,slight; ± very slight; – unrecognizable. Number of organisms: ###,very many; ##,many; +,few; –,negative in culture.

FIG. 2. Summary of the histopathological and morphological findings of the gastro-intestinal tract of germfree mice monoassociated with *C. albicans* alone, with cortisone treatment, and with amphotericin B administration.

mobilization of Kupffer's cell in the liver; enlargement of follicles in the spleen; and ischemic disorder of ganglion cells in the brain. These lesions were, in general, rather moderate in grade. In the kidneys and pancreas no lesions were detected. Contrary to this, the group treated with cortisone showed a tendency toward more intensified lesions in all organs examined. In particular, the stomach was characterized by a marked proliferation of epithelial cells and a vigorous multiplication of the hyphal form of candida in the horny layer of the epithelium at a relatively limited site between the forestomach and glandular stomach with invasion into the spindle cell layer (1, 4, 5). This is indicative of the establishment of candida infection in the epithelium. The yeast-like and germ-tube forms were present in large numbers in the contents taken from the stomach, but few were present in the tissues. These forms were similarly observed at other sites of the intestinal tract, not only in this group but also in the two others. In addition, in the cortisone-treated group, hemosiderosis in the spleen, congestion in the kidneys and ischemic change of Purkinje's cell in the cerebellum were noted. On the other hand, in the amphotericin B-administered group, those lesions caused by the challenging organisms showed a tendency toward rapid healing. However, more severe hemosiderosis in the spleen was observed, which might be due to an additional side effect of the antibiotic itself. Very few poorly stained (by periodic-acid Shiff stain) or no cells of the yeast form were seen in the stomach contents. In other parts of the intestinal tract and viscera, no candida growth was observed. These findings are summarized in Figure 2.

PART II – Diassociation with *C. albicans* and *S. flexneri.* A series of experiments was carried out on diassociation of germfree mice by challenging them with *C. albicans* and *S. flexneri*. In particular the gastrointestinal tract route was selected from the above viewpoints, after confirming the possible presence of the test strain of *S. flexneri* 2a in the tract (10).

Diassociation with *C. albicans* and subsequent challenge with *S. flexneri*. To each of the mice evacuating in their feces the maximum number of candida following oral challenge of 10^3 viable cells, 10^5 cells of shigella were seeded a week later by the same route.

As shown in Figure 3, the number of shigella in the feces increased rapidly, reaching the maximum number ($10^8 - 10^9$ cells/g) around 2 weeks later. This figure was maintained for a long period of time, whereas candida gradually decreased (6). Almost similar results were obtained in the case when a smaller inoculum of shigella (10^3 cells) was used.

At autopsy, candida were not recovered upon culture or, if so, were noted in small numbers ($10^2 - 10^3$ cells/g) in the contents obtained from various segments of the gastrointestinal tract. Shigella, on the other hand, was found in much larger numbers ($10^8 - 10^9$ cells/g) as in the monoassociated group. From the upper part of the small intestine, however, organisms were cultured in small numbers (10^4 cells/g) or not at all. Invasion of either organism was not observed in any other visceral organs.

Diassociation with *S. flexneri* and subsequent challenge with *C. albicans*.

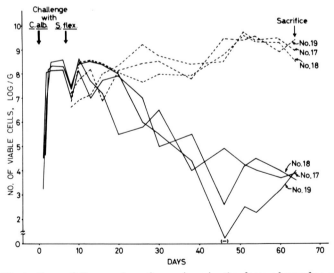

FIG. 3. Fluctuations of the number of organisms in the feces of germfree mice orally diassociated with *C. albicans* and subsequent challenge with *S. flexneri*. Organism: *C. albicans* 6713, 10^3 cells; *S. flexneri* 2a 5505, 10^5 cells.

335

In turn, the effects of diassociation were examined by reversing the order of challenge with the two organisms. Doses of 10^3 cells of shigella were followed a week later by 10^7 cells of candida. Even by introduction of such large numbers of candida cells, shigella monoflora was not affected at all. The number of candida cells increased moderately at the early stage, while maintaining a smaller plateau number for a relatively longer period than in the case of mono-association. However, the number of cells showed a tendency toward gradual reduction (6).

At autopsy, the numbers of both organisms found in the contents of the gastrointestinal canal were similar to those in the candida and shigella diassociation group described above. No organisms were demonstrated in the tissues of other organs.

Histopathological and morphological findings. Figure 4 summarizes the

Experimental group and inoculum (viable cells) per mouse	Results							
	Stomach		S. intest.		Cecum		L. intest.	
	L	M	L	M	L	M	L	M
C. alb. 10^3	++	++ / + / +	+	++ / −	+	++ / ++ / −	+	++ / −
S. flex. 10^3	−		±		±		−	
S. flex. 10^5	±		±		±		±	
C. alb. 10^3 + S. flex. 10^{3} *	++	+ / − / −	+	++ / − / −	±	+ / − / −	+	+ / − / −
C. alb. 10^3 + S. flex. 10^{5} *	±	+ / − / −	±	+ / − / −	±	+ / − / −	±	+ / − / −
C. alb. 10^3 + S. flex. 10^{3} ***	++	++ / − / −	±	+ / − / −	±	+ / − / −	±	+ / − / −
S. flex. 10^3 + C. alb. 10^{7} *	+	+ / − / −	±	+ / − / −	±	+ / − / −	±	+ / − / −
S. flex. 10^3 + C. alb. 10^{5} *	+	+ / − / −	+	+ / − / −	±	+ / − / −	+	+ / − / −
S. flex. 10^3 + C. alb. 10^{5} **	+++	++ / + / +++	+	+ / − / −	+	+ / − / −	±	+ / − / −
S. flex. 10^5 + C. alb. 10^{5} **	+++	++ / + / +++	±	+ / + / −	±	+ / + / −	±	+ / + / −
S. flex. 10^3 + C. alb. 10^{3} ***	++	++ / −	±	++ / −	±	+ / −	+	+ / −

See the footnote in **FIG. 2**

The subsequent inoculation was done after a week (*), after 5 weeks (**), and after 24 hr (***), respectively.

FIG. 4. Summary of the Histopathological and morphological findings of the gastrointestinal tract of germfree mice diassociated with *C. albicans* and *S. flexneri*. See the footnote in Figure 2. The subsequent inoculation was done after a week (*), after 5 weeks (**), and after 24 hr (***), respectively.

findings in the histopathology and morphogenesis of the mice at sacrifice in the above experiments. It should be noted that lesions, seemingly caused by candida, especially in the stomach, were more intensified by the persistence of shigella. Moreover, the predominant growth of the hyphal form of candida in the stomach epithelium was much more pronounced than in those monoassociated with the fungus and more so than in the cortisone-treated group. Neither were organisms detected in the tissues of any other viscera.

Conclusions

The CF No. 1/H strain of germfree mcie was demonstrated to be useful in colonization and infection experiments at least through oral inoculation of *C. albicans* or *S. flexneri.*

Cortisone treatment enhanced the candida infection in the hosts, whereas amphotericin B administration dramatically suppressed its colonization and/or infection.

The challenge with shigella proved to play an inhibitory role in candida colonization and/or infection in the gastrointestinal tract of gnotobiotic mice, being independent of the order of inoculation.

Morphogenesis of candida proved to be closely related to the severity of lesions in the tissues. The major site of the fungus infection was found to be the epithelium between the forestomach and glandular stomach; the infection was characterized by predominant growth of the hyphal form.

Acknowledgements

The authors are grateful to Dr. Y. Shukuda and his colleagues, the Hikari Plant, Takeda Chemical Industries, Ltd., for supplying the breeding stock of the CF No. 1/H strain.

References

1. Phillips, A. W., and Balish, E., *Appl. Microbiol. 14:* 737 (1966).
2. Iwata, K., *Proc. Jap. Med. Congr., 17th Gen. Assbl. 2:* 221 (1967).
3. Nishikawa, T., Ohnishi, N., and Sasaki, S., *Japan. J. Med. Mycol. 10:* 63 (1969).
4. Balish, E., and Phillips, A. W., *J. Bact. 91:* 1736 (1966).
5. Balish, E., and Phillips, A. W., *J. Bact. 91:* 1744 (1966).
6. Sasaki, S., *Japan. J. Bact. 25:* 79 (1970).
7. Shukuda, Y., Fujii, S., and Shibuki, M., a report at *ICLA Pacific Meeting on Laboratory Animals,* Tokyo, (1971).
8. Cherr, G. H., and Weaver, R. H., *Bact. Rev. 17:* 51 (1953).
9. Blyth, W., *Mycopath. Mycol. Appl. 10:* 269 (1959).
10. Formal, S. B., Dammin, G., Sprinz, H., Kundel, D., Schneider, H., Horowitz, R. E., Forbes, M., *J. Bact. 82:* 284 (1961).

DEVELOPMENT OF KANAMYCIN-RESISTANT *SERRATIA MARCESCENS* IN GNOTOBIOTIC MICE

George H. Bornside, Bette B. Bornside, and *Isidore Cohn, Jr.*
Department of Surgery, Louisiana State University Medical Center
New Orleans, Louisiana 70112, U.S.A.

Introduction

Gibbons and colleagues (1) have already demonstrated successful establishment and persistence in the intestinal tract of germfree mice of some fastidious bacterial species indigenous for humans. In a previous study we colonized germfree mice with a tetracycline-sensitive strain of *Staphylococcus aureus* and treated the mice with oral tetracycline (2). Colonization of germfree animals, maintained in flexible plastic isolators, with a single strain of an antibiotic-sensitive microorganism provides a unique experimental model in which to study the development of antibiotic resistance *in vivo* under controlled conditions. The gastrointestinal tract of a living animal is thus utilized as an *in vivo* pure culture system.

The results of our previous study (2) revealed that resistance developed in staphylococci following a single exposure of gnotobiotic mice to tetracycline, and that resistant staphylococci persisted for the two months of the experiment. Moreover, the isolation of tetracycline-resistant staphylococci from treated mice only, and not from untreated mice in adjacent cages within the same isolator, was of particular interest regarding clinical problems related to the transmission of hospital-acquired infections.

Serratia marcescens is one of the species of gram-negative bacteria in the family *Enterobacteriaceae* which is currently causing serious hospital-acquired infections. Although many isolates of *S. marcescens* are sensitive to kanamycin, 33 of 95 strains isolated at one hospital were found to be resistant to kanamycin, and to belong to serotypes endemic in the hospital (3). Others reported that most of their 20 strains of *S. marcescens* were resistant to kanamycin, and of these more than half resisted concentrations of kanamycin in excess of 12.5 mcg/ml (4).

Materials and Methods

Mice. A germfree line of CFW albino mice, established by Carworth Farms,

New City, N.Y., and maintained by the Louisiana State University Germfree Facility since 1963, was used. Plastic cages housing two mice were kept in flexible, plastic, germfree isolators. Initial culture for bacteria and fungi confirmed the sterility of the animals and the isolators. Weekly sterility cultures of each isolator ascertained that the strain of *S. marcescens* used for colonization was the only microorganism in the isolator and in the mice. Mice were given water and the commercial pelleted diet used at the Germfree Facility.

Antibiotic. Kanamycin sulfate (Sigma Chemical Company, St. Louis, Mo.) was used for both therapy and assay. A filter-sterilized solution (60 ml containing kanamycin at 5 mg/ml) in a rubber-stoppered bottle was passed into the isolator, and substituted for drinking water. Solutions were prepared on the same morning they were administered to the mice.

Microorganism. *S. marcescens* ATCC 274, a red pigmented strain, was used. Mice were colonized by swabbing their mouths with a broth culture which was passed into the isolator in a screw-capped tube.

Recovery of microorganisms from feces. Only fresh feces were collected for culture. The mouse was placed on the cage top within the isolator and held by the tail. A pair of cotton swabs was used to collect the fecal specimen as it was eliminated. The specimen and swabs were placed in a screw-capped tube, passed out of the isolator, and cultured immediately on blood agar and on peptone glycerol (PG) agar (5g/l Difco peptone, 10 ml/l glycerol, and 20g/l agar) according to the serial dilution method described by Lindsey (5). A portion of the fecal suspension was also inoculated into Trypticase Soy Broth (TSB) in case there was no growth on the blood agar plates. The TSB and blood cultures were incubated overnight at 37C; PG agar cultures were incubated at room temperature. The plates were examined, and quantitative counts of colonies recorded. A representative of each type of morphologically different colony on each agar plate was subcultured to a Trypticase Soy Agar (TSA) slant, incubated at 37C, stored in the refrigerator, and later assayed for sensitivity to kanamycin. Each subculture to TSA was numbered so that its description and source were not known at the time of assay. A total of 569 different isolates were collected and assayed.

Assay. Each microorganism to be tested was grown in TSB, and diluted so that a 0.1 ml aliquot (containing approximately 5×10^4 cells) was inoculated into 1 ml broth solutions containing 25, 15, 14, 12, 9, 8, 7, 6, 5, and 4 mcg kanamycin, respectively. A tube of TSB containing no antibiotic served as a positive control for each isolate tested, and a set of uninoculated tubes of each concentration of kanamycin served as a sterility check for each run of assays. The original strain of *S. marcescens* was reassayed at each run. It was initially resistant to kanamycin at 10 mcg/ml, but its resistance increased to 25 mcg/ml (i.e., sensitive to 15 mcg/ml) halfway through the study. Accordingly, kanamycin resistance was defined as resistance to more than 25 mcg/ml (i.e., growth in each assay tube).

Design of experiment. A single, flexible plastic isolator containing eight plastic cages, each housing a pair of germfree mice, was used. Inasmuch as pretreatment with antibiotic influenced the development of antibiotic resistance in our previous study, germfree mice in four cages were pretreated with kanamycin (5 mg/ml) in their drinking water on days 0 and 2; mice in the other four cages were untreated. On day 5, mice in six cages were treated with kanamycin, or colonized, or both, as indicated in Figure 1. Those cages receiving antibiotic were also treated on days 7 and 9. Feces were collected on days 6, 7, 8, 9, 12, 14, 16, 19, and subsequently on nine occasions during the six months of the experiment.

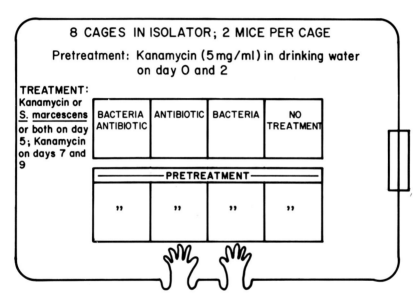

FIG. 1. Design of experiment.

Results

Mice challenged with bacteria alone on day 5 became colonized by the next day. Similarly, control mice receiving neither direct challenge with *S. marcescens* nor treatment with kanamycin became colonized by the next day. In this latter situation, colonization was indirect due to cross-contamination between cages as a result of air flow within the isolator, servicing activities, and collecting specimens for culture. Pretreatment with kanamycin delayed colonization of mice in the **control** and **bacteria only** cages an additional day or two. Paradoxically, mice pretreated with kanamycin and further treated on days 5, 7, and 9, became colonized from three to five days after their last exposure to antibiotic, whereas mice receiving no pretreatment became colonized 10 days after their last exposure (Table I). Thus, mice in cages treated with antibiotic became colonized indirectly despite concomitant bacterial challenge on day 5. The bacterial count in feces of colonized, untreated mice ranged from 10^7 to 10^8 per gram. During treatment with antibiotic, no bacteria were isolated.

TABLE I. **Effect of Kanamycin on Colonization of Mice with** *S. marcescens*

Pretreatment −Days 0&2	Bacteria − Day 5: Treatment− Days 5,7,&9	Day of Exp.	Colonization	
			Days After Bacteria on Day 5	Days After Antibiotic on Day 9
−	Control (none)	6	1	
−	Bacteria only	6	1	
−	Antibiotic only	19	14	10
−	Bacteria, Antibiotic	19	14	10
+	Control (none)	8	3	
+	Bacteria only	7	2	
+	Antibiotic only	12	7	3
+	Bacteria, Antibiotic	14	9	5

However, after subsequent indirect colonization counts of 10^7 to 10^8 per gram were also obtained from mice that had been treated.

Kanamycin-resistant mutants were isolated from mice in all cages (Table II. We cannot explain the occurrence of fewer resistant isolates from mice

TABLE II. **Effect of Kanamycin on Resistance of** *S. marcescens*

Pretreatment − Days 0&2	Bacteria − Day 5; Treatment− Days 5,7,&9	Kanamycin Resistance (⟩ 25 mcg/ml)		
		Isolates		
		Resistant	Total	Frequency
−	Control (none)	4	64	6%
−	Bacteria only	4	53	8%
−	Antibiotic only	34	58	59%
−	Bacteria, Antibiotic	9	45	20%
+	Control (none)	4	47	9%
+	Bacteria only	3	58	5%
+	Antibiotic only	8	53	15%
+	Bacteria, Antibiotic	1	56	2%

receiving kanamycin during both pretreatment and treatment. Among mice receiving antibiotic only during treatment, the 59% and 20% frequencies of resistant isolates are significantly greater than the control (P⟨0.1% and ⟨5%, respectively). The combined frequency of resistant mutants isolated from all antibiotic treated mice is also significantly greater than the combined frequency of mutants from untreated mice (P<0.1%). Isolates from mice treated with antibiotic were resistant to higher levels of kanamycin than were isolates from untreated mice (Table III). A collection of mutants resistant to kanamycin was

TABLE III. Effect of Kanamycin on Resistance of *S. marcescens* from Gnotobiotic Mice

Level of Kanamycin Sensitivity (mcg/ml)	Number of Isolates	
	Kanamycin Cage	Control Cage
>25	17	0
10−15	1	5
5−9	0	7
<5	0	6

reassayed to define its level of resistance more precisely. The majority of these resistant mutants was resistant to 25 mcg/ml and sensitive to 50 mcg/ml; the remainder was sensitive to 100 mcg/ml or more (Table IV).

S. marcescens readily produced spontaneous color-variant colonies on PG agar. Throughout the study representative red, pink, and white colonies were picked from each PG agar plate and assayed for sensitivity to kanamycin. There

TABLE IV. Distribution of Mutants Resistant to More than 25 mcg Kanamycin

Level of Kanamycin Sensitivity (mcg/ml)	Number of Isolates	Frequency
50	22	76%
100	5	17%
>150	2	7%

was no relationship between colonial pigmentation and kanamycin resistance of isolates from feces. However, at the termination of the study, the intestinal distribution of *S. marcescens* in several mice was determined. A striking relationship between colonial pigmentation and the site sampled was observed in each mouse (Table V). Clearly, pigmented colonies predominated in specimens from the ileum and nonpigmented colonies predominated in those from the cecum and colon. Previous exposure of mice to antibiotic did not affect this relationship. Representative colonies from each site in each animal were picked and assayed (Table VI). There was no relationship between resistance and site sampled. However, there was a relationship between pigmentation and resistance. Although a red or pink colony might be resistant to kanamycin, almost all nonpigmented colonies were resistant to kanamycin at levels of 25 mcg/ml or

TABLE V. Intestinal Distribution of S. marcescens In Three Gnotobiotic Mice

| Colony | Number of Colonies Per Gram of Contents | | |
	Ileum	Cecum	Colon
RED	83×10^5	6×10^7	4×10^7
PINK	73×10^5	33×10^7	47×10^7
WHITE	18×10^5	75×10^7	93×10^7
RED	31×10^5	4×10^7	3×10^7
PINK	23×10^5	18×10^7	10×10^7
WHITE	5×10^5	78×10^7	85×10^7
RED	93×10^5	42×10^7	25×10^7
PINK	77×10^5	17×10^7	12×10^7
WHITE	13×10^5	192×10^7	74×10^7

higher.

Conclusions

Direct colonization of germfree mice with a kanamycin-sensitive strain of S. marcescens was suppressed only in mice treated with kanamycin. Treated mice were subsequently colonized indirectly by cross-contamination from other mice.

Mutants of S. marcescens resistant to kanamycin (25 mcg/ml or higher) developed sporadically in untreated gnotobiotic mice. Nevertheless, significantly greater numbers of resistant isolates were obtained from treated mice. Pretreatment with kanamycin did not enhance this effect.

Although antibiotic-resistant mutants became the dominant flora in some treated mice, they did not become established in untreated mice sharing the closed community within the gnotobiotic isolator during six months. This is an

TABLE VI. Distribution of Kanamycin-resistant S. marescens In Four Gnotobiotic Mice

| Colony | Kanamycin Sensitivity (mcg/ml) | | |
	Ileum	Cecum	Colon
RED	10,10,12,12	8,10,15,)25	8,12,15,15,15
PINK	10,10,12,15	8,8,10,12,25	8,10,12,15,15,)25
WHITE	12,25,)25,)25,)25,)25	10,10,25,25,25, 25,25	10,12,12,12,12, 12,15,25,)25

example of bacterial interference or infection immunity (6). This phenomenon was also revealed in our previous study in which initial colonization with tetracycline-sensitive staphylococci interfered with subsequent colonization by resistant staphylococci (2).

Spontaneous color variant-colonies (red, pink, or white) of *S. marcescens* appeared on peptone-glycerol agar. Pigmented colonies predominated in specimens from the ileum of gnotobiotes, and nonpigmented colonies predominated in specimens from the cecum and colon. This relationship was not different in mice previously exposed to antibiotic. Although an occasional pigmented colony was kanamycin-resistant, most nonpigmented colonies were resistant to kanamycin.

The appearance of antibiotic-resistant bacteria involves either (a) development by mutation and selection, or (b) suppression of susceptible bacteria followed by replacement with resistant strains of unrelated origin. It is frequently difficult or impossible to distinguish between these possibilities in clinical or epidemiological settings. Studies with gnotobiotic animals allow the role of mutation to be disassociated from that of replacement, and afford a direct experimental approach for evaluating some epidemiological consequences of the use of antibiotics.

Acknowledgements

This investigation was supported in part by contract N00014-66-C-0189 from the Office of Naval Research and by grant RR-00272 from the Division of Research Resources of the National Institutes of Health.

References

1. Gibbons, R. J., Socransky, S. S., and Kapsimalis, B., *J. Bacteriol. 88:* 1316 (1964).
2. Bornside, G. H., Bornside, B. B., and Cohn, I., Jr., *Infect. Immunity 5:* 505 (1972).
3. Wilfert, J. N., Barrett, F. F., Ewing, W. H., Finland, M., and Kass, E. H., *Appl. Microbiol. 19:* 345 (1970).
4. Thornton, G. F., and Cramer, J. A., *Antimicrob. Ag. Chemother. 1970:* 514 (1971).
5. Lindsey, D., *J. Lab. Clin. Med. 53:* 299 (1953).
6. Dubos, R., *J.A.M.A. 184:* 1038 (1963).

ERYSIPELOTHRIX RHUSIOPATHIAE INFECTION IN HYPERSENSITIZED GNOTOBIOTIC PIGS AND SEM EXAMINATION OF THE LESIONS

H. D. Geissinger, O. P. Miniats and *D. G. Djurickovic*
Department of Biomedical Sciences and Clinical Studies
Ontario Veterinary College, University of Guelph
Guelph, Ontario, Canada

Introduction

The pathogenesis of swine erysipelas arthritis and endocarditis is controversial. It is agreed that following an initial bacteremia, the organism localizes most commonly in the skin, the joints and the heart valves. A difference of opinion exists on the question of whether *Erysipelothrix rhusiopathiae* has a special affinity for these organs and localizes there immediately following the initial infection (1, 2), or if the lesions are allergic manifestations which would occur as a result of previous sensitization to *E. rhusiopathiae* antigen (3, 4, 5). It has been found previously (6) that *E. rhusiopathiae* infection in gnotobiotic pigs resulted in a septicemia, which was often associated with bacteriologically positive lesions of arthritis and endocarditis. The present study was undertaken to elucidate any effects of hypersensitivity on the development of swine erysipelas arthritis and endocarditis.

Methods

Thirty-four gnotobiotic pigs which had or had not been immunized one or more times at weekly intervals with swine erysipelas bacterin were challenged with live cultures of septicemic (I) or endocarditic (A or B) strains of *E. rhusiopathiae*. Three immunized nonchallenged pigs served as controls. Pigs which did not die due to the infection were killed from 2 to 10 days after exposure. The surfaces of selected heart valves were scanned according to procedures described elsewhere (7). Tissues also were prepared for routine histopathology and, after preliminary examination with the light microscope, were re-examined with the scanning electron microscope (SEM). Details of histological section preparation for the SEM have been described previously (8).

347

Results and Discussion

Experiment 1. Three pigs which had been inoculated with strain I (which had been originally isolated from a septicemic case of swine erysipelas) died after 3 to 5 days. *E. rhusiopathiae* could be isolated from most organs; 2 pigs had arthritis in the tarsal joints, and one had a small lesion of valvular endocarditis on the tricuspid valve.

Another 2 pigs which had been inoculated with the same strain, but had been immunized 4 times before challenge, developed serological titers (1/320) high enough to protect them against the challenge of this highly virulent strain. When they were killed 5 days after exposure, organ cultures were bacteriologically sterile and no lesions were seen on gross pathological examination. Histopathological examination revealed a chronic glomerulonephritis in one pig.

Experiment 2. Six pigs which had been inoculated with live cultures of strain A, originally isolated from the lesions of endocarditis in a chronic case of swine erysipelas, reacted quite differently. None died, but elevated temperatures (above 105.0°F) were noted in all. At necropsy, 6 days after exposure, *E. rhusiopathiae* was isolated from some of the organ cultures and from most of the joints. Mural endocarditis, which was bacteriologically negative, was demonstrable in 1 pig. Lesions in the joints were present in 5 of these pigs.

In 7 pigs which had been sensitized to *E. rhusiopathiae* with a single injection of bacterin (titers of 1/40) similar results were noted at necropsy 3 to 6 days later with the exception that more heart lesions were demonstrable. Three of the 4 heart lesions observed were bacteriologically positive.

Hypersensitization of 4 pigs with 4 injections of bacterin (titers of 1/160) afforded protection against the clinical illness to subsequent challenge with strain A, although lesions of valvular endocarditis were noted in 2 pigs killed six days after exposure.

Three other pigs, which were immunized 6 times with the bacterin before challenge with strain A showed high serological titers (1/320) and did not react clinically to the inoculation of the live organism. At necropsy 4 days later, *E. rhusiopathiae* was isolated from the heart and joints of one pig, which also had lesions of myocarditis and arthritis. One pig in this group had bacteriologically positive lesions of arthritis.

Experiment 3. Two pigs which had been inoculated with strain B, originally isolated from an endocarditis in a pig, reacted clinically to the inoculations. One pig showed typical skin diamond lesions 3 days after exposure. *E. rhusiopathiae* was isolated from the tarsal joints and the heart valves of both pigs when they were killed seven days after exposure. Acute arthritis, petechiated kidneys and minimal lesions of endocarditis were present in one pig.

Seven pigs were vaccinated three times before they were challenged with strain B, which afforded protection against the clinical disease. No organisms could be isolated from the organs at necropsy 7 to 10 days later, however lesions of endocarditis and arthritis were seen in 3 pigs.

Experiment 4. Lastly, 3 gnotobiotic pigs were inoculated 4 times with swine erysipelas bacterin and not subsequently challenged with live bacteria. When they were killed 13 days after the last inoculation, bacterial organ cultures were negative, but thrombotic endocarditis and chronic glomerulonephritis were demonstrated microscopically.

SEM Examination. Figs. 1 and 2 are SEM-micrographs of the surface of a heart valve viewed *en face*. It is evident in both figures that the constituents of early deposits of crenated red blood cells or thrombi are easily defined with this mode of microscopy.

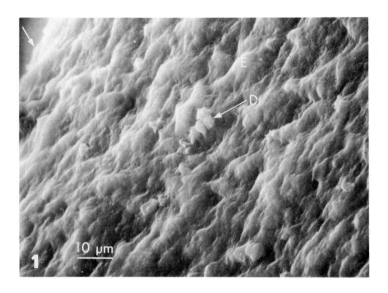

FIG. 1. Edge of heart valve (arrow) of hypersensitized pig infected with strain B. Note uneven endothelial cells (E) and deposit (D) consisting of crenated red blood cells. SEM x 900.

Fig. 3a is a light micrograph of a typical lesion of endocarditis found in the pigs which had been hypersensitized. It will be apparent from this low power light micrograph that the heart valve *per se* appears relatively normal. The lesion on top of the valve is a sterile thrombus. Fig. 3b is a scanning electron micrograph of the same area in the same section as Fig. 3a. The inclusion of it in this paper merely serves to demonstrate that the same area was scanned. Figs. 3c and 3d contain information which had not been apparent in light optical

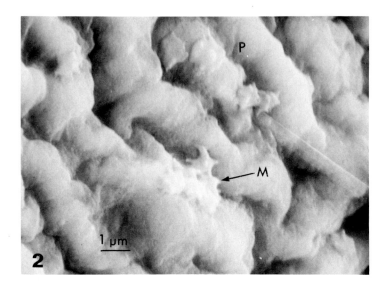

FIG. 2. Auricular surface of heart valve from a similar pig showing platelet microthrombus (M) and individual blood platelets (P). SEM x 8100.

micrographs of the same lesion even at the highest magnifications. It is shown in Fig. 3c that the attachment of the thrombus resulted in a desquamation of endothelial cells and subsequent exposure of the subendothelial connective tissue of the heart valve. In Fig. 3d the different components of the thrombus (blood platelets, fibrin, white and red blood cells) are stereoscopically defined with the SEM.

Figs. 4a, b and c are micrographs of a kidney glomerulus from the same pig. In Fig. 4a it is apparent that basophillic material is present in one of the glomerular capillaries. The damage in the capillaries of the entire glomerulus is not evident in the light micrograph, but is clearly brought out in the SEM-micrographs (Figs. 4b and c).

Conclusions

1. Since lesions of endocarditis were produced in pigs which were hypersensitized to erysipelothrix antigen and not followed by a challenge of live bacteria, we suspect that these lesions were non-specific, i.e. that they would have occurred in pigs hypersensitized to any (non-erysipelothrix) antigen.

2. As far as could be ascertained, the level of induced immunity to

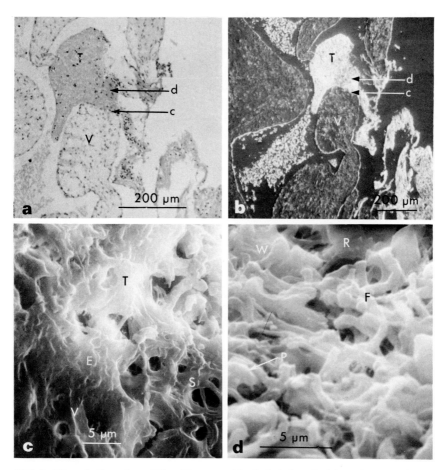

FIG. 3. Thrombotic endocarditis of hypersensitized pig infected with strain A. (a) Survey light micrograph showing heart valve (V) and thrombus (T). Areas of SEM-micrographs "c" and "d" are indicated H & E x 100. (b) SEM-micrograph of identical area. Tilt 0°, x 60. (c) Attachment of thrombus (T) to valve (V), showing damaged endothelial cells (E) and exposed subendothelial connective tissue (S). Tilt 45° x 2400. (d) Constituents of thrombus. Blood platelets (P), fibrin (F), white (W) and red (R) blood cells are shown. Tilt 45°, x 4300.

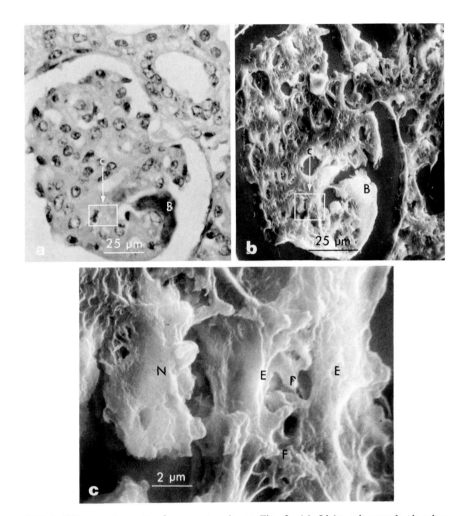

FIG. 4. Kidney glomerulus from same pig as Fig. 3. (a) Light micrograph showing basophilic deposit (B) in a glomerular capillary. Area of micrograph "c" indicated. H & E x 480. (b) Corresponding SEM-micrograph x 600. (c) Damaged area showing nucleus (N), glomerular capillary walls (E), and microthrombus consisting of platelets (P) and fibrin (F). SEM x 6000.

erysipelothrix in these pigs did not influence the severity of lesions of endocarditis and arthritis.

3. The SEM was a very useful tool for the *en face* examination of early endocarditic heart valves.

4. Used in conjunction with light microscopy, the SEM supplemented histological information, because structural detail in sections which had not been

seen before became apparent. This also led to a better appreciation of spatial relationships in the tissue of interest.

Acknowledgements

Supported by N.R.C. Grant A-3899, M.R.C. Grant MA-2082, and Grants from the Ontario Department of Agriculture and Food. We thank J.E.O.L. (Canada) for the loan of the SEM to the laboratory of one of us (H.D.G.).

References

1. Renk, W., and Wellman, G., *Zentbl. Vet. Med. B 10:* 551 (1963).
2. Shuman, R. D., Wood, R. L., and Monlux, W. S., *Cornell Vet. 55:* 378 (1965).
3. Michalka, J., *Wien tierarztl. Mschr. 26:* 449 (1939).
4. Freeman, M. J., Segre, D., and Berman, D. T., *Am. J. Vet. Res. 25:* 135 (1964).
5. Freeman, M. J., and Berman, D. T., *Am. J. Vet. Res. 25:* 145 and 151 (1964).
6. Geissinger, H. D., Miniats, O. P., and Quinn, P. J., *Zentbl. Vet. Med. B 16:* 689 (1969).
7. Shimamoto, T., Yamashita, Y., and Sunaga, T., *Proc. Jap. Acad. 45:* 507 (1969).
8. Geissinger, H. D., *J. Microsc. (Oxford) 93:* 109 (1971).

THE EFFECT OF ANTIBIOTICS AGAINST THE INTESTINAL BACTERIAL FLORA

T. Kikuchi, T. Oikawa, K. Inoue, M. Sakai,
N. Hara, K. Sunagawa and *Y. Ichihashi*
Department of Pediatrics
School of Medicine, Keio University
Tokyo, Japan

Introduction

When antibiotics are used clinically, it is expected that they eliminate pathogenic bacteria. However, antibiotics affect the normal bacterial flora as well as the pathogenic microorganisms. This problem is especially important when antibiotics are administered to the newborn infant, whose intestinal bacterial flora is just on the way to development.

In the treatment of infectious disease, it has often occurred that antibiotics were not clinically effective, even when they were proved to be effective *in vitro*. In order to investigate these problems, we have studied the changes in the intestinal bacterial flora of the infant and other experimental animals by the introduction of antibiotics. We have also studied the effect of antibiotics against bacterial flora in gnotobiotic mice, investigating the peculiarity of the intestinal bacterial flora and the pattern of resistance against antibiotics in intestinal infections.

Results

In these studies, as the culture medium of the intestinal bacteria, we used such media as DHL for coliforms, PEA azide for enterococcus, mannitol salt agar for staphylococcus, LBS for lactobacillus, BP for bacteroides and the cooked meat for the total bacterial counts.

When we administered erythromycin (EM) (50 mg/kg), chloramphenicol (CP) (50 mg/kg) and tetracycline (TC) (50 mg/kg) to infants, we found that the fecal bacterial counts did not change much. But when colistin sodium methansulfonate (CL) was administered, the number of gram negative bacilli decreased on the day following administration, but it soon recovered to the former level of bacterial flora when the administration of CL was stopped. In these results, it is recognized that the intestinal bacterial flora in the infant was

355

slightly affected by the usual dose of antibiotics except with CL.

Next we administered the antibiotics to the guinea pig, the rabbit and the monkey. These were chosen as experimental animals because the intestinal bacterial flora of the guinea pig is very different from that of human beings, and the flora of the monkey is almost the same as human beings. When 100 mg EM was administered orally to the guinea pig, a remarkable change was obtained. The guinea pig usually has coliforms less than 10^2 in the intestinal bacterial flora, but the coliforms increased in number and gradually increased up to 10^7 by the sixth day after EM was administered. Furthermore, the guinea pigs died in 10 to 14 days. When we administered EM to the monkey, whose intestinal bacterial flora is similar to human beings, no remarkable change was obtained. It is concluded that the effect of the antibiotics against the intestinal bacterial flora varies according to the species of animals and the composition of the intestinal bacterial flora. Because it is difficult to study the relationship between the bacteria and the antibiotics in conventional animals with so many affecting variables, we used germfree mice rendered gnotobiotic by contaminating them with various microorganisms.

When CL was administered to gnotobiotic mice associated with *Escherichia coli,* 026 K60 (MIC to CL3 .17γ), the number of *E. coli* decreased in some series, but there are other cases in which the bacteria did not decrease at all. Figure 1 shows the cases in which *E. coli* did not decrease at all. The survival curve shows that *E. coli* acquired resistance in 72 hours after introduction of CL, but there are some cases in which *E. coli* were still sensitive to CL. But when we administered CL to the gnotobiotic mice with pseudomonas, the bacteria did not decrease at all, even if they proved to be sensitive *in vitro* to CL. When we administered CL to gnotobiotes associated with *E. coli,* 026 K60 and pseudomonas, neither decreased in number, and it was noticed that *E. coli* acquired resistance in 24 hours, but not pseudomonas.

In these experiments, there are numerous observations which are not understood. The number of pseudomonas did not decrease at all in 120 hrs after administration when sensitive to antibiotics. There are some strains of *E. coli* which were not decreased in number by the antibiotics, even when still sensitive to the antibiotics *in vitro.*

When we administered CL to the inbred DK1 conventional mice, which are recognized to have CL sensitive *E. coli* at $10^4 - 10^6$ level in their fecal bacterial flora, the number of *E. coli* decreased on the day following administration. After the antibiotics were stopped, the number of *E. coli* was still less than 10^2 in the following 10 days. On the 17th day, the number was 4×10^2; and on the 23rd day 1×10^2. Later it was still less (Figure 2). In this experiment, antibiotics seem to have eliminated *E. coli* from the intestinal bacterial flora of the DK1 conventional mice.

Next we changed the antibiotics and studied the changes in the intestinal

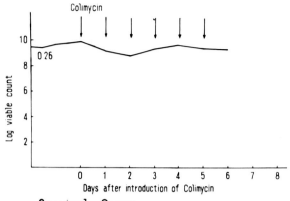

Survival Curve

(I) Gnotobiote (E. Coli. 0 26)

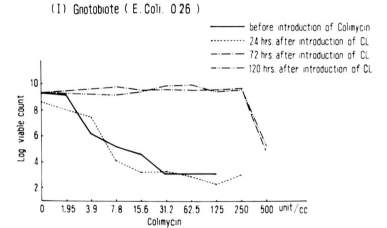

FIG. 1. The effect of colimycin on gnotobiotic mice – *E. coli* 0.26

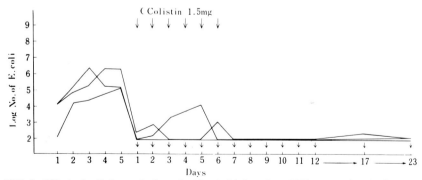

FIG. 2. Effect of colistin on the intestinal bacterial flora from DK1 conventional mice.

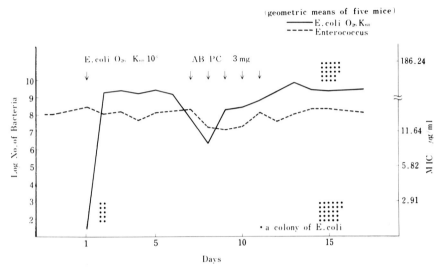

FIG. 3. Effect of AB-PC on the intestinal bacterial flora from ICR gnotobiotes (*E. coli* and enterococcus) and the change of the minimal inhibitory concentration of *E. coli* to AB-PC.

bacterial flora and the minimal inhibitory concentrations of the antibiotics before and after administration.

When we used AB-PC, the number of *E. coli* decreased and soon returned to the previous level after AB-PC was stopped without showing any resistance against antibiotics.

In the next experiment, we contaminated germfree mice with an enterococcus which was resistant to AB-PC. Then we superinfected with *E. coli*, 026 K60. When we administered AB-PC to them, the number of *E. coli* did not decrease sufficiently as in monoflora cases. It was established that some strains of the *E. coli* were resistant against AB-PC *in vitro*. However, in 2 mice out of 5, the number of *E. coli* decreased without showing any resistance to antibiotics (Figure 3).

Next we administered AB-PC to the gnotobiotic mice with *E. coli*, enterococcus and pseudomonas. The bacterial count of *E. coli* decreased about 10^2 cells during the administration of AB-PC, but soon recovered the previous level after AB-PC was stopped.

Conclusions

In these experiments, we found that there are many problems and discrepancies about the effect of antibiotics *in vitro*, and *in vivo*, even in the intestinal canal.

The effect of the antibiotics appears to depend not only upon the

358

sensitivity of the bacteria, but also on many factors involving the bacteria, the constitution of the intestinal bacterial flora and many other circumstances.

Recently there are many reports on increasing the resistant strains against many antibiotics. It is very important to investigate the effect of the antibiotics against the intestinal bacterial flora and to analyze the mechanism, so that we could avoid the unwilling side effects as much as possible.

References

1. Oikawa, T., Inoue, K., Sakai, M., Kikuchi, T., Ichihashi, Y, Ozawa, A., and Sasaki, S., *Progress in Antimicrobial and Anticancer Chemotherapy 1:* 290 (1970).
2. Kikuchi, T., Oikawa, T., Inoue, K., Sakai, M., Hara, N., and Ichihashi, Y., *XIII Int. Congr. Pediat. Infectious Disease 6:* 145 (1971).

INFLUENCE OF NUTRITIONAL LEVELS OF SPIRAMYCIN AND VIRGINIAMYCIN ON THE BACTERIAL METABOLITES IN THE GASTROINTESTINAL TRACT AND URINE OF ARTIFICIALLY REARED EARLY WEANED PIGLETS

H. Henderickx and *J. Decuypere*
Department of Nutrition and Hygiene
F. L., Rijksuniversiteit
Gent, Belgium

Introduction

The theory of a relation between microorganisms and metabolites in the gastrointestinal tract is a very old one. Suffice it to recall Metchnikoff's (1) theory on the saccharolytic and putrefactive bacterial action and the still older hypothesis by Bouchard (2) and Senator (3) on intestinal autointoxication. Despite its originality and value this older work has been criticized by Gyorgyi (4) because of its limited experimental evidence and its overgeneralization from too few biochemical measurements. This results from the fact that the older work was almost exclusively confined to humans. A better understanding of the relationship between the intestinal flora and host metabolism was mainly obtained with laboratory animals and with germfree and gnotobiological techniques. The growth promoting effect of antibiotics in animal production extended the research to domestic animals but introduced at the same time the antibiotic as a new parameter. Despite an overwhelming number of experiments on the action of antibiotics on the gut flora and its metabolism during the last fifteen years, it is still not possible as indicated by Francois and Michel (5) and by Ghesquiere (6) to put forward a clear and definite theory of the action of antibiotics on animal growth.

In our experiments with piglets fed an artificial diet, eventually supplemented with virginiamycin or spiramycin and kept in battery cages in very clean conditions, we tried to measure as many bacteriological and biochemical parameters as possible. This paper deals with the results of the measurements of some biochemical parameters.

Materials and Methods

Experimental details on animals, feed, treatment and slaughter are described by Decuypere and Van der Heyde (7). The analytical determinations started from a 10% homogenized suspension of gastrointestinal contents. The determinations carried out were: The dry matter content was obtained by drying at 105°C and minerals by ashing at 450°C. The pH and Eh of the suspensions were measured respectively with glass-calomel electrodes and with platinium-calomel electrodes. Soluble and reducing sugars were analyzed for by a copper reduction method (8); results, however, are expressed as mg glucose. Lactic acid, ammonia and urea were determined by microdiffusion techniques as described by Conway (9). The same technique was used for hydrogen sulphide. The colorometric determination however was based on the methylene-blue production (10). Nitrogen, soluble in 10% trichloroacetic acid, was obtained with a micro Kjeldahl procedure. Uric acid was assessed by phosphotungstic acid as described by de Vries and van Daatselaar (11). Volatile fatty acids were determined by gas-liquid-chromatography (12).

In addition, urinary creatine and creatinine were analyzed with picrate as described by de Vries and van Daatselaar (11).

Because of the necessity of concentrating free amino acids, amines and other ninhydrin-positive compounds from intestinal contents, the following procedure was adopted. One volume 10% suspension was mixed with one volume 1% picric acid. After centrifuging, washing, discarding the picrate with Dowex x 8, the supernatant was dried in a rotating evaporator. The dried residue was solubilized and an aliquot injected in a Technicon Automatic Analyzer. Elution was made with a lithium-citrate gradient buffer (13). The very basic compounds were chromatographed on a Zeocarb 226 column with a potassium-citrate buffer (14). The urinary compounds were concentrated on a strong cation exchange resin (Merck n°1). After elution and concentration at the required volume, an aliquot was chromatographed as previously described.

Results

Results are given in Tables I through V; the following abbreviations are used for the treatments: C for the control, V for the virginiamycin and S for the spiramycin treated group. The results in most cases are averages of nine animals per group.

As shown in Table I, differences were found between the treatments in compounds or parameters not directly related to microbial action. The dry matter percentage of the S-group was higher in every section of the tract; the mineral percentage was only different in the large intestine, again the S-group having the highest percentage. The pH was not different in the first part of the tract. In the last part of the large intestine the values of the S-piglets were always lower. For the soluble sugars, expressed as glucose, no differences were found in the stomach and the small intestine. The S-animals, however, showed less of

362

TABLE I. Concentration of some Metabolites in the Gastrointestinal Tract

		Stom.	I Sm. In.	2 Sm. In.	3 Sm. In.	Cec.	L. In.
DM %	C	15.6	5.1	6.5	8.4	10.8	24.2
	V	15.4	4.1	6.3	8.6	9.4	24.9
	S	16.1	—	11.6	8.9	12.8	31.0
ASH %	C	0.7	0.8	0.8	0.9	3.3	6.7
	V	0.9	—	0.7	0.9	3.1	7.5
	S	0.7	—	0.8	1.4	2.9	9.5
pH	C	4.6	5.6	6.1	7.4	7.1	8.3
	V	4.7	6.1	6.4	7.3	7.3	8.1
	S	4.6	6.0	6.2	7.2	7.4	7.9
Glucose	C	1214	—	538	1005	206	350
mg/100 g	V	1420	—	730	995	252	289
	S	1313	—	808	550	103	189
Σ vfa	C	0.84	0.98	0.53	1.23	15.56	6.66
mmol/100 g	V	0.88	0.53	0.45	1.52	13.82	5.07
	S	1.50	0.45	0.79	1.39	12.06	4.52
H Lact.	C	0.45	0.61	0.60	0.75	0.35	0.37
mmol/100 g	V	0.43	1.61	0.62	0.81	0.41	0.34
	S	0.66	0.91	1.00	1.21	0.60	0.36
Soluble N	C	10.9	20.4	39.7	20.1	15.5	18.6
mmol/100 g	V	13.5	—	26.3	30.7	12.8	20.9
	S	13.0	30.5	47.9	32.2	15.0	22.1
NH_3	C	0.11	0.11	0.13	0.16	3.11	2.06
mmol/100 g	V	0.03	0	0.03	0.24	1.50	1.47
	S	0	0.10	0.07	0.13	1.55	0.99
H_2S	C	0	0	0	0	1.09	1.60
mmol/100 g	V	0	0	0	0	1.31	1.86
	S	0	0	0	0	0.74	1.34
Urea	C	0.79	1.33	1.29	1.21	0.80	0.83
mmol/100 g	V	0.64	1.06	0.88	1.07	0.74	0.64
	S	0.61	1.30	1.13	0.99	0.72	0.61
Uric acid	C	0.44	0.36	0.30	0.48	1.28	1.86
mmol/100 g	V	0.48	0.50	0.30	0.54	1.07	1.52
	S	0.48	0.29	0.44	0.56	1.08	1.28

TABLE II. Percentage Composition of the Volatile Fatty Acids in the
Contents of Cecum and Large Intestine (Molar Percentage)

	Control		Virginiamycin		Spiramycin	
	C	L. In.	C.	L. In.	C.	L. In.
Acetic	63.9	52.4	59.5	54.5	67.2	60.5
Propionic	21.6	16.4	23.4	14.1	20.0	12.8
Isobutyric	2.7	16.0	7.9	14.8	2.3	2.8
Butyric	9.0	9.3	6.8	9.2	7.1	16.2
Isovaleric	1.4	3.0	1.1	3.8	1.9	4.5
Valeric	1.4	3.0	1.4	3.6	1.5	3.2

these sugars in the large intestine and the last part of the small intestine. Nitrogen, soluble in trichloroacetic acid, showed no differences within the treatments, although in every segment this parameter was always higher in the S-animals.

In the concentration of compounds which could be metabolized by microorganisms, differences arose between the treatments. Urea was always higher in the control group, while the antibiotic influence was variable. The values of uric acid were not very different in the small intestine, but in cecum and large intestine the lowest values were found in the S-group.

With the products directly produced by the microflora, differences were more pronounced. Lactic acid was present in a higher concentration in the antibiotic treated animals. In cecum and large intestine the experimental groups had a lower concentration of volatile fatty acids. In Table II, it can be seen that small differences existed among the major compounds and that virginiamycin in general gave a concentration between that of the control and that of spiramycin. An important difference was the lower concentration of iso-acids with the S-piglets, which reflected a lower deamination of amino acids. The ammonia level was always lower in the experimental groups, but the most striking differences were found in the last part of the intestinal tract. Hydrogen sulphide, which was absent in the stomach and small intestine, was found in the large intestine in lower concentration in the S-piglets. In the intestinal content a maximum of 78 ninhydrin-positive compounds were detected, of which 41 could be identified, while in the urine 103 compounds were found of which 43 could be identified.

The unknown peaks could be tentatively identified in comparison with the chromatograms obtained by Hamilton (15) and by King (16). No uniform trend could be detected in analyzing the figures of Table III. Some compounds were present in higher amounts in the control than in the experimental groups; e.g. the sulphur containing amino acids. With other compounds the opposite was observed, e.g. glutanic acid. When differences existed the virginiamycin treatment group always fell between the control and the spiramycin groups. With

TABLE III. Concentration of Free Amino Acids and Related Compounds
In the Intestinal Contents (in μmol/100 g)

	Control		Virginiamycin		Spiramycin	
	Sm. In.	C. + L. In.	Sm. In.	C. + L. In.	Sm. In.	C. + L. In.
CYSO$_3$H	11.8	15.2	9.4	10.2	2.0	4.6
TAUR	9.9	0	2.7	0.5	1.8	TR
ASP	TR	0	0.1	0	9.4	4.3
THR	TR	0	0.9	0	10.9	TR
SER	TR	0	TR	0	8.1	TR
GLU	0	0	1.4	1.6	21.4	2.1
PRO	0	0	0	0	6.3	0
VAL	TR	TR	21.5	1.1	16.3	0.8
CYSH	51.6	21.3	20.6	18.5	6.1	TR
MET	21.9	15.1	23.8	13.7	3.0	TR
ILEU	24.0	TR	23.2	0	11.3	0.9
TYR	7.8	3.4	13.7	TR	10.7	1.1
PHE	12.0	5.0	12.6	3.1	10.1	1.1
ETH-NH$_2$	4.4	0	2.5	TR	3.7	2.1
γ-NH$_2$-BUT	3.6	1.7	4.8	2.3	3.3	TR
TRY	3.9	0.2	0.8	0.5	0.8	TR
LYS	3.0	TR	2.0	TR	1.4	0.2
HIS	3.7	1.0	5.9	0.3	5.3	0.8
3-CH$_3$-HIS	3.7	TR	1.9	1.0	0.4	0.1
ARG	5.5	1.2	3.1	0.4	5.0	0.5
PEA	1.6	1.8	0.5	1.0	0.3	0.7
TYRA	1.1	1.1	0.4	1.0	TR	TR
CAD	0.2	0.6	TR	TR	0.1	TR
PUT	0.3	0.3	TR	TR	0.1	TR
HISTA	0.3	0.5	TR	0.1	TR	TR
AGMA	0.1	0.1	0	TR	0	TR
TRYPTA	TR	TR	TR	TR	0	0

metabolites such as 3-CH$_3$-histidine, and tyramine, the concentration was always lowest in the S-animals. The measurements in the urine (Table IV) demonstrated that with spiramycin in most cases a higher excretion of the ninhydrin-positive compounds was obtained. In Tables III and IV only the compounds which were identified and which were present in a different concentration were inserted.

With the other urinary compounds (Table V), spiramycin increased the elimination of total nitrogen and urea, but a marked difference was found in the creatine excretion: the amount excreted in the treated animals was half that of the control piglets.

In general it can be stated that, if differences were encountered in our measurements, the most extreme values were obtained in most cases with spiramycin.

365

TABLE IV. Concentration of Free Amino Acids and Related Compounds
In the Urine (in μmol/mg creatinine)

	Control	Virginiamycin	Spiramycin
CYSO$_3$H	4.4	8.0	7.3
TAUR	1.5	4.4	10.0
HYPRO	3.1	13.1	10.8
THR	6.5	14.9	15.4
SER	3.0	8.6	12.1
SARC	1.3	2.5	11.3
GLU	4.5	8.8	10.1
GLY	29.3	56.9	36.4
α-NH$_2$-BUT	1.2	0	2.3
VAL	1.2	1.2	2.5
GLUC-NH$_2$	0.2	0.3	1.0
CYSH	3.5	5.5	11.2
MET	0.9	1.5	TR
ILEU	0.7	3.8	7.1
LEU	1.8	2.0	5.4
TYR	3.2	8.4	2.3
PHE	0.3	1.6	10.4
ETH-NH$_2$	1.0	4.1	12.5
γ-NH$_2$-BUT	0.6	11.3	11.0
TRY	2.1	5.9	7.8
LYS	4.9	2.3	17.1
ORN	1.7	3.3	4.5
TYRA	0.1	0.1	0.2
PUTR	0.1	0.1	0.2
CAD	TR	TR	TR
HISTA	TR	TR	TR

TABLE V. Excretion of Urinary Compounds (mg/mg creatinine)

	Total N	Urea	Uric Acid	Creatine
Control	15.97	31.1	0.35	0.79
Spiramycin	14.52	27.2	0.37	0.39
Virginiamycin	19.26	36.7	0.34	0.40

Conclusions

In our experiments the influence of antibiotic treatment can be measured in two areas: a) the action of the gut flora and b) the general metabolism as evidenced in the urine.

In regard to the first point, the concentration of a metabolite in the intestinal content is the result of different factors of which the most important are: production and metabolism, absorption through the gut wall and eventually excretion in the lumen, inflow from the foregoing part of the tract and outflow to the following part. Some of these processes are probably influenced by antibiotics. Therefore it can be that relating the concentration of a metabolite to microbial action is a simplification which for some metabolites or for some intestinal areas is not valuable. The most important observations are the following: The influence of spiramycin is always more pronounced than virginiamycin, an influence which is opposite to the bacterial count and distribution where virginiamycin seemed to be responsible for a change in the microbial picture. The change in metabolites by spiramycin and eventually by virginiamycin is more distinct in cecum and large intestine, where an economy of nutrients is only possible after absorption in this area, a process which is not yet fully understood. Although the inhibition of the production of some metabolites can clearly be attributed to a modified microbial action (e.g., for ammonia, hydrogen sulphide, some amines and ninhydrin positive compounds, isobutyric acid), the differences between the groups of other compounds can not be caused only by the intestinal flora. The dry matter percentage, the mineral percentage, and the concentration of some of the free amino acids are very clear illustrations of this. Therefore the influence on some physiological processes by the antibiotics can not be excluded.

In regard to the second point, the higher excretion of nitrogen, urea and amino acids in the urine of S-animals leads to the supposition of a lower nitrogen retention. This can be obtained by a higher supply of valuable nitrogen, caused by a suppression of microbial catabolic action or by an action of the antibiotic on the intermediate metabolism of the animal. Of this no confirmation can be found in our experiments. However the lower creatine excretion with the antibiotic treatment is consistent with this possibility.

The growth promoting effect by the two antibiotics in this study is therefore more complex than relating this effect to the presence of some compounds in the intestinal content.

References

1. Metchnikoff, E., *Mem. Proc. Manchester Lit. and Phil. Soc. 45:* 1 (1901).
2. Bouchard, C. J., *Comp. Rend. Soc. Biol. I:* 665 (1884).
3. Senator, H., *Berl. Klin. Wschr. 5:* 254 (1880).
4. Gyorgyi, P., *Ann. Nutr. Alim. II:* A189 (1957).
5. Francois, A. C., and Michel, M. C., *Nutr. et Dieta 10:* 35 (1968).
6. Ghesquiere, L, Thesis, University of Gent, Belgium (1970).
7. Decuypere, J., and Van der Heyde, H., *Zbt. Bakt. I Orig.* (In Press).
8. Somogyi, M., and Nelson, N., in "Klinische Diagnostiek," (E. Gorter and W. C. De Graaff, eds), Kroesse, Leiden, The Netherlands, (1955).
9. Conway, E. J., in "Microdiffusion and Volumetric Error," (Crosby, ed.), Lockwood, London, (1957).

10. Boltz, D. F., in "Colorimetric Determination of Nonmetals," *Interscience Publ.*, New York (1958).

11. de Vries, J. and van Daatselaar, D., in "Klinische Diagnostiek," (E. Gorter and W. C. De Graaff, eds.), Edit. Kroesse, Leiden, The Netherlands, (1955).

12. Cottyn, B. G., and Boucque, C. V., *J. Agr. Food Chem. 16:* 105 (1968).

13. Vega, A., *Technicon Symposium,* London, (1968).

14. Wall, R. A., *Technicon Symposium,* London, (1967).

15. Hamilton, P. B., *Anal. Chem. 35:* 2055 (1963).

16. King, J. S., *Clinica Chimica Acta 9:* 441 (1964).

STUDY OF THE GASTROINTESTINAL MICROFLORA OF SUCKLING AND EARLY WEANED PIGLETS USING DIFFERENT FEEDING SYSTEMS AND FEED ADDITIVES

J. Decuypere, H. Van der Heyde and *H. Henderickx*
Department of Nutrition and Hygiene
F. L., Rijksuniversiteit
Gent, Belgium

Introduction

The gastrointestinal flora of early weaned artificially reared piglets has been studied at this institute for the last ten years. This was done primarily to find a rearing method resulting in satisfactory growth and welfare of the piglets which is believed to result in a stable gastrointestinal microflora. Indeed, the flora of suckling piglets shows considerable variation between litters (1, 2), probably caused by variations in the sow's milk yield and milk composition as well as by variations in environmental conditions.

In order to obtain a stable flora, a rearing method was developed (3) mainly based on a very clean housing (wire cages) in a controlled environment (temp. $27 \pm 2°C$, r.h. $60 \pm 10\%$). This technique allowed us to wean the piglets at the mean age of 5 to 7 days, which minimized sow dependent variations. Different feeding systems were tested during the first 5 years of the experiments. These results are summarized in the first part of this communication. It was only on a dry *ad libitum* feeding system based on milk powder that a reproducible flora was built up. Digestive disorders were much more frequent with the other methods studied. With this milk powder feeding method, we started the study of the effect of certain so-called growth promoters (mainly antibiotics) on the gastrointestinal microflora. The antibiotics chosen were virginiamycin (RIT, Belgium) and spiramycin (Specia, France) administered at doses of 50 ppm. As many aspects as possible were studied on a relatively large number of animals. Included were the quantitative and topographical composition of the gastrointestinal microflora, some physico-chemical characteristics of the contents (pH, Eh, dry matter) and the endproducts resulting from the carbohydrate and protein fraction of the diet. These determinations were carried out with the hope of finding a basis for the explanation of the growth promoting action of dietary additives previously documented extensively in the literature. Extensive reviews on this subject were published recently (4, 5). These authors pointed out that the results of all experiments described so far, show no good accordance at all. One author (5) looks for an explanation related more to the systemic action of these additives. The other group (4) holds that addition of such compounds primarily results in a change of the metabolic action of the intestinal flora, which results in a more economic utilization of the nutrients by the animal, eventually combined with a diminished production of toxic or pharmacologically active substances.

Material and Methods

All the piglets in these experiments were of the Belgian Land race. They were weaned at the mean age of 7 days and reared in cages. The detailed rearing method has been described previously (3). More details about the feeding systems tested are given in Table I. When the influence of the antibiotics was studied, the dry *ad libitum* feeding method, with the same food composition, was used except that the citric acid was omitted. The antibiotics were mixed into the diet at a concentration of 50 ppm. Three times 9 piglets were used in these experiments, which consisted of 3 replications of three treatments: C = control, V = virginiamycin and S = spiramycin. After about one month for the feeding trials and after 14 days for the antibiotic treatments, the animals were slaughtered and the gastrointestinal tract was removed and unfolded on a table. The whole intestinal tract was divided into several segments of which the first

TABLE I. Composition of the Experimental Groups, According to Feeding Management

Feeding Management	No.	Code
Suckling piglets (no creep feed)	26	S.R.
Condensed cow milk: 20% dry matter		
2 times a day, *ad libitum,* in cups	5	C.M. 2 t/d. AL.
4 times a day, *ad libitum,* presented in bottles with a dummy	10	C.M. 4 t/d. AL.
Prepared ration (a)		
20% dry matter, 4 times a day, scale fed (b)	5	M.A. 20%, 4 t/d. SF
33% dry matter, 3 times a day, scale fed (c)	4	M.A. 33%, 3 t/d. SF
95% dry matter, dry *ad libitum*	7	M.A. Dry AL.

(a) ½ full cream powder, ½ skim milk powder, 1% citric acid, vitamins and minerals.
(b) Beginning with 50 cm^3 per meal and increasing 5 cm^3 per meal per day.
(c) First and second week, 100 cm^3 per meal; third week, 150 cm^3 per meal.

contained the stomach, segments 2 to 8 were 6 equal parts of the small intestine, with the most proximal segment sub-divided again into two equal parts. Segment 9 contained the cecum, while segments 10 to 12 were three equal parts of the large intestine. For the examination, segments 1, 3, 5, 7, 9 and 12 were selected. The contents were stripped out, weighed and serial dilutions were prepared after homogenization. The bacteriological methods were described elsewhere (1, 6-8) and were based on the drop count quantitative procedure (9). The selective media used, characteristics of the colonies and nomenclature are given in Table II.

TABLE II. Cultivation Procedures, Colony Characteristics and Nomenclature of Organisms Isolated

Media used	Time and type of incubation	Characteristics of the colonies	Nomenclature
Eosin Methylene Blue Agar (Difco)	18 hr aerobic	Dark or dark centered	Coliforms
Simmons Citrate Agar (Difco)	48 hr aerobic	Blue	Citrate-fermenting coliforms
Streptococcus faecalis Agar (Difco)	48 hr aerobic	Yellow	Enterococci
Staphylococcus Medium 110 (Difco)	48 hr aerobic	Yellow, white or orange	Micrococcaceae
Rogosa SL Agar (Difco)	48 hr anaerobic + aerobic	All	Lactobacilli
Blood Agar Base I (Oxoid) + 5% sheep blood	48 hr anaerobic	All	Total number of anaerobes
Blood Agar Base I (Oxoid) + 5% egg yolk	18 hr anaerobic	Large, surrounded by a large white ring	*Clostridium perfringens*

The colonies were counted under binocular magnification and the logarithmic number of viable organisms in one gram of fresh content was calculated. The averages in the tables were calculated as the mean of the individual logarithmic values.

Results

Results of the bacteriology of different feeding managements. The results of the experiments concerning the different feeding systems are summarized in

TABLE III. Mean Log Number of Viable Organisms per Gram Fresh Contents in the Gastrointestinal Tract of Piglets Reared on Different Feeding Managements

Feeding	Segments					
managements	1	3	5	7	9	12
COLIFORMS						
SR	3.7	3.7	4.6	7.2	8.4	8.5
CM 2t/d. AL.	5.5	5.3	5.8	6.9	7.5	7.6
CM 4t/d. AL.	5.3	4.7	5.0	6.4	8.8	9.0
MA 20% 4t/d. SF	5.0	4.3	4.2	6.1	9.3	8.2
MA 33% 3t/d. SF	4.4	3.5	3.6	5.5	8.8	8.3
MA dry AL.	6.2	5.2	5.5	7.0	8.1	8.2
CITRATE-FERMENTING COLIFORMS						
SR	3.0	3.1	3.1	3.4	4.1	3.8
CM 2t/d. AL.	4.4	4.5	4.8	5.7	6.4	6.4
CM 4t/d. AL.	5.0	4.5	4.8	5.7	5.7	3.9
MA 20% 4t/d. SF	4.8	3.6	4.2	4.6	4.8	3.7
MA 33% 3t/d. SF	3.9	3.0	3.3	3.0	4.6	3.0
MA dry AL.	3.0	3.0	3.0	3.0	3.1	3.0
ENTEROCOCCI						
SR	3.5	3.6	3.7	5.0	5.6	5.8
CM 2t/d. AL.	5.0	4.8	5.2	5.8	7.5	7.9
CM 4t/d. AL.	5.8	4.7	5.1	6.3	8.4	7.9
MA 20% 4t/d. SF	4.5	3.5	3.3	4.8	7.3	7.8
MA 33% 3t/d. SF	4.5	3.3	3.6	4.4	7.5	7.7
MA dry AL.	3.2	3.1	3.0	4.1	5.8	5.8
LACTOBACILLI: AEROBIC COUNT						
SR	7.5	6.9	7.2	7.9	8.4	8.1
CM 2t/d. AL.	3.5	3.2	3.5	4.2	4.1	4.0
CM 4t/d. AL.	6.7	5.7	5.3	7.4	8.9	8.1
CM 20% 4t/d. SF	4.2	3.2	3.2	4.2	6.6	4.0
CM 33% 3t/d. SF	5.4	4.5	4.3	5.5	8.3	7.5
MA dry AL.	7.5	7.2	7.2	7.5	8.2	7.5
ANAEROBIC LACTOBACILLI						
(SR)	(9.1)[a]	(8.6)	(8.6)	(9.6)	(9.6)	(8.4)
CM 2t/d. AL.	4.3	3.9	4.3	5.3	7.6	7.4
CM 4t/d. AL.	7.4	6.2	5.9	7.8	9.4	8.5
MA 20% 4t/d. SF	4.5	3.5	3.5	4.6	7.1	4.6
MA 33% 3t/d. SF	5.8	4.7	5.0	6.0	8.5	7.4
MA dry AL.	8.3	7.8	7.8	7.9	8.5	7.6
TOTAL NUMBER OF ANAEROBES						
SR	8.5	8.0	8.5	9.0	9.6	9.7
CM 2t/d. AL.	7.6	7.3	7.7	8.4	10.1	10.1
CM 4t/d. AL.	7.7	6.7	6.8	8.1	10.5	9.8

TABLE III. Continued

Feeding	Segments					
managements	1	3	5	7	9	12
MA 20% 4t/d. SF	6.5	5.5	5.8	7.1	10.2	9.6
MA 33% 3t/d. SF	6.2	5.5	6.1	7.1	10.2	9.8
MA dry AL.	8.3	7.7	7.7	8.2	9.5	9.8
CLOSTRIDIUM PERFRINGENS						
SR	3.0	3.0	3.0	3.0	7.0	7.5
CM 2t/d. AL.	3.2	3.0	3.0	3.0	8.2	8.3
CM 4t/d. AL.	3.0	3.0	3.0	3.0	6.9	7.5
MA 20% 4t/d. SF	3.0	3.0	3.0	3.0	6.4	7.3
MA 33% 3t/d. SF	3.0	3.0	3.0	3.0	7.2	7.4
MA dry AL.	3.0	3.0	3.0	3.1	4.8	4.9

[a]Data in parentheses since only four piglets were cultured for anaerobic lactobacilli.

Table III. Although no real comparison can be made between the several feed trials, because the experiments were done with animals of different origin and at different times, some marked influences can be noted as follows.

Coliforms. As pointed out by other authors, only a low number of coliforms is normally present in the stomach and upper segments of the small intestine of suckling piglets (10-12). In the artificially reared piglets, on the other hand, the number of coliforms in the upper segments seems related to the nutrient intake as the highest numbers are found in the *ad libitum* fed piglets. Indeed, in the dry-*ad libitum*-fed piglets, the highest numbers are noted. The lowest count is found in the most restricted group (MA 33%, 3t/d. SF).

Citrate-fermenting coliforms. Citrate-fermenting coliforms are rarely isolated in suckling piglets (2). In artificially reared piglets fed a liquid diet relatively high numbers are noted. In the dry-fed piglets, as in the suckling piglets, these bacteria could only be isolated occasionally.

Enterococci. In the suckling piglets, the enterococci closely follow the pattern of distribution of the coliforms, but in the lower parts of the intestine their number is about 100 times lower. Also in the liquid-fed piglets, the distribution of the coliform population is followed and the same differences between *ad libitum* and scale-fed animals is noted. However, this similarity is not observed for the dry-fed piglets where their number is relatively scarce in the small intestine.

Lactobacilli and total number of anaerobes. In the suckling piglets the anaerobic lactobacilli were counted only for 4 animals so that no real comparison with the mean aerobic count is possible. In the stomach and the small intestine of nearly all the piglets, the anaerobic lactobacillus count is about

½ to 1 log. unit higher than the aerobic one. However, all were facultative anaerobes as seen by inoculation on agar slants.

The same differences between the two counts is noted normally in the cecum and large intestine, except for the piglets who were fed twice a day *ad libitum* where high numbers of strict anaerobic lactobacilli of the bifidus type could be isolated. In further experiments, however, such organisms were never found again. Comparing the anaerobic lactobacillus count with the total count of anaerobes, it can be seen that in the stomach and small intestine of suckling piglets, lactobacilli are the predominating organisms while in the cecum and large intestine other organisms outnumbered the lactobacilli by a factor 100 to 1000. On further examination it was seen that the dominant organisms in the lower segments were strict anaerobic Gram-negative pleomorphic rods probably belonging to the *Bacteroides* group.

The same pattern of dominance is seen in the dry-fed piglets, in which the number of lactobacilli is quite identical with the number found in the suckling piglets.

In the liquid-fed piglets on the other hand, the general finding is a very sharp reduction of the number of lactobacilli, most pronounced in the stomach and the small intestine. The lowest numbers again are found in the piglets that were only fed twice a day and thereby consumed very large amounts at once. In the piglets fed 4 times a day *ad libitum*, the number of lactobacilli in the stomach and small intestine was about 100 times higher than in the above cited group. Limiting the amount of milk to a certain scale again resulted in lower numbers of lactobacilli. In these piglets on the other hand, we found that the difference of anaerobic lactobacilli and the total anaerobic count was already pronounced in the small intestine and gradually reached a maximum of 3 log. units difference in the cecum and rectum. This again was most pronounced in the group fed twice a day. This suggests that in these liquid-fed piglets, organisms other than lactobacilli dominated the microflora. Some preliminary examinations revealed high numbers of streptococci in these segments.

Clostridium perfringens. In all the piglets, it is only in the cecum and large intestine that clostridia can be isolated. There are no real differences between the experimental groups. Indeed, the low value found in the dry-fed piglets is not a real mean value since in 3 of the 7 piglets no clostridia were found at all. In the others, numbers equal to the suckling piglets were noted.

Results of feeding antibiotics. The results of the experiments with nutritional doses of virginiamycin and spiramycin are summarized in Table IV. The antibiotics were given during a period of 14 days after which the animals were slaughtered for analysis. In these experiments, only virginiamycin gave a growth response of about 10%. The changes in the gastrointestinal microflora can be summarized as follows:

TABLE IV. Mean Log Number of the Viable Organisms per Gram Fresh Contents in the Gastrointestinal Tract of Early Weaned Piglets as Influenced by Nutritional Doses of Virginiamycin and Spiramycin.

Treatment		Segments					
		1	3	5	7	9	12
COLIFORMS	C (a)	4.3(b)	4.0	4.5	5.8	7.4	7.1
	V	5.4	4.4	4.7	6.5	7.9	7.6
	S	4.8	4.1	4.9	5.8	7.2	7.4
CITRATE-FERMENTING							
COLIFORMS	C	3.1	3.1	3.1	3.6	3.9	3.3
	V	3.6	3.3	3.4	4.5	5.0	4.0
	S	3.9	3.7	4.2	4.3	4.8	3.8
ENTEROCOCCI							
	C	4.1	3.9	4.1	5.0	6.7	6.9
	V	5.1	4.2	4.8	6.5	7.7	6.8
	S	5.2	4.6	5.3	5.9	7.5	7.2
ANAEROBIC LACTOBACILLI							
	C	8.2	7.6	7.7	7.9	8.4	7.7
	V	6.8	6.1	6.6	7.3	7.9	6.2
	S	7.6	7.2	7.7	8.0	8.3	7.0
TOTAL NUMBER OF ANAEROBES							
	C	8.2	7.3	7.7	8.1	10.1	9.8
	V	7.4	6.8	7.0	7.8	10.3	9.8
	S	7.9	7.3	7.8	8.2	10.1	9.8
CLOSTRIDIUM PERFRINGENS							
	C	3.0	3.0	3.0	3.0	4.3	4.7
	V	3.0	3.0	3.0	3.0	3.1	3.1
	S	3.4	3.1	3.0	3.2	4.3	4.7

(a) C = control, V = 50 ppm Virginiamycin, S = 50 ppm Spiramycin
(b) n = 9

Coliforms and citrate-fermenting coliforms. Little differences are found except perhaps a small increase for both antibiotics.

Enterococci. Here again the enterococci closely follow the trend of the coliforms; a small increase is noted for both antibiotics.

Lactobacilli and total number of anaerobes. In the virginiamycin treated piglets a marked fall in the number of lactobacilli is noted in the stomach and

375

small intestine. In the spiramycin treated piglets on the other hand the same number as in the control animals could be isolated.

As cited previously the total anaerobic count of the stomach and small intestine of dry-fed piglets is nearly a reflection of the anaerobic lactobacillus count, suggesting that lactobacilli are dominant in those segments. This is a fact in the control and spiramycin group while in the virginiamycin treated group the difference between the two values reaches values of the order of ½ to 1 log. unit, which suggests that other organisms may be dominating here again. Indeed in further experiments which are currently going on, it was found that anaerobic streptococci can be isolated also.

In the cecum and large intestine, again *Bacteroides sp.* are the dominating bacteria and no differences between the experimental groups can be found.

Clostridia. The virginiamycin treatment resulted in the elimination of the clostridia in nearly all of the piglets while spiramycin did not.

Conclusions

From the above feed management experiments, it can be deduced that not only feed composition but also the way of giving the feed can have pronounced effects on the gastrointestinal flora of piglets.

A liquid feeding system resulted in a sharp decrease in the number of lactobacilli combined with a shift in the dominating bacteria of the stomach and small intestine. Indeed instead of lactobacilli other organisms could be isolated in the largest numbers (streptococci). Also the coliform population became more important. These changes were also observed by others (13) in pigs with a disturbed gastrointestinal microflora. This might suggest that in our liquid-fed piglets a certain degree of dysbacteriosis, caused by unphysiological feeding methods, was present. This could be an explanation for the frequent gastrointestinal disorders seen in these piglets.

In the dry-fed piglets on the other hand, gastrointestinal disorders are seldom observed and the growth is quite good. It is thereby noteworthy that the gastrointestinal microflora is quite identical (except for the coliforms) with the flora seen in the suckling piglets.

The changes observed in the antibiotic experiments, such as a rise in the number of coliforms, the decrease of the number of lactobacilli, the elimination of the clostridia are changes that have been reported for other growth promoting antibiotics (14-16).

The shift in the dominating bacteria of the small intestine in virginiamycin treated piglets was never observed before. The meaning of this change is not well understood. Perhaps it is only a secondary effect caused by the depression of the lactobacilli, since the same effect occurred with the milk feeding.

References

1. Van der Heyde, H., and Henderickx, H., *Zbt. Bakt. I, Orig. 195:* 80 (1964).
2. Van der Heyde, H., and Henderickx, H., *Zbt. Bakt. I, Orig. 195:* 215 (1964).
3. Van der Heyde, H., *Het. Ingenieursblad. 10:* 1 (1970).
4. Francois, A. C., and Michel, M. C., *Nutr. et Diet. 10:* 35 (1968).
5. Ghesquiere, L., Thesis, University of Gent, Belgium, (1970).
6. Van der Heyde, H., *Zbt. Bakt. I, Orig. 189:* 224 (1963).
7. Van der Heyde, H., Thesis, University of Gent, Belgium, (1967).
8. Decuypere, J., and Van der Heyde, H., *Zbt. Bakt. I, Orig.*, (In Press).
9. Miles, A. A., and Misra, S. S., *J. Hyg. 38:* 732 (1938).
10. Pesti, L., *Act. Vet. Hung. 12:* 299 (1962).
11. Kenworthy, R., and Crabb, W. E., *J. Comp. Path. 73:* 215 (1963).
12. Namioka, S., Murata, M., Osada, H., Ishizawa, T., and Kuro-Oka, R., *Jap. J. Vet. Sci. 27:* 221 (1965).
13. Ogata, M., and Morishita, Y., *Jap. J. Vet. Sci. 31:* 71 (1969).
14. Larson, N. L., and Hill, E. G., *J. Animal Sci. 14:* 674 (1955).
15. Bridges, J. M., Dyer, I. A., and Powers, J. J., *J. Animal Sci. 12:* 96 (1953).
16. Kellogg, T. F., Hays, V. W., Catron, D. V., Quinn, L. Y., and Speer, V. C., *J. Animal Sci. 23:* 1089 (1964).

377

STUDIES WITH *LACTOBACILLUS CASEI* IN GNOTOBIOTIC MICE

Philip B. Carter
Trudeau Institute, Inc., Saranac Lake, New York 12983, U.S.A.

and

Morris Pollard
Department of Microbiology and Lobund Laboratory
University of Notre Dame, Notre Dame, Indiana 46556, U.S.A.

Introduction

Various members of the indigenous microflora of man and of other animals appear to demonstrate low immunogenicity in their host (1). Such characteristics of the "normal" microflora have often been reported as controls for studies with pathogenic organisms and their significance was "masked" by the effects of other microorganisms. Host-parasite interactions of individual members of the "normal" microbial flora can be examined more precisely by use of the clean, uniform, and "low profile" tissue systems of axenic animals. Changes demonstrated in these animals would have a more clearly defined causal relationship to the microorganism under study than in conventional animals. We report herein interactions of gnotobiotic mice with *Lactobacillus casei,* a representative nonpathogenic and persistent member of the so-called "normal" microflora of mice, which will serve to define more clearly the nature of the "normal" flora.

When germfree (GF) mice are conventionalized by exposure to the environment of the animal quarters, they manifest activation of the immunogenic mechanisms: lymph nodes, spleen, and Peyer's patches increase in size and germinal centers and plasma cells appear in them; the lamina propriae of the intestine become thicker and contain more cells; and serum gamma globulin levels become elevated (2, 3). After being monoassociated with pathogenic microorganisms, gnotobiotic mice manifest many of the cellular and serological conversions seen in conventionalized mice (2). However, when nonpathogenic members of the "normal" intestinal flora of the mouse are associated with GF mice, they do not initiate any of these changes (4).

Materials and Methods

Sixty-two six week old Lobund GF mice of both Swiss-Webster and CFW strains (both random bred) were monoassociated orally with 18 hour cultures of *L. casei* propagated in thioglycolate broth. (This strain was isolated from the human oral cavity in 1937.) Thereafter, they were maintained monoassociated in the germfree isolator system. Three GF mice of each strain were necropsied as controls just prior to monoassociation, and thereafter, three mice of each strain were necropsied at three days, one week, and at weekly intervals for eight weeks. Feces and blood from all animals were cultured for bacterial content in thioglycolate broth at 37° C. Tissues were collected and processed for histological examination, these included: all of the Peyer's patches and the cecal tonsil, the axillary and mesenteric lymph nodes, spleen, pancreas, liver, kidney, adrenal, lung, and thymus. Blood serum was collected from each mouse and stored at −20°C until tested.

Sera were examined for specific antibody using the indirect fluorescein-tagged antibody technique described by Horowitz *et al.* (5). This technique was employed because of its high sensitivity to low titers of antibody and to avoid the complications of auto-agglutination which occurs with lactobacilli.

Groups of *L. casei* monoassociated mice were subjected to the immuno-suppressive effects of whole body X-irradiation or to treatment with cyclophosphamide (*Cytoxan,* Mead Johnson, Evansville, Indiana) to study the possible modifying effects of immunosuppression on the host-parasite inter-action.

The administration of X-rays followed a previously described scheme (7). The X-ray source was a 260-kVp Picker therapy X-ray machine operated at 250 kV and 18 ma with a filtration of 1.0 mm Al and 0.25 mm Cu. This gave a rate of approximately 40 R/min as measured in air with a Victoreen condenser R-meter. A single dose of 700 R (approximately 700 rads) X-irradiation was given to twenty 11 week old CFW mice of both sexes which had been associated with *L. casei* at 6 weeks of age. This X-ray dose corresponds to an $LD_{50(30)}$ for conventional CFW mice but only an $LD_{10-20(30)}$ for GF CFW mice at 11 weeks of age.

Cyclophosphamide was given to gnotobiotic CFW mice monoassociated at birth with *L. casei* and treated with the drug at 54 days of age. Three i.p. injections were given, each on every other day for a 4 day period. Each dose (200 mg/kg body weight) was approximately twice the LD_{100} for Lobund-reared conventional mice. Cyclophosphamide has a low organotropic toxicity (8), so the cause of death has been attributed to secondary infection following immunosuppression (9).

An attempt was made to induce disease with nonpathogenic members of the indigenous microflora by circumventing some of the immune defense mechanisms of the host via intracerebral inoculation. Conventional weanling mice were inoculated intracerebrally with 0.03 ml of an 18 hour culture of either *L. casei, Streptococcus faecalis,* or *Enterobacter aerogenes* in saline (approximately 10^6 cells).

Results

Serology. Sera from mice monoassociated with *L. casei* during the experimental period were negative for *L. casei* antibody. Sera from *L. casei* hyperimmunized rats served as a positive control for the test as well as sera from *Clostridium difficile* monoassociated mice.

Histology. Throughout the period of monoassociation, the tissues in both strains of gnotobiotic mice were unchanged from those observed in the GF controls. The Peyer's patches and cecal tonsils remained small and contained only rare germinal zones. The lamina propriae remained thin and relatively acellular. The histology of the spleens and lymph nodes were within the structural parameters of normal GF mice: they were small and contained rare germinal zones and plasma cells.

Bacteriology. *L. casei* was recovered from the intestines throughout the course of the experiment; however, bacteremia could not be demonstrated.

Effects of X-irradiation. The group of gnotobiotic mice monoassociated with *L. casei* and subjected to the immunosuppressive effects of whole body X-irradiation were run because previous work (6) attributed the high mortality rate in irradiated conventional mice to systemic infection by members of the indigenous microbial flora. It was of interest to determine whether the presence of *L. casei* in gnotobiotic mice would enhance the damaging effects of X-irradiation.

Sixteen of twenty irradiated monoassociated mice survived the thirty day test period. The other mice had succumbed on day 13 post-irradiation which coincided with the time of most severe hematopoietic depletion. Blood and liver samples from the surviving mice were bacteria-free at the end of the test period (at 40 days post-irradiation) and their tissues appeared normal.

Cyclophosphamide treatment. As an additional study on the effect of immuno-suppression, CFW mice, monoassociated at birth with *L. casei,* were treated with cyclophosphamide. Twelve out of thirteen mice survived until 32 days after the last injection of the drug. At necropsy, all the experimental animals showed dramatic involution of the lymph nodes and spleen but no signs of pathology caused by *L. casei* were observed.

Intracerebral inoculation. In an attempt to induce disease with non-pathogenic members of the indigenous microflora, conventional weanling mice were inoculated intracerebrally with viable *S. faecalis* in saline (approx. 10^6 cells). This procedure induced neither illness nor death throughout a four day postinoculation observation period. At this time, *S. faecalis* was recovered from the brain tissues of the six inoculated mice. Weanling mice similarly inoculated with *L. casei* showed neither illness nor death during a two week observation period subsequent to inoculation, at which time *L. casei* was recovered from all of the brains (8/8). Total bacterial counts were not determined. Weanling mice inoculated with *E. aerogenes* resulted in a 93% (14/15) mortality rate by the end of the observation period.

Conclusions

The host response to *L. casei* resembles that reported with *S. faecalis* (2). The organism colonized the intestinal tract but the immunogenic mechanisms remained unaltered from the axenic state. Thus, the above two organisms of the so-called "normal" flora have been shown to persist in the mouse without eliciting a detectable host response and without producing disease even when host defenses were depressed by either whole body X-irradiation or cyclophosphamide or when circumvented by intracerebral inoculation. Examinations directed at other members of the "normal" microbial flora (4) indicate that the negative host responses to *L. casei* and *S. faecalis* are not exemplary of the "resident" flora. These organisms may belong to what could be termed the true normal flora whose presence in the intestine may be beneficial to the animal (10).

Acknowledgement

This work was supported by funds from the U.S. Office of Naval Research and from Title IV Fellowship funds of the National Defense Education Act (Carter).

References

1. Rosebury, T., "Microorganisms Indigenous to Man," McGraw-Hill, New York, p. 360, p. 435, (1962).
2. Pollard, M., and Sharon, N., *Infect. Immunity 2:* 96 (1970).
3. Wagner, M., and Wostmann, B. S., *Ann. N.Y. Acad. Sci. 94:* 210 (1962).
4. Carter, P. B., and Pollard, M., *J. Reticuloendothel. Soc. 9:* 580 (1971); Carter, P. B., "Host Responses to Normal Intestinal Microflora," Ph.D. Thesis, Univ. of Notre Dame, Indiana, p. 110, (1971).
5. Horowitz, R. E., Bauer, H., Paronetto, F., Abrams, G. D., Watkins, K. C., and Popper, H., *Amer. J. Pathol. 44:* 747 (1964).
6. Vincent, J. G., Veomett, R. C., and Riley, R. F., *J. Bacteriol. 69:* 38 (1955).
7. Wilson, B. R., *Radiat. Res. 20:* 477 (1963).
8. Brock, N., and Hohorst, H. J. *Cancer 20:* 900 (1967).
9. Sharbaugh, R. J., "Cyclophosphamide-induced Immunosuppression and Its Effects on Host Resistance to Invasion," Ph.D. Thesis, Medical Center, Univ. of Mississippi, p. 148, (1969).

10. Klainer, A. S., Gorbach, S., and Weinstein, L., *J. Bacteriol. 94:* 383 (1967); Rettger, L. F., and Cheplin, H. A., "A Treatise on the Transformation of the Intestinal Flora with Special Reference to the Implantation of *Bacillus acidophilus*," Yale University Press, New Haven, p. 135, (1921).

IMMUNOLOGIC CONVERSION OF *VIBRIO CHOLERAE* IN GNOTOBIOTIC MICE

C. E. Miller,* K. H. Wong, J. C. Feeley,** and *M. E. Forlines*
Laboratory of Bacterial Products, Division of Biologics Standards
National Institutes of Health, Department of Health, Education and Welfare
Bethesda, Maryland 20014, U.S.A.

Introduction

Three convalescent carriers of *Vibrio cholerae* were identified in a group of 81 patients admitted to a hospital in the 1967 cholera season in Calcutta (1). Cultures of *V. cholerae*, identified as biotype El Tor vibrios, were recovered by purging with MgSo4 or by evacuation of the gall bladder and sampling the intestinal fluids. One patient shed only rough vibrios during the 331 days of study before treatment with antibiotics.

V. cholerae grows well in gnotobiotic bacteria-free mice (2). The serotype changes in response to immunologic pressure. After a few weeks, the cholera vibrios become rough and persist for many months. Inoculation of a rough colony into uninoculated gnotobiotic mice led to the recovery of smooth vibrios. In a few weeks, however, the rough forms predominated again. It was suggested that the rough cholera vibrios from chronic carriers may revert to the smooth form under appropriate conditions (1). The results of studies on a rough strain from a carrier are presented here.

Results

After inoculation through a stomach tube, *V. cholerae* readily became established in the intestines of gnotobiotic, bacteria-free mice. The total bacterial count soon stabilized near 10^8 cells/ml of fecal extract (Fig. 1). Selective treatment of a gelatin buffered saline extract of infected mouse feces with guinea pig complement and anti-rough serum effectively reduced rough organisms and facilitated the recovery of smooth forms (3). The bacteria recovered did not agglutinate in anti-rough serum, but were still agglutinable in 1:1,000 acriflavine. Two additional passages of these organisms in uninoculated

---

*Present address: National Cancer Institute, NIH, Bethesda, Maryland 20014, U.S.A.
**Present address: Center for Disease Control, Atlanta, Georgia 30333, U.S.A.

385

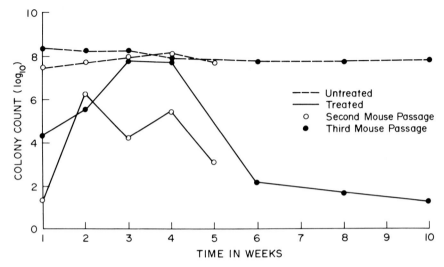

FIG. 1. Relative counts of *Vibrio cholerae* in mouse feces.

gnotobiotic mice resulted in the recovery of completely smooth *V. cholerae*. Cultures belonging to the serotypes of Ogawa, Inaba and Hikojima were identified. These cultures, as well as two rough strains recovered later from these mice, were saved for further study.

The results of serological and biochemical tests are shown in Table I. All isolates were Heiberg Group I, El Tor cholera vibrios and similar to the *V. cholerae* isolated from the convalescent carrier (1). Their ability to produce cholera-like fluid and death in infant rabbits (4) is shown in Table II. The original rough culture from the convalescent carrier caused no fluid production,

TABLE I. Serologic and Biochemical Reactions of *V. cholerae* Isolates from Mice

Culture	Gp I	Slide Agglutinations Og	In	X	Ac[b]	Polymyxin B Sensitivity	Chick Cell Agglut.	Fermentation Suc[c]	Man[c]	Arab[c]
Original	+	ND[a]	ND	+	+	−	+	+	+	−
Ogawa	+	+	−	−	−	−	+	+	+	−
Inaba	+	−	+	−	−	−	+	+	+	−
Hikojima	+	+	+	−	−	−	+	+	+	−
Rough O	+	+	−	+	+	−	+	+	+	−
Rough X	+	+	+	+	+	−	+	+	+	−
VC-12[d]	+	+	−	−	−	+	−	+	+	−

a ND = not done
b Acriflavin, 1:1,000
c Sucrose, mannose, arabinose
d *V. cholerae* "classical" strain (positive control)

TABLE II. Mortality in Infant Rabbits Given *V. cholerae* Isolated from
Gnotobiotic Mice

V. cholerae Strain	48 hour mortality (D/N)
Original culture	0/6
Ogawa	1/6
Inaba	5/6
Hikojima	2/6
Rough O	2/6
Rough X	1/6
Negative Control (Syncase medium)	0/6
Positive Control (Ogawa VC-12)	6/6

while all the isolates from gnotobiotic mice caused one or more rabbits to die
with cholera-like fluid in the intestines.

Conclusions

Rough forms of *V. cholerae* could revert to any of the typical, smooth
forms when established in gnotobiotic, bacteria-free mice. The conversion was
gradual and progressive. The ability of these smooth forms to produce diarrheal
fluid in infant rabbits was markedly increased over the original rough culture. All
of the isolates from the third mouse passage caused some mortality in the infant
rabbits. The smooth Inaba isolate was nearly as virulent as the positive control
"classical" strain VC-12 (5) killing five of six rabbits in 48 hours.

V. cholerae appears to be very adaptable to environmental pressures.
Changes similar to that observed in the mice may occur in endemic areas of
cholera. In a rural area of East Pakistan, many inapparent infections with *V.
cholerae* were detected from serum samples (6). These infections were more
common in the segment of the population with low antibody titers, and they
could serve as a mechanism for *V. cholerae* to adjust to the type of antibody in
the general population.

References

1. Pierce, N. F., Banwell, J. G., Gorbach, S. L., Mitra, R. C., and Mondall, A., *Ann. Intern. Med. 72:* 357 (1970).
2. Sack, R. B., and Miller, C. E., *J. Bacteriol. 99:* 688 (1969).
3. Pollitzer, R., in "Cholera," W.H.O. Geneva, p. 246, (1959).
4. Finkelstein, R. A., Norris, H. T., and Dutta, N. K., *J. Inf. Dis. 114:* 203 (1964).
5. McIntyre, O. R., and Feeley, J. C., *J. Inf. Dis. 114:* 468 (1964).
6. Mosley, W. H., Benenson, A. S., and Barui, R., *Bull. W.H.O. 38:* 335 (1968).

SIGNIFICANCE OF INTESTINAL BACTERIAL FLORA TO INFECTION

S. Sasaki, N. Ohnishi, T. Shimamura, R. Maeda, K. Mizuno, and *T. Takahashi*
Department of Microbiology, School of Medicine
Keio University, Tokyo, Japan

Introduction

Among the several physiological roles of normal bacterial flora in the intestines, many reports concerning the resistance to intestinal infection has been presented. In these reports, the mechanism of this phenomenon has been attributed to a single agent, for example, nutritional competition, antibiotic production, change of redox potential, long chain unsaturated fatty acids, etc.

In this report, the significance of both antibody and bile acid and their role in the adjustment of the intestinal flora will be discussed. In all experiments, ICR germfree mice which were bred in our laboratory were provided as the host. The artificial flora established in these animals was composed of *Escherichia coli* and *Streptococcus faecalis,* while *Shigella flexneri* 2a was used as the representative pathogen.

Many researchers have experienced the persistence of bacteria in the intestines for long periods of time when inoculated into germfree animals per os without the occurence of any symptoms. Even pathogens such as *Shigella sp.* or *Vibrio sp.* were not exceptions to this rule. For example, *Shigella sp.* can persist in the intestines of mice for more than 200 days.

Hitherto, it was believed that coproantibody was produced in the intestines following an intestinal infection with a pathogen and that the antibacterial activity of the antibody was useful in eliminating the bacteria. However, to confirm this idea, and to understand the fact mentioned above, the bacterial should persist if: a) the coproantibody is not produced or b) though the antibody is produced, the phenomenon requires another substance to realize the eradicating activity of this antibody.

On the other hand, we have reported that the number of *S. flexneri* 2a in the feces of monoassociated mice decreased following superinfection with *E. coli* and *S. faecalis.* Within 80 days after the superinfection, shigella became undetectable when feces were cultured on SS agar. The question of evaluation of the coproantibody activity becomes an issue in this case and will be considered in this report.

In order to investigate the participation of the intestinal flora in the shigella eradication phenomenon, bile salt metabolism was studied in the past. It is well known that bile acids are secreted from the liver in conjugated form and certain species of bacteria, for example, *S. faecalis, Lactobacillus bifidus, Clostridium perfringens, Bacteroides fragilis* etc., have the ability to metabolize and deconjugate them. As a result of this process, free bile acid is produced. Additionally, free bile acid is transformed to other intermediate metabolites by *Bacillus cereus, C. perfringens, Bacteroides sp., E. coli* etc. In these processes, more attention should be paid to the antibiotic activity of these metabolites to exogenous bacteria. For example, one of these metabolites, 7-keto-deoxycholic acid, produced by *E. coli* from cholic acid, has specific antibiotic activity for pathogens. However there is no evidence whether these metabolic pathways exist independently or not.

In this study berberin hydrocholoride, a well known cholagogue, was used. In this case, the increase of bile secretion does not only mean an increase of total secretion volume of bile but also an increase in the absolute volume of bile acid.

Then, following the administration of berberin to mice at a rate of 500 mg/kg/day per os, bile acid contents in the small intestines and liver were examined successively using thin layer chromatography.

Results

On the 3rd day after administration of berberin to germfree mice, cholic acid and chenodeoxycholic acid were found in the free form in the small intestines. On the 7th day, the same bile acids were detected in the small intestines, cecum and liver. In contrast, free bile acid was not detected in the untreated control group.

The biological activity of these free bile acids were examined. After 2 weeks of monoassociation with *S. flexneri* in germfree mice, *E. coli* was given orally and berberin was given at a rate of 500 mg/kg/day simultaneously. The number of shigella in the feces decreased gradually and disappeared in about 70 days. This pattern was the same as in the case in which *E. coli* and *S. faecalis* were superinfected simultaneously. However, in the combination of *S. faecalis* and berberin, dimunition of the shigella infection was not recognized. Berberin administration alone did not have any effect on the persistence of *S. flexneri*. The results of this experiment suggest that the significance of the existance of excessive amounts of free bile acid was not sufficient to cause a reduction in the shigella infection. Under normal circumstance, the presence of *S. faecalis* is considered important for the deconjugation of the liver secreted bile acids (conjugated form) to make them available to *E. coli*. The *E. coli* can then further metabolize the free bile acids so produced to maintain the proper enterohepatic circulation of the bile acids. The *S. faecalis* function can be by-passed by the administration of berberin which causes an increase in the production and release of free bile acids.

On the other hand, although excess bile acid was present with *S. faecalis*, normal bile salt metabolism might have been disturbed, because this microorganism does not have the ability to transform free bile acid to the next step in the metabolic pathway. In other words, the result of deconjugation by the streptococcus had the same effect as berberin administration. From these data, existence of a continuous system between *E. coli* and *S. faecalis* as members of the normal flora was recognized and the significance of the characteristic distribution of flora becomes more clear.

At this point, the presence of antibody in these mice should be considered. As preliminary information, the experiment concerning antibody production in mice monoassociated with *S. flexneri* is presented.

After 2 weeks of challenge with shigella in ICR germfree mice, serum, bile and intestinal contents were examined for the various immunoglobulins using the gel-precipitation technique. Only IgA was detected in bile and contents of the intestines after challenge and it continued to persist for several weeks. This IgA was considered to have a close relationship to the so-called coproantibody, as shown in the experimental data obtained through Sephedex G 200 gel filtration and DEAE cellulose chromatography. Though the secretory component of the IgA was not examined, from the effluent pattern of gel filtration it was presumed to be polymerized secretory IgA. In reference to this, it is preferable to be conservative and not express any ideas regarding the subject of coproantibody as to whether it might be IgA or IgE. However, the fact that some antibody appeared in the intestines following the infection can not be disregarded.

Germfree mice were divided into 4 groups with persisting *S. flexneri* infections of 1, 2, 3, and 4 weeks in each group respectively. Each group was superinfected per os with *E. coli* and *S. faecalis* and the shigella infection was checked periodically. In the one-week group, the host-parasite balance may not have been established and the shigella infection was rejected easily by the antagonists. But in the two-week group, a balance was established gradually and thus able to persist against the antagonistic power of the flora. Therefore, the rejection of the shigella infection was not recognized. However, in the three-week group, the production of antibody became significant and its influence upon the shigella organisms became apparent and rejection of the shigella clearly appeared. This tendency was even more pronounced in the four-week group.

In these types of experiments, long periods are required and therefore it is not possible to avoid the aging process of the animals. Because of this, one must be careful in evaluating the experimental data, because aged animals have shown nonspecific resistance at times.

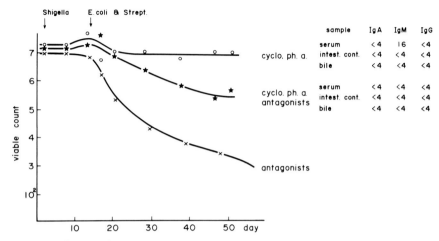

FIG. 1. Influence of cyclophosphamide on persistence of *Shigella flexneri* in germfree mice.

To confirm this hypothesis, another experiment was devised. Mice at 2, 4, 8 and 16 weeks of age were prepared, thus making 4 groups according to age. All mice were inoculated per os with *S. flexneri* and after one week, a challenge with *E. coli* and *S. faecalis* was given. Then the fate of the shigella infection was checked. The dimunition of the shigella infection was recognized in all groups without exception. Under this condition there was no need to consider the production of antibody in the various groups. Thus this phenomenon of rejection of the shigella organisms might be considered as the influence of the antagonists regardless of age.

Furthermore, the attempt was made to check the rejection phenomenon under the condition of suppression of antibody production. For this purpose we used cyclophosphamide (Endoxan) at a rate of 40 mg/kg/day subcutaneously. From previous experience, it was known that this substance can inhibit the production of coproantibody to *Vibrio* in germfree mice. It was expected that the same activity to shigella monoassociation in germfree mice would occur. *E. coli* and *S. faecalis* were given per os to mice that had previous persisting shigella. Endoxan was given in parallel and shigella infection was followed by fecal examination.

The results are shown in Fig. 1. Administration of Endoxan did not show any influence on the persistence of shigella which stayed at the level of 10^7 throughout the experiment in monoassociated mice. When the antagonists were added to this condition, rejection of shigella occurred slowly and slightly, and the number of shigella at 5 weeks remained at the level of 10^5. This pattern of rejection was clearly different from that of the non-Endoxan-treated control group in which the antagonists coexisted with antibody.

Conclusions

From these data, the phenomenon of the suppression and reduction of shigella infection appears to be the result of the combined activity of both antibody and bile acids.

References

1. Sasaki, S., Ohnishi, N., Suzuki, R., Adachi, K., Miyashita, M., Shimamura, T., Tazume, S., Maeda, R., and Takahashi, T., *J. Inf. Dis. 121:* 124 (1970).
2. Sasaki, S., *Keio J. Med. 19:* 87 (1970).
3. Suzuki, R., *Keio J. Med. 19:* 73 (1970).

EXPERIMENTAL AIRBORNE INFLUENZA PR8-A INFECTIONS IN GERMFREE MICE

C. G. Loosli, R. D. Buckley, S. Y. Hwang-Kow, J. D. Hardy,
D. P. Ryan, R. Serebrin, J. A. Joyce and *M. S. Hertweck*
Departments of Pathology, Medicine and Biochemistry
The University of Southern California
School of Medicine
Los Angeles, California 90033, U.S.A.

Introduction

Epidemic influenza in man is generally considered to be an airborne infection. While influenze virus infections in germfree mice have been studied by others (1-3), the virus was introduced directly into the lungs by intranasal instillation. However, the inhalation of the virus as fine particles, compared to intranasal instillation, is quantitatively more accurate as a means of infecting mice (4). This laboratory has employed for many years the aerosol procedure for the study of the pathogenesis and pathology of influenza PR8-A virus infections in conventional specific pathogen-free (SPF) mice (5-8). This report gives the result of similar studies using the germfree mouse.

Materials and Methods

The germfree mice (CD-1 strain) were either purchased (Charles River Breeding Laboratories, Wilmington, Massachusetts) or raised from germfree stock at the USC Germfree Animal Facility. Five separate exposures were made involving 461 mice (279 female, 182 male) which varied in age from 2½ to 5½ months at the time of onset of infection. All were infected and maintained in isolets except for one experiment when conventional and germfree mice were simultaneously infected with airborne virus.

The animals were exposed to aerosolized virus in a sterile 16 liter desiccator jar inside a sterile plastic isolet, following which they were then returned to their respective isolets. A DeVilbiss 40 atomizer was used to nebulize the virus suspension at one atmosphere pressure by filtered compressed air. In each experiment mice of approximately the same age were subjected to a sublethal cloud of a 10^{-5} dilution of mouse-lung suspension of PR8-A mouse adapted virus over a 10 minute period, the details of which have been described (5-8).

Sufficient animals were employed so that smaller groups, after exposure, could be sacrificed at close intervals of time, namely at 0 hour, 1, 2, 3, 4, 5, 7, 10, 14, 21 and 30 days. At each interval 3 mice were sacrificed for lung-virus growth and blood antibody determinations; 5 for light (hematoxylin-eosin-azure II stain (HEA)) and electronmicroscopic study; and 3 for histochemical examination employing lactate dehydrogenase (LDH) and glucose-6-phosphate dehydrogenase (Gl-6-PDH) as cell markers. At the time of sacrifice lung-virus homogenates using trypticase soy broth (TSB) and blood agar plates and fecal specimens of individual mice using thioglycollate broth were cultured for the presence of bacteria. The details of the procedures employed in this study have been given in reported studies of viral influenzal infections in conventional mice (7-11).

Results

Lung virus and serum antibody responses. As was the case with conventional SPF mice, germfree mice, following exposure to aerosolized virus, developed pulmonary infections. Influenza virus in high titers can be demonstrated in the lungs at 24 hours and up to 14 days after onset (Table I). The lung

TABLE I. Lung Virus Titers (Egg Infectivity Doses)*

				Days After Onset					
Exp.	1	2	3	4	5	7	10	14	21
M 18	10^3	10^4	10^5	10^5	10^5	10^3	–	–	–
M 19F	–	–	10^6	10^6	10^6	10^4	10^3	–	–
M 19M	–	–	10^6	10^6	10^6	10^4	10^4	–	–
M 19FC	–	–	10^5	10^5	10^5	10^3	10^3	–	–
M 29	10^3	–	10^6	–	10^7	10^5	10^4	10^4	–
M 30	10^4	–	10^4	–	10^5	10^5	10^3	10^4	–
M 7FC	10^5	10^6	10^6	10^6	10^5	10^4	10^4	0	0

*Pooled lungs of three mice.

virus titers were similar to those of conventional mice (M19FC, M7FC) exposed under similar conditions. Likewise, serum antibody responses were essentially the same in germfree, monocontaminated, and conventional pathogen-free mice. Hemagglutination inhibition (HI) antibodies were detected at 7 days and were present in sera of mice sacrificed at 30 days. In experiments (M29, M30) where the germfree mice were not contaminated, the HI antibody response was somewhat lower (Table II). Although not shown in Table II, neutralizing antibodies were detected in low titers after 7 days in sera of mice in experiments M19, M29 and M30, the only sera tested. Cultures of the lung-virus homogenates

396

TABLE II. Hemagglutination Inhibition (HI) Antibody Titers as Serum Dilutions*

Exp.	Days After Onset								
	2	3	4	5	7	10	14	21	30
M 18	0	0	0	0	40	80	—	40	—
M 19F	0	0	0	0	0	40	80	—	—
M 19M	0	0	0	0	20	80	40	—	—
M 19FC	0	0	0	0	20	40	160	—	—
M 24	—	—	—	—	—	80	—	—	—
M 29	0	0	0	0	0	10	10	0	0
M 30	0	0	0	0	0	10	10	20	—
M 7FC	0	0	0	0	10	20	20	40	80

*Pooled sera from three mice.

of conventional and germfree mice for the presence of bacteria were invariably sterile, and bacteria were never seen in the pneumonic exudate at any stage after onset of infection. Thus, the lung reactions described below can be considered as being due specifically to the airborne influenza virus.

Light microscopy. The mouse lung is simply constructed and had no respiratory bronchioles. The bronchial passages are lined by an epithelial membrane composed of ciliated and non-ciliated (Clara) cells with prominent cytoplasmic blebs (Fig. 1a). The alveoli are lined by membraneous (type I) and large granular (type II) cells. All the above cells were susceptible to invasion and destruction by the influenza virus.

Following sublethal exposure to airborne influenza virus, microscopic pulmonary lesions were seen as early as 24 to 48 hours. They were small and involved only a few areas in different parts of the lung (Fig. 1b). In such areas the bronchial lining cells were greatly swollen and the alveolar walls thickened with inflammatory exudate cells (Fig. 1c). Through the electron microscope, the cells had marked degenerative change and influenza virus particles were seen being shed from the membraneous surfaces of the cells (Fig. 1d).

The influenza virus spreads by direct extension from bronchus to bronchus by aspiration of infectious exudate. By 4 days after onset, focal areas of pneumonitis were seen both grossly and microscopically (arrow, Fig. 2a). The lesions were characterized by destruction of the bronchial and alveolar lining cells, cellular thickening of the alveolar walls, alveolar exudate cells from the blood, and cellular debri containing numerous viral particles (Fig. 2b). At 7 days one or more lobes may be uniformly involved in the pneumonic process (arrow, Fig. 2c). The bronchial lining membrane was reduced to a single layer of flattened, nonciliated cells with cell debri in the lumen and alveolar spaces (Fig. 2d). Seven to 8 days after onset, HI and neutralizing serum antibodies developed, after which the virus rapidly disappeared from the infected lungs resulting in no further spread.

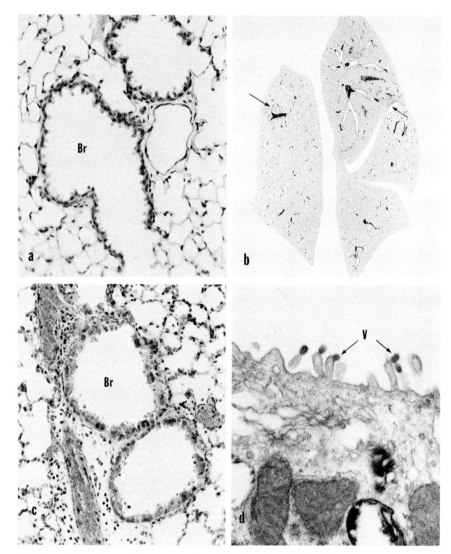

FIG. 1. a. Normal germfree mouse lung showing bronchiole (Br), HEA stain x 250.
b. Forty-eight hour influenzal lung lesions (arrows), HEA x 6. c. Forty-eight hour bronchial
(Br) lesion (arrow, left lobe in b) HEA x 250. d. EM photograph, type II cell shedding virus
(arrows, V), 72 hours x 40,000.

By 10 days the involved lobes had extensive atelectasis and could not be
completely re-expanded with the fixative (Fig. 3a). The bronchial lining
membranes now exhibited rapid regeneration with the ciliated and non-ciliated
cells being replaced by a metaplastic layer several cells in thickness (Fig. 3b).

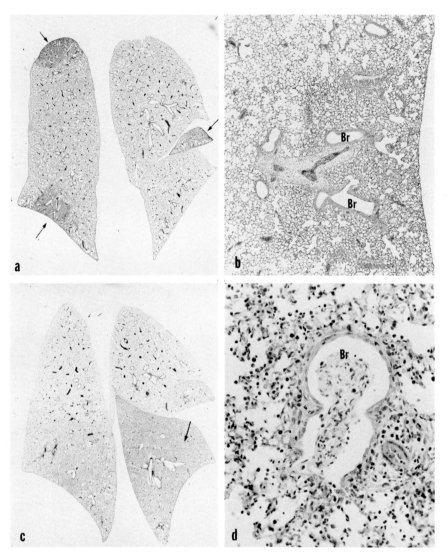

FIG. 2. a. Four day influenza lung lesions (arrows), left lobe, HEA x 6. b. Four day lesion (arrow, left lobe in a), HEA x 45. c. Seven day influenzal lesion, right lower lobe, HEA x 6. d. Seven day lesion (arrow in c), HEA x 250.

These cells or membranes then grew peripherally as syncytial masses into the surrounding collapsed alveolar ducts and alveoli producing epithelial nodules and permanent collapse of the involved lobes (arrows, Fig. 3c & 3d). Lung lobes not showing epithelial proliferation underwent resolution with residual scarring (Fig. 3d).

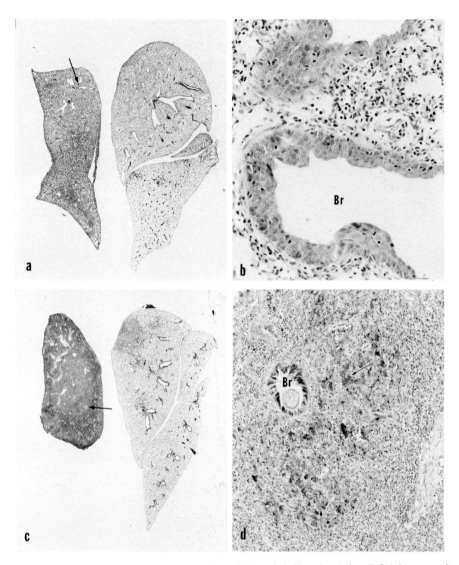

FIG. 3. a. Ten day influenzal lung lesions, HEA x 6. b. Ten day lesion (left lobe, arrow in a), HEA x 250. c. Twenty-one day influenzal lesion, left lobe, HEA x 6. d. Twenty-one day lesion (arrow in c), HEA x 250.

Enzyme staining. The lactate dehydrogenase (LDH) procedure stained both the bronchial lining cells and thy large type II cells on the alveolar walls (Fig. 4a). It can be seen in the 7 day lesion (Fig. 4b) that these cells were destroyed by the virus. By 10 days, the regenerating bronchial lining membranes

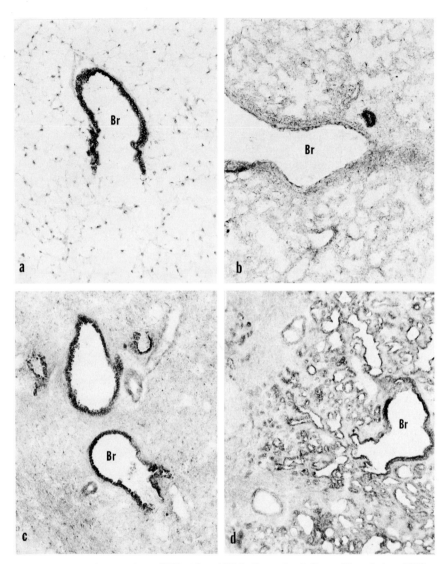

FIG. 4. a. Normal mouse lung, LDH stain x 125. b. Seven day influenzal lung lesion, LDH x 125. c. Ten day influenzal lung lesion, LDH x 100. d. Twenty-one day influenzal lung lesion, LDH x 75.

again stained heavily, but the surrounding collapsed lung parenchyma had no staining or regeneration of the type II cells (Fig. 4c). The epithelial nodules seen in the 21 day lesions also stained heavily, but not the collapsed lung tissue (Fig. 4d).

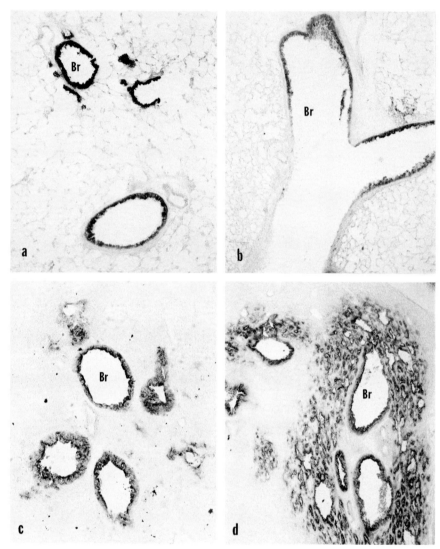

FIG. 5. a. Normal mouse lung, Gl-6-PDH stain x 75. b. Seven day influenzal lung lesion, Gl-6-PDH x 55. c. Fourteen day influenzal lung lesion, Gl-6-PDH x 75. d. Twenty-one day influenzal lung lesion, Gl-6-PDH x 55.

The glucose-6-phosphate dehydrogenase (Gl-6-PDH) procedure stained heavily the bronchial lining cells with only minimal to no staining of the type II cells (Fig. 5a). The 7 day lesion had the bronchial lining membrane partially destroyed by the virus (Fig. 5b). By 10 days, the regenerating membranes had intense staining with Gl-6-PDH, but not the surrounding collapsed tissue (Fig. 5c). Likewise, the epithelial nodules seen in the 21 day lesions also stained heavily, indicating that the cells were derived from the regenerating bronchial lining cells which had grown peripherally into the surrounding alveolar spaces (Fig. 5d).

Discussion

Dolowy and Muldoon (1) and Wescott *et al.* (2) found that germfree mice were more susceptible respectively to mouse adapted PR8-A and A/2/Japan/170/62 influenza viruses when compared to conventional strains. Tennant, Parker and Ward (3), on the other hand, could find no difference in susceptibility of germfree mice to infection with influenza PR8-A virus compared to susceptibility of conventional mice of the same genetic origin. The findings reported here are in agreement with these investigators. Dolowy and Muldoon (1) could find no HI antibody response in germfree mice following intranasal inoculation of PR8-A virus. In our study, these were shown to be present, but in lower titers in the germfree mouse compared to conventional and monocontaminated mice. Dolowy and Muldoon (1) observed bacteria in some of the pulmonary lesions indicating a mixed infection. Such contamination with bacteria was not encountered in this study due, probably, to the fact that the aerosol procedure was employed for infecting the mice with influenza virus (6-8).

The pathogenesis and pathology of airborne influenza virus infection in germfree mice (CD-1 strain) were similar in every way to those seen in the lungs of conventional pathogen-free mice of the same genetic strain. The marked atelectasis of the lung lobes following infection with the influenza virus resulted, in all probability, from the destruction of the type II alveolar cells, the principal source of surfactant (8). As was the case with conventional mice, the epithelial nodules seen in the germfree mouse in the 21 day lesions were derived from the peripheral growth of regenerating bronchial epithelium (6, 7, 8). Preliminary studies indicated that the pathological changes in the lungs following airborne influenza virus infections in vitamin A-deficient germfree and conventional mice were significantly different in that the epithelial nodules had extensive squamous metaplasia and keratinization. Such lesions were not seen in animals on regular or high vitamin A diets (12).

Summary

Pulmonary changes in germfree, monocontaminated and conventinal mice provoked by inhalation of influenza PR8-A virus are similar. When germfree mice were exposed simultaneously with conventional mice to airborne virus, the growth of virus in the lungs and the HI and neutralizing antibody responses in the two groups were the same. Germfree and monocontaminated mice showed similar lung virus growth. Germfree mice infected only with the airborne virus showed more persistent lung virus titers and less pronounced HI antibody response. Neutralizing antibody also was present in sera of germfree mice sacrificed at 7 days and later after onset of infection.

Acknowledgements

This study was supported in part by the Division of Research Resources, National Institutes of Health, RR00407; Environmental Protection Agency, AP01075; The Council for Tobacco Research-USA; The Hughes Employees Give Once Club; the Eli Lilly Company; and the Hastings Fund of the University of Southern California.

We wish to thank Miss Edna Stone for expertly preparing the histological sections.

References

1. Dolowy, W. C., and Muldoon, R. L., *Proc. Soc. Exp. Biol. Med. 116:* 365 (1964).
2. Wescott, R. B., Todd, A. C., and Easterday, B. C., *Amer. J. Vet. Res. 26:* 192 (1965).
3. Tennant, R. W., Parker, J. C., Ward, T. G., *J. Nat. Cancer Inst. 34:* 381 (1965).
4. Bowers, R. H., Davies, O. L., Hurst, E. W., *Brit. J. Exp. Path. 33:* 601 (1952).
5. Loosli, C. G., Robertson, O. H., and Puck, T. T., *J. Infect. Dis. 72:* 142 (1943).
6. Loosli, C. G., *J. Infect. Dis. 84:* 153 (1949).
7. Loosli, C. G., Hertweck, M. S., Hockwald, R. S., *Arch. Environ. Health 21:* 332 (1970).
8. Loosli, C. G., Buckley, R. D., Hardy, J. D., *et al., Trans. Assoc. Amer. Phy. 89:* 182 (1971).
9. Robinson, R. Q., and Dowdle, W. R., in "Diagnostic Procedures for Viral and Rickettsial Infections," 4th edition, (E. H. Lennette and N. J. Schmidt, eds.), APHA, Inc., New York, p. 414, (1969).
10. Tyler, W. S., and Pearse, A. G., *Thorax 20:* 149 (1965).
11. Pearse, A. G. E., in "Histochemistry: Theoretical and Applied," 2nd edition, Little, Brown & Co., Boston, pp. 568, 911, (1961).
12. Loosli, C. G., Buckley, R. D., Joyce, J. A., *et al.,* (In Press).

PATHOGENICITY OF *CANDIDA ALBICANS* AS INFLUENCED BY *ESCHERICHIA COLI,* GENTAMICIN THERAPY, AND THERMAL INJURY IN THE GERMFREE MOUSE

E. J. Oestreicher, R. P. Hummell, M. P. Maley and *B. G. MacMillan*
Department of Surgery of the University of Cincinnati Medical Center and
the Shriners Burns Institute, Cincinnati, Ohio 45219, U.S.A.

Introduction

A series of *in vitro* studies performed in our laboratories have demonstrated that approximately 20% of *Escherichia coli* isolates obtained from burn patients had an inhibitory effect when streaked across *Candida albicans* on Brain Heart Infusion (BHI) agar (Baltimore Biological Laboratories, Inc.). Inhibition was defined as a lack of growth of the *C. albicans* at the intersections with the *E. coli* (1, 2).

As reported by other investigators (3-5), it was found that oral contamination of mice with 10^6 cells/ml of drinking water resulted in the recovery of *C. albicans* from the feces at 10^8 cells/g over a 90 day period. Similar to the findings of Nishikawa (4), it was further discovered that *E. coli* would colonize at 10^{12} cells/g stool in germfree mice monocontaminated with this organism. With these *in vivo* findings and base line data, the following experiments were undertaken.

Materials and Methods

Stock cultures of *C. albicans* (11952), an inhibitory *E. coli* (11922), and a noninhibitory *E. coli* (11) were maintained on standard trypticase soybean agar (TSA) slants at $-20°F$. Cultures for infecting the animals were grown in standard BHI broth for 18 hours at $37°C$. The cultures were serially diluted to determine the number of viable cells. Approximately 10^6 cells/ml of drinking water for *C. albicans* and 10^8 cells/ml of both types of *E. coli* were administered to each animal.

Over 300 mice of ICR strain obtained from A. R. Schmidt Co., Wisconsin, were used. Each mouse was housed individually on wire mesh bottom cages to minimize coprophagy. Purina chow (5010-C) and water were given *ad lib*, except for 24 hours prior to oral contamination when water was withheld.

405

Groups of monocontaminated mice were divided as follows: *C. albicans*, inhibitory *E. coli,* and noninhibitory *E. coli.* Bicontaminated mice received either *C. albicans* or one of the types of *E. coli* as the primary organisms. Fourteen days were alloted for the first organism to establish before the second organism was introduced. Each of these categories were subdivided into: controls, burned, gentamicin treated, and burn plus gentamicin therapy mice.

For the evaluation of a thermal injury, a nylon burn restrainer was constructed according to the calculations of Walker (6). Animals were anesthetized with methoxyflurane (Penthrane, Abbott), shaved, and given a 10% third degree water immersion burn of the back (100°C for 10 seconds).

Animals treated with gentamicin (Schering Corp.) received daily intramuscular doses of 3mg/kg (7). Gentamicin was also incorporated into the drinking water at later stages (20 mg/kg) to reduce the levels of gastrointestinal *E. coli.*

A dialysate was prepared from each *E. coli* strain by growing the bacteria on BHI agar in dialysis membranes for 24 hours at 37°C, before vacuum dialysis into a dry flash for another 24 hours at 4°C. The dialysates were passed through a 0.2μ filter (Nalgene millipore) to remove viable organisms. Drops of each dialysate were placed on BHI agar plates previously seeded with *C. albicans* and incubated at 37°C for 24 hours to determine inhibition. The BHI media was also dialysed and tested as a control.

Dialysates obtained *in vitro* were given orally to 40 mice monocontaminated with *C. albicans* in the following groups of 10 mice each: BHI media, inhibitory *E. coli*, noninhibitory *E. coli* and water.

Pooled stools from a minimum of five animals in each category were taken three times a week. The stool was weighed to 1×10^{-4} gram (wet weight), diluted and plated on BHI agar containing gentamicin for the isolation of *C. albicans.* Eosin Methylene Blue agar was employed for the isolation of *E. coli.* Stool containing *E. coli* was previously subjected to mild probe sonication for 30 seconds at 75% output to avoid a clumping of *E. coli* cells. Larger particles were then removed from the solution by centrifugation at 500 RPM for 5 minutes (8).

All animals were euthanized from 60-90 days after oral contamination. Sections of kidneys, spleen, liver, heart, lungs, burn scar (where applicable) and intestine were cultured in thioglycolate media and plated. Sections of these tissues were also fixed in 10% formalin. The tissues were then stained using the Grittley and hematoxylin-eosin stains.

Results

Inhibition of candida was observed on all plates to which the inhibitory *E. coli* dialysate had been added. The media alone and noninhibitory *E. coli* dialysate had no reaction against candida.

TABLE I. Fecal *C. albicans* Levels in Monocontaminated and Bicontaminated Mice

Group	Mean	t-Value*
C. albicans only	1.8×10^8	
Inhibitory *E. coli* and *C. albicans*	1.0×10^6	0.001
C. albicans and inhibitory *E. coli*	8.0×10^6	
Non-inhibitory *E. coli* and *C. albicans*	7.5×10^7	0.100
C. albicans and non-inhibitory *E. coli*	5.1×10^7	

*t-values as compared to *C. albicans* only levels at 95% confidence limits.

In bicontaminated animals containing the inhibitory *E. coli,* the candida counts decreased significantly (t=<.001) from 1.8×10^8 to 10^6 cells/g stool, independent of which organism had been administered first (Table I). The noninhibitory *E. coli,* however, did not decrease candida significantly (t = .10).

TABLE II. Fecal *E. coli* Levels in Monocontaminated and Bicontaminated Mice

Group	Mean	t-Value*
Inhibitory *E. coli*	1.4×10^{12}	
Inhibitory *E. coli* and *C. albicans*	1.1×10^{12}	⟩0.500
C. albicans and inhibitory *E. coli*	1.5×10^{12}	
Non-inhibitory *E. coli*	5.6×10^{11}	
Non-inhibitory *E. coli* and *C. albicans*	3.2×10^{11}	0.100
C. albicans and non-inhibitory *E. coli*	3.0×10^{11}	
Inhibitory *E. coli*	1.4×10^{12}	0.100
Non-inhibitory *E. coli*	5.6×10^{11}	

*t-values as compared to inhibitory or non-inhibitory *E. coli* levels at 95% confidence limits.

TABLE III. Fecal *E. coli* and *C. albicans* Levels in Monocontaminated and Bicontaminated Mice (Treated with Gentamicin and /or Burn)

Group	Control	Gentamicin	Burn	Burn + Gentamicin
C. albicans	1.8×10^8	1.8×10^8	9.6×10^9	1.9×10^8
E. coli	1.4×10^{12}	5.4×10^9	1.2×10^{12}	4.9×10^9
C. albicans + Inhibitory	8.0×10^6	2.9×10^6	5.7×10^6	8.5×10^6
E. coli	1.5×10^{12}	6.9×10^9	5.0×10^{11}	1.9×10^{10}
C. albicans + Non-inhibitory	5.1×10^7	4.0×10^7	3.5×10^6	7.8×10^7
E. coli	3.0×10^{11}	5.8×10^{10}	4.2×10^{11}	5.0×10^{10}

Both types of *E. coli* remained at approximately the same level as when present as a monocontaminant (Table II). As seen in Table III, the levels of candida were not affected by either the burn or gentamicin therapy as compared to the *C. albicans* control. *E. coli* was also unaffected by the burn, whereas gentamicin therapy reduced its levels significantly ($t = <.001$). The lower than expected level of *C. albicans* in the presence of a noninhibitory *E. coli,* in burned mice, to date, cannot be explained.

Mice fed the inhibitory *E. coli* dialysate had significantly lower candida levels compared to mice fed other dialysates (Table IV).

There were no fatalities from candida in any of the groups tested. All mice had positive gastrointestinal tract cultures for *C. albicans,* but cultures from other organs revealed no definite pattern. Groups containing viable *E. coli* had similar results. Histologic examination revealed no intraorgan dissemination by

TABLE IV. Fecal *C. albicans* Levels in Mice Fed Monocontaminated Dialysate

Group	Mean	t-Value*
C. albicans only (water)	1.0×10^8	
BHI Media	3.6×10^8	0.400
Non-inhibitory *E. coli*	1.1×10^8	>0.500
Inhibitory *E. coli*	3.0×10^6	<0.001

*t-value as compared to *C. albicans* at 95% confidence limits.

C. albicans or *E. coli.* Candida cells were observed in the budding phase adhered to the intestinal wall and tracheobronchial tree. On only two animals were these cells found to exist in the pseudohyphal phase in the intestine.

Discussion

Nishikawa (4) reported complete elimination of candida from mouse feces when *E. coli* had previously been administered. Clark (3) reported that animals monocontaminated with candida would shed the fungus more abundantly than mice with diflora of *E. coli* and candida.

In our study, *C. albicans* was found to readily colonize in the presence of two separate types of *E. coli.* However, the inhibitory *E. coli* caused a significant reduction of candida *in vivo* and a zone of inhibition against candida *in vitro.* The noninhibitory *E. coli* did not reduce the levels of candida significantly *in vivo* and had no zone of inhibition against candida *in vitro.* Further, a substance (heat stable above 100°C; molecular weight less than 12,000) has been isolated from the inhibitory *E. coli* and shown to be active in reducing candida levels *in vivo.* Lack of complete elimination of the candida by the metabolic by-product of *E. coli* by gentamicin could be due to the reingestion of these organisms enhanced by the closed environment of barrier isolation systems. It has been demonstrated that different microorganisms can also reduce the gastrointestinal levels of *C albicans* while others increase colonization (9).

Gentamicin is currently being employed both topically and systemically in the treatment of burns (7, 10). Although *C. albicans* has become a threat to the extensively burned and debilitated patient, from the results shown, it can be seen that neither 10% third degree burn nor gentamicin therapy effected the pathogenesis of *C. albicans* in the germfree mice. Other immune mechanisms or bacterial interactions may be responsible for *C. albicans* invasion in burned patients.

Summary

The recent rise in fatal *C. albicans* infections occurring in seriously ill burn patients has stimulated a study of *C. albicans* as influenced by various strains of *E. coli*, gentamicin therapy, and thermal injury. *In vitro* and *in vivo* studies have indicated that some isolates of *E. coli* will inhibit growth of *C. albicans* while other *E. coli* isolates will not. Further results suggested the existence of a substance isolated from *in vitro* grown inhibitory *E. coli* cells as the causative agent in reducing *C. albicans* levels in the gastrointestinal tract of germfree mice.

Gentamicin therapy decreased *E. coli* in the gastrointestinal tract of animals but had no effect on the *C. albicans* levels in the stool. Thermal injury had no effect on the level of *C. albicans* and *E. coli* cultured from the intestine. In these experiments, with otherwise healthy gnotobiotic animals, there were no fatalities from *C. albicans* or *E. coli.* Further pathological study revealed no evidence of intraorgan dissemination of *C. albicans* or *E. coli.*

Acknowledgements

Supported in part by Trauma Grant 5-P01-GM15428-05. The authors wish to express their gratitude to Phillip Miskell and Roger West for technical assistance rendered in these experiments.

References

1. Hummel, R. P., Oestreicher, E. J., Maley, M. P., and MacMillan, B. G., in "10th Annual Meeting of the Association for Gnotobiotics," Columbus, Ohio, (1971).
2. Maley, M. P., MacMillan, B. G., and Hummel, R. P., in "American Burn Association Meeting," San Antonio, Texas, 1971, (In Press).
3. Clark, J. D., *Inf. and Immun. 4:* 731 (1971).
4. Nishikawa, T. H., Hatano, N., Ohnishi, N., Sasaki, S., and Nomura, T., *Jap. J. Microbiol. 13:* 263 (1969).
5. Phillips, A. W., and Balish, E., *Appl. Micro. 14:* 737 (1966).
6. Walker, H. L., and Mason, A. D., *J. Trauma 8:* 1049 (1968).
7. MacMillan, B. G., *J. Infect. Dis. 119:* 492 (1969).
8. Gutman, H., and Pattee, P. A., *Can. J. Microbiol. 16:* 1371 (1970).
9. Luckey, T. D., *Am. J. Clin. Nutrition 23:* 1430 (1970).
10. Hummel, R. P., MacMillan, B. G., Altemeier, W. A., *Ann. of Surg. 172:* 370 (1970).

SECTION VIII

MICROBIOLOGY: "NORMAL" FLORA

EQUILIBRIUM BETWEEN TEN STRICTLY ANAEROBIC BACTERIAL STRAINS IN THE DIGESTIVE TRACT OF "GNOTOXENIC" MICE AND RATS. ROLE OF THE DIET.

P. Raibaud and *R. Ducluzeau*
Laboratoire d'Ecologie Microbienne
I.N.R.A., C.N.R.Z.
78-Jouy-en-Josas, France

Introduction

The microbial flora of the digestive tract of "holoxenic" (conventional) rats and mice includes a number of genera of bacteria (1, 2), particularly the strictly anaerobic bacteria which usually constitute the dominant population. The interactions which regulate the equilibrium between these strictly anaerobic bacteria are, as yet, poorly understood. Ducluzeau and his colleagues (3) have studied the equilibrium which is established in the "gnotoxenic" (gnotobiotic) mouse between 12 bacterial strains, including 3 strictly anaerobic strains. In the present work, we have studied the equilibrium which is established between 10 strictly anaerobic strains in the digestive tract for adult "gnotoxenic" mice, as a function of the mode of inoculation of the strains and of the dietary regimen of the animals. We have also compared the equilibrium thus established in mice with that observed in axenic rats inoculated with the same strains.

Materials and Methods

The 10 strictly anaerobic strains, originally isolated from the digestive tract of "holoxenic" rats, are: two strains of *Streptococcus, S. intermedius* RO3x8 (S_1) and *S. putridus* 1xOx914 (S_2); a strain of *Eubacterium parvum* ROx29; a strain of *Zymobacterium* sp. ROx31; a strain of *Pasteurella vulgata* ROx20; a strain of *Ristella putredinis* ROx23; a strain of *Veillonella alcalescens* ROx19; a strain of *Clostridium difficile* ROx30; a strain of *Inflabilis mangenoti* R^dIx10x2; and a strain of *Acuformis perennis* ROx24.

Adult axenic C_3H mice and Fischer rats were supplied by E. Sacquet (C.N.R.S. France) and were maintained in Trexler type isolators. They were housed in groups of 6 mice or 3 rats per cage. The diets used were: a commercial (Duquesne-Purina) diet, "D"; a semi-synthetic diet, "S", (4); and cows' milk

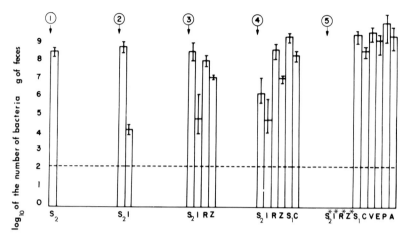

FIG. 1. Equilibria of the fecal microflora of 6 "gnotoxenic" mice fed a commercial diet (diet "D") after the successive introduction of each of the following 5 bacterial inocula: 1. *Streptococcus* 1xOx914 (S$_2$); 2. *Inflabilis* R^{d}Ix10x2 (I); 3. *Ristella* ROx23 (R) + *Zymobacterium* ROx31 (Z); 4. *Streptococcus* RO$_3$x8 (S$_1$) + *Clostridium* ROx30 (C); 5. *Veillonella* ROx19 (V) + *Eubacterium* ROx29 (E) + *Pasteurella* ROx20 (P) + *Acuformis* ROx24 (A).

*A strain is considered to be absent when the count is $\langle 10^2$ per g of feces.

sterilized by an ultra-high-temperature procedure. The animals were supplied either with water or with a solution of lactose, 20% weight/volume, sterilized by filtration. The latter solution was administered to one of the groups receiving diet "D." Inoculation with the bacterial strains was accomplished either directly per os, or via the atmosphere. In the latter case, the axenic animals were introduced into an isolator already containing the "gnotoxenic" animals, but in separate cages. Enumeration of the bacteria was accomplished using selective media, to be described elsewhere, with inoculation of the media performed according to previously described anaerobic techniques (5). Bacterial numbers were reported per gram of fresh feces or per gram of fresh organ including contents. Counts were performed on stomach, 3 equal portions of small intestine, cecum, and colon. Samples from the animals of a given group were pooled.

Results

Figure 1 shows that 4 strains (*Inflabilis, Ristella, Zymobacterium* and *Streptococcus,* S$_2$), previously established in the digestive tract of the "gnotoxenic" mice are eliminated when the other strains become established. Even when *Inflabilis* is present in the feces, the number is always low. Among the strains which become established at numbers ranging from $10^8 - 10^{10}$ per gram, *Pasteurella* is the most abundant, and *Clostridium* the least. The

414

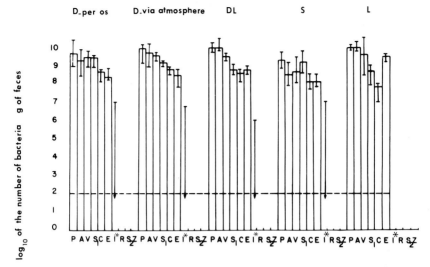

FIG. 2. Influence of the dietary regimen of the animals and the mode of inoculation of the bacterial strains on the final equilibrium between bacteria in the feces. Each group includes 6 "gnotoxenic" mice. D = commercial diet; DL = diet "D" supplemented with lactose; S = semi-synthetic diet; L = cows' milk. The symbols designating the various strains are the same as in Figure 1.

*A strain is considered to be absent when the count is $\langle 10^2$ per g of feces.

equilibrium which is established becomes stable in a few days.

Figure 2 illustrates the effects of the dietary regimen and the mode of inoculation upon the equilibrium between the 6 permanently established strains. When the animals are inoculated via the atmosphere, the equilibrium obtained is the same as when the bacterial strains are introduced directly per os. Lactose causes a decrease in the number of *Streptococcus,* S_1, and an increase in the number of *Acuformis.* Milk produces the same changes in the numbers of *Streptococcus*, S_1, and *Acuformis,* but in addition causes a reduction in the number of *Clostridium* and an increase in the number of *Eubacterium.* Diet "S" produces a decrease in the numbers of bacteria of all of the established strains.

Figure 3 shows that after inoculation via the atmosphere, the maximum number of bacteria in the feces is reached either rapidly (1 day or less) or gradually (approximately 5 days). The delay in the establishment of various strains differs depending on the diet, even within a given strain; but a given diet does not have the same effect on all of the strains.

Figures 4 and 5 illustrate, for each of the bacterial strains, the number attained by the end of the experiment (approximately 3 months) in the various portions of the digestive tract. The results are shown as a function of the dietary regimen and of the mode of inoculation. The cecum and the colon contain approximately the same numbers of bacteria. Only *Acuformis* is more abundant

415

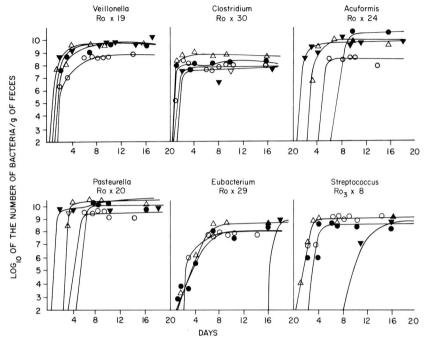

FIG. 3. Kinetics of the implantation, via the atmosphere, of various bacterial strains in the feces of "gnotoxenic" mice as a function of the dietary regimen of the animals. D = commercial diet; DL = diet "D" supplemented with lactose; S = semi-synthetic diet; L = cows' milk. The point of origin of each curve corresponds to the last day on which the bacterial count is less than 10^2 per g of feces.

△—△ = D   ○—○ = S
▼—▼ = DL   ●—● = L

in the cecum than in the colon. The stomach and the small intestine contain fewer bacteria than the cecum. For *Eubacterium* the regional differences are slight whatever the dietary regimen. For *Clostridium* and *Acuformis* the regional differences and the differences due to diet are much more marked.

Figure 6 contrasts the numbers of viable bacteria in various parts of digestive tract of axenic mice inoculated with single strains, and the numbers in mice inoculated per os with a mixture of strains. (All animals received diet "D"). The differences observed between the "monoxenic" and "polygnotoxenic" animals are slight, except for *Clostridium*. Three of the 4 strains that are eliminated by the other strains grow better in the cecum and colon than in the small intestine (of "monoxenic" mice). For the 4th, *Inflabilis,* the number of viable cells is approximately equal in all levels of the digestive tract.

Figures 7 and 8 illustrate the equilibrium obtained, in the feces and the digestive tract, respectively, when the 10 strains are inoculated per os in axenic

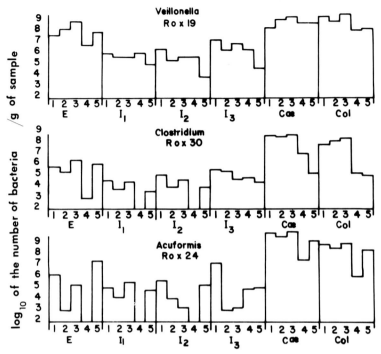

FIG. 4. Variation in the number of each of the strains of bacteria that become established in "gnotoxenic" mice after simultaneous inoculation. The counts in each level of the digestive tract are shown as a function of the dietary regimen and of the mode of inoculation. Also see Fig. 5. 1. Diet "D," inoculation per os. 2. Diet "D," inoculation via the atmosphere. 3. Diet "DL." 4. Diet "S." 5. Diet "L." E = stomach, I_1, I_2, I_3 = superior, middle and inferior thirds of the small intestine; Cae = cecum; Col = colon.

rats receiving diet "D." In these animals, as contrasted to the mice, *Ristella*, *Zymobacterium*, and strain S_2 of the *Streptococcus* persist at various levels in the feces and in the different segments of the digestive tract. Only *Inflabilis* does not become established. Therefore, this strain does not appear in Figures 7 and 8. The other 6 strains are established in approximately the same numbers in rats as in mice.

Discussion and Conclusion

These experiments demonstrate that certain associations of strictly anaerobic bacteria may play a barrier role vis-a-vis other strictly anaerobic bacteria. This role, however, depends upon the host. In addition, the dietary regimen can have a significant effect on the total number of viable bacteria, which may be altered as much as 100-fold in the feces and 1,000-fold at the

417

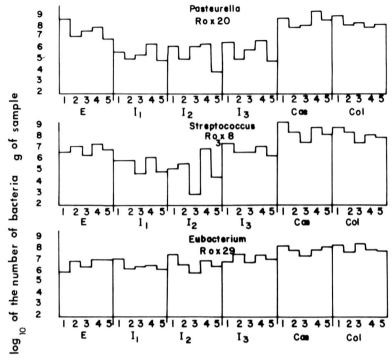

FIG. 5. Variation in the number of each of the strains of bacteria that become established in "gnotoxenic" mice after simultaneous inoculation. The counts in each level of the digestive tract are shown as a function of the dietary regimen and of the mode of inoculation. Also see Figure 4. 1. Diet "D," inoculation per os. 2. Diet "D," inoculation via the atmosphere. 3. Diet "DL." 4. Diet "S." 5. Diet "L." E = stomach, I_1 I_2, I_3 = superior, middle and inferior thirds of the small intestine; Cae = cecum; Col = colon.

uppermost level of the small intestine. The dietary regimen, however, does not significantly modify the balance between the dominant and the subdominant bacteria.

The number of viable bacterial cells sometimes remains low along the entire digestive tract, even in a "monoxenic" animal. This is the case for the mouse harboring *Inflabilis*. It could be argued that this strain is sensitive to atmospheric oxygen to the extent that the number recovered does not represent the actual number present in the sample. However, the fact that the numbers were found to be approximately equal in the small intestine and in the cecum suggests that most of the cells of *Inflabilis* may actually lose their viability within the cecum. The 6 bacterial strains which become permanently established in mice, when inoculated singly or in a mixture, were always more abundant in the cecum than in the small intestine. In the stomach, their numbers were the

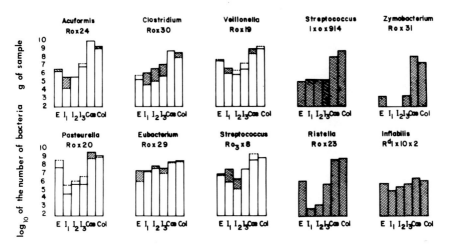

FIG. 6. Comparison between the numbers of ten bacterial strains in different segments of the digestive tract of "gnotoxenic" mice fed diet "D" when the strains are inoculated either alone ("monoxenic" animals) or simultaneously with all of the others ("polygnotoxenic" animals). White bars: "polygnotoxenic" animals. Grey bars: "monoxenic" animals. The symbols designating the various segments of the digestive tract (E, I₁, I₂, I₃, Cae, Col) are the same as in Figure 4.

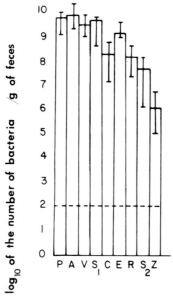

FIG. 7. Final equilibrium established between 9 bacterial strains in the feces of a group of 3 "gnotoxenic" rats fed diet "D." The symbols designating the various strains are the same as in Figure 1. A strain is considered to be absent when the count is $\langle 10^2$ per g of feces.

419

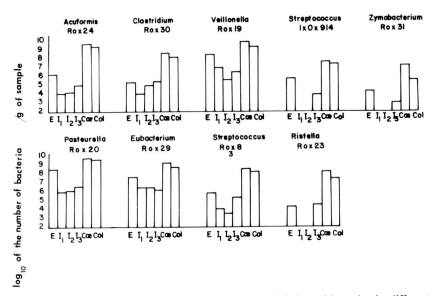

FIG. 8. Comparison between the numbers of each of 9 bacterial strains in different segments of the digestive tract of "polygnotoxenic" rats fed diet "D," following simultaneous inoculation of the strains. The symbols designating the various segments of the digestive tract (E, I₁, I₂, I₃, Cae, Col) are the same as in Figure 4.

same or higher than in the small intestine, but lower than in the cecum or feces. Since coprophagy was not prevented, it cannot be concluded that there was multiplication of these strains in the stomach.

Finally, it should be noted that, in an isolator, strictly anaerobic bacteria even if not spore-forming are able to establish themselves in axenic animals, even though these animals are not in direct contact with the "gnotoxenic" animals.

References

1. Raibaud, P., Dickinson, A. B., Sacquet, E., Charlier, H., and Mocquot, G., *Ann. Inst. Pasteur 110:* 861 (1966).
2. Gordon, J. H., and Dubos, R., *J. Exp. Med. 132:* 251 (1970).
3. Ducluzeau, R., and Raibaud, P., *Ann. Inst. Pasteur 116:* 345 (1969).
4. Sacquet, E., Raibaud, P, and Garnier, J., *Ann. Inst. Pasteur 120:* 501 (1971).
5. Raibaud, P., Dickinson, A. B., Sacquet, E., Charlier, H., and Mocquot, G., *Ann. Inst. Pasteur 110:* 568 (1966).

KINETICS OF THE ESTABLISHMENT OF A STRICTLY ANAEROBIC MICROFLORA IN THE DIGESTIVE TRACT OF "GNOTOXENIC" MICE BETWEEN BIRTH AND WEANING

Robert Ducluzeau, Pierre Raibaud and *Monique Ladire*
Laboratoire d'Ecologie Microbienne, I.N.R.A.
78 – Jouy -en-Josas, France

Introduction

At the time of birth, the infant mouse is axenic. However, facultatively anaerobic bacteria implant rapidly in the digestive tract after birth. In contrast, the strictly anaerobic species, particularly the gram-negative forms which constitute the dominant microflora of the terminal intestine of the adult, appear much later, approximately at the time of weaning (1-4).

In the present study we have attempted to learn if this delay in the establishment of strictly anaerobic bacteria is dependent upon an antagonistic effect of the facultatively anaerobic bacteria which are established first. For this purpose we have used mice born to "gnotoxenic" mothers bearing only a defined strictly anaerobic microflora, and have followed the rate and sequence of appearance of the different strains present in the mothers.

Materials and Methods

For these experiments, 10 different mothers were used. They produced a total of 130 young in 1-4 successive litters.

These infant mice were sacrificed between 3 and 21 days of age. The schedule of sacrifice was such as to provide a minimum of 4 infant mice from different mothers for each of the days of the first week, and 6-15 mice for each of the days of the second week, during which time the variation in the microflora is more pronounced.

The equilibrium of the microflora in the digestive tract of the "gnotoxenic" mothers has been described in the preceding paper by Raibaud and Ducluzeau (5). Their fecal microflora is composed of the following numbers of bacteria per gram of fresh feces: *Pasteurella*, 8×10^9; *Acuformis*, 3×10^9; *Streptococcus* RO 3 x 8, 5×10^8; *Clostridium*, 7×10^8; *Eubacterium*, 4×10^8.

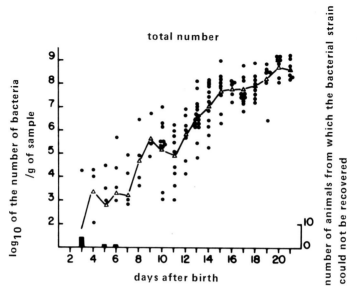

FIG. 1. Evolution of the total number of bacteria in the digestive tract of "gnotoxenic" infant mice between birth and weaning. Each black circle represents an individual bacterial count. The black bars represent the numbers of mice from whose digestive tract no bacteria could be recovered with the techniques utilized. The open triangles represent the arithmetic means of the values obtained for all individuals in a particular age group.

Results

The maximum numbers of viable bacteria in the digestive tract of the infant mice are shown in Figure 1, without regard to the identity of the dominant species. Bacteria are found in the digestive tract of even very young animals, but always in small numbers until the tenth day of age. Beyond that time in all animals there is an increase in the number of bacteria which is rapid until day 15, and slower thereafter. Even on the twenty-first day, the day of weaning, no more than 10^9 viable bacteria per gram of digestive tract are found, in contrast to the usual number of 8×10^9 in the adult.

The data in Figures 2 through 4 indicate that the 6 strains originally present in the feces of the mothers are markedly different from one another with respect to the kinetics of their appearance.

Veillonella is the only strain which can be found in the digestive tract very early, although always in low numbers. This strain grows progressively to reach a maximum at about day 15. *Pasteurella, Clostridium* and *Acuformis* are practically absent until about the eleventh or twelfth day of life, and then abruptly reach their respective maximum levels, which are always lower than those in the mother. *Eubacterium* and *Streptococcus* are the most delayed

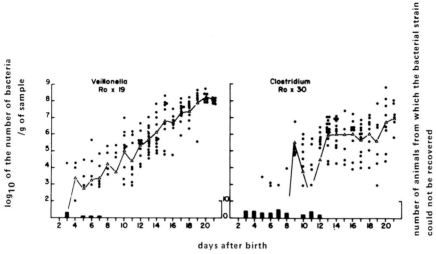

FIG. 2. Evolution of the number of *Veillonella* and *Clostridium* in the digestive tract of "gnotoxenic" infant mice between birth and weaning.

in their appearance, and subsequently multiply slowly and irregularly, reaching levels of only approximately 10^6 and 10^5, respectively, at the time of weaning. In fact, these two strains may yet be absent from the digestive tract of some animals at the time of weaning.

In the experiments reported in Figures 5 and 6, the 6 bacterial strains are compared with respect to the kinetics of their implantation within individual

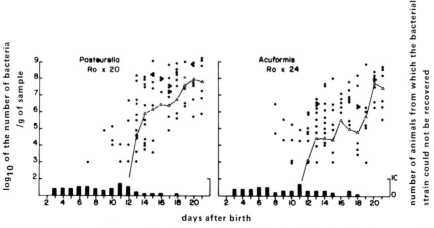

FIG. 3. Evolution of the number of *Pasteurella* and *Acuformis* in the digestive tract of "gnotoxenic" infant mice between birth and weaning.

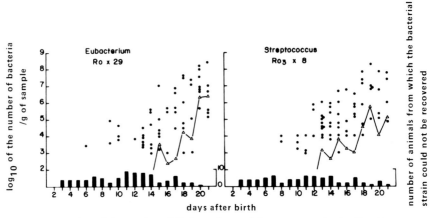

FIG. 4. Evolution of the number of *Eubacterium* and *Streptococcus* in the digestive tract of "gnotoxenic" infant mice between birth and weaning.

litters. As shown in Figure 5, three successive litters from the same mother are compared to reveal the possible effects of litter-order. As shown in Figure 6, the second litters of three different mothers are compared to reveal the possible unique effects of a particular mother on her litter.

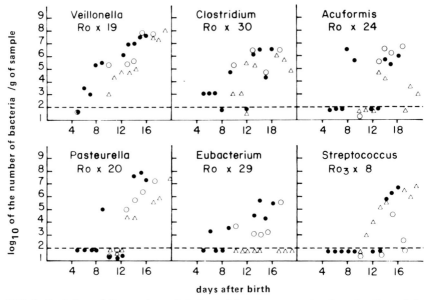

FIG. 5. Evolution of the numbers of six bacterial strains composing the microflora of the mother, compared in different litters of infant mice. Three successive litters from the same mother. ● = litter 1; ○ = litter 2; △ = litter 3.

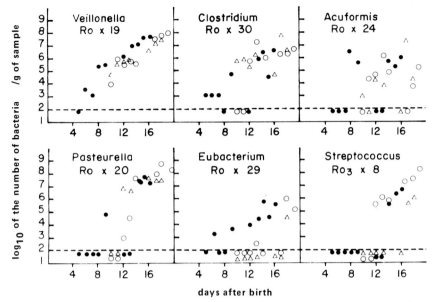

FIG. 6. Evolution of the numbers of six bacterial strains composing the microflora of the mother, compared in different litters of infant mice. Second litters from three different mothers. • = litter 1; ○ = litter 2; △ = litter 3.

In the case of *Veillonella, Pasteurella, Eubacterium* and *Streptococcus,* the appearance of the bacteria is quite regular **within** each litter, in the sense that when a particular strain appears in one member of the litter, that strain can be recovered in equal or greater numbers from each of the remaining members of the litter sacrificed thereafter. However, various litters differ **from one another**, thus explaining the spread of counts shown in Figures 2 through 4.

In contrast, for *Clostridium* and particularly for *Acuformis*, one can find, in a single litter at almost any age, some animals carrying the bacteria and some not. In contrast to the other four strains then, the spread of counts shown in the Figures for *Clostridium* and *Acuformis* is due to variations even between animals of a single litter.

None of the observed variations, however, seems to be related to litter-order or to the characteristics of a particular mother.

Discussion and Conclusions

Our results show clearly that even in the absence of facultatively anaerobic bacteria, there is a long delay in the establishment of a strictly anaerobic microflora in the digestive tract of infant mice. The antagonistic role of

Lactobacillaceae such as *Lactobacillus, Bifidobacterium,* and *Streptococcus*, so often invoked to explain the absence of strictly anaerobic species, cannot exist in this situation, since *Lactobacillaceae* are absent.

How, then, can one explain such a delay in the appearance, in the young, of bacteria so numerous in the mother? It appears that the bacteria studied fail to grow because of the lack of favorable physico-chemical conditions in the digestive tract of the young.

The milk of the mother is the only food of the infants during the first weeks of life. So, this milk and products of its digestion in the stomach and intestine constitute the main source of nutrition for the bacteria of infant mice. Then gradually the suckling mice begin to ingest particles of solid food supplied for the mother. At $20 - 21$ days, an abundance of such food particles is present in the stomachs of the young, and probably ingestion of solid food begins even earlier, perhaps around the fifteenth day of life. Thus, it is reasonable to suggest that the mother's milk is deficient in certain growth factors essential to the strictly anaerobic bacteria, factors which subsequently are supplied by the solid food ingested by the mice.

We found no influence of individual mothers or of litter-order upon the kinetics of appearance of the bacteria in infant mice. This can be explained by the fact that the mice are inbred and are fed a diet of constant composition, which results in the production of milk of similarly constant character.

During the first weeks of life of infant mice, many physical, chemical, and morphological characteristics of the digestive tract are changed progressively. The passage of immunoglobulin in the colostrum and milk of the mother decreases, various digestive enzymes become functional, and the cecum develops gradually, with an increase in volume at the end of the second week of life. The appearance of alimentary stasis at the cecal level possibly contributes to a decrease in oxidation-reduction potential, rendering the content more similar to that of the axenic adult, in which each of the bacterial strains studied can become established. It is not yet clear which among these, and possibly among other physiologic characteristics of the host, are important in influencing the establishment and regulation of strictly anaerobic bacteria.

It has become evident, however, that the indigenous strictly anaerobic microflora constitutes a vital mechanism of antibacterial defense of the host. The absence of this microflora during the first weeks of life probably explains the great susceptibility of the very young animal, including the human infant, to bacterial infection of the digestive tract.

References

1. Schaedler, R. W., Dubos, R., and Costello, R., *J. Exp. Med. 122:* 59 (1965).
2. Savage, D. C., Dubos, R., and Schaedler, R. W., *J. Exp. Med. 127:* 1 (1968).

3. Lee, A., Gordon, J., Lee, C. J., and Dubos, R., *J. Exp. Med. 133:* 339 (1971).
4. Lee, A., and Gemell, E., *Infect. Immunity. 5:* 1 (1972).
5. Raibaud, P., and Ducluzeau, R., in "Germfree Research: Biological Effect of Gnotobiotic Environments," (J. B. Heneghan, ed.), Academic Press, New York, p. 413, (1973).

PATTERNS OF INTERACTION IN GNOTOBIOTIC MICE AMONG BACTERIA OF A SYNTHETIC "NORMAL" INTESTINAL FLORA

Rolf Freter, Gerald D. Abrams and *Alexander Aranki*
The University of Michigan
Ann Arbor, Michigan 48104, U.S.A.

Introduction

The long-range goal of this study is to investigate the mechanisms by which the normal intestinal flora maintains its ecological balance and by which it inhibits the growth of invading pathogens. Earlier studies from this laboratory (1), which utilized a simplified "normal" flora that consisted only of *Escherichia coli*, had implicated metabolic competition as the mechanism which controlled the growth of Shigella in this system. In contrast, other workers postulated control mechanisms involving inhibitory fatty acids (2), bile salts (3) or colicines (4) as the agents responsible for control of intestinal flora. This problem has not been resolved to date.

These problems were investigated further in this laboratory by recent studies with precisely defined synthetic "normal" floras which were implanted into germfree mice by feeding strains of bacteria isolated in pure culture from the intestine of conventional mice. As reported earlier (5) gnotobiotic mice associated with 5 facultatively anaerobic bacteria plus 50 strict anaerobes (designated as "N-strains") resembled conventionalized control animals (i.e., germfree mice fed cecal homogenates from conventional mice) with respect to the following criteria: 1) size of the *E. coli* population in the cecum, 2) size of the cecum, 3) histology of the intestine, and 4) development of the mucosa — associated layer of bacteria in stomach and large intestine.

Later studies showed that these results changed when the usual refined diet (L-356) was replaced by a crude diet (Charles River Formula 7RF, or L-485, Telklad). With the latter type of diet, mice associated with the N-strains had larger ceca and a higher *E. coli* population as compared to conventionalized controls on the same diet (6).

Results

A second collection consisting of 100 strictly anaerobic gram negative

TABLE I. Efficiency of a Collection of 100 Anaerobic Bacteria (F-strains) In Reducing the Population of *E. coli* C25 and the Cecal Size of Gnotobiotic Mice Receiving Diet L-485

Germfree mice associated with	n*	Cecum % of body wt**	No. of *E. coli* C25 per cecum $(x\ 10^{-6})$**
F-strains + *E. coli* C25	24	1.51 (0.54 − 2.18)	5.62 (0.70 − 15.1)
Cecal homogenate from conventional mice + *E. coli* C25	20	1.48 (0.88 − 1.97)	3.78 (0.30 − 21.4)
E. coli C25 only	16	5.0 (3.00 − 7.0)	5,700 (2,000 − 11,000)

*Number of mice tested
**Mean and (range)

bacteria (designated "F-strains") has been isolated from normal mice. Gnotobiotic mice, associated with this flora plus *E. coli* strain C25, became normal, i.e., they had similar cecal size and *E. coli* populations as control animals conventionalized by feeding cecal homogenate from conventional mice (Table I). The parameters shown in the table became stabilized within 3 weeks after feeding the bacteria to germfree mice, and remained constant indefinitely thereafter (the longest period tested was 6 months). Total microscopic bacterial counts in the ceca of F-strain or N-strain associated mice, conventionalized controls and conventional mice were identical (in the order of 2×10^{10} per cecum). Consequently, the effect of the F-strain population on intestinal *E. coli* levels could not have been due to the mechanical flushing action of a transient diarrhea.

In order to study the mechanisms of bacterial interactions in a controlled environment, continuous flow cultures were established in anaerobic glove boxes in an atmosphere of 10% H_2, 5% CO_2 and 85% N_2, containing less than 5 ppm oxygen. Veal infusion broth enriched with yeast extract (5%), hemin (100 mg/l), and menadione (0.5 mg/l) was used as the growth medium. The volume of the growth tubes was 7 ml and the flow rate was maintained at 1.17 ml/hr. In view of our earlier finding (1) that *in vitro* culture methods do not readily reproduce *in vivo* interactions of bacteria, a number of experiments were carried out to determine whether the *in vivo* interactions of the various bacterial populations tested in the mouse intestine may be duplicated in this continuous flow culture system. To date, the system has reproduced the following *in vivo* interactions: 1)

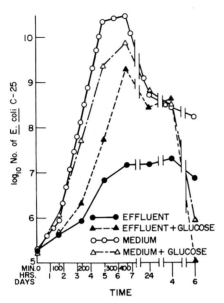

FIG. 1. Effect of glucose on the growth of *E. coli* in filtered effluent from a continuous flow culture of *E. coli* plus homogenate of normal mouse cecum.

E. coli C25 plus cecal homogenate from conventional mice: the presence of the homogenate resulted in a reduction of the *E. coli* population as shown in Table I; 2) *E. coli* C25 plus the N-strain collection of anaerobes; 3) *E. coli* C25 plus the F-strain collection of anaerobes (Both 2) and 3) resulted in a reduction of the *E. coli* population as compared with an *E. coli* population in monoassociated mice or in pure continuous flow cultures); 4) Shigella plus F-strains; 5) Shigella plus cecal homogenate from conventional mice; 6) Shigella plus F-strains plus *E. coli* C25 (populations 4) to 6) yielded various characteristic degrees of suppression of the Shigella population); and 7) *E. coli* C25 plus various single strains of gram negative anaerobic bacteria, produced no reduction in *E. coli* populations (i.e., they were as high as those found in monoassociated mice or in pure continuous flow cultures). In addition to the above correlations, we have shown that a continuous flow culture inoculated with cecal homogenates from normal mice preserved the composition of the normal flora for at least 3 months. When effluent from such a 3-month-old culture was fed to germfree mice the animals became conventionalized (with respect to the criteria enumerated previously) in the same manner as after feeding fresh cecal homogenates.

The determination of the above correlations suggests that the mechanisms of bacterial interaction in anaerobic continuous flow cultures may indeed resemble those occurring in the mouse intestine, at least in the large intestine where the flora is most numerous. Consequently, attempts were made to define

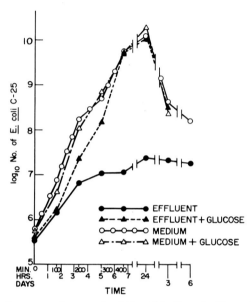

FIG. 2. Effect of glucose on the growth of *E. coli* **in filtered effluent from a continuous flow culture of** *E. coli* **plus the F-strain collection of intestinal anaerobes.**

inhibitory mechanisms limiting the growth of *E. coli* populations in continuous flow cultures. Populations of a) *E. coli* C25 plus the F-strain collection of anaerobes, or b) *E. coli* C25 plus homogenate of normal mouse cecum, were established in continuous flow cultures for at least 4 weeks. At this time the *E. coli* population had leveled off at about $10^6 - 10^7$ per ml, as compared to $10^8 - 10^9$ per ml in pure *E. coli* cultures. Effluent from the mixed cultures was then collected into a flask placed on a cold plate, which effected immediate freezing of the material. After two days of collection the material was thawed and filtered through Millipore membranes (0.30 μ pore size). The sterile filtrates were then inoculated with *E. coli* C25. Small amounts (10% of volume) of either distilled water or 10% glucose solution were added. Control cultures using Millipore filtered sterile medium instead of culture filtrates were also prepared. The entire experiment was carried out in the anaerobic chamber.

Figures 1 and 2 show the growth of *E. coli* C25 under the above conditions. As may be seen, the growth of *E. coli* in the culture filtrates was minimal, as compared to growth in the original medium. Significantly, normal growth of *E. coli* could be obtained by adding glucose to the filtrates.

Conclusions

The data shown in Table I, taken together with those published earlier (6), indicate that important functions of the intestinal flora (e.g., those controlling cecal size and *E. coli* population) are carried out by different groups of bacteria, depending on the diet fed.

Figures 1 and 2 indicate that competition for nutrients (replaceable by glucose) was at least a major factor which controlled the *E. coli* population in mixed continuous flow cultures of intestinal bacteria. The data which showed correlations between *in vivo* and *in vitro* interactions of intestinal bacterial populations suggest that a similar mechanism may also be operating *in vivo*. This corroborates earlier observations from this laboratory (6) which showed a lack of correlation between *in vivo* suppression of *E. coli* populations and the concentration of intestinal fatty acids. Obviously, further *in vivo* studies will have to confirm these conclusions before they can be accepted as definite. Relevant work is in progress.

Acknowledgement

This investigation was supported by U.S. Public Health Service Grant AI 07328.

References

1. Freter, R., *J. Infect. Dis. 110:* 38 (1962).
2. Bohnhoff, M., Miller, C. P., and Martin, W. R., *J. Exp. Med. 120:* 817 (1964); Meynell, C. G., *Brit. J. Exp. Path. 44:* 209 (1963).
3. Floch, M. H., Gershengoren, W., Diamond, S., and Hersch, T., *Am. J. Clin. Nutr. 23:* 8 (1970).
4. Ikari, N. S., Kenton, D. M., and Young, V. M., *Proc. Soc. Exptl. Biol. Med. 130:* 1280 (1969).
5. Syed, S. A., Abrams, G. D., and Freter, R., *Infect. and Immun. 2:* 376 (1970).
6. Freter, R., *Recent Progr. Microb. 10:* 333 (1970).

CONTROL OF STAPHYLOCOCCI IN THE GUT OF MICE

*R. Orcutt** and *R. W. Schaedler*
Department of Microbiology
Jefferson Medical College of Thomas Jefferson University
Philadelphia, Pennsylvania 19107, U.S.A.

Introduction

Although most humans harbor staphylococci on their body surfaces, these bacteria are seldom cultured from stools. Similarly, it is difficult to establish staphylococci in the nares or gut of experimental animals presumably due to interference by pre-existing normal flora. On the other hand, alteration of the gut flora by broad spectrum antimicrobial therapy often allows the re-colonization of the gastrointestinal tract with staphylococci which may result in enterocolitis (1).

This phenomenon of bacterial interference has recently been applied in clinical situations. Colonization of newborn infants with a non-virulent *Staphylococcus aureus* strain 502A has been successful in curtailing epidemics in nurseries caused by virulent strains of *S. aureus* 80/81 (2). *In vivo* studies of bacterial interference have been hampered by the lack of a suitable animal model (3, 4). Therefore, the investigation of the control of staphylococci in the gut was undertaken in gnotobiotic mice.

Materials and Methods

Male axenic and COBS mice of the CD-1 strain (The Charles River Breeding Laboratories, Inc.) 3 to 4 weeks of age were utilized in this study. The animals were associated with staphylococci and *Escherichia coli* by *per os* administration of 0.2 ml of 18 hour trypticase soy broth cultures using a blunt-ended needle. The fusiform-shaped bacteria were colonized in gnotobiotic mice, previously associated with staphylococci, in the following manner. Inside an anaerobic glove box a heavy suspension of the bacteria was obtained by harvesting abundant growth from the surface of agar plates (Schaedler agar from BBL supplemented with 5 percent defibrinated sheep's blood) using a 5×10^{-4}

*Present address: The Charles River Breeding Laboratories, Inc., Wilmington, Massachusetts, 01887, U.S.A.

M solution of Cysteine·HCl (pH 7.0) as the diluent. The dense cell suspension was placed in a test tube, stoppered with a rubber medicine bottle cap, and then taken out of the anaerobic chamber. After introducing the cell suspension into the germfree isolator, the mice were made to defecate as many fecal pellets as possible, i.e., usually 3 or 4. A 1.0 cc syringe, fitted with a 20 gauge needle, was filled with the suspension through the rubber stopper. The 20 gauge needle was then quickly replaced with a blunt-ended needle, and 0.5 cc was administered past the anal sphincter directly into the large intestine. The remaining 0.5 cc was given *per os* immediately afterwards. Even single strains of fusiform-shaped bacteria could be colonized in mice, monoassociated with staphylococci, using this protocol. Bacteroides could be established merely by *per os* administration of 0.5 cc of 24 hour broth cultures (Schaedler broth from BBL) into mice precolonized with an aerobic organism such as one of the staphylococci.

Individual stool samples from at least 4 and usually 6 animals from each isolator were homogenized in charcoal water within the anaerobic glove box, serially diluted, and plated on the appropriate media. Schaedler agar plus sheep's blood was used to assay for the fusiform-shaped and bacteroides bacteria. *S. aureus* strain 502A was differentiated from strain 80/81 in that the former was β-hemolytic on blood agar and the latter could be selectively grown on trypticase soy agar plus 0.05 μg of potassium penicillin G. Strain 502A is sensitive to the antibiotic, whereas strain 80/81 is resistant. When *E. coli* and staphylococci were associated in the same isolator, tergitol-7 agar plus triphenyltetrazolium chloride

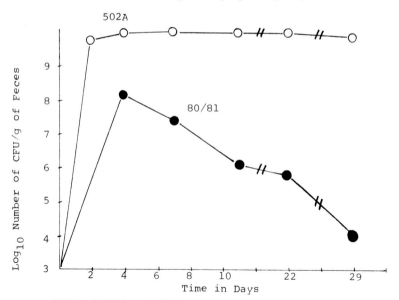

FIG. 1. Inhibition of 80/81 in 502A associated gnotobiotic mice.

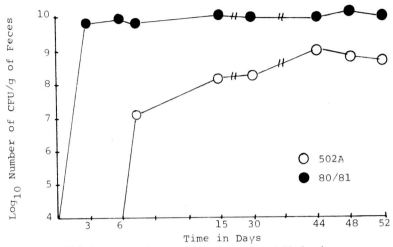

FIG. 2. Fate of 502A in 80/81 associated gnotobiotic mice.

was used to assay for *E. coli* and mannitol salt agar for the staphylococci.

Results

When either *S. aureus* strain 502A or strain 80/81 was administered *per os* to germfree mice, populations of 5 x $10^9 - 10^{10}$ CFU/g of feces were obtained within 48 hours (Figs. 1 and 2). However, if strain 80/81 was given to mice that were previously colonized with strain 502A, the former did not proliferate to high numbers and was eventually eliminated from the gastrointestinal tract (Fig. 1). Conversely, as illustrated in Fig. 2, strain 502A was able to gradually increase to almost its value in monoassociated animals when administered to mice that had been previously associated with 80/81 strain. The data in Figure 3 further demonstrate that when mice are associated with these two staphylococci simultaneously, both strains multiply to approximately the same concentrations they attain in their monoassociated states. Thus, it becomes apparent that pre-establishment of the less virulent 502A is a necessary condition for the interference to take place.

The indigenous flora plays a major role in the prevention of establishment of foreign bacteria in the gut (5). Therefore, various bacteria of the normal flora of COBS CD-1 mice were assayed for their ability to eliminate staphylococci from the gut of gnotobiotic mice. Figure 4 shows that *E. coli* is able to inhibit the growth of *Staphylococcus epidermidis* but not that of *S. aureus.* The data plotted in Figure 4 were compiled from two different experiments, one in which germfree mice were colonized by *S. epidermidis* and subsequently challenged with *E. coli,* and the other in which Giorgio strain of *S. aureus* was tested in an identical manner.

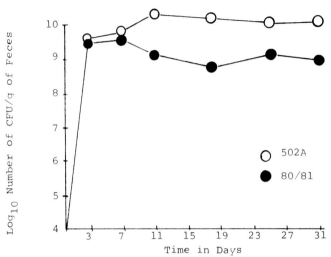

FIG. 3. The co-existence of *S. aureus* **strains 502A and 80/81 when associated simul-taneously in gnotobiotic mice.**

It appears that a relatively simple flora can control the less virulent organism, but the major "overall" control in the gut is exerted by the anaerobic organisms, especially the fusiform-shaped bacteria. When five strains of these bacteria were introduced into animals monoassociated with *S. aureus* the staphylococci were reduced to barely detectable numbers (see Fig. 5) in the

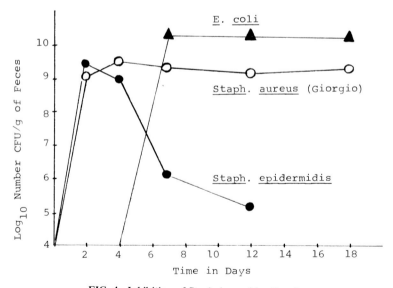

FIG. 4. Inhibition of Staphylococci by *E. coli.*

438

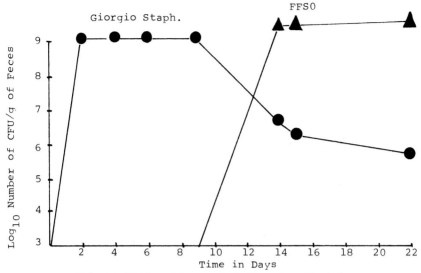

FIG. 5. Inhibition of *S. aureus* by fusiform-shaped bacteria.

feces and were completely eliminated from the stomach and small bowel. Although strain Giorgio is shown in Figure 5, the same results were obtained with strain 502A, 80/81 and *S. epidermidis.*

Conclusions

The "non-virulent" *S. aureus* strain 502A was shown to prevent the multiplication of the virulent hospital strain 80/81 in the gastrointestinal tract of gnotobiotic mice. The interference occurs only if 502A is fully established before challenging with strain 80/81. Consequently, colonization of infants with 502A as soon as possible is a crucial factor for subsequent protection against virulent staphylococci. Previous attempts to use mice were unsuccessful due to interfering normal flora. The use of germfree animals eliminated this problem.

Much of the early work dealing with enteric pathogen-normal flora interactions centered around the ability of *E. coli* to inhibit a variety of pathogens *in vitro* and *in vivo* (6). It should be noted, however, that high concentrations of *E. coli* in the gut are necessary to exert such an inhibition. Such numbers of coli are only present in the infant mouse gut from the 10th to the 16th days of life (7). It should also be noted that *E. coli* itself is greatly reduced in number in the gut of weanling and adult Specific Pathogen-Free (SPF) mice upon the establishment of the obligately anaerobic bacteria in the large intestine. Recent evidence has implicated the fusiform-shaped bacteria as the major group of organisms responsible for this inhibition (8).

Figure 4 shows that a strain of *E. coli,* isolated from COBS CD-1 mice, is capable of reducing the numbers of *S. epidermidis* in the gut of gnotobiotic mice. However, when the virulent Giorgio strain of *S. aureus* was challenged with this coliform, no inhibition was observed. On the contrary, several strains of fusiform-shaped bacteria were shown to effectively suppress the growth of *S. aureus* strain Giorgio in gnotobiotic mice. The same results were obtained when strain 502A, 80/81, and *S. epidermidis* were tested in an identical manner.

Based on these studies with *E. coli* and staphylococci, it seems possible that the degree of pathogenicity may correlate with the facility or ease of inhibiting these bacteria in the gut of mice. Nevertheless, many more strains of staphylococci would have to be tested before such a generalization could be considered credible. In any event, it is clear that the obligately anaerobic fusiform-shaped organisms, which greatly outnumber all other bacteria in the feces of mice, are fully capable of inhibiting the more pathogenic species of staphylococci in the gut of gnotobiotic mice, whereas *E. coli* is not. An important consideration is the realization that *E. coli* only attains high concentrations in the germfree and infant (SPF) mouse gut. These large populations of coliforms are reduced to $10^4 - 10^5/g$ of feces in the adult mouse and at these low numbers their role in suppressing the growth of exogenous pathogenic bacteria would seem to be negligible.

Acknowledgement

This investigation was partially supported by N.I.H. Grant No. AI-08758.

References

1. Dearing, W. H., Boggenstoss, A. H., and Weed, L. A., *Gastroenterology 38:* 441 (1960).
2. Shinefield, H. R., and Ribble, H. C., *Amer. J. Dis. Child. 121:* 148 (1971).
3. Antony, B. F., and Wannamaker, L. W., *J. Exp. Med. 125:* 319 (1967).
4. Tsang, K., and Welker, G. W., *Bacteriological Proceedings*, p. 48, (1971).
5. Bohnhoff, M., Miller, C. P., and Martin, W. R., *J. Exp. Med. 120:* 805 (1964).
6. Hengtes, D. J., *Amer. J. Clin. Nut. 23:* 1451 (1970).
7. Schaedler, R. W., Dubos, R., and Costello, R., *J. Exp. Med. 122:* 59 (1965).
8. Lee, A., and Gemmel, E., *Infect. and Imm. 5:* 1 (1972).

THE SLOW-TO-RAPID LACTOSE FERMENTATION SHIFT IN THE COLIFORM BACTERIAL POPULATION OF THE GERMFREE-LIKE CECA OF ANTIBIOTIC-TREATED RATS

Ralph F. Wiseman
University of Kentucky
Lexington, Kentucky 40506, U.S.A.

Introduction

In 1965, Schaedler, Dubos and Costello (1) reported that when germfree mice were associated with a slow lactose fermenting coliform bacillus (SLF), the bacterium reached 10^8 to 10^9 per gram of tissue in the intestinal tract, while in NCS (conventional) mice the level stabilized at 10^3 per gram. After 11 weeks residence only the SLF was recovered from the NCS mice, while a larger percentage of the population recovered from the gnotobiotes fermented lactose rapidly (RLF). Franzese and Wilkins (2), using a known SLF (*Paracolobactrum coliforme*) culture, supported these findings. Their results showed not only the appearance of RLF mutants, but also that the RLF had a faster growth advantage in all areas of the intestinal tract of the gnotobiotes, except in the ileum. They proposed that, if the increased growth rate in the cecum was the result of more carbohydrate utilization, the substrate was probably of host origin.

Since our previous studies of the germfree-like characteristics in antibiotic-treated rats revealed the emergence of a predominantly antibiotic-resistant SLF coliform cecal population, a study was designed to determine if the SLF to RLF shift also occurred in antibiotic treated animals.

Results

When CDF (Fischer 344 strain, Charles River Breeding Laboratories, Wilmington, Mass.) rats were administered a mixture of bacitracin (4 mg/ml), streptomycin (4 mg/ml) and nystatin (0.1 mg/ml) in acidified drinking water, the appearance of a modified cecal flora was evident in 1 day (Table I). Antibiotic resistant SLF constituted the "total" microflora of the treated animal at this time, reaching levels to 10^4 per gram of content. The RLF, which reached 10^6 per gram in untreated controls, was not detected in the treated rats at 1 and

441

TABLE I. Slow (SLF) to Rapid (RLF) Lactose Fermentation Shift Among Coliform Bacteria in Cecal Content of Antibiotic*-Treated Rats**

Days of treatment	Range of Bacterial Counts Per Gram Wet Cecal Content	
	SLF	RLF
0	$4 \times 10^3 - 1 \times 10^4$	$1 \times 10^3 - 2 \times 10^6$
1	$\langle 10^3 - 1 \times 10^4$	$\langle 10^3$
2	$2 \times 10^9 - 4 \times 10^9$	$\langle 10^3$
7	$2 \times 10^9 - 4 \times 10^9$	$6 \times 10^8 - 2 \times 10^9$***
14	$3 \times 10^8 - 8 \times 10^8$	$2 \times 10^8 - 4 \times 10^9$
21	$4 \times 10^8 - 1 \times 10^9$	$2 \times 10^8 - 4 \times 10^9$
28	$2 \times 10^8 - 4 \times 10^8$	$2 \times 10^7 - 4 \times 10^9$
42	$2 \times 10^8 - 2 \times 10^9$	$3 \times 10^7 - 3 \times 10^9$

*Streptomycin and bacitracin (4 mg each/ml), nystatin (0.1 mg/ml) in pH4 drinking water
**5 rats per treatment group
***Higher values in range usually mucoid-type colonies

2 days. Lactobacilli, enterococci, staphylococci, fungi and anaerobic bacteria were not detected in the treated animals at any assay period, when cecal content was diluted to 10^{-3}.

While the SLF population in the treated rats reached 10^9 per gram of cecal content at 2 days, the shift was not evident until 7 days, at which time RLF colonies appeared on the Tergitol-7 (Difco) culture plates. Two types of RLF colonies were apparent, a smaller irregular colony (*Escherichia*-type) and a larger, very mucoid colony (*Aerobacter*-type). While the RLF persisted during the 42 days of this study, the SLF did not disappear from the cecum.

In one trial, several SLF colonies (observed on T-7 agar, after 14 days of antibiotic treatment) exhibited RLF "wedge" sectors. This phenomenon was also detected in later studies, but was not apparent until after 3-4 weeks of treatment.

The SLF to RLF shift was paralleled by the appearance of germfree-like characteristics in the treated rats (Table II). Cecal size (content weight) continued to increase during the 42 day study. The initial germfree-like liquidity of the content, returned to near conventional values on day 7, while the pH of the content remained between the conventional and germfree values. The K^+ and Cl^- concentrations of the content while exhibiting some fluctuations, remained nearer the germfree level.

At day 1 the pCO_2 (34.9 mm Hg) and the E_h (−77mV) of content from treated rats were in the range of germfree values. At 7 days, the pCO_2 (93.2 mm Hg) and E_h (−148 mV) returned to the conventional range.

Preliminary studies of content from antibiotic-treated animals also indicated the presence of macromolecular colloidal substances which are similar to those present in germfree cecal content.

TABLE II. Some Germfree-like Characteristics of Cecal Content from Antibiotic-
Treated Rats (CDF Male, 200-250 g)

Days of Treatment	Content weight (g/100 g bwt)	Dry weight (%)	pH	K$^+$ (mM/L)	Cl$^-$ (mM/L)
	range		range		
0	1.5* (1.3 − 1.6)	20-25	6.1 (5.8 − 6.2)	26.2	17.4
2	2.9 (2.5 − 3.5)	12.3	7.0 (6.6 − 7.8)	−	−
7	4.2 (3.7 − 4.8)	21.3	6.5 (6.3 − 6.7)	23.0	4.0
14	6.2 (5.4 − 6.8)	21.2	6.5 (6.4 − 6.6)	22.5	2.3
21	7.3 (7.0 − 7.7)	21.6	6.5 (6.4 − 6.6)	19.9	4.0
28	7.8 (6.7 − 9.6)	18.7	6.3 (6.3 − 6.4)	15.5	5.5
42	9.0 (6.3 − 10.6)	22.4	6.4 (6.1 − 6.5)	18.3	3.2
Gf**	(6 − 10)	17	(7 − 7.5)	17	⟨1

*Average values of 5 rats per treatment group
**Average observation of germfree counterparts

Conclusion

This study indicates that the shift from a SLF coliform bacterial population to one that contains a significant number of RLF, which occurs in the intestinal tract of germfree animals monoassociated with a SLF, also occurs among the resistant SLF modified flora of antibiotic-treated animals. The appearance of sectoring colonies among the modified flora on T-7 agar reflects a mutational event, which in association with the acquisition of antibiotic resistance, releases (or transfers) genetic factors that are required for lactose fermentation. In addition to the segregation event, it is also possible that low levels of resistant RLF mutants which are selected by the antibiotic-containing environment, eventually become a major segment of the modified flora.

Acknowledgement

Supported in part by U.S.P.H.S. Grant 14621.

References

1. Schaedler, R. W., Dubos, R., and Costello, R., *J. Exptl. Med. 122:* 77 (1965).
2. Franzese, J. A., and Wilkins, T. D., in *Proc. 9th Annual Meeting, Assn. for Gnotobiotics,* Notre Dame, Indiana, June, (1970).

SECTION IX

GNOTOBIOTIC ENVIRONMENTS IN PARASITOLOGY

ASPICULURIS TETRAPTERA NIETSCH, 1821, IN GERMFREE AND CONVENTIONAL MICE

Zdzislaw W. Przyjalkowski
Institute of Parasitology
Polish Academy of Sciences
Warszawa, Poland

Introduction

Aspiculuris tetraptera, a pinworm of mice, is a parasitic nematode, belonging to the family Oxyuridae. It is commonly found in the colon of wild and laboratory mice. *A. tetraptera* is very similar to the human pinworm, *Enterobius vermicularis* Linnaeus, 1758, for which it serves as a model in therapeutic studies. *E. vermicularis* does not develop in hosts other than man.

Artificial infection of *A. tetraptera* in conventional laboratory mice is easily produced (1). It is important to incubate fertile *A. tetraptera* eggs as described by Anya (2). Further development of infective eggs takes place in the mouse intestine. This development depends to a great degree on the presence and composition of intestinal bacterial flora (3). The influence of intestinal bacteria on the establishment of *A. tetraptera* was described in experiments of Stefanski and Przyjalkowski (1) and Przyjalkowski (4).

The purpose of the experiments reported here was to study the influence of normal intestinal flora by comparing the establishment of *A. tetraptera* in conventional and in germfree mice.

Materials and Methods

Ten germfree and 10 conventional 16 week old C3H were used. All conventional and 7 germfree mice were males. Three of the germfree mice were females. All mice were free of parasites at the start of the study. The bacteria-free status of germfree mice was determined as in previous work (5). Infective eggs were sterilized with benzalkonium chloride (Zephiran) in a 1:3,000 solution for 10 minutes. They then were washed 3 times in sterile Earle's solution and finally resuspended in sterile Earle's solution. The suspension also was treated with 300 units of penicillin, 3 μg of streptomycin and 100 units of nystatin per ml of liquid.

447

The inocula of 100 *A tetraptera* eggs per host were taken into the isolator in sterile, sealed 1 ml ampules through the entry port. These suspensions of eggs were administered to the mice directly into the esophagus with a blunt needle and a sterile 1 ml syringe.

Three gnotobiotic and 3 conventional mice were sacrificed 2 weeks after exposure and 7 mice from both groups were killed 3 weeks after exposure to infective eggs of *A. tetraptera.* During the experiments all mice were fed the same diet, and kept under similar conditions regarding temperature and humidity.

Results and Discussion

The bacteria-free status of gnotobiotic mice infected with *A. tetraptera* was maintained throughout the course of experiments and no adult worms were found in these hosts. Conventional mice harbored an average of 13.8 worms per mouse with a range of 1-31. The difference between the results obtained from these groups of mice, gnotobiotic and conventional, is striking.

Many workers have shown (6, 7) that incubation of *A. tetraptera* eggs to the infective stages requires oxygen and suitable temperature $(20 - 30°$ C.). Further development takes place in the lower intestine or cecum of the host, where the first larvae appear. After molting the larvae migrate into the crypts of the colon. Only larvae reaching the crypts undergo the further development (8). Later they return to the lumen of the colon where they grow into adults.

Mathies (9) reported female mice more resistant to infection with the mouse pinworm than male mice. With age both sexes became more refractory to infection but complete resistance has not been observed even in mice older than used in these experiments.

Stahl (10) showed that 25% of *A. tetraptera* eggs developed into adult worms in 18 week old mice. In the present experiments, development of 13.8% of eggs in C_3H conventional mice was more than in previous experiments (1) in which an average of about 10% development per mouse was obtained.

It is difficult to discuss the results obtained in gnotobiotic mice, because no experiments of this kind have been reported previously in such hosts with *A. tetraptera.* However, many experiments have been carried out on gnotobiotic animals with parasitic nematodes of the small intestine (4, 11, 12, 13, 14). Wells (15) has shown that conventional mice given terramycin had fewer pinworms than untreated controls. Perhaps the effect was indirect. Alteration of the bacterial flora may have disturbed the nutrition of the worm.

Summary

The experiments reported here support the hypothesis of Stefanski (3) that bacterial flora is necessary for the establishment of some worm infection.

They also suggest that the human pinworm, *E. vermicularis,* needs intestinal bacterial components for establishment. Further experiments are necessary to confirm the results of the present study and to determine the interrelation between intestinal flora and parasites in different sections of digestive tract.

References

1. Stefanski, W., and Przyjalkowski, Z. W., *Acta Parasitol. Polon. 15:* 285 (1967).
2. Anya, A. O., *J. Helminth. 40:* 253 (1966).
3. Stefanski, W., *Acta Parasitol. Polon. 13:* 1 (1965).
4. Przyjalkowski, Z. W., *Bull. Acad. Sci. Pol. Cl. II. Ser. Sci. Biol. 16:* 433 (1968).
5. Przyjalkowski, Z. W., and Wescott, R. B., *Acata Parasitol. Polon. 17:* 265 (1970).
6. Hsü, K. C., *J. Helminth. 25:* 131 (1952).
7. Chan, K. F., *J. Parasitol. 41:* 529 (1955).
8. Anya, A. O., *J. Helminth. 40:* 261 (1966).
9. Mathies, A. W., *Expl. Parasitol. 8:* 39 (1959).
10. Stahl, W., *J. Parasitol. 47:* 939 (1961).
11. Wescott, R. B., and Todd, A. C., *J. Parasitol. 50:* 138 (1964).
12. Wescott, R. B., *Expl. Parasitol. 22:* 245 (1968).
13. Przyjalkowski, Z. W., and Wescott, R. B., *Bull. Pol. Acad. Sci. Ser. Sci. Biol. 17:* 57 (1968).
14. Przyjalkowski, Z. W., and Wescott, R. B., *Expl. Parasitol. 25:* 8 (1969).
15. Wells, H. S., *J. Infect. Dis. 89:* 190 (1951).

COMPARATIVE PATHOLOGY AND LESIONS OF EXPERIMENTAL INFECTIONS WITH *EIMERIA TENELLA* IN GERMFREE, SPECIFIC PATHOGEN-FREE AND CONVENTIONAL CHICKENS

C. V. Radhakrishnan and *R. E. Bradley, Sr.*
Department of Veterinary Science, University of Florida
Gainesville, Florida 32601, U.S.A.

Introduction

Eimeria tenella (Railliet and Lucet, 1891; Protozoa: Eimeriidae) is the most common and pathogenic of the 9 species of eimeria occurring in the chicken (1). These sporozoans occur as intracellular parasites of the epithelial cells of the intestinal tract producing the disease known as coccidiosis. Coccidiosis with sudden onset and a high rate of mortality is regularly associated with infection due to *E. tenella* and since the lesions are confined to the ceca the disease is often referred to as acute cecal coccidiosis. Outbreaks usually occur in young chickens 3-8 weeks of age (2) following ingestion of large numbers of the infective stage of *E. tenella,* the sporulated oocysts. Like other species of eimeria, both schizogony and gametogony occur within the same host. The maturation of numerous second generation schizonts within the epithelial cells and subsequent liberation of the second generation merozoites from schizonts causes extensive destruction of the epithelial cells. Severe hemorrhage occurs into the cecal lumen followed by tissue necrosis and thickening of the cecal wall. The hemorrhage is the most important effect of the parasitism and is one of the factors causing mortality. All these changes occur during the 6th to 7th day after ingestion of oocysts. The disease is at its peak on the 7th day postexposure and 90% of the mortality occurs within 9 days following initial exposure to the oocysts.

The effect of normal bacterial flora on the biology and immunology of the host and possible relationship between this flora and certain diseases have been investigated by many workers. Phillips *et al.* (3), using germfree guinea pigs, proved that the presence of bacterial flora is essential for the survival of *Entamoeba histolytica* and pathogenesis of amebiasis. Based on these findings, Wittner and Rosenbaum (4) studied the role of bacteria in modifying the virulence of *E. histolytica.* Bradley and Reid (5) demonstrated a dual etiology involving a protozoan *(Histomonas meleagridis)* and a single species of bacteria

451

(Escherichia coli, Clostridium perfringens or *Bacillus subtilis)* for infectious enterohepatitis in turkeys. Several other studies have been made on the role of bacterial flora affecting the course of infection in infectious enterohepatitis (6, 7, 8). Hegde *et al.* (9) studied the pathogenicity of *Eimeria brunetti* in bacteria-free chickens and showed that the parasite can develop and produce disease in bacteria-free chickens. The knowledge regarding the role of cecal flora in the initiation, development, or severity of cecal coccidiosis is limited. The cecal bacterial flora constitutes 90% of the total gastrointestinal flora and is of great biological importance to the health of chickens (10, 11). Johansson and Sarles (12) reported that during *E. tenella* infection growth of *C. perfringens* is stimulated while the growth of *Lactobacillus sp.* is suppressed. Clark *et al.* (13) found no difference in the course of *E. tenella* infection in bacteria-free and conventional chickens. There was, however, a delay of 12 to 15 hours in the appearance of the 2nd generation merozoites in the feces of chickens. Kemp *et al.* (14) reported a delayed development of endogenous stages of *E. tenella* in germfree chickens especially 2nd generation schizonts, gametocytes and oocysts. They also found a striking lack of reticuloendothelial cells in the lamina propria and submucosa and substantially low numbers of mononuclear inflammatory cells in germfree chicks exposed to *E. tenella.* Radhakrishnan (15) reported a more frequent isolation of *C. perfringens* from non-infected SPF chickens than from non-infected conventional chickens. A stimulation of growth of *C. perfringens* and coliforms occurred with a concomitant reduction in the growth of *Lactobacillus sp.* in SPF and conventional chickens suffering from typical cecal coccidiosis. The observations on the development of cecal coccidiosis and the pathological manifestations in germfree, specific pathogen-free and conventional chickens when inoculated with a standardized dose of surface sterilized infective oocysts of *E. tenella* are reported herein.

Methods

One hundred thousand oocysts of *E. tenella* were used for inoculation into each chicken. The experimental chickens were kept under observation for 7 days and then necropsied. The gross cecal lesions were scored following the method of Johnson and Reid (16).

Results and Discussion

The comparative pathology and lesions of experimental infection with *E. tenella* in germfree, SPF and conventional chickens are reported in Table 1. In a total of 32 germfree chickens inoculated with *E. tenella* alone, no clinical signs or mortality were observed. Gross examination of the cecum revealed no thickening, hemorrhage, core formation or sloughing of the mucosa. Cecal enlargement was also not noticed. Other visceral organs were also normal in

452

TABLE I. Comparison of Pathology Due To *Eimeria tenella* In 3 Week-Old Germfree, SPF, and Conventional Chickens Following Inoculation with 100,000 Surface-Sterilized Sporulated Oocysts.

Environment	Number of Chickens	Clinical Signs	Mortality	Macroscopic Grading of Lesions (mean)	Histopathology
Germfree	32	No bleeding; no decrease in hematocrit value; no weakness or loss of appetite	0/32 (0%)	0	Endogenous stages (immature schizonts and macrogametocytes) were seen rarely; No tissue damage or inflammatory reaction
Specific Pathogen-Free	88	Bleeding started 96 hours post-inoculation; hematocrit value decreased from a mean of 28.3% to a mean of 23.7%; weakness and loss of appetite	33/88 (38%)	2.6	Sloughing of mucosa, hemorrhage, and inflammatory reaction; numerous second generation schizonts
Conventional	104	Bleeding started 96 hours post-inoculation; decrease in hematocrit value from a mean of 30.3% to 20.1%.	23/104 (22.1%) cr	3.1	Sloughing of mucosa, hemorrhage, and inflammatory reaction; numerous second generation schizonts

appearance and identical with those from non-exposed control chickens. Histopathologically, there was no tissue damage, hemorrhage, sloughing or thickening of the mucosa. However, *E. tenella* appeared to survive and undergo a delayed development since a few endogenous stages such as immature schizonts and early gametocytes were seen in the epithelial cells of the mucosa. But the large second generation schizonts and inflammatory cells were not seen. Cecal coccidiosis as described by Tyzzer (17) and Tyzzer *et al.* (18) was not seen in these chickens.

Pathological manifestations in SPF chickens inoculated with *E. tenella* were typical of cecal coccidiosis. Clinical signs like bleeding, anorexia, droopiness and mortality were noticed. Thirty-three of the total 88 chickens inoculated died establishing a mortality rate of 38%. Macroscopic as well as microscopic lesions were observed in all inoculated chickens establishing an infection rate of 100%. The mean hematocrit value dropped from a pre-exposure value of 28.3%

to 23.7% on the 7th day post-exposure.

In conventional chickens, clinical symptoms were identical with those seen in SPF chickens. Infection rate was 100% and mean gross lesion score was 3.1. Twenty-three out of 104 inoculated chickens died due to cecal coccidiosis registering a mortality rate of 22.1%. The mean hematocrit value dropped from a pre-exposure value of 30.3% to 20.1% on the 7th day post-exposure. The clinical symptoms, gross lesions in the cecum and the presence of large numbers of 2nd generation schizonts, extensive denudation of the cecal mucosa and hemorrhage on histopathological examination of SPF and conventional chickens inoculated with *E. tenella* confirmed the presence of cecal coccidiosis as described by Tyzzer (17) and Tyzzer *et al.* (18).

Conclusions

Typical cecal coccidiosis did not develop in germfree chickens inoculated with a standard dose of infective oocysts of *E. tenella.* However, small numbers of *E. tenella* were able to develop at a slower rate in germfree chickens as compared with the rate seen in SPF and conventional chickens. The typical cecal coccidiosis syndrome and its pathological manifestations developed in SPF and conventional chickens inoculated with a standard dose of infective oocysts of *E. tenella.* Higher mortality but lower mean score of gross lesions due to coccidiosis were seen in SPF chickens compared to that seen in conventional chickens. Indigenous bacteria seem to aid the rapid development of the endogenous stages of *E. tenella* and production of typical cecal coccidiosis.

References

1. Davies, S. F. H., Joyner, L. P., and Kendall, S. B., *Coccidiosis,* Oliver and Boyd, Edinburgh, (1963).
2. Gardiner, J. L., *Poultry Sci. 34:* 415 (1955).
3. Phillips, B. P., Wolfe, P. A., Rees, C. W., Gordon, H. A., Wright, W. H., and Reyniers, J. A., *Am. J. Trop. Med. & Hyg. 4:* 675 (1955).
4. Wittner, M., and Rosenbaum, R. M., *Am. J. Trop. Med. & Hyg. 19:* 755 (1970).
5. Bradley, R. E., and Reid, W. M., *Exp. Parasit. 19:* 91 (1966).
6. Doll, J. P., and Franker, C. K., *J. Parasit. 49:* 411 (1963).
7. Franker, C. K., and Doll, J. P., *J. Parasit. 50:* 636 (1964).
8. Springer, W. T., Johnson, J., and Reid, W. M., *Exp. Parasit. 28:* 383 (1970).
9. Hegde, K. S., Reid, W. M., Johnson, J., and Womack, H. E., *J. Parasit. 55:* 402 (1969).
10. Coates, M. E., Ford, J. E., and Harrison, G. F., in "Advances in Germfree Research and Gnotobiology," (M. Miyakawa and T. D. Luckey, eds.), Chemical Rubber Co. Press, p. 110, (1968).
11. Timms, L., *Br. Vet. J. 124:* 470 (1968).
12. Johansson, K. R., and Sarles, W. B., *J. Bact. 56:* 635 (1948).
13. Clark, D. T., Smith, C. K., and Dardas, R. B., *Poultry Sci. 41:* 1635 (1952).
14. Kemp. R. L., Reid, W. M., and Johnson, J., *Am. Soc. Parasit. A87,* a (1971).
15. Radhakrishnan, C. V., Doctoral dissertation, Univ. of Florida, (1971).

16. Johnson, J., and Reid, W. M., *Exp. Parasit. 28:* 30 (1970).
17. Tyzzer, E. E., *Am. J. Hyg. 10:* 269 (1929).
18. Tyzzer, E. E., Theiler, H., and Jones, E. E., *Am. J. Hyg. 15:* 319 (1932).

THE DEVELOPMENT OF *EIMERIA TENELLA* IN GERMFREE CHICKENS

Joyce Johnson and *W. M. Reid*
University of Georgia, Athens, Georgia 30601

and

R. L. Kemp
Iowa State University, Ames, Iowa 50010, U.S.A.

Introduction

Investigations of host-parasite relationships in germfree chickens has shown varying degrees of dependency of different parasites on the intestinal microflora of the host. *Histomonas meleagridis,* a protozoan parasite capable of causing death in turkeys must have certain bacteria present to produce such pathogenicity (1, 2). On the other hand, no differences in the development of the chicken tapeworm, *Raillietina cesticillus,* was observed in germfree compared to conventional chickens (3). Johnson and Reid (In Press) found that while *Ascaridia galli* could survive in the absence of bacteria, a significantly larger number of larvae established themselves in conventional chickens.

Limited work has been reported on the effect of the germfree environment on the etiology of coccidiosis in chickens. Hegde *et al.* (4) found no substantial difference in the weight gains and lesion scores of germfree and conventional chickens infected with *Eimeria brunetti.* Pathogenicity induced by *Eimeria tenella* was reported by Clark *et al.* (5) to be similar in germfree and conventional chickens. They did find a delay in the life cycle of the parasite infecting the germfree birds. Second generation merozoites were released 12 to 15 hours later than in conventional chickens. Visco and Burns (6) working with the same species, did not record a delay in the life cycle, but they did find a big difference in pathogenicity with 77 percent mortality occurring in the conventional chickens and none in the germfree.

This present study was undertaken to more fully understand the relationship existing between *E. tenella* and normal intestinal microflora. The delay in the life cycle and the conflicting reports on pathogenicity were investigated.

Materials and Methods

All chickens were hatched and housed in plastic film isolators and tested

457

for sterility by bacteriological methods. The chickens of Experiment 1 were divided into four treatment groups: 1) conventional infected, 2) conventional uninfected, 3) germfree infected, and 4) germfree uninfected. Two isolators containing 10 chickens were included in each treatment group. When the chickens were five days of age, the chickens were each orally inoculated with 40,000 oocysts which had been sterilized with peracetic acid (7). One chicken from each treatment group was necropsied on days 3, 4, 5, 6, and the remainder on day 7 when the trial was terminated. All cecal lesions were scored visually for pathology (8) on a scale of 0 to +4 and tissues for histopathologic studies were fixed in 10 per cent buffered formol-saline.

A second trial was completed using 5 isolators containing germfree infected chickens, 1 with germfree uninfected, 4 conventional infected, and 1 conventional uninfected. Two chickens were killed daily from day 4 through 10 for examination of gross lesions and histopathologic studies.

Results

Gross lesions in the germfree chickens were less severe than those found in conventional infected chickens in both trials (Table I). A mortality rate of 39 per cent occurred in the conventional chickens and no deaths occurred in the germfree.

Histopathologic studies showed that the cecal mucosa was deeper in the conventional chickens than in the germfree and contained numerous glands. Differences in tissue response of the gnotobiotes were reflected in a paucity of reticuloendothelial cells in the **lamina propria** and **submucosa**. Numbers of mononuclear inflammatory cells were substantially lower in germfree chickens. Core formation was seen in the conventional chickens, but was absent in the germfree infected.

In Experiment 1 there was a 24 to 36 hour delay in the release of the second generation merozoites in the germfree chickens, and a 24 hour delay occurred in Experiment 2.

Discussion

Infections of *E. tenella* did occur in the germfree chickens but pathogenicity was not severe. The delay in the life cycle of the parasite may be related to changes in the cecal mucosa, but it is not known why the development of the second generation schizonts is affected. Patillo (9) has reported that the sporozoites of *E. tenella* are transported to the epithelial cells lining the gland fundi by macrophages. The sparcity of such cells (10) in the unstimulated germfree mucosa may be responsible for the lower number of endogenous stages in the germfree ceca. No cecal core formation was noted in the germfree chickens. This is another indication of the lack of tissue response.

TABLE I. Comparison of the Lesion Scores in the Conventional and Germfree Chickens in Experiments 1 and 2.

Exper. No.	Treatment of Isolator	No. Chicks	Average lesion scores days post-infection						
			4	5	6	7	8[a]	9	10
1	Conv.	10	0.0	3.0	3.0	2.8			
	Conv.	10	1.0	3.0	3.0	3.0			
	Average		0.5	3.0	3.0	2.9			
	G-F	10	0.0	2.0	3.0	2.0			
	G-F[b]	10	0.0	1.0	1.0	1.7			
2	Conv.	14	1.5	2.5	3.8	3.7	3.0	2.0	2.0
	Conv.	12	0.5	3.0	4.0	4.0	3.0	–	–
	Conv.	14	1.5	3.0	4.0	3.8	3.0	2.0	3.0
	Conv.	12	1.0	3.5	3.8	3.7	3.0	–	–
	Average		1.1	3.0	3.9	3.8	3.0	2.0	2.5
	G-F	14	0.0	2.0	3.0	3.0	2.0	2.5	0.0
	G-F	14	1.5	1.5	3.0	2.5	2.0	2.5	1.0
	G-F	14	0.5	1.0	3.0	2.5	3.0	3.0	1.5
	G-F	14	0.0	1.5	3.0	2.5	2.5	3.0	1.0
	G-F[b]	14	0.5	1.5	3.0	3.0	3.0	2.5	1.0
	Average		0.5	1.5**	3.0**	2.6**	2.4	2.8*	0.9**

[a]Scores of conventional groups from day 8 are represented by one bird.
[b]Isolator became monocontaminated with *Bacillus subtilis* and not included in mean.
*Significantly different (P<.05) from corresponding value within time period.
**Significantly different (P<.01) from corresponding value within time period.

The results confirm the report of Clark *et al.* (5) that a delay in the life cycle does occur. They reported a delay of only 12 to 15 hours as compared to one of 24 to 36 hours found in this study. These results do not confirm, however, that there is no difference in pathogenicity between the germfree and the conventional infected chickens. Mortality is an indication of pathogenicity and 39 percent was recorded in the conventional infected chickens compared with none in the germfree. These data closely correlate with the work of Visco and Burns (6) who found 77 per cent mortality in the conventional infected chickens.

There is a close relationship between the cecal microflora and the pathogenicity of *E. tenella*. Whether the microflora serve to stimulate the reticuloendothelial system or act as secondary invaders, they play a role in the etiology of cecal coccidiosis. Bacterial microflora must be present in the chicken for *E. tenella* infections to produce full pathogenicity.

Acknowledgements

This work was supported in part by N.I.H. Grant No. R01 A109323 03.

References

1. Bradley, R. E., Ph.D. Dissertation, Univ. of Georgia, (1965).
2. Franker, C. K., and Doll, J. P., *J. Parasitol 50:* 636 (1964).
3. Bradley, R. E., Botero, H., Johnson, J., and Reid, W. M., *Exp. Parasitol. 21:* 403 (1967).
4. Hegde, K. S, Reid, W. M., Johnson, J., and Womack, H. E., *J. Parasitol. 55:* 402 (1969).
5. Clark, D. T., Smith, C. K., and Dardas, R. B., *Poultry Sci. 41:* 1635 (1962).
6. Visco, J. R., and Burns, W. C., *J. Parasitol. 52:* 31 (1966).
7. Doll, J. P., Trexler, P. C., Reynolds, L. I., and Bernard, G. R., *American Midland Naturalist 69:* 231 (1963).
8. Johnson, J., and Reid, W. M., *Exp. Parasitol. 28:* 30 (1970).
9. Patillo, W. H., *J. Parasitol. 45:* 253 (1959).
10. Reyniers, J. A., Gordon, H. A., Ervin, R. F., and Wagner, M., in "Lobund Reports," Univ. Notre Dame Press, Notre Dame, Indiana, p. 182, (1960).

EIMERIA MAXIMA INFECTIONS IN GERMFREE AND GNOTOBIOTIC CHICKENS

John T. Rice, W. M. Reid, and *Joyce Johnson*
University of Georgia
Athens, Georgia 30601, U.S.A.

Infections of an intestinal species of coccidia, *E. maxima,* were studied in germfree and conventional chickens. Development of immunity following several immunizing infections in both types of hosts was compared. Comparison of weight gains, lesion scores and duration of oocyst production showed no differences between the germfree and conventional birds. Neither were differences found in coccidial immunity to *E. maxima* judged by comparing weight gains and lesion scores 7 days after a challenge infection. The prepatent period in both groups was 135 hours. Histopathological studies showed that the parasites developed in the same time sequence in germfree and conventional hosts.

These findings are in agreement with similar studies carried out on other intestinal species, *E. brunetti* and *E. necatrix* (Hegde, 1968, Ph.D. Diss., University of Georgia). However, they contrast with reports by Visco and Burns (1966, 41st Ann. Meeting Amer. Soc. Parasitol.) and Kemp and Johnson (personal communications) indicating reduced mortality and delay of the life cycle in germfree chickens parasitized with the cecal coccidium, *E. tenella.* (Supported by NIH Grant 5 ROI A109323-03).

461

SECTION X

RADIATION AND IMMUNOLOGY

INFLUENCE OF ANTIBIOTIC DECONTAMINATION ON THROMBOCYTOPENIC BLEEDING IN IRRADIATED RATS

R. Hohage, H. Meyer and *T. M. Fliedner*
Center of Internal Medicine and Pediatrics, Division of Hematology and
Center for Basic Clinical Research, Division of Clinical Physiology,
University of Ulm, Ulm, Germany

Introduction

The physiological microbial flora of the gut is often responsible for the manifestation of infections following bone marrow destruction after ionizing radiation. This bone marrow destruction also results in a thrombocytopenia and so bleeding is observed. There is evidence that bacterial infections may enhance the extent of the bleeding. From clinical experience, the extent and intensity of thrombocytopenic bleeding does not directly correlate to the platelet count in cases of bone marrow failure. In fact, patients may tolerate very low platelet counts, but when microbial infection occurs, severe bleeding may commence. Heit *et al.* (1) observed that germfree mice not only have a longer survival time following whole-body-X-irradiation that is lethal to conventional mice, but also observed a reduced bleeding tendency of these animals in comparison to the conventional controls.

The main problem of studying the influence of a microbial flora on bleeding tendency, however, is the lack of suitable techniques to measure hemorrhage quantitatively in animals in different gnotobiotic states. In this study an attempt has been made to quantitate hemorrhage by measuring the appearance of red cells in the thoracic duct lymph and by measuring the hemoglobin concentration of mesenteric lymph nodes following whole-body-X-irradiation. Ross *et al.* (2) demonstrated that there is a constant rise of red blood cell counts in the thoracic duct lymph at the 7th day after X-irradiation in rats. Later on, Jackson *et al.* (3) were able to correlate the red cell concentration in lymph of dogs with their platelet count after lethal whole body irradiation and showed that platelet substitution was able to stop this evidence of bleeding almost instantaneously.

Materials and Methods

Female Sprague-Dawley rats were decontaminated by means of antibiotics and maintained under sterile conditions in a laminar-flow-bench. Initially each rat was fed 40 mg of Bacitracin, Neomycin and Streptomycin once by stomach tube. For another 10 days the rats received the antibiotics with their drinking water, containing 4 mg/ml each of Bacitracin, Neomycin and Streptomycin. The gut became bacteria-free within three to four days, but antibiotics were given throughout the whole experiment. The conventional control rats were kept under the same conditions, but they were given water without antibiotics. The animals were given whole-body-X-irradiation with 700 R at 250 KV and 15 mA.

At 7, 9 and 12 days after irradiation, the animals were anesthetized with thiobarbitate and the red blood cells and the platelets were counted after cutting the tip of the tail. The thoracic duct was then cannulated according to a technique described by Bollman *et al.* (4).

When about 0.5 ml of lymph was collected, the erythrocyte count of the lymph sample was determined.

To compare the extent of hemorrhage in lymph nodes, the animals were sacrificed. Immediately after death, all lymph nodes of the radix mesenterii were removed and the wet weight measured. The lymph nodes were homogenized in 10 ml of distilled water, until the erythrocytes were completely lysed. The homogenate was then centrifuged and the hemoglobin of the supernatant determined using the Bencidine method according to Crosby and Furth (5).

Results

Figure 1 demonstrates the average red blood cell counts and the platelet counts of decontaminated and conventional rats after irradiation and the

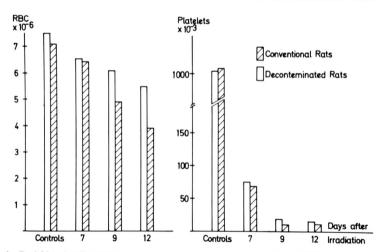

FIG. 1. Red blood cell counts and platelet counts in groups of 700 R-X-irradiated rats and of nonirradiated controls (n = 8).

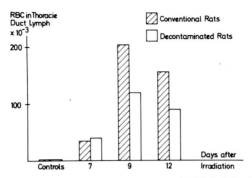

FIG. 2. Red blood cells in the thoracic duct lymph of 700 R-X-irradiated rats and of nonirradiated controls (n = 8).

non-irradiated controls. Each group represents the average of 8 animals. There is a progressive fall in the red blood cell count, beginning with the 7th day after irradiation. The decrease appears to be more pronounced, however, in the conventional rats than in the decontaminated ones. The platelet count in both groups of animals was markedly reduced by the 7th day after irradiation. The thrombocytopenia continued throughout the experiment. However, the counts appear to be somewhat lower in the conventional rats.

The erythrocyte count in the thoracic duct lymph of conventional and decontaminated rats is shown in Figure 2. In the nonirradiated controls, the counts vary from $500/\mu l$ to $2000/\mu l$. In the irradiated animals, the erythrocyte count reaches a peak at the 9th post-irradiation day, both in decontaminated and in conventional rats; but in the latter, the red cell content of the lymph at

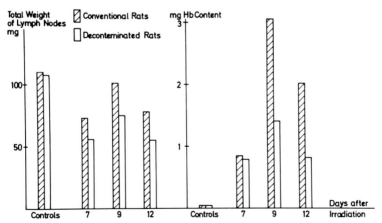

FIG. 3. Hemorrhage of mesenteric lymph nodes following 700 R-X-irradiation. Left side: Wet weight of the mesenteric lymph nodes in irradiated animals and in nonirradiated controls. Right side: hemoglobin content of the homogenized lymph nodes (n = 8).

the peak was much higher.

Figure 3 presents the results of the hemoglobin measurements of lymph nodes. The hemoglobin content was nearly zero in the nonirradiated controls. In the irradiated animals, the hemoglobin content reached top values at the 9th post-irradiation day and decreases thereafter. In this figure too, the hemoglobin content of lymph nodes was much higher in conventional than in decontaminated rats.

However, it is important to recognize that the averages of the total weight of all mesenteric lymph nodes were somewhat higher in the conventional group than in the decontaminated group. Thus, the higher hemoglobin content in the first group may partly be explained by the greater amount of lymph node tissue. But even if the hemoglobin content is expressed in percent of the total lymph node tissue, there remains a striking difference between lymph nodes of the conventional and decontaminated animals (Figure 4).

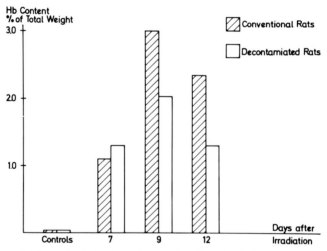

FIG. 4. Hemoglobin content of the extirpated lymph nodes in irradiated animals and in controls, calculated as percent of the total weight of the lymph nodes (n = 8).

Conclusions

These data indicate that the lymph node hemorrhage following whole-body-X-irradiation is more intensive in conventional rats than in animals with a bacteria-free gut.

Bleeding due to thrombocytopenia after radiation exposure at this dose level seems to peak at the 9th day after irradiation. The question arises as to why the hemoglobin content of the mesenteric lymph nodes decreases between day 9 and 12. However, one has to consider the fact that using our technique only the water-soluble hemoglobin of the lymph nodes can be measured. Hemoglobin deposited in the reticulo-endothelial system will not appear in our determinations, and these deposits may be larger at day 12 than at day 9. Regarding the decline of platelet counts in irradiated rats, it seems unlikely that the increased bleeding tendency of conventional rats is due only to a reduced platelet count. The differences in platelet counts of both groups were too minimal.

On the other hand it is not easy at the moment to explain the mechanisms behind the reduced bleeding tendency in decontaminated animals. Waaler *et al.* (6) studied some parameters of the plasmatic coagulation system as FV, VII, VIII, IX, X, XII, thromboplastin time, and the prothrombin level; and they found no striking differences between germfree and conventional rats. In previous experiments, we were unable to demonstrate differences in bleeding time, platelet aggregation and platelet retraction, between nonirradiated conventional and decontaminated animals, nor did we find differences in the euglobulin lysis time, or plasminogen and antiplasmin levels of the fibrinolytic system. Therefore, it is unlikely that there were changes in the normal coagulation state in the course of decontamination or during the germfree state.

In 1970, however, Wilson *et al.* (7) were able to demonstrate evidence of circulating vasoactive substances of bacterial origin, perhaps endotoxins, which caused an increased permeability of the vessel wall in X-irradiated mice. In axenic mice, such increased permeability could not be observed. These vasoactive substances may also be responsible for the enhancement of bleeding tendency in conventional rats. Bacterial endotoxins may pass the intestinal wall, which is more or less damaged following X-irradiation with lethal doses. The integrity of the vessel wall is much reduced by the thrombocytopenia. Additional damage, whether it was caused by the release of kinins, or by the toxic substances themselves, could lead to increased bleeding.

This hypothesis is supported by the observation that nearly all signs of hemorrhage observed in the animals were close to the intestinal wall or to the associated blood and lymph vessels. Whether or not the invasion of bacteria into tissues and blood stream causes another kind of vessel damage, is still an open question.

References

1. Heit, H., Fliedner, T. M., Fache, I., and Schnell, G., *Rad. Research 41:* 163 (1970).
2. Ross, M. H., Furth, J., and Bigelow, R. R., *Blood 7:* 141 (1952).
3. Jackson, D. P., Sorensen, D. K., Cronkite, E. P., Bond, V. P., Fliedner, T. M., *J. Clin. Invest. 38:* 1689 (1959).
4. Bollman, J. L., Cain, J. C., Grindlay, J. H., *J. Lab. Clin. Med. 33:* 1349 (1948).
5. Crosby, W. H., and Furth, F. W., *Blood 11:* 380 (1956).
6. Waaler, B. A., Gustafsson, B. E., Hauge, A., Nilsson, D., Amundsen, E., *Proc. Soc. Exp. Biol. Med. 117:* 444 (1964).
7. Wilson, R., Barry, T. A., Bealmer, P. M., *Rad. Research 41:* 89 (1970).

EVIDENCE FOR GRAFT VS. HOST REACTION IN THE GERMFREE ALLOGENEIC RADIATION CHIMERA

P. M. Bealmear,* B. E. Loughman, A. A. Nordin and *R. Wilson**
Lobund Laboratory, University of Notre Dame
Notre Dame, Indiana 46556, U.S.A.

Introduction

The graft-versus-host (GVH) reactions that constitute the secondary disease seen in allogeneic radiation chimeras are usually fatal within the 60 days following bone marrow transplantation when animals are maintained in a normal environment. As we have shown previously, the elimination of the microflora of the host delays, but does not avert, the fatal effects of GVH; it also mitigates the pathology of secondary disease (1, 2).

That the secondary disease that develops in the conventional radiation chimera is complicated by infection has been shown by earlier studies by Van Bekkum and Vos (3) and by Connell (1), who either reduced the microflora or eliminated it in an attempt to ameliorate the syndrome. Van Bekkum and Vos (3) treated xenogeneic radiation chimeras with aureomycin, and their diarrhea disappeared; the diarrhea was absent only when the chimeras were treated with the antibiotics, and reappeared when treatment was discontinued. Connell (1) treated lethally irradiated germfree mice with allogeneic bone marrow and maintained surviving animals through a 120-day post-irradiation observation period. These animals were survivors of a dose-response study, and they had not all received the same dose of radiation. Furthermore, the bone marrow inoculum had been only roughly quantitated as "femur equivalents."

Through a more appropriate experimental design Jones *et al.* (2) tested the hypothesis suggested by these earlier studies that the absence of a microflora in allogeneic radiation chimeras results in a greatly reduced mortality from secondary disease and a modification of the symptoms characteristic of this syndrome.

*Present address: Division of Experimental Biology, Baylor College of Medicine, Houston, Texas 77025, U.S.A.

Materials and Methods

Inbred C3H/He and DBA/2 mice, which differ at 14 specificities and are alike at two specificities of the H-2 locus, were used. C3H/He has the H-2^k allele, and the DBA/2 has the H-2^d allele. These two strains differ also at the H-1, H-6, and H-7 loci.

All animals were fed a diet of sterilized Teklad pellets (4) and tap water *ad libitum.* The water of conventional mice was maintained at a pH of about 2.5.

Germfree mice were housed in shoe box plastic cages in Trexler flexible film isolators (5), and were maintained under the routine procedures developed at the Lobund Laboratory (6). Bacteriological surveillance (7) was made biweekly and at the termination of an experiment. Conventional mice were housed in the same type cages on the shelves of the animal room.

The x-radiation source was a 260-kVp therapy x-ray machine operated at 250 kV and 15 mA with a filtration of 1.00 mm Al and 0.25 mm Cu (HLV, 1.05 mm Cu). Germfree and conventional mice of approximately 11 weeks of age were irradiated dorsoventrally with a skin-target distance of about 50 cm. The procedure for irradiation of germfree mice has been described previously (8). Conventional mice were given 825 rads, and germfree mice were given 1000 rads in single exposures. Since these two doses, which exceed the LD$_{100}$ for the C3H/He strain, produce similar mortality curves and a comparable post-irradiation hematological response, they are considered equivalent in this laboratory (9).

It was determined by a dose response curve that 5×10^6 bone marrow cells i.v. were necessary to give 100% survival after the above doses of radiation; double that dose was given in all further experiments (10). A 0.5 ml sample containing 10^7 nucleated bone marrow cells was injected i.v. into the tail vein approximately 24 hrs post-irradiation. C3H/He mice were the recipient strain for all experiments; C3H/He mice were the donor strain for all syngeneic experiments; DBA/2 mice were the donor strain for all allogeneic transplants; and inbred Fischer 344 rats were the donors for the xenogeneic transplants.

Results

Germfree C3H/He mice x-irradiated with 1000 R and given 10^7 histoincompatible DBA/2 bone marrow cells i.v. did not demonstrate gross symptoms of the graft-vs.-host reaction, and 98% survived the 15-month period of observation. By contrast, conventional C3H/He mice irradiated with 825 R and given 10^7 conventional DBA/2 bone marrow cells i.v. had 64% survival at 30 days and no survivors at 120 days post-irradiation (2). The conventional allogeneic chimeras presented the usual symptoms of secondary disease observed in other laboratories.

A histopathological study of the apparently healthy germfree allogeneic

472

chimeras revealed GVH reactions characterized by lymphoid cell infiltration and subsequent tissue degeneration in the lymph nodes, spleen, thymus, and Peyer's patches. Liver, kidney, and lung tissue damage seemed to be associated with the perivascular infiltration of mononuclear cells; damage to these 3 organs seemed to be a late feature of the disease, often occurring after the 3rd post-transplant month (10). In sections stained with H & E, the GVH reaction was not detectable during the early days post-transplant (10), therefore, methyl green and pyronin stain was used to try to find the large pyroninophilic cells associated with GVH at an earlier time period. These large pyroninophilic cells appeared as early as 4 days post-transplant, and their numbers increased with time. This indicated that GVH begins immediately after transplant, but is usually not fatal until the animal has lived out about three fourths of its normal life span. This also indicates that any successful treatment for GVH must begin at the time of transplant.

We then questioned the immunological capabilities of the germfree allogeneic radiation chimera undergoing GVH. An indirect test for chimerism by means of challenge with skin grafts from the donor strain of mice and from a third party strain revealed that the allogeneic chimeras were tolerant to donor strain skin and rejected third party skin (10). This indicated that they were really chimeric and were immunologically competent, at least for skin graft rejection.

Both allogeneic and syngeneic chimeras were immunized with sheep red blood cells, then their responses were measured by the plaque assay (11). By use of the appropriate isoantisera, it was determined that the cells responsible for the response to sheep red blood cells were always of donor origin. The magnitude of the response was depressed and delayed in the allogeneic chimeras as compared to the syngeneic chimeras. An *in vitro* immunization and challenge of spleen cells from allogeneic chimeras gave comparable results; the response of the allogeneic chimeras was greatly reduced.

When challenged with the antigen flagellin from *Salmonella adelaide*, which measures B cell response, both syngeneic and allogeneic chimeras responded comparably.

The T and B cell response of the chimeras was tested further by the response to phytohemagglutinin (PHA) and to pokeweed mitogen (PWM). Stockman *et al.* (12) showed that the response to PHA is a T cell response and a to PWM is a B cell response. Allogeneic chimeras approximately 1 year post-transplant did not respond to PHA during the normal period for stimulation, whereas syngeneic chimeras gave a PHA response comparable to that of untreated control mice. Allogeneic chimeras, however, did respond to PWM with the same magnitude as the syngeneic chimeras and the untreated control mice.

Additional tests for cell mediated immunity (CMI) or the T cell response included the response to third party tumor cells. The allogeneic chimeras gave a delayed and greatly reduced response to third party tumor cells as measured by the chromium release assay.

Conclusions

The absence of a microflora delays, but does not avert the fatal effects of GVH; the pathology of secondary disease, however, is mitigated. The germfree allogeneic radiation chimera has a greatly reduced or absent T cell response as demonstrated by its lack of response to third party tumor cells. The responses which are supposed to be both T and B cell mediated are reduced in the chimera, but not absent. The B cell response of the allogeneic chimera is almost normal. Though morphologically the thymus of the allogeneic chimera appears to be normal, it would seem that the stroma of the thymus and the cells that reconstitute it must be of the same H-2 locus for the T cells to function normally.

Though the germfree state did not eliminate GVH in the allogeneic chimera, it did permit the animal to live out three fourths of its normal life span without obvious symptoms of the disease. The germfree state also enables investigators to have a prolonged time period in which to study GVH and hopefully to find a method for eliminating it.

Acknowledgements

We are grateful for the technical assistance of Dr. Ellen Richie, Mr. Michael Dauphinee, Mr. Michael Gallagher, and Mr. Michael Magliolo.

This research was supported by Grants No. 1 R01 A1 10990-01, No. EC-00080, and No. 5R01 A 107659-06 from the U.S.P.H.S.

References

1. Connell, S. M. S. J., and Wilson, R., *Life Sci. 4:* 721 (1965).
2. Jones, J. M., Wilson, R., and Bealmear, P. M., *Radiat. Res. 45:* 577 (1971).
3. Van Bekkum, D. W., and Vos, O., *Int. J. Radiat. Biol. 3:* 173 (1961).
4. Kellogg, T. F., and Wostmann, B. S., *Lab. Anim. Care 19:* 812 (1969).
5. Trexler, P. C., *Ann. N.Y. Acad. Sci. 78:* 29 (1959).
6. Reyniers, J. A., *Ann. N.Y. Acad. Sci. 78:* 47 (1959).
7. Wagner, M. , *Ann. N.Y. Acad. Sci. 78:* 89 (1959).
8. Wilson, R., *Radiat. Res. 20:* 477 (1963).
9. Bealmear, P. M., unpublished observations.
10. Jones, J. M., "A Study of Secondary Disease in Gnotobiotic Mouse Radiation Chimeras," Doctoral Dissertation, U. Notre Dame, Notre Dame, Indiana, p. 205, (1970).
11. Loughman, B. E., "A Study of the Humoral Immune Response of Mouse Radiation Chimeras: Thymus Cell Function in Allogeneic Radiation Chimeras," Doctoral Dissertation, U. Notre Dame, Notre Dame, Indiana, p. 153, (1972).

12. Stockman, G. D., Gallagher, M. T., Heim, L. R., South, M. A., and Trentin, J. J., *Proc. Soc. Exp. Biol. & Med. 136:* 980 (1971).

MORTALITY OF SECONDARY DISEASE IN ANTIBIOTIC-TREATED MOUSE RADIATION CHIMERAS

H. Heit, R. Wilson, T. M. Fliedner and *E. Kohne*
Center of Basic Clinical Research, University of Ulm
Ulm, Germany

Introduction

It has been known for more than 10 years that antimicrobial treatment has a suppressive effect on secondary disease and mortality of allogeneic bone marrow chimeras (1). The role of the microflora gained new interest, however, since Jones *et al.* in 1971 published that the germfree state virtually eliminates the symptoms and mortality associated with graft-versus-host disease in allogeneic mouse chimeras and prolongs the mean survival time of xenogeneic chimeras (2).

It is the purpose of this presentation to give our preliminary data about allogeneic bone marrow transplantation in mice that were reared in a conventional microbial environment but then rendered "germfree" by means of antibiotic treatment.

Materials and Methods

All studies were performed using $C_{57}Bl$ mice as bone marrow donors and CBA mice as lethally irradiated recipients. This combination guarantees a high mortality from secondary disease since $C_{57}Bl$ and CBA mice differ in all genetic specificities of H-2 locus except at H_5 (3).

Fifty CBA mice, 8-10 weeks old, were given Bacitracin, Neomycin, and Carbenicillin disodium, which are poorly absorbed from the gastrointestinal tract, in their drinking water at a concentration of 4 g/liter. As a fungistatic 1 g Pimaricin was added per liter. Sterile food and water was offered *ad libitum*. From day 3 of antibiotic treatment all bacteriological swabs from feces and bedding material were negative; a general sterility was achieved 4 − 5 weeks thereafter.

As irradiated and bone marrow treated but not decontaminated controls, a comparable number of conventional CBA mice of the same age were used. A secondary contamination of the animals was prevented by maintaining them in a laminar flow bench or sterile containers.

Two weeks after the onset of antibiotic treatment, the decontaminated and the conventional control CBA mice received 800 rads wholebody irradiation using a 250 KVP 15 mA Stabilipan X-ray generator (Siemens) with a filtration of 0.1 mm Cu. Twenty-four hours later 1×10^7 bone marrow cells from female, 10 weeks old $C_{57}Bl$ mice were injected intravenously.

All transplanted animals were proved to be bone marrow chimeras by Hb-electrophoresis. Complete chimerism was proved to be established from week 7 onwards; the first signs were noticed between weeks 4 and 5.

After transplantation the animals were randomized and divided into 2 groups of 25 mice each, one of them to determine the mean survival time over a period of 120 days, the other to look for possible differences in the expression of graft-versus-host reaction. For this purpose 2 animals per week were sacrificed and examined over a period of 9 weeks.

Results

In Figure 1, the per cent survival of conventional and decontaminated allogeneic bone marrow recipients as well as of irradiated controls without bone marrow transfusion is shown. All CBA mice not given a bone marrow transfusion died within 2 and 3 weeks after irradiation. No recipient of allogeneic bone marrow, however, died before the fourth week. In the course of week 4, 40% and by week 9, 100% of the conventional allogeneic chimeras died of secondary disease.

No decontamined bone marrow recipient died before week 5. At the end of the 9th week 80% of the animals were still alive and a little less than 50%

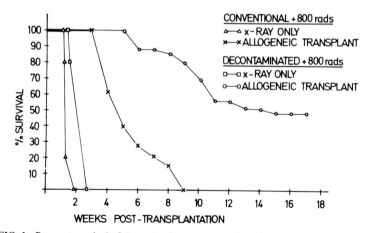

FIG. 1. Per cent survival of decontaminated conventional bone marrow chimeras.

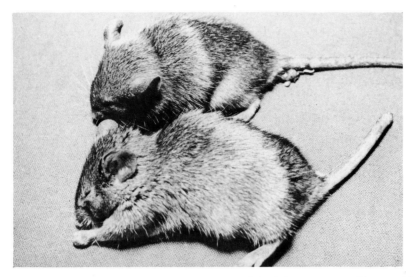

FIG. 2. Conventional (above) and decontaminated (below) bone marrow chimeras, 6th week.

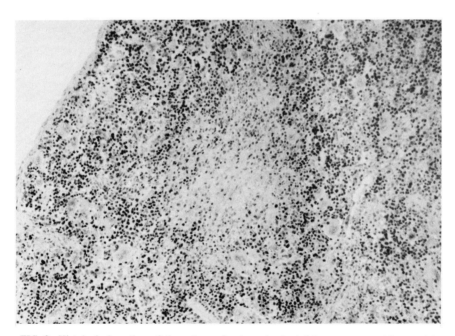

FIG. 3. Histological section of the spleen of a decontaminated bone marrow chimera: 6th week.

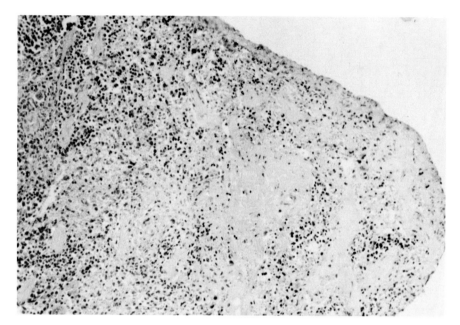

FIG. 4. Histological section of the spleen of a conventional bone marrow chimera: 6th week.

survived the observation period of 120 days.

Figure 2 shows a conventional and a decontaminated CBA mouse 6 weeks after 800 rads whole body irradiation and allogeneic bone marrow transplantation. While the conventional allogeneic bone marrow recipients showed all symptoms of secondary disease such as diarrhea, wasting, and hair loss, the decontaminated animals appeared to be in good physical condition, except for some weight reduction. Those of this group which died, however, showed a comparable cachexia and adynamia as the conventional did, but never diarrhea.

The results of autopsy in the two animal groups during the first 9 weeks after irradiation and bone marrow transplantation indicated the typical symptoms of the organ manifestations of allogeneic bone marrow grafting.

Compared with unirradiated controls, the lymphatic organs in both groups were obviously enlarged within the first 3 weeks after transplantation. Thereafter they decreased in size and became atrophic by week 5. No lymphatic regeneration was noticed in the course of the subsequent 4 weeks. A difference between decontaminated and conventional recipients could not be established.

From week 6 onwards the conventional chimeras showed signs of bacteremia. Disseminated abscesses and necrotic foci of liver and spleen were a characteristic finding in this period; in addition, infectious ascites was repeatedly

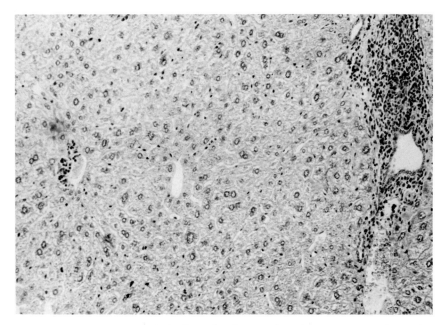

FIG. 5. Histological section of the liver of a decontaminated bone marrow chimera: 9th week.

found.

In contrast, no comparable observations could be made in the decontaminated chimeras; in particular, there were no macroscopic visible necrosis nor abscesses.

Histological sections of different organs such as lymph nodes, spleen, liver, kidney, thymus, skin and small intestine had been made of all animals autopsied.

It appeared that the findings in the spleen were particularly typical for the characteristic changes due to secondary disease in both animal groups and were demonstrated as representative of all lymphatic organs. In the first two weeks, the spleen histology was characterized by increasing hemopoietic activity; nodules of erythropoiesis were present, and a high content of myelopoietic activity was obvious in the conventional mouse spleen, whereas lymphopoietic cells were rare.

At week 3, there was first evidence of the development of necrotic lesions in both animal groups. They were present during the entire 9 week observation period with a maximum during the 5th and 6th week (Figs. 3, 4). Hemopoiesis persisted although less pronounced compared to the first 2 − 4 weeks.

Necrotic foci in the liver of both decontaminated and conventional animals at week 9 are seen in Figs. 5 and 6. No marked difference between

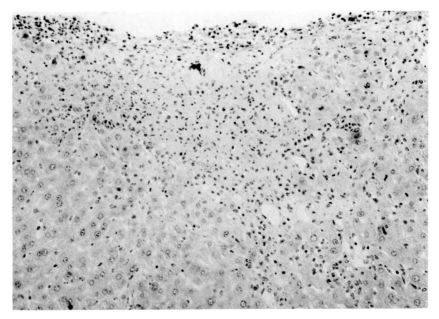

FIG. 6. Histological section of the liver of a conventional bone marrow chimera: 9th week.

decontaminated and conventional chimeras was seen in any of the organs examined. It appeared, however, that the extent and the frequency of necrotic foci were a little more prominent in the conventional mice.

These data — although preliminary — demonstrate that mortality due to secondary disease is based at least on two components: the immunological processes of graft-versus-host reaction and the manifestation of bacterial infections. Thus the possibility of surviving secondary disease seems to depend in part on the gnotobiotic status of the animals. In this context, it was of interest to study whether or not a reassociation with the usual microbial flora will reduce the chance of survival of allogeneic chimeras. In earlier experiments germfree allogeneic chimeras died with signs of secondary disease if bacterial contamination was performed. In the present study, 10 of the decontaminated chimeras surviving 120 days were conventionalized stepwise. All of them tolerated the association with bacteria and showed no symptoms of relapse of secondary diseases over a period of 20 additional weeks to date.

Summary

1) Animals, rendered "germfree" by antibiotic treatment and given allogeneic bone marrow transplantation develop histological signs and symptoms of graft-versus-host reaction, but 80% survive 9 weeks, at which time all

conventional controls have died. After 120 days, 50% of the decontaminated chimeras were still alive.

2) Reconventionalization beginning 175 days after irradiation and allogeneic bone marrow grafting — at a time of established chimerism — did not produce any mortality for 20 additional weeks.

References

1. Van Bekkum, D. W., and Vos, O., *Int. J. Radiat. Biol. 3:* 173 (1961).
2. Jones, J. M., Wilson, R., and Bealmear, P., *Radiat. Res. 45:* 577 (1971).
3. Snell, G. D., and Stimpfling, J. H., in "Biology of the Laboratory Mouse," by the Staff of the Jackson Memorial Laboratory, (E. L. Green, ed.), 2nd Ed., McGraw-Hill, New York, p. 457, (1966).

INFLUENCE OF A DEFINED FLORA ON THE SERUM PROTEINS OF GNOTOBIOTIC RATS

E. Balish, C. E. Yale and *R. Hong*
Departments of Surgery, Medical Microbiology, and Pediatrics
University of Wisconsin Medical School
Madison, Wisconsin 53706, U.S.A.

Introduction

Shortly after birth, the immunologic systems of conventional animals are stimulated by the microbial flora. This stimulation plays a vital role in increasing the cellular and humoral defense of the host and yet we know very little about the relative contributions of the various microorganisms toward the development of this increased immunity. The germfree animal provides us with a unique experimental tool to determine the role of specific intestinal bacteria in activating cellular and humoral immunologic systems after oral challenge. In this study, cellulose acetate electrophoresis and immunoelectrophoresis were used to study the serum proteins of germfree Sprague-Dawley rats before, and four weeks after, oral monoassociation with common intestinal microorganisms.

Results

Each species established itself in the intestinal tract of the gnotobiotic rat within 48 hrs. During the 4 weeks of monoassociation there was no apparent illness, weight loss or change in cecal size. At the time of sacrifice, i.e., 4 weeks after challenge, bacteria were cultured from all sections of the gastrointestinal tract. The largest viable populations were found in contents from the cecum and colon ($10^{10} - 10^{11}$/g for *Streptococcus faecalis, Bacillus fragilis*, and *Lactobacillus acidophilus*).

In order to be sure that the alterations in serum proteins were due to the test bacteria and not the commercial diet, we assayed the serum proteins of 90 and 180 day old rats. Except for what appeared to be an increase in the alpha-2 fraction of serum from 180 day old rats the serum proteins did not appear to be altered by the commercial diet. Immunoelectrophoresis patterns of serum from 3 and 6 month old germfree rats and a 90 day old conventional rat are shown in Fig. 1.

GERM-FREE
180 days old

GERM-FREE
90 days old

CONVENTIONAL
90 days old

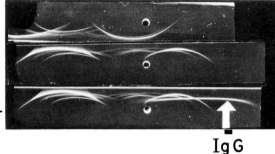

IgG

FIG. 1. Immunoelectrophoresis pattern of serum from germfree and conventional Sprague-Dawley rats fed an autoclaved 5010C crude diet.

In comparison to conventional rats, the germfree rats appeared to have lower values for total protein, alpha-1, beta and gamma globulins (Table I). In comparison to germfree rats, monoassociation appeared to increase the total serum protein values. Of the four gram-positive bacteria studied, only *Staphylococcus aureus* 80/81 and *Clostridium perfringens* caused an apparent increase

GERM-FREE

Lactobacillus
   acidophilus

Staphylococcus
   aureus

Streptococcus
   faecalis

Clostridium
   perfringens

Candida
   albicans

CONVENTIONAL

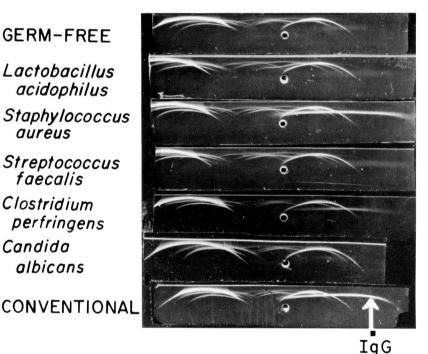

IgG

FIG. 2. Immunoelectrophoresis patterns of serum from 118 day old germfree, conventional and monoassociated rats.

Table I. Serum Proteins of Germfree, Monoassociated and Conventional 120 Day Old Sprague-Dawley Rats

Microbial Status	No. Rats	Total Protein	Albumin	Serum proteins (g/100 ml)[*]			
				Alpha-1	Alpha-2	Beta	Gamma
Germ-free	6	6.0 (5.8-6.2)	2.8 (2.6-3.0)	1.68 (1.44-1.85)	0.46 (0.41-0.51)	0.85 (0.77-0.88)	0.20 (0.2-0.2)
Monognotobiotic S. aureus	3	6.86 (6.8-6.9)	3.26 (3.1-3.4)	1.51 (1.44-1.71)	0.42 (0.35-0.44)	1.12 (1.06-1.16)	0.52 (0.5-0.6)
S. faecalis	3	6.33 (6.3-6.4)	2.76 (2.7-2.8)	2.10 (2.04-2.13)	0.45 (0.40-0.49)	0.84 (0.80-0.91)	0.13 (0.1-0.2)
L. acidophilus	3	6.40 (6.4-6.4)	2.88 (2.8-2.9)	2.03 (2.01-2.05)	0.37 (0.36-0.39)	0.95 (0.91-0.98)	0.16 (0.1-0.2)
C. perfringens	2	6.50 (6.4-6.6)	3.70 (3.5-3.9)	1.19 (1.08-1.30)	0.59 (0.57-0.63)	0.91 (0.89-0.93)	0.40 (0.4-0.4)
C. albicans	13	6.50 (5.0-7.2)	2.70 (2.2-3.0)	1.61 (1.13-2.16)	0.98 (0.54-2.04)	1.15 (0.51-1.25)	0.19 (0.1-0.4)
Conventional	4	6.7 (6.4-7.0)	2.8 (2.7-3.0)	2.8 (2.7-3.0)	0.34 (0.24-0.41)	1.20 (1.13-1.27)	0.68 (0.5-0.9)

[*]Mean and range of values observed.

in gamma globulin (Table I). This is even more evident in Fig. 2 where the serum protein patterns, of rats monoassociated with each of the four gram-positive bacteria used in this study, are compared with serum protein patterns of conventional and germfree rats of the same age. It can be seen that, within 4 weeks, *C. perfringens* and *S. aureus* were able to stimulate IgG. Table I shows that *S. aureus* also caused increased in total protein, albumin, and beta globulin. *C. perfringens* caused an increase in all serum proteins except alpha-1 globulin. *S. faecalis* was associated with an apparent increase in alpha-1 globulin whereas *L. acidophilus* increased alpha-1 and beta globulins. *Candida albicans* (Fig. 2 and Table I) did not cause any appreciable increase in gamma globulins, but the opportunistic yeast did increase the total protein, alpha-2, and beta globulin fractions.

Pseudomonas aeruginosa, *Klebsiella penumoniae* and *Enterobacter aerogenes* were able to increase the level of gamma globulins within 4 weeks after an oral challenge (Table II and Fig. 3). *P. aeruginosa* increased all protein

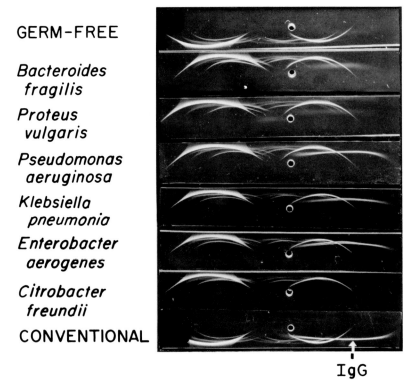

GERM-FREE

Bacteroides fragilis

Proteus vulgaris

Pseudomonas aeruginosa

Klebsiella pneumonia

Enterobacter aerogenes

Citrobacter freundii

CONVENTIONAL

IgG

FIG. 3. Immunoelectrophoresis patterns of serum from 118 day old germfree, conventional and monoassociated (with gram-negative bacteria) Sprague-Dawley rats.

Table II. Serum Proteins of Germfree, Monoassociated and Conventional 120 Day Old Sprague-Dawley Rats

Microbial Status	No. Rats	Serum proteins (g/100 ml)[*]					
		Total Protein	Albumin	Alpha-1	Alpha-2	Beta	Gamma
Germ-free	6	6.0 (5.8-6.2)	2.8 (2.6-3.0)	1.68 (1.44-1.85)	0.46 (0.41-0.51)	0.85 (0.77-0.88)	0.20 (0.2-0.2)
P. aeruginosa	3	6.66 (6.6-6.8)	3.2 (3.1-3.3)	1.57 (1.50-1.66)	0.49 (0.41-0.56)	1.07 (1.02-1.12)	0.36 (0.3-0.4)
P. vulgaris	3	9.4 (6.8-11.9)	4.03 (3.4-5.1)	3.1 (2.56-4.12)	0.77 (0.54-0.81)	1.40 (1.14-1.79)	0.16 (0.1-0.2)
B. fragilis	3	6.3 (6.2-6.4)	2.96 (2.8-3.2)	2.06 (1.78-2.29)	0.49 (0.38-0.57)	0.93 (0.83-1.04)	0.10 (0.1-0.1)
C. freundii	2	7.8 (7.8-7.8)	4.1 (4.1-4.1)	2.3 (2.1-2.5)	0.45 (0.44-0.46)	0.89 (0.67-1.11)	0.10 (0.1-0.1)
K. pneumoniae	2	6.2 (6.0-6.4)	3.3 (3.1-3.6)	1.07 (1.07-1.08)	0.51 (0.48-0.54)	0.86 (0.83-0.89)	0.45 (0.4-0.5)
E. aerogenes	2	6.4 (6.2-6.6)	3.1 (3.1-3.1)	1.05 (1.02-1.08)	0.51 (0.47-0.55)	0.76 (0.78-0.75)	0.45 (0.3-0.6)
Conventional	4	6.7 (6.4-7.0)	2.8 (2.7-3.0)	2.8 (2.7-3.0)	0.34 (0.24-0.41)	1.20 (1.13-1.27)	0.68 (0.5-0.9)

[*]Mean and range of values observed.

fractions except alpha-1 and alpha-2 globulins, whereas *B. fragilis* was associated only with an increase in alpha-1 globulin. *Proteus vulgaris*, although unable to stimulate gamma globulin, did cause very noticeable increases in all other protein fractions (Table II). In addition to increasing gamma globulin, *K. pneumoniae* and *E. aerogenes* were also associated with larger levels of total protein, albumin and alpha-2 globulin and a decrease in alpha-1 protein. *E. aerogenes* decreased the level of beta globulin. *Citrobacter freundii* appeared to be associated mainly with increases in total protein, albumin and alpha-1 globulin.

Although germfree rat serum had good agglutination titers for *S. aureus*, very low levels of agglutinins were present for the other microorganisms used in this study. Four weeks of monoassociation with *S. faecalis* or *C. albicans* did not stimulate agglutinin production. However, monoassociation with all of the other bacteria (listed in Tables I and II) caused an increase in serum agglutinins. A large increase in agglutinins (256-512) was apparent in serum from rats colonized with *S. aureus* and *P. aeruginosa* for 4 weeks.

Conclusions

Studies in this laboratory and others (1) have demonstrated a very noticeable hypogammaglobulinemia in the germfree rat. Our immuno-electrophoretic studies failed to show qualitative differences in the serum protein patterns of 90 and 180 day old rats fed a commercial, steam-sterilized diet, *ad libitum*. It was previously demonstrated that feeding germfree rats a synthetic, filter-sterilized diet did not result in any drastic increase or decrease in the serum proteins of germfree rats (2). Thus, assuming that the pure bacterial cultures did not increase the antigenicity of dietary components, the changes in serum proteins observed in this study were probably due to the viable bacteria in the intestinal tract.

In this study it was evident that microorganisms are capable of altering serum proteins. However, not all microorganisms were able to increase the level of gamma globulins. The extreme variations in the serum proteins of monoassociated rats, along with the failure of serum protein values to return to germfree levels, as described in other studies with *Salmonella typhimurium* (3), indicates that intestinal bacteria can induce a variety of alterations in serum proteins. The composition of an animals's microbial flora could play a key role in the development of both humoral and cellular immunity. Flora-induced alterations in serum proteins could account for the observed differences in the susceptibility of various animal species to certain microbes and their resistance to others. In addition to microbial antagonisms in the intestinal tract, the inability of bacteria to induce significant alterations in serum proteins may be a partial explanation of why certain bacteria are able to persist in very large numbers in the intestinal tract and other microorganisms, which cause a more intense humoral response, are present in much smaller numbers.

Acknowledgement

This research was supported in part by Public Health Service Grant AI06956 from the National Institute of Allergy and Infectious Diseases.

References

1. Wostmann, B. S., *Ann. N.Y. Acad. Sci. 94:* 272 (1961).
2. Wostmann, B. S., Olson, G. B., and Pleasants, J. R., *Nature 206:* 1056 (1965).
3. Wostmann, B. S., *Proc. Soc. Exp. Biol. Med. 134:* 294 (1970).

COMPARISONS OF NATURAL AND IMMUNE ANTIBODIES TO TEICHOIC ACIDS IN GERMFREE AND CONVENTIONAL GUINEA PIGS

G. T. Frederick and *F. W. Chorpenning*
The Ohio State University
Columbus, Ohio 43210, U.S.A.

Introduction

A great deal of conflicting data have been published regarding immunological comparisons between germfree and conventional animals. Generally, the germfree animal has exhibited a less well-defined lymphoid tissue (1-4) and lower immunoglobulin levels (4-7) than the conventional animal. In some instances, lower specific responses to antigen have been reported in the germfree animal (8-12). In others, responses were comparable to the conventional animal (13-16). The majority of immunological comparisons have employed injection of whole red blood cells or microbial cells, while a few have used soluble proteins. Such complex stimuli may yield confusing results due to individual differences in prior exposure to cross-reacting antigens. For clarity of interpretation, systems of narrow specificity and sensitive testing methods must be employed. We feel also that natural antibody systems can be an important tool for assessing the immunological status of germfree animals. Therefore, we have investigated antibodies in germfree and conventional guinea pigs to a glycerol teichoic acid antigen present in a number of gram-positive bacteria.

Materials and Methods

For our test system, we used purified and chemically defined teichoic acid extracted from a *Bacillus species* (OSU No. 372). The specificity of passive hemagglutination (PHA) tests with this antigen resided in its poly-glycerophosphate (PGP) backbone, insuring that the reactions involved a single antibody specificity (17). Furthermore, 100% of the adult conventional guinea pigs tested exhibited natural anti-PGP antibodies (17), providing an ideal system for study of their immunological status in an otherwise natural, unstressed animal.

Forty-two random-bred conventional guinea pigs, fed Purina Guinea Pig Chow (Ralston-Purina Co., St. Louis, Mo.) and 48 germfree guinea pigs, fed a

493

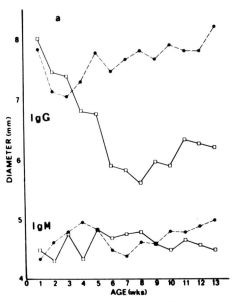

FIG. 1a. Relative levels of total IgG and IgM in germfree (□—□) and conventional (●—●) whole sera. Average diameters of radial immunodiffusion patterns of whole sera tested with rabbit anti-guinea pig IgM and rabbit anti-guinea pig IgG.

nutritionally identical diet (No. 010999, General Biochemicals, Chagrin Falls, Ohio) were studied from birth. Individual sera from consecutive weekly bleedings were tested by radial immunodiffusion (RID) versus rabbit anti-guinea pig IgM and IgG.

Results

Figure 1a shows the average of the total levels of IgM and IgG classes of immunoglobulins in these animals, as measured by diameters of RID patterns, illustrated in Figure 2. Throughout the early life of both groups, comparable levels of IgM were present, as reported by Arnason in mice (18). But the levels of IgG were lower in the germfree animals. Consecutive sera, tested for anti-PGP antibodies by PHA with guinea pig red cells to which teichoic acid had been adsorbed, exhibited average levels of natural antibody as shown in Figure 1b. Whole sera were fractionated on Sephadex G-200 (Pharmacia Fine Chemicals, Piscataway, N.J.) and fractions were characterized by 2-mercaptoethanol susceptibility, immunoelectrophoresis (IE) and immunodiffusion. Both IgM and IgG antibodies of this specificity were present at birth, apparently being of maternal origin since the titers fell for the first 4 weeks. Then IgM antibodies rose in both groups, the rise in germfree animals being much more rapid, reaching a higher titer, and remaining constant thereafter. This observation of

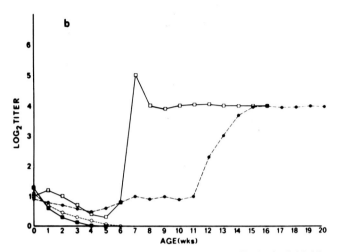

FIG. 1b. Average titers of specific anti-PGP natural antibody in IgM (Germfree □—□, Conventional ●—●) and IgG (Germfree ■—■, Conventional ○—○) classes of immunoglobulins as measured by passive hemagglutination.

sustained levels of antibody to a bacterial antigen in germfree animals is similar to the observations of Wostmann and Olson (12) who employed injections of BSA. The conventional rise occurred more slowly, eventually reaching the same level.

The surviving germfree pigs, and 6 of the conventional animals, were each injected i.p. with 500 micrograms of teichoic acid antigen. Figure 3 shows a comparison between germfree and conventional responses to this injection. The

TABLE I. Presence of Anti-PGP Antibody Activity in IgG Subclasses

Age Group (weeks)		Immunoglobulin Present		Anti-Teichoic Acid (PHA) in	
		gamma one	gamma two	gamma one	gamma two
0-5 GF	(20)	+	+	+	—
0-6 C	(20)	+	+	+	—
5-16 GF	(20)	+	+	—	—
6-16 C	(20)	+	+	—	—
16-20 C	(14)	+	+	—	—
)21 C	(30)	+	+	+	—
16-18*GF	(2)	+	+	+	—
16-18*C	(6)	+	+	+	—

GF — germfree
C — conventional
( ) — number of animals in group in parentheses
* — injected with 500 micrograms of teichoic acid

495

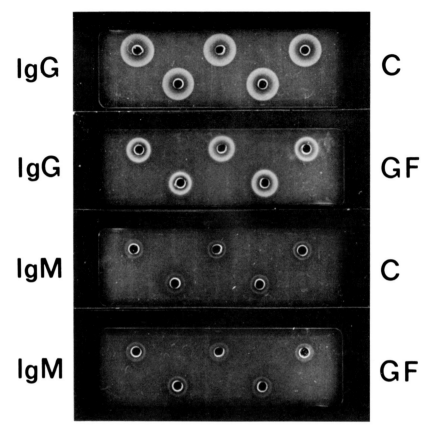

FIG. 2. Radial immunodiffusion patterns of germfree (GF) and conventional (C) whole sera at 8 weeks of age. Twelve microliter aliquots of whole sera were placed in wells cut in 1% Noble agar in barbital buffer, pH 8.6, containing 5% rabbit anti-guinea pig IgG (IgG) or rabbit anti-guinea pig IgM (IgM).

average rise in titer of the conventional animals had the same slope as the average rise of the germfree animals. Also, anti-PGP antibody activity appeared in the IgG class in both groups of immunized animals, while none was present in this class in the normal animals. The IgG immunoglobulins of both natural and immune sera were further fractionated by ion-exchange chromatography using tris buffers of increasing molarities. The two major subclasses, $\gamma_1 G$ and $\gamma_2 G$, were tested by PHA for antibodies to PGP. Figure 4 shows the characterization of the ion-exchange fractions by IE. A comparison of results in the germfree and conventional groups at various ages is shown in Table I. It is clear that whether the guinea pigs were germfree or not, anti-PGP antibodies appeared only in the $\gamma_1 G$ subclass. In conventional animals, natural IgG anti-PGP antibodies were also

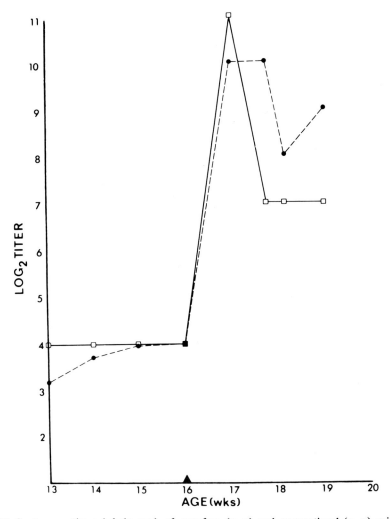

FIG. 3. Average titers (whole sera) of germfree (□—□) and conventional (●—●) animals following injection (▲) with 500 micrograms of teichoic acid.

restricted to the $\gamma_1 G$ subclass, appearing at 20-21 weeks. Since the germfree animals could not be maintained longer than 16 weeks, we have no data on natural IgG in these animals.

Conclusions

A number of previous investigators have suggested that germfree animals respond more slowly than conventional animals (7-11). The lower IgG levels

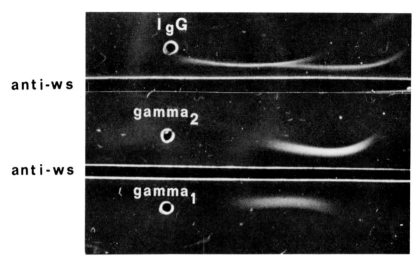

FIG. 4. Immunoelectrophoresis patterns of IgG-, gamma$_2$G-, and gamma$_1$G-containing serum fractions versus rabbit anti-guinea pig whole serum (anti-ws).

shown in Figure 1a could be interpreted in this manner. However, the accelerated IgM anti-PGP response in the germfree animals (Fig. 1b) contradicts this assumption. The lower IgG levels in the germfree animals could have resulted from exposure to fewer antigens and to lower dosages than in the conventional animals, if we assume that greater dosages are required to elicit secondary responses. The early rapid rise of natural IgM anti-PGP suggests that the germfree animal may actually be responding to teichoic acid antigen under less antigenic competition than its conventional counterpart. This is in agreement with the observation of Kim and Watson (19), who have demonstrated a more rapid rate of antibody production during the "true" primary response in germfree piglets. Failure of IgG antibody production in both groups may be indicative of a prolongation of the primary response due to a low level antigenic stimulus. Once a level is reached, either by buildup of a constant low dosage or by artificial immunization, the host's secondary response is triggered. This conservation of the immune response seems quite plausible when one considers the large number of natural antigens constantly challenging the immune system. We are presently injecting young animals to determine how early this anamnestic-like response can be elicited and to determine if the response can be correlated with antigen dosage.

The observation that IgG anti-PGP antibodies, whether natural or immune, were restricted to the γ_1G subclass is interesting apart from the germfree-conventional comparison, since it has been shown that guinea pigs, artifically immunized with other antigens, produced antibodies in both subclasses (20-22).

Perhaps some aspect of the natural stimulus, such as type of antigen, dosage, or oral route, is responsible for this restriction of anti-PGP antibodies to the γG subclass.

The similarities observed between responses of both germfree and conventional animals to i.p. injection of teichoic acid suggests that they were equally capable of a secondary response when both dosage and route were adequate. This fact, in addition to the previously mentioned identical occurrence of γ₁G antibodies in the two groups and the high levels of natural antibody in the germfree group indicates that they probably do not differ in immunological competence.

Acknowledgement

We wish to acknowledge the work of Major Harry Rozmiarek during the initial stages of this investigation.

References

1. Miyakawa, M., *Ann. N. Y. Acad. Sci. 78:* 221 (1959).
2. Gordon, H. A., Bruckner-Kardoss, E., Staley, T. E., Wagner, M., and Wostmann, B. S., *Acta. Anat. 64:* 367 (1966).
3. Bealmear, P., and Wilson, R., *Anat. Rec. 154:* 261 (1966).
4. Thorbecke, G. J., Gordon, H. A., Wostmann, B. S., Wagner, M., and Reyniers, J. A., *J. Infect. Dis. 101:* 237 (1957).
5. Sell, S., *J. Immunol. 93:* 122 (1964).
6. Wostmann, B. S., Pleasants, J. R., Bealmear, P., and Kincade, P. W., *Immunol. 19:* 443 (1970).
7. Sell, S., and Fahey, J. L., *J. Immunol. 93:* 81 (1964).
8. Horowitz, R. E., Bauer, H., Paronetto, F., Abrams, G. D., Watkins, K. C., and Popper, H., *Am. J. Path. 44:* 747 (1964).
9. Michael, J. G., Whitby, J. L., and Landy, M., *J. Exp. Med. 115:* 131 (1962).
10. Bauer, H., Horowitz, R. E., Watkins, K. C., and Popper, H., *J. Am. Med. Assoc. 187:* 715 (1964).
11. Wostmann, B. S., and Olson, G. B., *J. Immunol. 92:* 41 (1964).
12. Olson, G. B., and Wostmann, B. S., *Fed. Proc. 24:* 381 (1965).
13. Sell, S., *J. Immunol. 95:* 300 (1965).
14. Landy, M., Whitby, J. L., Michael, J. G., Woods, M. W., and Newton, W. L., *Proc. Soc. Exp. Biol. Med. 109:* 352 (1962).
15. Nordin, A. A., *Proc. Soc. Exp. Biol. Med. 129:* 57 (1962).
16. Bosma, M. J., Makinodan, T., and Walburg, H. E., *J. Immunol. 99:* 420 (1967).
17. Decker, G. P., Chorpenning, F. W., and Frederick, G. T., *J. Immunol. 108:* 214 (1972).
18. Arnason, B. G., Salomon, J. C., and Grabar, P., *C. R. Acad. Sci. Paris 259:* 4882 (1964).
19. Kim, Y. B., and Watson, D. W., *Bacteriol. Proc. 21:* 75 (1968).
20. Sandberg, A. L., Oliviera, B., and Osler, A. G., *J. Immunol. 106:* 282 (1971).
21. Benacerraf, B., Ovary, Z., Bloch, K. J., and Franklin, E. C., *J. Exp. Med. 117:* 937 (1963).
22. Nussenweig, V., Green, I., Vassalli, P., and Benacerraf, B., *Immunol. 14:* 601 (1968).

VIRAL ENTERIC INFECTION AND LOCAL IgA ANTIBODY: STUDIES IN GERMFREE MICE THYMECTOMIZED AND/OR INFECTED WITH A MOUSE ADENOVIRUS

Kazuo Hashimoto, Nobuhiko Onishi, Takashi Tajiri,
Yasuo Okada, Ryozo Maeda, Yumiko Sugihara and *Shogo Sasaki*
Department of Microbiology, School of Medicine
Keio University, Tokyo, Japan

Introduction

We have developed an experimental model suitable for analyzing a viral enteric infection and its corresponding immune response. The biological combination utilized consisted of a mouse adenovirus, strain K87 as the infecting agent, and an inbred conventional mouse, strain DK1 as the host (1, 2). In mice orally challenged with this strain of virus, the agent grows in cells scattered throughout the epithelial layer of the mucous membrane of the small intestine and is excreted in the feces for 2 – 3 weeks without any symptoms of the disease. In mice which have experienced such an enteric infection, a strong "intestinal resistance" is established. This is a kind of local immunity and a defense mechanism of the first order against the infection after oral challenge.

Although the virus-neutralizing antibody increases in the serum during and after the course of the infection, the same antibody, elevated in the serum as the result of a vaccination with inactivated virus or passive transfer of serum containing antibody, gives no such intestinal resistance. In mice subjected to this type of enteric infection, the virus-neutralizing substance is found in the intestinal tract for several months thereafter, while this substance can not be detected in the intestinal tract of serum-transferred mice (3). The substance in the intestinal tract has now been recognized as an IgA antibody against the virus (4). On the other hand, virus-neutralizing antibody in the serum was predominantly associated with IgG.

These facts may indicate that the serum IgG antibody plays no role in the resistance, and that the intestinal IgA antibody possibly does have an important role in this process. The possible importance of the intestinal IgA antibody has been supported by some unpublished data which indicate the parallelism between the presence of intestinal IgA antibody and intestinal resistance. One experiment using cyclophosphamide and another observing the establishment of

501

reinfection a long time after the first infection give evidence supporting the role of IgA antibodies.

First of all, in the experiments using conventional mice, the intestinal IgA — though not specific to the virus — was detectable even when mice were uninfected with the virus. The reason for this might have been because the IgA was produced in response to antigens derived mainly from the normal bacterial flora, for it was undetectable in our germfree mice. Thus we felt that the IgA response might better be analyzed in germfree mice. Using such an experimental model, differentiation between the cell mediated immune response and the antibody response might possibly be accomplished. For this purpose, a neonatally thymectomized germfree mouse could be the most suitable model. No wasting syndrome occurs in germfree mice as it does in conventional mice prepared in this manner, and the inhibition of the cell mediated immune response could be differentiated from the antibody response.

Results

The present study was initiated to compare the process of the adenovirus-enteric infection and the appearance of antibodies in germfree ICR mice with those in conventional DK1 mice, which had been fairly well defined as previously reported (3, 4). When germfree mice, 4 — 6 weeks of age, were infected orally, the infection proceeded in the same manner as observed in the conventional animals. This is shown graphically by the shaded area in Figure 1 which designates the virus titer calculated by a tube method. Examination by the fluorescent antibody technique gave evidence that the sites of viral growth were limited to the cells in the epithelial layer of the mucous membrane, similar to that observed in conventional animals. Patterns of the appearance of

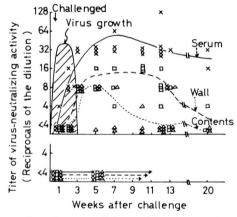

FIG. 1. The mouse adenovirus-neutralizing activity in germfree ICR mice after oral challenge of the virus. x = Serum, □ = Intestinal wall, △ = Intestinal contents.

virus-neutralizing antibodies in the serum, intestinal wall, and intestinal contents are also shown in Figure 1. The titers were slightly lower and the duration of their appearance shorter, but they were very similar to those of conventional mice. These facts indicated that a comparable response would take place in germfree mice as occurred in conventional animals. No noticeable symptoms were observed in these germfree mice.

Patterns of viral growth in the intestinal tract of the neonatally thymectomized germfree mice are illustrated in Figure 2 and compared with

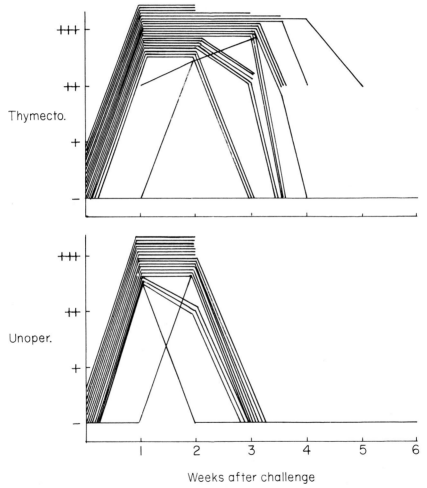

FIG. 2. Comparison of viral growth in thymectomized and in unoperated germfree ICR mice. +++, ++, + indicate respectively large, medium, and small amounts of the virus recovered in the feces.

those of the unoperated control mice. A clear prolonged growth of the virus could be observed with a few exceptions.

The neutralizing antibody and the immunoglobulins of these mice were examined. As shown in Figure 3, the appearance of neutralizing antibodies both

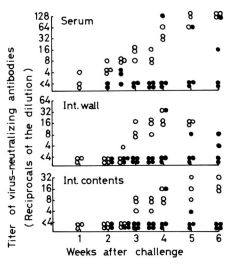

FIG. 3. Virus–neutralizing antibody in the serum, intestinal wall and intestinal contents of thymectomized (•) and unoperated (○) germfree ICR mice after oral challenge of the virus.

in the serum and in the intestinal tract (wall and contents) was retarded in the thymectomized mice. Considering the independence of the viral growth on the presence of the serum antibody from our former studies, it seems that the delayed appearance of the local neutralizing antibody in thymectomized mice prolonged the viral growth. Retardation of the appearance of IgA was also observed in thymectomized mice, thus supporting the fact that the neutralizing antibody belonged to the IgA class of immunoglobulin.

To confirm these observations, detailed examinations were performed in two representative, No. 4G1 and No. 4G2, thymectomized mice. Virus recovery was positive in No. 4G1 continually for 5 weeks after the virus challenge, while in No. 4G2 virus was present for only 2 weeks, as illustrated in Figure 4. Neutralizing antibodies in the intestinal tracts as well as in the sera measured after the animals were sacrificed were lower in No. 4G1 than in No. 4G2. Histopathological examinations of both mice were performed and the results were summarized in Table I. The complete absence of the thymus was definite in No. 4G1, but its partial presence was observed in No. 4G2. Neonatal thymectomy was unsuccessful in the latter. Also the absence of thymus-dependent lymphocytes was prominent in the spleen and in the mesenteric

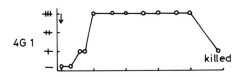

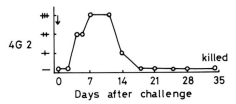

FIG. 4. Viral growth in 2 representatives of thymectomized germfree ICR mice after oral challenge of the virus. +++, ++, + indicate respectively large, medium, and small amounts of the virus recovered in the feces.

lymph nodes of the former, but not in the latter.

Conclusions

Neonatal thymectomy, which is known to affect the cell mediated immunity more than the humoral immunity in some cases, influenced the local antibody level as well as the circulating antibody level in our experimental model of the mouse-adenovirus and the mouse. We have failed to dissociate the cell mediated immune response from the antibody response in our system; however, observed facts may offer additional evidence to support the idea that intestinal resistance is acquired through IgA antibody produced locally in the intestinal tract.

TABLE I. Histopathological Examinations of Two Representatives of Thymectomized Germfree ICR Mice 5 Weeks After Oral Challenge of the Virus

Mouse No.	Presence of thymus	Mesenteric lymph nodes			Spleen		
		Thymus dependent lymphocytes	Germinal center	Plasma cells	Thymus dependent lymphocytes	Germinal center	Plasma cells
4G1	−	Greatly reduced	+	+	Greatly reduced	+	++
4G2	+ Partial	Normal numbers	+	±	Normal numbers	+	±

505

Acknowledgement

This research was partly supported by a grant (No. 69117) from The Naito Foundation, Japan.

References

1. Hashimoto, K., Sugiyama, T., and Sasaki, S., *Japan. J. Microbiol. 10:* 115 (1966).
2. Sugiyama, T., Hashimoto, K., and Sasaki, S., *Japan. J. Microbiol. 11:* 33 (1967).
3. Hashimoto, K., Sugiyama, T., Yoshikawa, M., and Sasaki, S., *Japan J. Microbiol. 14:* 381 (1970).
4. Hashimoto, K., Yoshikawa, M., Sugihara, Y., and Sasaki, S., *Japan. J. Microbiol. 15:* 499 (1971).

ASCORBIC ACID AND GLUCOCORTICOID LEVELS IN RELATION TO UNDERDEVELOPED LYMPHATIC TISSUE IN GERMFREE GUINEA PIGS

Otar V. Chakhava

Laboratory of Gnotobiology, The Gamaleya Institute for Epidemiology and Microbiology, Academy of Medical Sciences, Moscow, U.S.S.R.

Introduction

Germfree animals have their own phenotypic characteristics (1). It is well known that the germfree state causes very significant underdevelopment of the lymphatic tissue. In regard to the wet weight of adrenals, germfree guinea pigs showed conventional characteristics (2, 3).

This paper presents evidence for a secondary mechanism, resulting from

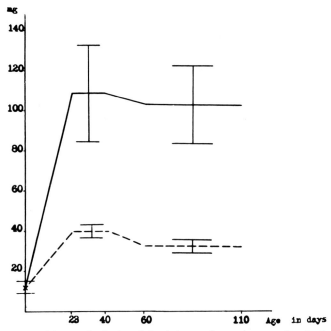

FIG. 1. Relative weights (mg) of adrenal glands in germfree and conventional guinea pigs of different ages. Newborn (x); Germfree (−); and Conventional (- - -) animals.

TABLE I. Plasma and Adrenal Ocsicorticosteroids (OCS) in Gnotobiotic and Conventional Guinea Pigs

Animals No. of animals		Gnotobiotic[a] 14[a]	Conventional 26	P
11-OCS in plasma μg%	Total	275 + 16	44 + 3	<0.001
	Free	153 + 18[b]	27 + 2	<0.001
	Bind	24 + 6[b]	17 + 3	0.25
11-OCS in adrenals, μg% per 100 mg		1.6 + 0.2	2.3 + 0.2	0.02

Animals No. of animals	Germfree 11	Conventional 11	
17-OCS in plasma, μg%	346 (260 − 432)	58 (44 − 72)	<0.001

[a]Germfree (10) and *Staphylococcus albus* monoflora (4) animals.
[b]Observed 5 germfree guinea pigs.

the absence of a normal microflora, that exerts an additional effect on the lymphatic tissue of germfree guinea pigs.

Materials and Methods

The following groups of animals of both sexes were used; germfree, monocontaminated, and conventional. These guinea pigs were up to 3½ months of age, and were fed a practical type diet, supplemented with vitamins (B-mix, A, D_2, mixed tocopherols, K_3), salt mixture, arginine, and cystine. Ascorbic acid autoclaved in bidistilled water was added to the drinking water: 10 to 30 mg per

TABLE II. Ascorbic Acid in Adrenals of Germfree, Monocontaminated and Conventional Guinea Pigs

Animals No. of animals	Germfree 10	Monocontaminated 8[a]	Conventional 8
Ascorbic acid μg per relative wt of adrenals	147 (105 − 189)	(131 (73 − 189)	34 (23 − 45)
Ascorbic acid, μg%	144 + 11	93 + 11	94 + 15

[a]Contaminated with *Staphylococcus albus* (4) or sporeforming bacillus (4).

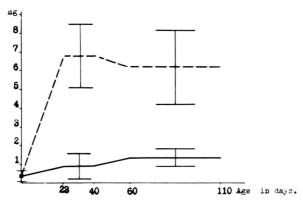

FIG. 2. Relative weights (mg) of ileocecal lymph nodes in germfree and conventional guinea pigs of different ages. Newborn (x); Germfree (−); and Conventional (- - -) animals.

guinea pig, depending on the age. Sterility test media were: fluid thioglycolate medium, a "C" medium, Sabouraud's broth, and blood agar.

Results

The relative wet weight of the adrenals in germfree guinea pigs reached the maximal level at the end of the third week after birth and remained unchanged during the entire period of observation (Fig. 1). Hypertrophy of the adrenals was accompanied with hyperproduction of glucocorticosteroids, as has been shown in collaboration with G. A. Shapiro and N. A. Oseretskovski. Levels of 11- and 17-ocsicorticosteroids in plasma of the germfree animals was approximately 6 times higher than in the conventional controls (Table I). It is important to note that an increase in the hormone concentration in the blood of the germfree

TABLE III. Globulin Containing (GC) Cells in Lymph Nodes and Spleen and the Relative Weight of These Organs in Germfree (GF) and Conventional (CV) Guinea Pigs

No. of GC cells in:		One field of vision[a]	Middle section	Relative weight (mg)
Ileocecal	GF	2.2 + 4.3	5 − 20	1.1 (0.8 − 1.3)
lymphnode	CV	29.2 + 6.0	200 − 500	6.4 (5.4 − 7.4)
Popliteal	GF	2 − 3	2 − 4	1.0 (0.7 − 1.3)
lymph node	CV	12.6 + 6.8	20 − 100	2.6 (2.3 − 2.8)
Spleen[b]	GF	28.9 + 4.9	100 − 200	147 (132 − 162)
	CV	22.4 + 2.5	200 − 400	143 (130 − 156)

[a] x 400.
[b] 21 germfree, 71 conventional animals.

guinea pigs was conditioned mainly by free physiologically active fractions.

The adrenals of the gnotobiotic guinea pigs contained more ascorbic acid than the conventional controls, although both groups of animals received equal amounts of the vitamin. These data obtained with V. Y. Vissarionova indicate that the germfree state favors the accumulation of vitamin C in the adrenals, thus providing hyperfunction of the adrenal cortex (Table II).

Humoller *et al.* (4) have established that ceruloplasmin is an oxidizer of ascorbic acid. Therefore, it may be suggested that the decreased level of this glycoprotein in the germfree guinea pig serum, as detected by disc-electrophoresis (5), stimulates the accumulation of ascorbic acid in the adrenals. In this regard, Jayle and Boisier (6) reported that cortisone acts as a depressor of the glycoprotein level in blood.

Underdevelopment of the lymphatic tissue in the germfree guinea pigs coincided in time with hypertrophy of the adrenals (compare Figs. 1 and 2). It should be noted, too, that the lymphatic tissue was underdeveloped in the lymph nodes but not in the spleen.

Indeed, the amount of globulin-containing cells detected by the Coon's method in spleens of germfree guinea pigs was decreased insignificantly (7), and the relative weights of this organ in gnotobiotic and conventional animals were equal (Table III). It is known that the spleen is less sensitive to the effect of cortisone than the lymph nodes (8).

Figure 3 shows the relative weights of the adrenals and lymph nodes of

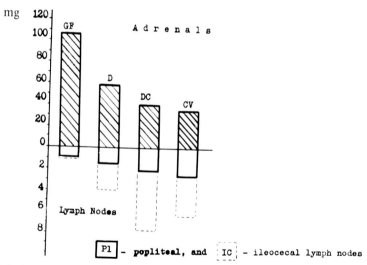

FIG. 3. Comparison of relative weights of adrenal glands and lymph nodes in germfree and conventional animals fed different diets. Germfree (GF); Conventional fed sterile diet (D); Conventional fed contaminated diet (DC); and Conventional fed regular diet (CV).

four groups of guinea pigs: germfree (GF), conventional (CV) on sterile diet, CV on diet contaminated with fecal flora of CV guinea pigs, and CV on regular diet.

In Figure 3 we see again the inversely proportional relationship between the weights of the adrenals and the lymph nodes. This relationship is in agreement with the findings of Berliner and Dougherty (9) that lymphocytes are biological inactivators of excessive amounts of cortisone.

Conclusions

These data support the hypothesis proposed by several investigators that decreased antigenic stimulation in germfree guinea pigs creates a vicious circle: underdeveloped lymphatic tissue → hypercorticism → hypoglycoproteinemia (ceruloplasmin) → increased deposition of ascorbic acid in adrenals → hypercorticism → secondary depression of underdeveloped lymphatic tissue.

References

1. Miyakawa, M., Wostmann, B. S., and Gordon, H. A., *Science 173:* 171 (1971).
2. Phillips, B. P., Wolfe, P. A., and Gordon, H. A., *Ann. N.Y. Acad. Sci. 78:* 183 (1959).
3. Pleasants, J. R., Reddy, B. S., Zimmerman, D. R., Bruckner-Kardoss, E., and Wostmann, B. S., *Aschr. Versuchstierk. 9:* 195 (1967).
4. Humoller, F. L., Holthans, J. M., and Mohler, D. J., in "V Intern. Biochem. Congr., Moscow, 1961," p. 14, Moscow (1962).
5. Chakhava, O. V., Chibisova, V. A., Shakhanina, K. L., and Zazenkina, T. I., *Bull. Exp. Biol. Med. 11:* 40 (1969).
6. Jayle, M. F., and Boisier, G., *Exp. Ann. Biochem. Med. 17:* 157 (1955).
7. Lebedev, K. A., Chakhava, O. V., and Zazenkina, T. L., *Zuzn. Microbiol., Epid. and Immun. 7:* 122 (1969).
8. Zdrodovski, P. F., "Problems of Infection, Immunity and Allergy," Moscow, (1969).
9. Berliner, M. L., and Dougherty, T. F., *J. Reticuloendothelial Soc. 5:* 567 (1968).

SECTION XI

PHYSIOLOGICAL EFFECTS OF GNOTOBIOTIC ENVIRONMENTS

TESTICULAR FUNCTIONS OF GERMFREE MICE

Tatsuji Nomura, Nakaaki Ohsawa, Kiyoko Kageyama,
Muneo Saito and *Yoshio Tajima*
Central Institute for Experimental Animals
Tokyo, Japan

Introduction

To better understand "germfree animals," their characteristics are being investigated from several different viewpoints. The results of one aspect of this work — the study of testicular function in mice through the endocrinological approach — are presented in this paper.

Materials and Methods

The animals used were as follows: conventional mice from ICR-JCL stock maintained in a barrier system, germfree mice of the same ICR-JCL stock maintained in vinyl isolators and gnotobiotic mice obtained by feeding bacterial cultures to the germfree mice. The pentacontaminated gnotobiotic parents were contaminated with *Escherichia coli, Staphylococcus sp., Lactobacillus sp., Streptococcus sp.* and *Bacteroides sp.* at the age of 4 weeks, and the 3 types of gnotobiotic F_1 mice and conventionalized F_1 mice were born of contaminated parents. Five animals of each age were used for each experiment.

The testicular endocrine function was measured by determining the testosterone content of the testes before and after stimulation with luteinizing hormone (LH).

The analysis of maximal activity of testosterone biosynthesis in mice testes was as follows. Under pentobarbital anesthesia, one unit of LH was given intravenously. Fifteen minutes later, both testes were removed and homogenized. The testicular homogenate was subjected to fluorometry for testosterone using red sulfuric acid fluorescence (1, 2). For the analysis of the resting levels, both testes are removed at 0 (zero) time without LH injection.

Table I gives the extraction and purification procedures for testosterone from the mouse testicular homogenate to be used in the fluorometric examinations.

Table II gives the procedure for the development of red sulfuric acid

**TABLE I. Preparation of Mouse Testes for Measuring Testosterone
by Fluorometric Examination**

1. Extraction
     2 ml of testis homogenate
     15 ml of CH_2Cl_2
2. Washing with alkali and distilled water
3. CH_2Cl_2 phase evaporated to dryness
4. Partition (2 times)
     5 ml of 70% CH_3OH
     2 ml of Petro. Ether
5. CH_3OH evaporated
6. Residual water phase extracted with 10 ml of CH_2Cl_2
7. CH_2Cl_2 phase evaporated to dryness
8. Thin layer chromatography (Benzene:Ethyl Acetate 1:1)
9. Testosterone fraction eluted with CH_3OH
10. CH_3OH evaporated to dryness
11. Extracts subjected to fluorometry (red sulfuric acid fluor).
     Excitation W.L. $-$ 595 mμ Emission W. L. $-$ 620 mμ

fluorescence of testosterone. Fluorescence characteristics were: activation maximum $-$ 595 mμ; fluorescence maximum $-$ 620 mμ. The minimum detectable amount of testosterone was 100 pg.

TABLE II. Procedure for Measuring Red Sulfuric Acid Fluorescence

1. 1 ml of sulfuric acid reagent (70% H_2SO_4, 30% C_2H_5OH) added to sample
2. Heated for 10 min. in a 60°C water bath
3. Cooled in an ice bath
4. Diluted with 2 ml of C_2H_5OH
5. Placed at room temperature for 30 min.
6. Red fluorescence determined in a spectrofluorophotometer

Activation	: maximum 595 mμ
Fluorescence	: maximum 620 mμ

Results

Figure 1 presents the results of investigations of testicular endocrine functions of conventional ICR-JCL mice from 3 to 13 weeks of age. The resting or base-line level of testosterone content in testis, shown as LH($-$), was low at 3 weeks, increased gradually through 8 weeks, reached a peak value at 9 weeks, and then decreased gradually.

The maximum capacity of testosterone biosynthesis after LH injection, shown as reserve function, LH($+$), started to increase rapidly at 5 weeks, reached the maximum level at 6 weeks and stayed at this level through 9 weeks of age. At 10 and 11 weeks of age, the reserve functions appear to decrease. The reason for this is not clear at present. After 12 weeks of age, the levels again started to

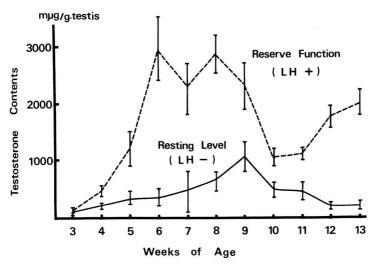

FIG. 1. Changes in testosterone content in conventional ICR mice testes according to age.

increase. The data clearly indicate that the time studies are very important for precise assessment of testicular endocrine functions.

Since the resting level of testosterone synthesis was low and tends to vary considerably, the reserve functions have been chosen as the parameter for the studies on testicular endocrine functions of germfree and gnotobiotic mice.

Figure 2 compares the testicular endocrine functions between the germfree

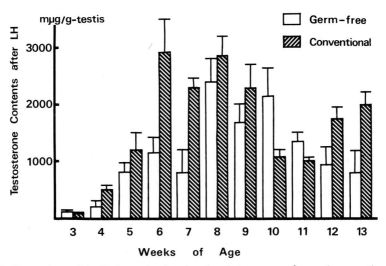

FIG. 2. Comparison of testicular endocrine function between germfree and conventional ICR mice.

and conventional mice. The activity of testosterone biosynthesis in conventional mice reached a maximum at 6 weeks of age and was maintained through 9 weeks of age. On the other hand, the activity in germfree mice reached a maximum at 8 weeks of age and stayed at the maximum through 10 weeks of age. There seemed to be no significant difference between the maximum levels of both groups. The data clearly indicate that the onset of increased activity of testosterone biosynthesis at puberty in germfree mice was about 2 weeks after that in conventional mice. The results suggest that there was some abnormality in the mechanism of sexual maturation of male germfree mice, when compared to conventional males.

The testicular endocrine functions in germfree mice were considerably lower than those in conventional mice after 12 weeks of age. The significance of the results remains to be clarified.

Figure 3 compares the testicular endocrine functions in germfree and gnotobiotic mice which were available in the laboratory. All mice were approximately 30 weeks of age, maintained in vinyl isolators and fed CL-2 diet sterilized at 126°C for 30 minutes. The testicular endocrine functions of germfree mice were very low (Fig. 3). Gnotobiotic parents which were pentacontaminated, also had low activity. On the other hand, three types of gnotobiotic F1 mice had high activity of testicular endocrine functions, which were probably not significantly different from those of conventionalized F1 mice.

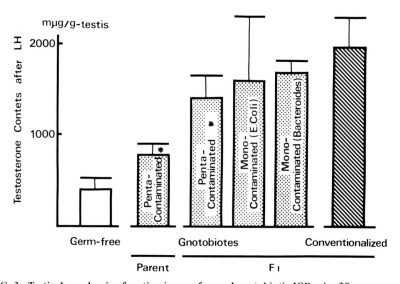

FIG. 3.   Testicular endocrine function in germfree and gnotobiotic ICR mice.**
   *E. coli, Staphylococcus sp., Lactobacillus sp., Streptococcus sp., and Bacteroides sp.
**All mice were reared in vinyl isolators and fed CL-2 diet sterilized at 126°C for 30 min.

Since the testicular endocrine functions of gnotobiotic parents were as low as those of germfree mice and the testicular endocrine functions of gnotobiotic F1 mice were as high as those of conventionalized mice, it might be possible to say that the time of contamination with bacteria plays an important role in determining the normal development of sexual functions in male mice.

Conclusions

Through comparative studies on the testicular endocrine functions of germfree, gnotobiotic and conventional mice, two different phenomena were observed.

First, the activity of testosterone biosynthesis under maximum stimulation of LH in germfree mice reached a maximum at 8 weeks of age and continued there through 10 weeks of age. This onset of increased activity was 2 weeks later than that in conventional mice.

Second, testicular endocrine functions of gnotobiotic F1 mice were higher than those of their parents and were similar to those of conventionalized mice. The functions in the gnotobiotic parents were low as in germfree mice.

Further investigations are needed to clarify the mechanisms of these phenomena.

References

1. Ohsawa, N., Kageyama, K., and Ibayashi, H., *Proc. Symposium on Chem. Physiol. and Pathol. 9:* (1969).
2. Ohsawa, N., Kageyama, K., and Ibayashi, H., *Excerpta Medica,* Third International Congress on Hormonal Steroids, No. 210, (1970).

STUDIES OF VASOPRESSIN IN GERMFREE
AND CONVENTIONAL RATS

Mitsuo Ukai and *Kenichi Kato*
Institute of Germfree Life Research and
Second Department of Surgery,
Nagoya University School of Medicine
Nagoya, Japan

Introduction

Vasopressin is one of the polypeptide hormones which is produced in the hypothalamus, transported to the posterior pituitary via the axons and stored there until stimulation. Once a stimulus arrives near a neurosecretory cell through the afferent fiber, the excited cell functions actively to release vasopressin into the systemic circulation from its part in the neurohypophysis. As soon as vasopressin enters the blood stream, it is widely distributed and inactivated by various organs such as the kidney and the liver. The inactivation by these organs is thought to be a result of enzymatic destruction of vasopressin. On the other hand, the rate of some metabolic process or hormone release has been known to be slower in the germfree animal (1). It would, therefore, be interesting to examine the question whether the release of vasopressin, which is physiologically important in the self-defense mechanism, or its inactivation can be modified by the complete absence of bacteria.

In the present study, the ability of the hypothalamic-neurohypophyseal system to secrete vasopressin and that of the liver to inactivate it were tested in adult germfree female rats of the Wistar strain as well as in their conventional counterparts. Blood and neurohypophyseal contents of vasopressin were used as parameters of the neurosecretory response to stress.

Methods

Within a few seconds after handling the animals, they were decapitated and their blood was collected into a heparinized centrifuge tube containing a minute amount of Trasylol, followed by removal of the pituitary. Blood was immediately precipitated with cold trichloroacetic acid (TCA) by the method of Moran *et al.* for bioassay of blood vasopressin (2). The posterior lobe was

521

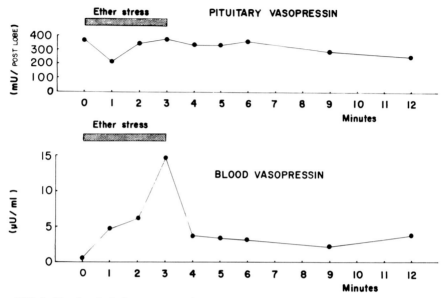

FIG. 1. Blood and pituitary vasopressin responses to a standard ether stress in conventional rats. Each dot represents the mean of the group of 4 rats.

separated from the anterior lobe, weighed, homogenized with 0.1 N acetic acid (1 ml/lobe) and precipitated by addition of dry TCA (50 mg/lobe). The ether-washed supernatant was diluted about 5,000 times with "injection solution" which consisted of 0.2% sodium chloride, 0.0285% acetic acid and 10^{-3} M disodium ethylenediaminetetraacetate.

In the course of bioassay procedures for blood and posterior pituitary vasopressin, 0.2 ml of injection solution which contained sample- or standard-vasopressin was alternatively infused into the femoral vein of ethanolized-hydrated rat. If the infused dose of vasopressin was more than 1 μU, there was an increase in urinary conductance and a decrease in urine flow (3). The former was used as an index for calculating the infused dose of vasopressin in relation to the dose of standard vasopressin.

Results

1) Vasopressin secretory response to a standard ether stress in conventional rats. The effect of a 3-minute ether stress on the content of blood and neurohypophyseal vasopressin was studied in 9 groups of 4 conventional rats (Fig. 1). One minute after exposure to ether, a considerable increase in blood vasopressin was observed in association with a remarkable decrease in neurohypophyseal vasopressin, which indicated that 140 mU or more of vasopressin was released within a minute. It would be worthy of note that the blood

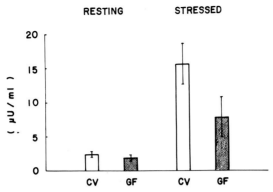

FIG. 2. Blood vasopressin levels before and 3 minutes after exposure to ether in germfree (GF) and conventional (CV) rats. M. ± S.E. in each group of 3 rats.

vasopressin showed the highest at the end of stress, when the neurohypophyseal content had already been restored to the prestimulatory level, which suggests a quick transport of vasopressin through the axons from the hypothalamus.

2) Blood and pituitary vasopressin content in germfree and conventional rats under resting and ether-stressed conditions. In the resting state of overnight 17-hour dehydration, the level of blood vasopressin in the germfree animal was 1.9 ± 0.3 μU/ml, which did not differ from that in the conventional animal, 2.4 ± 0.4 μU/ml (Fig. 2). Three minutes after exposure to ether, the blood vasopressin value in the germfree rat (7.8 ± 2.9 μU/ml) was significantly lower than that in the conventional rat (15.6 ± 3.0 μU/ml). It was also an unexpected matter that the neurohypophyseal content of vasopressin was less in the germfree rats who showed a smaller response of blood vasopressin (Fig. 3). These results suggest that there may be a difference in the secretory rate of vasopressin between the germfree and conventional stressed rats.

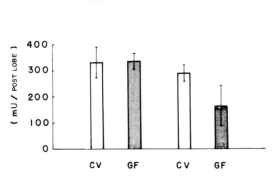

FIG. 3. Pituitary vasopressin content before and 3 minutes after exposure to ether in germfree and conventional rats. M. ± S.E. in each group of 3 rats.

TABLE I. Blood and Pituitary Vasopressin Content In A Germfree Rat with Intussuception (M. ± S.D.) and In Conventional Hydrated and Dehydrated Rats (M. ± S.E.)

	No. of rats	Status	Vasopressin in blood (μU/ml)	Vasopressin in pituitary (μU/post lobe)
GF	1	Ileus	6.4 + 1.7	162 + 49
CV	4	72h. Dehydration	8.1 + 1.2	271 + 35
CV	3	17h. Dehydration	2.4 + 0.4	332 + 58
CV	4	Hydration	0.9 + 0.2	490 + 53

3) Blood and pituitary vasopressin content in germfree and conventional rats under dehydrated conditions. The contents of vasopressin in the blood and neurohypophysis of a germfree rat with intussusception were compared to those in conventional rats with dehydration (Table I). The blood value in the germfree rat (6.4 ± 1.7 μU/ml) was close to that in the conventional rats (8.1 ± 1.2 μU/ml) with 3-day dehydration, while the neurohypophyseal content in the germfree rat was less than that in the dehydrated-conventional rats, who showed an increase in plasma osmolality (320 mOsm/kg) and a 17% loss of body weight in 3 days. Although plasma osmolality was not determined in this case, a considerable increase in blood vasopressin and a 51% decrease in pituitary vasopressin appear to be a result of plasma hyperosmolality due to dehydration (4) which suggests an important role for the osmoreceptors in the secretory mechanism of vasopressin in the germfree rat.

4) Inactivation of vasopressin by the liver of germfree and conventional rats. One mU lysine vasopressin was incubated with the supernatant of 10 mg liver homogenates from 4 germfree and 4 conventional rats. To determine the remaining dose of vasopressin in the medium at the end of incubation, the medium was passed through a CG-50 resin column and the purified eluate was bioassayed. As shown in Figure 4, more than 900 μU of vasopressin was

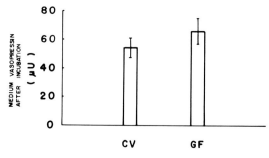

FIG. 4. Inactivation of lysine vasopressin (LVP) by the liver of germfree and conventional rats. 1 mU LVP was incubated with the supernatant of 10 mg liver homogenates of each group of 4 rats for 1 hour at 37°C. M. ± S.E.

inactivated by the 10 mg livers of the germfree and conventional rats within an hour at 37°C (5). The remaining dose of vasopressin appeared to be higher in the germfree rats, but the difference was not significant.

Conclusions

The secretory activity of vasopressin by the hypothalamic-neurohypophyseal system and the inactivating potency of vasopressin by the liver were studied in germfree and conventional adult rats.

In the resting state, there was no difference either in the blood vasopressin level or in the neurohypophyseal vasopressin content between the two groups of rats. However, ether stress revealed a difference in the pattern of the secretory response between the two groups. The blood vasopressin response was smaller in the germfree rats than in the conventional and the pituitary vasopressin content was less in the former 3 minutes after ether stress.

In a germfree rat with intussusception, an increase in blood vasopressin and a decrease in neurohypophyseal vasopressin were observed. These values resembled those in the dehydrated conventional rats, which suggests that the osmoreceptors may be involved in the control mechanism of vasopressin secretion in the germfree rat.

The liver of the germfree rat had a potency to inactivate vasopressin *in vitro*. No significant difference of such a potency was obtained between the two groups.

References

1. Wiech, N. L., Hamilton, J. G., and Miller, O. N., *J. Nutr. 93:*324 (1967).
2. Moran, W. H. Jr., Miltenberger, F. W., Shuayb, W. A., and Zimmermann, B., *Surgery 56:* 99 (1964).
3. Ukai, M., Moran, W. H. Jr., and Zimmermann, B., *Ann. Surg. 168:* 16 (1968).
4. Jones, C. W., and Pickering, B. T., *J. Physiol. (Lond.) 203:* 449 (1969).
5. Ginsburg, M., and Heller, H., *J. Endocr. 9:* 283 (1953).

RESPONSIVENESS OF JEJUNAL-ILEAL MESENTERY MICROVESSELS IN UNOPERATED AND CECECTOMIZED GERMFREE RATS TO SOME SMOOTH MUSCLE AGONISTS

S. Baez

Departments of Anesthesiology and Physiology,
Albert Einstein College of Medicine
Yeshiva University, New York, N. Y. 10461

and

G. Bruckner and *H. A. Gordon*
Department of Pharmacology
Medical Center, University of Kentucky
Lexington, Kentucky 40506, U.S.A.

Introduction

In contrast to the numerous, detailed reports of studies on diverse facets of the conditions and consequences of germfree life, those related to the cardiovascular and circulatory system remain scanty and incomplete. Although in an early report by Gordon *et al.* (1) it already was noted that, as compared to conventional controls, the weight of the heart, the total blood volume, and cardiac output of germfree rats were reduced, little further quantitative information can be found in the literature concerning the status of the circulatory systems in germfree life.

The evidence is accruing that the resistance and exchange segments of the circulation, i.e., the microvasculature and microcirculation, might be directly involved and/or possibly underlie many of the observed system-modifications in germfree animals. For example, the blood flow in organs that are normally in close contact with the flora was found reduced (1), and also a reduced oxygen partial pressure was reported in liver and subcutaneous tissues by Matsuzawa and Wilson (2). In addition, the slow compensatory rebound of systemic blood pressure after controlled bleeding, and the delayed achievement of maximal blood loss, first reported in anesthetized germfree rats by Zweifach *et al.* (3), and confirmed in similar experiments with unanesthetized animals by Heneghan (4) are indicative of a modified pattern of compensatory involvement of the resistance vessels of the microcirculatory system in gnotobiotic animals under

527

the stress of hemorrhagic hypotension. This view was substantiated by the recent report by Baez and Gordon (5) that germfree rats exhibit a significant decrease in vasomotor activity, and marked refractoriness of arterioles and precapillary sphincters to epinephrine, norepinephrine, and vasopressin, as compared to conventional control animals.

Our previously reported microcirculatory study was made in the mesentery immediately adjacent to the enlarged cecum, the mesoappendix. The cecum in the germfree rat has been found to accumulate active substances, some of which (α pigment) affect the tone of plain muscle as shown by Gordon *et al.* (6) and increase intestinal villus motility as reported by Gordon and Kokas (7). Therefore, we have repeated our microcirculatory study in the more distant ileal and jejunal regions of mesentery in non-operated germfree and conventional control rats. Also, because previous observations by Wostmann and Bruckner-Kardoss (8) show that cecectomy, early in the life of germfree rats, attenuated the depression of metabolic and cardiocirculatory variables in these animals, the present microcirculatory observation was extended to the jejunal-ileal micro-vasculature in cecectomized germfree and conventional rats.

Materials and Methods

All of the rats utilized in these experiments were of the Fischer 344 CD strain of both sexes. Eighteen of the twenty-one rats weighed 145-175 g, and the other 3 210-270 g. They were fed steam-sterilized L-462 diet (Lobund Institute, Notre Dame, Ind.) *ad libitum.* The germfree rats were maintained in flexible plastic isolators and the conventional controls in the open environment in the same air-conditioned room. The microscopic study of the microcirculation in jejunal-ileal mesentery was first made in a group of 10 unoperated (non-op.) rats, 4 conventional (Conv) and 6 germfree (GF). In another group of 12 animals, 5 Conv and 7 GF, a cecectomy (cec.) was performed in their respective environments, at 8 weeks of age, by procedures previously described (8). Microscopic observation and measurements, in approximately similar sites of jejunal-ileal mesentery, were carried out $6 - 8$ weeks later. The animals had free access to food and water until the day of the experiment. The germfree rats remained in the isolator until the injection of the anesthetic (Urethane 150 mg/100 g i.m.) required for surgery, at which time they were exposed to the laboratory environment. A segment (5-6 cm) of small intestine, upper ileum or jejunum, was exposed via a small (1 cm) supra-umbilical midline incision, and the attached mesentery gently spread over a suitable shaped lucite block. From the moment of exposure, the tissues were moistened by a continuous drip of mammalian Ringer's gelatin solution ($37.5 \pm 0.5°C$) of the following composition in mM/L: NaCl, 153.3; KCl, 5.63; CaCl$_2$, 2.16; gelatin (10 g/liter), adjusted to pH 7.4 with NaHCO$_3$. In order to prevent the usual slow ($0.05 - 0.1/15$ min) shift of perfusion fluid pH toward alkalinity, only a small amount (250 ml) of the fluid was placed in the supplying polysterene flask at a time, and the pH was periodically checked at 15 − 20 min intervals and adjusted if necessary. In all experiments, a 10 − 12 min period was allowed for the stabilization of the preparation before starting measurement and drug stimulation.

The smooth muscle stimulating drugs used were the catecholamine I-norepinephrine (levarterenol bitartrate, *Levophed*; Winthrop Laboratories, New York), diluted stock solution (100 μg/ml) with distilled water, and the polypeptides angiotensin amide (Hypertensin; CIBA Pharmaceutical Company, Summit, N.J.), and vasopressin (*Pitressin*; Parke, Davis & Co.) also diluted with distilled water in stock solution of 10 μg/ml and 1.0 IU/ml, respectively. Further dilutions of the stimulants were made as needed with warm Ringer's solution just before topical application in a 0.05 ml volume. For the observation and microphotography, we used a Leitz tri-ocular microscope equipped with x10, x20 U M metalurgical lenses, a x32 water immersion lense, and a x15 ocular. After observing the vasculature in the entire field, notations and micro-photography are made of: a) the presence or absence of vasomotion in precapillary vessels and sphincters, b) the pattern of blood flow through intervening capillaries, and c) the presence, if any, of foci of petechia. Only then was an arteriole (primary or secondary) target-selected for evaluating their responsiveness to the stimulants. For the vessel diameter measurements, we used the image-splitting method described by Baez (9). In brief, after three to four measurements of control vessel lumen size, the stimulating agent was delivered at 5 min intervals along the perfusing fluid in increasing doses, starting with doses not producing vessel response. This procedure was continued, separately with each drug, until a threshold concentration was achieved, which resulted in a 40 − 50 per cent decrease in arteriolar lumen.

All procedures were standardized as much as possible in all the experiments and the observations and measurements were completed within 50 − 60 min from the moment of the removal of the rats from their sterile environment.

Results

Observation at low (x100) power, in non-operated animals, showed a less frequent vasomotion and increased incidence of tortuosity prevailed in the mesentery microvasculature in germfree rats, distinguishing them from conventional control. This observation is consonant with previous findings in the mesoappendix of gnotobiotic rats. In contrast to this, no differences were found in the appearance of the microcirculation and microvasculature in jejunal-ileal mesentery of cecectomized germfree and conventional rats. In both types of animals, 4 − 6 weeks following operation, there was a brisk blood flow through

529

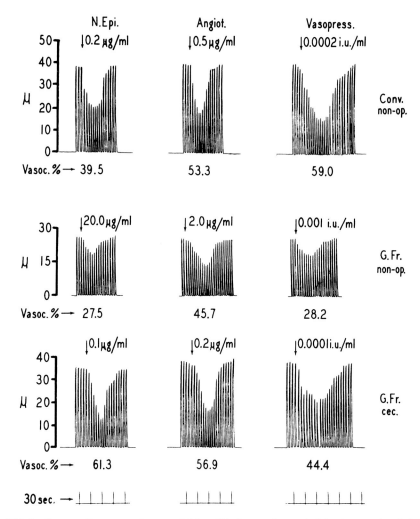

FIG. 1. Comparative responsiveness of jejunal-ileal mesentery arterioles to norepinephrine (N.Epi.), angiotensin (Angiot.) and vasopressin (Vasopress.) in rats. Conventional non-operated (Conv non-op) top, germfree non-operated (GF non-op) middle and germfree cecectomized (GF cec.) bottom. Each deflection is a measure of the vessel lumen, in micra, at the time. Greater concentrations of vasopressin (20-fold) norepinephrine (100-fold) and angiotensin (5-fold) were required to achieve threshold response in GF non-op rat when compared to Conv non-op control. Note that the minimal doses of all three drugs to achieve threshold response in GF cec. compares to Conv non-op Vasoc. % = arteriole lumen narrowing percent. Time marker (bottom) = 30 sec. intervals.

530

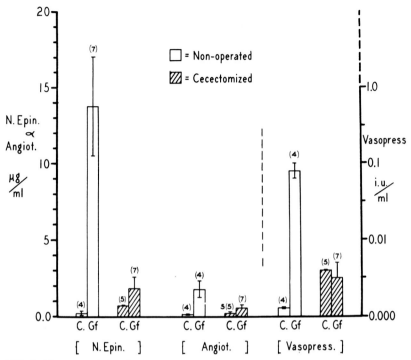

FIG. 2. Mean and S.E. of minimal doses of topical norepinephrine, angiotensin (μg/ml) vasopressin (IU/ml) required to achieve threshold (30 – 60%) arteriolar constriction in non-operated (white bars) and cecectomized (hatched bars), germfree (Gf, and conventional (C) rats. In parenthesis on top of bars = number of animals in each category.

the capillary bed and vasomotion was equally present in both groups of animals. No overtly tortuous vessels were found in the cecectomized germfree rats.

An example of typical experiments for determination of the relative level of responsiveness of smooth muscle in precapillary vessels to selected stimulants is shown in Figure 1. The protocol is a composite of separate experiments in rats: Conv non-op (top), GF non-op (middle) and GF cec. (bottom). The arteriole in Conv non-op rats readily constricted (39.5%) to the small (0.2 μg/ml) dose of topical norepinephrine (N.Epi.), whereas only a moderate (27.5%) arteriole lumen narrowing was obtained in GF non-op. rats with the much stronger (x100) solution (20.0 μg/ml) of the stimulant. In contrast to the latter, and in close similarity to the former, the target arteriole in GF cec. (4 wks. post-op) responded with a marked (61.3%) constriction to an even weaker (0.1 μg/ml) solution of the catecholamine. Although less marked, similar refractoriness of the arteriole in the GF cec. rat also vasoconstricted (56.9%) readily to the much weaker (0.2 μg/ml) solution of angiotensin. In the example

531

(Fig. 1)., a clear-cut difference in arteriolar responses to vasopressin was seen from one animal condition to another. The result of these and of all other experiments is presented in bar-graph form in Figure 2. The result of similar measurements in 4 Conv cec. rats is also included in the Figure. In spite of small variation from one animal to another, there was a clear-cut difference in the response of the vasculature of jejunal-ileal mesentery in each category group of animals, to the three vascular smooth muscle agonists employed. The doses (Mean and Standard Error, M & SE) of topical norepinephrine (N. Epi.), angiotensin (Angiot.) and vasopressin (Vasopress.) required to cause threshold response $(30 - 60\%$ vaso-constriction) in non-op. groups were: for N.Epi. (μg/ml, Conv 0.2 ± 0.16 and GF 13.75 ± 3.25 respectively; for Angiot. (μg/ml) Conv 0.1 ± 0.001 and GF 1.75 ± 0.30; and for Vasopress. (IU/ml), Conv 0.0012 ± 0.001 and GF 0.09 ± 0.001. Note, hatched bar-graphs in same Figure 2, that after cecectomy $(4 - 6$ weeks), the responsiveness of similar precapillary microvessels in jejunal-ileal mesentery compares well in the two groups of animals. The minimal doses (M & SE) producing vessel threshold responses were: for N.Epi. (μg/ml) Conv 0.32 ± 0.01, GF 1.78 ± 0.78; Angiot. (μg/ml) Conv 0.32 ± 0.066, GF 0.67 ± 0.30; and Vasopress. (IU/ml) Conv. 0.006 ± 0.000, GF 0.005 ± 0.002. Not included in Figure 2, there were 3 other GF rats weighing between $305 - 327$ gms at the time of examination of jejunal-ileal mesentery microvasculature. Two of these animals showed vascular responses to all three stimulants comparable to those in conventional controls, in spite of the presence of an enlarged cecum. In the third rat, hyporesponsiveness was found in the vasculature in ileal mesentery, but not in similar vessels of jejunal region.

Conclusions

The present data on the relative level of vascular responses to drugs, together with other observed and secured, by microphotography, micro-circulatory variables indicates: 1) Refractoriness of germfree rat microvasculature to the catecholamines epinephrine and norepinephrine and the polypeptide vasopressin is not a phenomenon restricted to mesocecal micro-circulation. It is also extended to the vasculature in the mesentery of jejunal-ileal region. 2) In contrast to our previous findings in mesoappendix vasculature, the arterioles of jejunal-ileal mesentery of GF rats were also hyporesponsive to topical angiotensin when compared to Conv control. 3) Surgical removal of the enlarged cecum reverses the modified microvascular characteristics of the germfree rat toward levels found in conventional control animals. These findings strongly suggest that the noted modification in microvascular smooth muscle responsiveness in germfree rodents might be related, in part, to the accumulated active substance in the enlarged cecum. The present data is too brief to account for the observed greater variability in the vessel responsiveness to the stimulant

532

used in jejunal-ileal mesentery than in the mesoappendix of the germfree rats.

Acknowledgements

Work supported in part by Grants HL-06736-11 and AM-14621-05, U.S. Public Health Service.

References

1. Gordon, H. A., Wostmann, B. S., and Bruckner-Kardoss, E., *Proc. Soc. Exp. Biol. Med. 114:* 301 (1963).
2. Matsuzawa, T., and Wilson, R., *Tohoku J. Exp. Med. 85:* 361 (1965).
3. Zweifach, B. W., Gordon, H. A., Wagner, M., and Reyniers, J. A., *J. Exp. Med. 107:* 437 (1958).
4. Heneghan, J. B., Peuler, M., Costrini, A., and Cohn, I. Jr., *Surg. Forum 21:* 232 (1970).
5. Baez, S., and Gordon, H. A., *J. Exp. Med. 134:* 846 (1971).
6. Gordon, H. A., Bruckner-Kardoss, E., Staley, T. E., Wagner, M., and Wostmann, B. S., *Acta Anat. 63:* 367 (1966).
7. Gordon, H. A., and Kokas, E., *Biochem. Pharmacol. 17:* 2333 (1968).
8. Wostmann, B. S., Bruckner-Kardoss, E., and Knight, P. L. Jr., *Proc. Soc. Exp. Biol. Med. 128:* 137 (1968).
9. Baez, S., *J. Appl. Physiol. 211:* 299 (1966).

EPINEPHRINE INHIBITORY SUBSTANCE IN INTESTINAL CONTENTS OF GERMFREE RATS

Geza G. Bruckner
Department of Pharmacology
College of Medicine
University of Kentucky
Lexington, Kentucky 40506, U.S.A.

Introduction

It has been found that germfree (GF) rats display reduced cardiac output and O_2 consumption in comparison to conventional (CONV) rats, but the surgical removal of the cecum early in GF life largely eliminates these anomalies (1). Recently it has been shown that GF rats show marked reduction in 1-epinephrine (EPI) sensitivity of mesocecal arterioles in comparison to CONV rats (2) and that GF cecal supernatant topically applied to mesocecal arterioles of CONV rats is highly EPI inhibitory as contrasted with CONV cecal supernatants (3).

The purpose of this study was to establish in GF and CONV rats: a) the distribution of the EPI inhibitory substance in the intestinal tract, including the remaining cecal segment of cecectomized rats (cecal button), and b) whether the terminal eluate from cecal supernatants applied on a weak cation exchange resin retain EPI inhibition.

Methods

The contents of the small intestine, cecum, large intestine, and of the cecal button of GF and CONV (unoperated and cecectomized at 2 months), 4 month old CDF male rats (Charles River Breeding Labs, Wilmington, Mass.) fed L-462 (8) diet were harvested, centrifuged (40,000 g 30 min). The supernatants were diluted 1:1 with distilled H_2O, Millipore filtered (0.45 μ), adjusted to pH 7.4 and 300 mOsm, and stored at $-20°C$. Primary fractionation of the cecal and button supernatants was carried out by elution with 0.25 N NaOH after application to a cation-resin column (Biorex 70, Bio Rad Labs., Richmond, Calif.). This permitted the separation of the supernatants into effluents which consisted of primarily negatively charged ("Initial Pool") and more positively charged ("Terminal Pool," TP) material. After reconstitution to the original volumes by flash evaporation at 37°C, all samples were adjusted to pH 7.4 and 300 mOsm.

Anesthetized (urethane, 1.5 g/kg body weight, subcutaneously) CONV male rats of the Holtzmann strain (180 – 240 g, 2 months old, fed Purina 5010C diet) were prepared by standard procedures for *in vivo* microscopic observation of the vascular bed of the mesocecal membrane (4, 5). Metarterioles were selected which yielded approx. 17 – 40% constriction (standard constriction) upon topically applied EPI (0.01 – 1.0 μg/ml) in Krebs-Henseleit solution with 1% gelatin added. The same metarterioles were then used for testing the effect of topical pretreatment with intestinal supernatants and purified fractions, which preceded by 60 – 90 sec the application of graded concentrations of EPI which caused constriction similar to the untreated control. Intestinal supernatants, purified fractions, and EPI were uniformly applied in 0.05 ml volumes.

Basal diameter of the vessels (10 – 40 μ) was determined during constant drip irrigation (1.0 ml/min) of the preparation with Krebs-Henseleit (warmed to 37.5°C). Flow was then interrupted for the pretreatment period (60 – 90 sec) (diameter recordings were continued) and then subsequently resumed for EPI standard constriction determinations (Fig. 1). After each pretreatment the untreated standard constriction was again verified with EPI before further tests were carried out.

Results

In the first series (Table I), metarterioles not pretreated (control) required an average of 0.4 (μg/ml) of EPI to yield a standard constriction of 20 – 40% (45 observations). As indicated earlier, the dosage for control standard constriction was obtained with concentrations of EPI in the range of 0.01 – 1.0 μg/ml. This method of bioassay requires that, for each material tested, the control value must be previously determined because the EPI sensitivity of CONV rat mesocecal arterioles ranges between 0.01 and 1.0 μg/ml (occasionally greater deviations occur) to result in the desired 17 – 40% constriction.

Table I indicates the results obtained by pretreatment with various intestinal supernatants (GF and CONV, non-operated "NON-OP," and cecectomized "CEC") from small intestine (SIS), cecum (CS), large intestine (LIS), and cecal button (BUS). These results indicate that the EPI inhibitory substance is found in both GF NON-OP and CEC rats in similar concentrations along the entire intestinal tract. CONV NON-OP or CEC rats, however, appear to have only approximately 1/8 the concentration of the EPI inhibitory substance in samples which are comparable to the GF rats.

Table II shows the results obtained from cecal and button supernatants which have been purified via cationic chromatography. The control value in this

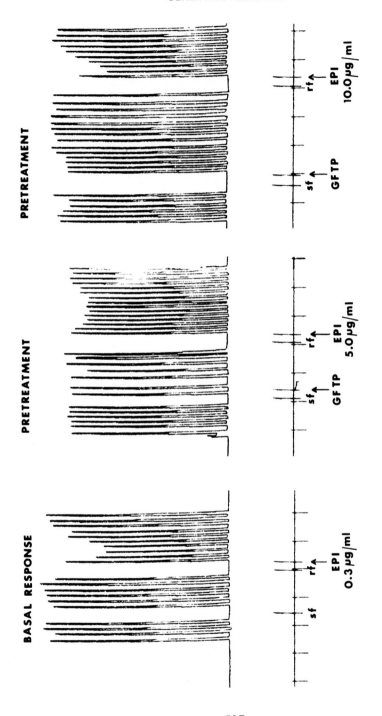

FIG. 1. Effect of germfree terminal pool (GFTP) on mesocecal arteriole (*in vivo*).

TABLE I. Dose-Response Relationships Between Topically Applied 1-Epinephrine and Constriction of Conventional Rat Mesocecal Arterioles; Untreated or Topically Pretreated with Various GF and CONV (non-operated or cecectomized) Intestinal Supernatants

DONORS	Untreated (n:45)		Pretreated with supernatants (samples dil. 1:1) from:							
	M	Range	SIS		CS		BUS		LIS	
(n: 3 − 5)	0.4	0.1 − 1.0	M	Range	M	Range	M	Range	M	Range
GF Non-Op			16	5 − 20	16	10 − 30		−	15	10 − 20
GF Cec			23	20 − 30		−	24	15 − 30	14	10 − 20
Conv Non-Op			2	1 − 5	2	2 − 2		−		N.D.
Conv Cec			2	2 − 2		−	3	1 − 5	3	1 − 5

n: No. of Observations. GF Non-Op: Germfree non-operated; GF CEC: Germfree cecectomized; SIS: Small intestine supernatant; C.S.: cecal supernatant; BUS: Button supernatant; LIS: Large intestine supernatant; N.D.: Not Determined.

series averaged 0.2 μg/ml EPI (17 observations), showing a more EPI sensitive test group than in the previous series. The results of the purified fractions, however, show the same overall 8 fold increase in EPI inhibition of GF NON-OP or CEC over CONV NON-OP or CEC. Two methods of calculating the results were carried out to detect any discrepancies which might occur by applying each rat as its own control. As Table III indicates, only slight variation occurs between averaging control and pretreatment values as μg/ml EPI or by equating the pretreatment value against its own control and expressing this as per cent

TABLE II. Dose-Response Relationships Between 1-Epinephrine and Conv Rat Mesocecal Arteriole Constriction, Untreated or Pretreated with Cecal (CS) or Button (BUS) Terminal Pools (TP)

DONORS	Untreated (n: 17)		Pretreated with TP (samples original concentration) from			
	M	Range	CSTP		BUSTP	
(n: 3 − 5)	0.2	.04 − .3	M	Range	M	Range
GF Non-Op			7.6	3.0 − 10.0		
GF Cec				−	3.5	3.0 − 5.0
Conv Non-Op			0.4	0.1 − 0.5		−
Conv Cec				−	0.3	0.1 − 0.5

Key: Same as Table I.

TABLE III. Significance of Differences* Found in Mesocecal Preparations, Pretreated or Untreated with Various "Terminal Pools"

I. Values expressed in μg/ml EPI required to cause 17 − 39% metarteriole constriction

	n	M	Range	P
GF Non-Op CSTP	5	7.6	3.00 − 10.0	.017
Conv. Non-Op CSTP	3	0.4	0.1 − 0.5	
GF Cec BUSTP	4	3.5	3.0 − 5.0	.015
Conv Cec BUSTP	4	0.3	0.1 − 0.5	
Conv Cec BUSTP	4	0.3	0.1 − 0.5	NS**
Untreated Control	17	0.2	0.04 − 0.3	

II. Values expressed as % increase of EPI dose over untreated control dose required to cause 17 - 39% constriction

	n	M x 100	Range x 100	P
GF Non-Op CSTP	5	56.0	17.0 − 100.0	.017
Conv Non-Op CSTP	3	1.5	1.0 − 1.7	
GF Cec BUSTP	4	52.5	10.0 − 75.0	.015
Conv Cec BUSTP	4	1.4	1.0 − 1.7	

*Calculated by the method of Wilcoxant's as described by Mann and Whitney (7).
**Non significant

increase of EPI required to produce the desired 17 − 39% constriction.

Discussion and Conclusions

These findings suggest that the signs of EPI refractoriness which were observed in the mesenteric microvessels of GF rats may be linked to the presence of EPI inhibitory substance in the intestines of these hosts. The TP obtained from GF rat cecal supernatants has been found to contain "α-pigment" after passage through columns of anion exchange resin; this pigment was found to cause reduced EPI sensitivity of vascular and intestinal muscles (6). From this standpoint, one may speculate that the EPI inhibitory substance found by the mesocecal bioassay method in this experiment is the same as α-pigment, and that it is not only found in the cecal supernatant of GF rats, but also along the entire intestinal tract. The fact that cecectomy of germfree rats brings cardiac output and O_2 consumption values within the range of CONV can possibly be attributed to a reduction of circulating EPI inhibitory substance through the elimination of the "main reservoir" available for absorption and not to a reduction of the inhibitory substance concentration. In this sense, α-pigment may be a link to understanding the anomalies of the GF rat regarding the previously stated parameters.

References

1. Wostmann, B. S., Bruckner-Kardoss, E., and Knight, P. L. Jr., *Proc. Soc. Exp. Biol. Med. 128:* 137 (1968).
2. Baez, S., and Gordon, H. A., *J. Exp. Med. 134:* 846 (1971).
3. Bruckner, G. G., Abstract 9th Annual Meeting of the Association for Gnotobiotics, Notre Dame, Ind., U.S.A. (1970).
4. Zweifach, B. W., and Metz, D. B., *Ergeb. Anat. Entwicklungsgesch 35:* 181 (1956).
5. Baez, S., *J. Appl. Physiol. 211:* 299 (1966).
6. Gordon, H. A., and Kokas, E., *Biochem. Pharmacol. 17:* 2333 (1968).
7. Mann, H. B., and Whitney, D. R., *Ann. Math. Statist. 18:* 50 (1947).
8. Wostmann, B. S., *Ann. N.Y. Acad. Sci. 78:* 175 (1959).

HEMORRHAGIC SHOCK IN CECECTOMIZED GERMFREE RATS

James B. Heneghan
Departments of Surgery and Physiology
Louisiana State University Medical Center
New Orleans, Louisiana 70112, U.S.A.

Introduction

Previous experimentation in our laboratory (1) and in other laboratories (2, 3) has tended to minimize the importance of the microbial flora in the shock syndrome, since both germfree (GF) and conventional (CONV) rats were equally susceptible to hemorrhagic shock. However, compared to the CONV animal, the GF rat's cecum contains increased quantities of vasoactive substances (4). The purpose of this investigation was to determine the influence of the GF rodent's enlarged cecum on its response to hemorrhagic shock.

Materials and Methods

Gnotobiotic Techniques. All of the rats utilized in these experiments were L.S.U. Strain Fischer 344 CDF rats (Charles River Breeding Laboratories, Wilmington, Mass.) of both sexes which weighed between *250* to *350* g at 14 weeks of age. These rats were reared in clear plastic cages on corn cob bedding and were fed *ad libitum* water and diet, Purina 5010-C (Ralston Purina Co., St. Louis, Mo.) which was sterilized for 25 minutes at 121°C in standard sterilizing cylinders. GF animals were maintained in flexible film isolators and the CONV animals were maintained in the open laboratory. Standard sterility testing was performed every two weeks by using the techniques outlined by Wagner (5).

Experimental Techniques. Ten litters with 8 GF rats each were divided randomly into 4 groups: 2 CONV control, 2 GF control, 2 CONV cecectomized, and 2 GF cecectomized. Littermates were conventionalized (exposed to a "normal" flora) at 4 weeks of age, cecectomized at 7 weeks, and bled at 14 weeks.

Under open drop anesthesia, methoxyflurane, the rat's femoral arteries were cannulated with polyethylene tubing. The rats were then heparinized, placed in a restraining cage, and allowed to awaken. Blood pressure and heart rate were measured with a low volume displacement transducer and recorded on a polygraph. Transducer cables were passed through a rubber stopper in the wall of the isolator; this provided for transmission of electrical signals through an air-tight connection between the transducer inside the isolator and the recorder which was outside. Blood pressure was maintained, at 60 mm Hg for 1 hr and at 50 mm Hg for 3 hrs, by adjusting the height of the burette reservoir.

Results

The results of these experiments are summarized in Table I. Nineteen out of 20 GF cecectomized rats survived following exposure to graded hypovolemia, whereas an average of only 10 out of 20 rats survived in the other 3 experimental categories. This shock model (60 mm Hg for 1 hr and 50 mm Hg for 3 hrs) was chosen because it produced a 50% survival in CONV control rats and thus positive or negative changes could be observed.

The minor differences in the per cent body weight shed between the 4 experimental categories indicated that each group was subjected to approximately the same hemorrhagic insult, i.e., each group lost similar quantities of blood.

As hypovolemia progressed, the rat's ability to compensate by decreasing the relative size of its vascular system diminished and a point was reached when the animal had lost the maximum amount of blood. The time that this occurred measured from the time blood loss began was another parameter which indicated the cecectomized GF rat's increased resistance to hypovolemia. These animals were still able to compensate an average of 72 minutes longer than the other 3 experimental categories.

Finally, after shedding the maximum volume of blood, the relative size of the animal's vascular system began to increase and blood was taken back from the reservoir in order to maintain blood pressure at the given level. Again the cecectomized GF rats required only 3% of their shed blood, whereas the other 3 groups required 3 to 5 times as much. This again emphasized the increased

TABLE I. Response of Littermate Rats with Graded Hemorrhage to Blood Pressures of 60 mm Hg for 1 hr and 50 mm Hg for 3 hrs

Category	Survival No. Survived/ No. Shocked	% Body Wt. Shed	Time Maximum Blood Loss (min)	% Shed Blood Retaken
CONV Control	9/20	2.7 + 0.7*	115 + 38*	15 + 3*
GF Control	13/20	2.4 + 0.3	135 + 27	10 + 2
CONV Cecectomized	6/20	2.8 + 0.6	117 + 58	12 + 5
GF Cecectomized	19/20	2.2 + 0.4	194 + 32	3 + 1

*Mean + standard deviation

ability of cecectomized GF rats to resist hemorrhagic shock.

Possible explanations of the protective effect of cecectomy are as follows. First, as shown by Gordon *et al.* (4), the presence of a 5 times greater quantity of bioactive and vasoactive substances in the GF rat cecum may cause certain changes observed in basic cardiovascular parameters of normal GF rats: decreased cardiac output, decreased blood volume, decreased heart weight and increased hemoconcentration and blood viscosity. In addition, Bruckner (6) has shown that the mesenteric microvessels of GF rats are much more refractory to epinephrine than those of CONV rats. These changes, which return to more normal values following cecectomy, tend to make the normal intact GF rat more susceptible to hemorrhagic shock. Second, the enlarged cecum of the GF rat represents a substantial increase in the size of the splanchnic vascular bed into which blood can pool following reinfusion. Indeed petechial hemorrhage in the mucosa as well as frank hemorrhage into the gut lumen have been common findings at necropsy.

Summary and Conclusions

To summarize, the increased resistance of cecectomized GF rats to hemorrhagic shock indicates that the enlarged cecum of GF rodents tends to offset the advantages of the absence of an intestinal flora. This is the first investigation to show an increased resistance to hemorrhagic shock in GF animals and tends to reemphasize the importance of the flora in the shock syndrome. The mechanisms underlying this increased resistance may be related to the quantities of bioactive substances in the intestinal tract or the size of the vascular bed in the GF rat's cecum.

Thus the cecectomized GF rat has been shown to be significantly resistant to hemorrhagic shock and will be a good model to study further the effects of the flora in hemorrhagic shock.

Acknowledgements

This research was supported in part by U.S.P.H.S. Grant RR-00272, from Animal Resources Branch, Division of Research Resources, National Institutes of Health.

The technical assistance of Martin Peuler, while a medical student at L.S.U., was greatly appreciated.

References

1. Heneghan, J. B., in "Advances in Germfree Research and Gnotobiology," (M. Miyakawa and T. D. Luckey, eds.), Chemical Rubber Co. Press, Cleveland, Ohio, p. 166, (1968).
2. Zweifach, B. W., Gordon, H. A., Wagner, M., and Reyniers, J. A., *J. Exp. Med. 107:* 437 (1958).

3. McNulty, W. P. Jr., and Linares, R., *Amer. J. Physiol. 198:* 141 (1960).
4. Gordon, H. A., *Ann. N.Y. Acad. Sci. 147:* 83 (1967).
5. Wagner, M., *Ann. N.Y. Acad. Sci. 78:* 89 (1959).
6. Bruckner, G., in "Germfree Research: Biological Effect of Gnotobiotic Environments," (J. B. Heneghan, ed.), Academic Press, New York, p. 535, (1973).

CECAL REDUCTION IN "GNOTOXENIC" RATS

Edmond Sacquet, Michel Lachkar and *Catherine Mathis*
Centre National de la Recherche Scientifique
71 — Gif-Sur-Yvette, France

and

Pierre Raibaud
Centre National de la Recherche Zootechnique
I.N.R.A.
78 — Jouy-en-Josas, France

Introduction

Terminology. The terms coined by Raibaud *et al.* (1) are used in this paper. The germfree animal is called "**axenic.**" The animal which is associated with a known bacteria or with several known bacteria is called "**gnotoxenic.**" Conventional animal is called "**polyxenic.**"

Two kinds of polyxenic animals are distinguished: the "**holoxenic**" animal is the animal which has never been deprived of the microbial heritage received from its parents; the "**heteroxenic**" animal is the animal which has not been allowed to receive this microbial heritage (for instance, which was born through Cesarean section), and which is protected from any contact with the holoxenic animals (for instance, SPF animals).

Rationale. Cecum enlargement is one of the dominant features in axenic rodents. There are many reasons to study this anomaly: 1) It is a defect and one of the main causes of death (2, 3); 2) in spite of many studies, the way microbial flora prevents cecal enlargment in polyxenic rodents is partly unknown; 3) it has several important consequences: reduced basal metabolism and blood circulation in axenic rats have been proven to be related to cecal enlargement (4); 4) it is a source of difficulties in the use of axenic rodents in experimental work: cecal enlargement contributes to make axenic rodents different from their polyxenic homologues; comparison between axenic and polyxenic rodents is therefore difficult, and the understanding of experimental data is sometimes very uncertain; 5) it does not take place in all axenic animal species, namely pigs and birds; it, therefore, often makes impossible generalization of what is observed in rodents to other animal species.

In order to palliate the difficulties caused by cecal enlargement, two possibilities seem to be offered (2, 3). One possibility is to surgically remove the large cecum of axenic rodents (5) and to use these cecectomized rats. The other possibility is to associate the germfree rodents with a minimal bacterial flora which reduces the large cecum of axenic rodents to polyxenic values but which has no action upon the metabolic or physiologic character which is under study.

Cecectomy in axenic rats was found to restore blood circulation and basal metabolism to polyxenic values (4). However this surgical procedure was also found to modify two important physiological features of axenic rats: the speed of gastrointestinal transit and the speed of the renewal of intestinal epithelium (6, 8). These modifications induced by cecectomy were observed to be very different from the actions exerted by gastrointestinal flora upon these two features, actions which were observed when axenic and holoxenic rats were compared (7, 8).

In the holoxenic rat as in mice (9, 10), intestinal flora was observed to increase the small intestinal epithelium renewal, at all the levels of this organ. In axenic rats, cecectomy induced an alteration of mitotic activity at the level of lieberkühn glands. Mitosis became irregular and as a result, the length of the villi became very variable from one villus to the other, or from one side to the other side of the same villus. There was an increase of the speed of migration at the level of duodenum, no modification at the level of jejunum and a decrease at the level of ileum.

In holoxenic rats, as in mice (11), the presence of intestinal flora increased the speed of gastrointestinal transit at all the levels of the gastrointestinal tract (7). Cecectomy did not increase the slow stomach transit of axenic rats; it increased the transit speed at the level of the small intestine to values which were apparently nearer the values observed in holoxenic rats; it increased the speed of transit in the distal part of the digestive tract to values which were higher than the values observed in holoxenic rats.

The conclusions of these studies were that cecectomy had to be used with discrimination according to the objectives of the experimenter, and that the study of the reduction of cecal enlargement by a minimal number of bacterial strains should be undertaken. Our purpose is to describe the first results obtained in this study.

Experimental animals. The axenic and gnotoxenic rats were maintained in Trexler type isolators. The holoxenic rats were "open room animals."

The rats used in this study were random bred rats, received from Carworth Farm (C.F. rats) fifteen years ago, and inbred Fischer rats originated from Charles River Breeding Laboratories. Only males which weighed more than 150 g and less than 250 g were used.

Diets. Two diets were used: a commercial diet produced by Duquesne Purina (D.P. diet) and a semi-synthetic diet (S.N. diet). The ponderal composition of S.N. diet was as follows: casein 220, cornstarch 580, cellulose powder 50, corn oil 90, mineral mixture and vitamins 50, and water 200. The diet was steam-sterilized at 120°C for 20 min.

Bacteriological procedures. The procedures used to isolate bacteria from the gastrointestinal contents of polyxenic or gnotoxenic rats were according to Raibaud *et al.* (12).

The strains were established in the digestive tract of rats by stomach tubing and by rectum injection of broth cultures. When several bacterial strains had to be established in the gastrointestinal tract, the strains were cultivated separately, and the different cultures were mixed just before injection into rats. The rats were sacrificed at 9 a.m., 8 to 15 days later, for determination of cecal weights.

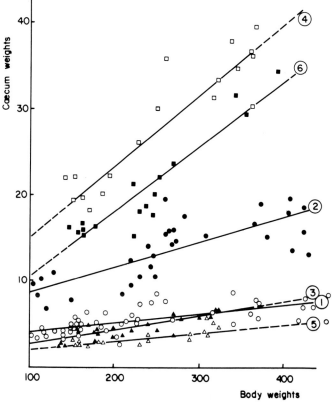

FIG. 1. Cecal weights expressed as a function of body weight. Ordinate: Cecal weight g. Abscissa: body weight g. Legend: 1: ○ C.F. holoxenic rats fed on D. P. diet; 2: ● C.F. axenic rats fed on D.P. diet; 3: ▲ Fischer holoxenic rats fed on D.P. diet; 4: □ Fischer axenic rats fed on D.P. diet; 5: △ Fischer holoxenic rats fed on S.N. diet; 6: ■ Fischer axenic rats fed on S.N. diet.

Statistical Methods. The results are expressed by the arithmetic mean (m), the standard deviation of the mean (SDM). Comparison between the means were made according to the t Student test.

Results

Figure 1 represents the values of cecal weight expressed as a function of body weights in axenic and holoxenic C.F. and Fischer rats. The C. F. rats were fed on D.P. diet. The Fischer rats were fed, one group on D.P. diet, another group on S.N. diet. From this Figure, one can conclude that: 1) within the limits of body weights observed, the relation between cecal weight and body weight is roughly linear; 2) the cecum in axenic Fischer rats is much heavier than in C.F. rats; 3) the cecal weight in Fischer rats which are fed on D.P. diet is heavier than when these rats are fed on S.N. diet. From these data, it was concluded that Fischer rats were better experimental animals to study the action of bacterial strains upon cecal weights.

Table I gives a nomenclature of the different bacterial strains which were isolated from holoxenic rats and which were used alone or in various combinations to seed the gastrointestinal tract of axenic Fischer rats.

Both S.N. and D.P. diets were used in these experiments because several bacteria [3, 4, 17, 18, 19, 21, 29] failed to establish themselves in the axenic rats fed on S.N. diet but proliferated in the digestive tract of rats fed on D.P. diet. Both diets were also used in order to appreciate a possible role of the composition of diet on the ability of bacteria to reduce cecum.

The action of the different bacterial strains upon cecal weight is presented

TABLE I. Numbering of Bacterial Strains and of a Strain of Yeast Used to Obtain "Gnotoxenic" Rats

Microbial strains	Number
Veillonella	1
Streptococcus (strict anaerobe)	2 to 9
Streptococcus (facultative anaerobe)	10 to 13
Sphaerophorus	14
Butyribacterium	15
Catenabacterium	16 to 20
Acuformis	11
Ramibacterium	22 and 23
Fusiformis	24
Endosporus	25
Clostridium bifermentans	26
Clostridium (facultative anaerobe)	27
Plectridium	28 and 29
Welchia perfringens	30

TABLE II. Cecal Weights in g per 100 g Body Weight in Gnotoxenic Fischer Rats Fed on Two Different Diets. M: Mean; SDM: Standard Deviation of the Mean; N: Number of Rats

Bacterial strains n°	S.N. diet			D.P. diet		
	M	SDM	n	M	SDM	n
2	11.7	0.25	4	9.1		1
4	6.0	0.31	4			
6	9.0	0.88	4			
7	16.5	0.69	3	14.4		1
14				8.2	0.53	7
15	6.3	0.24	5	10.0	0.40	5
16				13.6		1
17	8.5	0.37	6	11.8		2
19	10.0	0.21	4	16.1		1
22	9.0	0.50	4	12.3		2
23				8.9		3
24				12.9		1
26				7.5	0.25	8
27	9.0	0.66	4			
28				11.0		2
2+17	5.7	0.29	6	8.4	0.25	6
7+6	8.1	0.15	6			
14+15				8.7		1
14+26				7.8		1
14+28				7.8		2
15+26				6.4		1
15+28	5.9	0.60	5	8.5		1
26+28				7.5		1
14+15+26				7.4		1
14+15+28	4.5	0.30	5	6.4		1
14+26+28				6.6		1
15+26+28				5.4	0.28	6
2+6+7+17	5.0	0.30	8			
14+15+26+28	2.9	0.13	7	5.3		6
16+22+23+24				11.6		1
1+3+21+25+27+28	6.0	0.82	4			
2+14+15+17+26+28	1.9	0.06	6	4.1	0.13	6
14+15+16+22+23+24+26+28				4.8	0.42	8
1 to 9 +11+21+25+26+30				5.3	0.12	4
1+2+4 to 12+15 to 18+ 21+22+24+25+27 to 30	2.1		3			

in Table II. The results are to be compared with the cecal weights per 100 g of body weights in axenic and holoxenic Fischer rats (Table III).

Very few bacteria were able to decrease cecal enlargement when seeded singly ("monoxenic" rats). In the rats which received S.N. diet, only strain 4 and strain 15 produced a partial cecal reduction. In the rats which received D.P. diet

TABLE III. Cecal Weight in g per 100 g Body Weight in Axenic and Holoxenic
(Conventional) Rats Fed on S.N. and D.P. Diets

| | S.N. diet | | | D.P. diet | | |
	M	SDM	n	M	SDM	n
Axenic rats	9.1	0.36	9	10.9	0.53	12
Holoxenic rats (conventional)	1.6	0.09	8	2.0	0.15	12

only strain 14 and 26 had such an action. The most efficient strains only produced a partial reduction, 30 to 35% of the cecal weight in axenic rats.

When several strains were established together in axenic rats, a variety of results was observed. For instance, two strains which decreased the cecal weight when they were established singly, produced a reduction of similar magnitude when they were together; this was the case with strains 14 and 26. Strain 28, which was inefficient when single, increased the efficiency of all the bacterial strains to which it was added: 14, 15, 14 + 15, 14 + 26, 15 + 26, 14 + 15 + 26. Strain 15, which was inefficient when it was established singly in the rats fed on D.P. diet, also increased the efficiency of 26, 26 + 28, 14 + 26 + 28, but did not increase the efficiency of strain 14.

Some strains which did not reduce the cecum when they were single, remained inefficient when they were established together; so were strains 16, 22, 23, 24. The association of 16 + 22 + 23 + 24 with 14 + 15 + 26 + 28 did not increase the efficiency of the last mixture. But other strains which were inefficient when single, produced a strong cecal reduction when together; see for instance the association of strain 2 and 17 in rats fed on S.N. diet.

Diet was also found to be an important factor in cecal reduction. The influence of diet on cecal weight was observed in axenic and holoxenic rats (Figure 1 and Table III). It was also observed in gnotoxenic rats; strain 15, for instance, reduced the cecum of rats which were fed on S.N. diet and had no action upon the cecum of rats which were fed on D.P. diet.

Finally, the association of six strains, 2 + 14 + 15 + 17 + 26 + 28, produced a moderate cecal reduction in rats which were fed on D.P. diet and a very strong reduction of cecum in rats which were fed on S.N. diet. In these rats the cecal weight was 1.2 the cecal weight observed in holoxenic rats fed on S.N. diet. A more complex bacterial inoculum (see last line of Table II) did not give better results. However, rats which were born from parents which had received this more complex inoculum had similar cecal weights (mean weight per 100 g: 2.2; SDM: 0.11; number of rats: 7) and rats which were born from parents having received the six strains ("hexaxenic" rats) had somewhat bigger cecum (mean weight per 100 g: 2.5; SDM: 0.05; number of rats: 6).

These six bacterial strains also produced an important cecal reduction in mice (Table IV).

TABLE IV. Cecal Weights in g per 100 g Body Weight in Holoxenic (Conventional) and Six Bacterial Strains Associated C3H Mice

	S.N. diet			D.P. diet		
	M	SDM	n	M	SDM	n
Holoxenic (Conventional)	0.89	0.11	6	1.35	0.06	6
Hexaxenic (6 strains)	1.16	0.08	6	2.38	0.16	6

Discussion and Conclusions

Some attempts have been made in the past by various workers to reduce the enlarged cecum of axenic rats with bacterial strains (8, 14-16). The present study confirms earlier findings that associations of bacteria can produce an important cecal reduction. Moreover it shows that judicious choice of bacterial associations and of diet produces a cecal reduction of such a degree that cecal weights are very near holoxenic values.

The cecal weights obtained in C3H hexaxenic mice are similar to the cecal weights of CD-1 mice which were associated by Syed *et al.* with 50 strains of gram negative anaerobes plus 80 facultative anaerobes (16). In both experiments the mice were fed on a semi-synthetic diet, L-356 diet, which is very similar to S.N. diet.

The result of these experiments is a source of hope and of disappointment. A source of hope, because a great variety of combinations can be tried, with bacterial strains which have various properties. It is possible to hope that we shall have gnotoxenic rats which have basal metabolism, blood circulation, cecal volume, etc. . . . , similar to polyxenic values by the use of bacteria which do not deconjugate bile salts, do not produce coprostanol or have no uricase. Such gnotoxenic rats will be better hosts than the axenic rats for the study of the action of bacteria upon bile salts, cholesterol, uric acid metabolism.

A source of disappointment, because as the number of bacterial species which constitute an intestinal flora is very large, the number of possible combinations is beyond human power and some of the polyxenic rat features might never be reproduced.

References

1. Raibaud, P., Dickinson, A. B., Sacquet, E., Charlier, H., and Mocquot, G., *Ann. Inst. Pasteur III:* 193 (1966).
2. Gordon, H. A., in "Perspectives in Experimental Gerontology," Charles Thomas Publisher, p. 295, (1966).
3. Gordon, H. A., Bruckner-Kardoss, E., and Wostmann, B. S., *J. Geront. 21:* 380 (1966).
4. Wostmann, B. S., Bruckner-Kardoss, E., and Knight, P. L., *Proc. Soc. Exp. Biol. Med. 128:* 137 (1968).

5. Bruckner-Kardoss, E., and Wostmann, B. S., *Lab Anim. Care 17:* 542 (1967).
6. Guenet, J. L., Sacquet, E., Gueneau, G., and Meslin, J. C., *C. R. Acad. Sci. Paris 270:* 3087 (1970).
7. Sacquet, E., Guenet, J. L., Garnier, H., and Meslin, J. C., *C. R. Acad. Sci. Paris 272:* 841 (1971).
8. Sacquet, E., Garnier, H., and Raibaud, P., *C. R. Soc. Biol. 164:* 352 (1970).
9. Abrams, G. D., Bauer, N., and Sprinz, H., *Lab. Invest. 12:* 355 (1963).
10. Lesher, S., Walburg, H. E., and Sachez, G. A., *Nature 202:* 884 (1964).
11. Abrams, G. D., and Bishop, J. E., *Proc. Soc. Exp. Biol. Med. 126:* 301 (1967).
12. Raibaud, P., Dickinson, A. B., Sacquet, E., Charlier, H., and Mocquot, G., *Ann. Inst. Pasteur 110:* 568 (1966).
13. Loesche, W. J., *J. Bacteriol. 99:* 520 (1969).
14. Schaedler, R. W., Dubos, R., and Costello, R., *J. Exp. Med. 122:* 77 (1965).
15. Skelly, J. B., Trexler, P. C., and Tanami, J., *Proc. Soc. Exp. Biol. Med. 110:* 455 (1962).
16. Syed, S. A., Abrams, G. A., and Freter, R., *Infection and Immunity 2:* 376 (1970).

THE INFLUENCE OF GASTROINTESTINAL FLORA ON DIGESTIVE UTILIZATION OF FATTY ACIDS IN RATS

Y. Demarne and *J. Flanzy*
Station de Recherches de Nutrition
C.N.R.Z. — I.N.R.A.
78 — Jouy-en-Josas, France

and

E. Sacquet
Station des animaux sans germes
C.N.R.S.
91 — Gif-sur-Yvette, France

Introduction

The role of gastrointestinal flora in the apparent digestive utilization of fatty acids has been studied very little except for some pathological cases, and therefore is one of the least known factors. Progress in the production of germfree animals during the last 10 years now permits us to do research in this field.

The few studies reported in the literature were done with very unsaturated fat such as corn oil unsaturated homogenous triglycerides (1-4). As far as we know, saturated fat (tallow) was used only by Boyd and Edwards (1) in the chicken.

The authors show that in different species the germfree animal has a significantly higher apparent digestive utilization of corn oil than is recorded for the conventional animal. However, improvement is of low amplitude. Since corn oil contains about 50% linoleic acid and 30% oleic acid, and apparent digestibility of these fatty acids is always about 100%, we thought that if the germfree animal absorbed this oil better, it was perhaps because of a better absorption of long saturated fatty acids (palmitic and stearic). That is why we did a series of experiments on the rat to show the effect of an apparently non-pathogenic gastrointestinal flora on fatty acid absorption. In order to more easily estimate this action, we tested a series of fats, very rich in saturated fatty acids, on the germfree rat and the conventional rat (Fischer strain).

Materials and Methods

Germfree and conventional rats used in these studies were male Fischer strain rats. In experiments 1 and 2, the mean body weight at the beginning of the experimental period was 90 g. In experiment 3, due to the fact that a part of the tested animals were cecectomized at five weeks of age and that a recovery period was required, the mean body weight at the beginning of the experimental period was 250 g.

After an adaptation to the experimental diets, the rats were starved for 48 hours. Digestibility experiments were conducted for 2 weeks. The experimental diets were distributed *ad libitum.* Dry food consumption was calculated daily for each animal. Feces were collected daily and dried. At the end of the experimental period, the animals were starved until there was no fecal emission.

Fecal lipids were extracted in two steps. First, soluble lipids were extracted by a chloroform-methanol (2:1) mixture. Second, insoluble lipids (essentially calcium soaps) were extracted by distilled petroleum ether after acid hydrolysis. Fatty acids were separated by saponification, methylated, and were analyzed by gas liquid chromatography.

The apparent digestive utilization of fat or fatty acids was calculated as follows:

$$\text{Apparent Digestive Utilization (C.U.D.a.)} = \frac{\text{Ingestion (g)} - \text{Excretion (g)}}{\text{Ingestion (g)}} \times 100$$

Results

Experiment 1. Intake of fat mixture A. Presence of fatty acids ranging from C_{12} (lauric acid) to $C_{22:1}$ (erucic acid). The first experiment was done using a relatively complex mixture of fats. We covered all the series of medium and long-chain fatty acids commonly found in feeds, at the same time trying as much as possible to avoid having a large imbalance of one of them.

TABLE I. Component Fatty Acids of Fat A (%)

C_{12}	C_{14}	C_{16}	C_{18}	$C_{18:1}$	$C_{18:2}$	C_{20}	C_{22}	$C_{22:1}$
15.5	6.8	12.7	16.5	15.7	9.8	4.6	8.4	10

Table I shows the fatty acid composition of mixture A. More than 40% of the fatty acids present are long and saturated ($)C_{16}$).

During this experiment, we tested the apparent digestive utilization of the fat and of each one of the fatty acids composing it.

Figure 1 shows the different values we obtained. Thus, for apparent digestive utilization of fat A (CUD) we observed that: a) It is very low in all

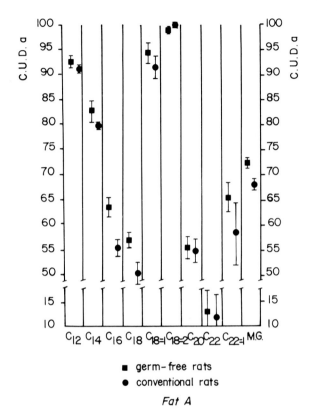

Fat A

FIG. 1. Apparent digestive utilization of fat A and of its fatty acids.

cases. This is to be expected due to the high proportion of saturated fatty acids in the mixture. b) Germfree rats absorb fat A significantly better than the conventional rats with intestinal flora. c) While the difference between the 2 lots is significant, it is low (73% against 68%). This represents an absolute improvement of 5% and a relative improvement of 7%.

For the apparent digestive utilization of fatty acids, we noted that: a) Apparent digestive utilization of the medium-chain saturated fatty acids, lauric (C_{12}) and myristic (C_{14}), and the unsaturated fatty acids, oleic ($C_{18:1}$) and linoleic ($C_{18:2}$), is not affected by intestinal flora; neither is that of the very long saturated fatty acids, arachidic (C_{20}) and behenic (C_{22}). We cannot estimate the difference of apparent digestive utilization of erucic acid ($C_{22:1}$) in either case because there is too wide a dispersion of values. b) Only the apparent digestive utilization of palmitic (C_{16}) and stearic (C_{18}) acids is significantly affected by the presence of intestinal flora.

Digestive utilization of palmitic acid ranges from 53% in the conventional animal to 63% in the germfree. Absolute improvement is 8% and relative improvement nears 14%. The digestibility of stearic acid does the same ranging from 50 to 57%.

If only the apparent digestibility of these 2 fatty acids is improved by the absence of flora, this may explain why there is so little increase of the digestive utilization of fat A in the germfree animal as compared to the conventional animal. Fat A contains only 29% of these fatty acids. The same result would surely be obtained when the animals receive very unsaturated fat such as corn oil which contains very low quantities of these fatty acids.

Experiment 2. Intake of saturated fat B, rich in palmitic and stearic acids. The second fat mixture tested had a more simple composition. Oils rich in very long fatty acids (rapeseed oil and hydrogenated rapeseed) were eliminated. As in the first experiment, the proportions of different fats were chosen so as to obtain almost 40% long saturated fatty acids ($\rangle C_{16}$). These types of fatty acids are represented only by palmitic (C_{16}) and stearic (C_{18}) acids, as shown in Table II.

TABLE II. Component Fatty Acids of Fat B (%)

C_{12}	C_{14}	C_{16}	C_{18}	$C_{18:1}$	$C_{18:2}$
15.4	6.2	23.6	19.8	29.3	5.7

Besides digestive utilization, this time we determined the fecal excretion of calcium soaps since several authors attribute bad digestive utilization of long saturated fatty acids partly to intraluminal synthesis of these types of components (5, 6).

Using fat B, we made the following observations (see Figure 2): a) Its digestive utilization is higher than that of fat A. This increase is certainly due to elimination of long saturated fatty acids. However, digestive utilization of palmitic (C_{16}) and stearic (C_{18}) acids is higher than for fat A. This illustrates the phenomenon of the reciprocal effect of fatty acids in absorption. b) Apparent digestive utilization of fat B is better in the germfree rat than in the conventional rat. The differences recorded are greater than in the previous experiment. Absolute improvement is almost 8% and relative improvement is 10% (87.7% against 80.8%).

This improvement of fat B digestibility goes along with a large increase in the digestive utilization of palmitic acid (12% absolute improvement) and stearic acid (16% absolute improvement). The results for oleic acid are not quite significant.

Figure 3 shows the percentage of fat B and each of its fatty acids ingested and then excreted in the form of calcium soaps. The highest percentage was

556

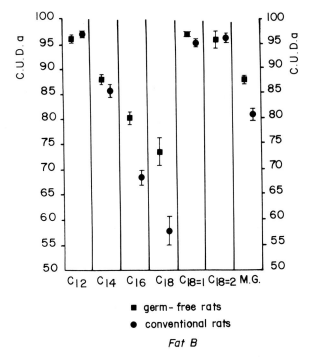

Fat B

FIG. 2. Apparent digestive utilization of fat B and of its fatty acids.

recorded for the conventional rat. For the same quantity ingested, the conventional rat excretes about twice as many insoluble soaps.

For the fatty acids, we observed that: a) No matter what the type of rat, the excretion percentage of insoluble soaps increases with the number of carbon atoms, and it drops suddenly when there is double binding. This phenomenon is of greater importance for palmitic and stearic acids. b) With the exception of lauric acid (C_{12}) and linoleic acid where there is no excretion, and which we do not show in the graph, all fatty acids have a tendency to be excreted in larger quantity in insoluble form in conventional animals than in germfree animals.

This phenomenon should be compared with results of the digestive studies shown above once we know the effect of intraluminal formation of soaps of these types on the digestive utilization of long saturated fatty acids.

Experiment 3. Accrued effects of cecectomy and the germfree state on the digestive utilization of fatty acids. In another series of experiments, we tested apparent digestive utilization of a simple fat C, cocoa butter, which is very rich in palmitic and stearic acids. However, instead of using 2 lots of animals as before, this time we used 4 lots of rats. Two lots were constituted, one composed of germfree rats and the other of conventional rats. Two more lots

557

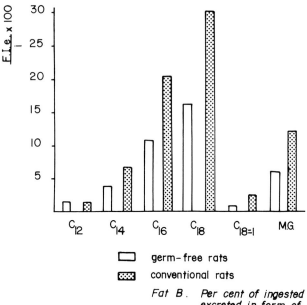

FIG. 3. Fecal excretion of insoluble soaps.

were also composed, one of cecectomized germfree rats and the other of cecectomized conventional rats. We wished to see what effect cecal hypertrophy in the germfree rat had on apparent digestive utilization of a saturated fat.

Fatty acid composition of the fat in the ration is shown in Table III. The

TABLE III. Component Fatty Acids of Fat C (%)

C_{16}	C_{18}	$C_{18:1}$	$C_{18:2}$
32.5	38.1	26.5	2.9

proportion of saturated fatty acids is extremely high (about 70%). The results of this experiment are shown in Figure 4, and it is apparent again that normal germfree rats have higher apparent digestive utilization than that observed for conventional rats (72% against 66%). However, improvement is less than that recorded with fat B.

The results are identical for digestive utilization of fatty acids. Digestive utilization is better in germfree animals than in conventional animals. However, improvement is lower than that observed for the fat B which contained only 40% long saturated fatty acids. This leads us to suppose that the ratio of

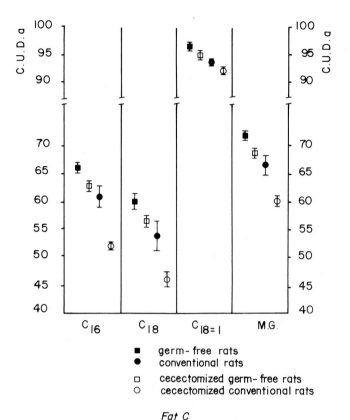

Fat C

FIG. 4. Influence on cecectomy on the apparent digestive utilization of fat C and of its fatty acids.

unsaturated fatty acid:saturated fatty acid has an effect on improvement of saturated fatty acid absorption in the germfree rat.

All rats with cecal excision have lower apparent digestive utilization than the normal controls. This operation in the germfree rat brings digestive utilization back to values which do not significantly differ from those reported for normal conventional animals.

However, the excision of a cecum 5 times smaller in the conventional rat decreases digestive utilization of fat C 2 to 3 times more. Thus, if systemic excision of the cecum in every case affects the conventional rat more although it has a much smaller cecum, cecal hypertrophy and the resulting transit modifications (7) cannot be responsible for the increase of digestive utilization of palmitic and stearic acids in the germfree rat.

Conclusions

From this first series of experiments, we may draw the following conclusions: 1) The germfree rat absorbs saturated fat better than the conventional rat. Since several authors (1-4) have already observed the same phenomenon with unsaturated fat, it is probable that this applies to all types of fats. 2) Differences of absorption between the two types of animals are greater for saturated fat, rich in palmitic and stearic acids, than for other fats. 3) The differences observed seem to be related to the ratio of unsaturated fatty acid:saturated fatty acid. The phenomenon seems to disappear when saturated fatty acid concentration in the fat reaches a certain point. 4) The germfree state mainly improves digestive utilization of palmitic and stearic acids. 5) As the digestive utilization of these fatty acids increases, the excretion of insoluble Ca^{++} soaps diminishes. 6) Removal of the voluminous germfree rat cecum, thus approximating intestinal transit in the conventional rat, also creates similar digestive utilization of the fatty acids. However, removal of the small cecum in the conventional rat reduces fatty acid absorption more than it does in the hypertrophied cecum of the germfree rat.

These results are still too fragmentary to be used to logically explain the phenomena described here. The results of other research paralleling this work in the field of germfree rat bile salts will orient our studies to understand differences of fatty acid absorption in germfree and conventional animals.

References

1. Boyd, F. M., Edwards, H. M. Jr., *Poultry Sci. 46:* 1481 (1967).
2. Evrard, E., Hoet, P. P., Eyssen, H., Charlier, H., Sacquet, E., *Brit. J. Exp. Pathol. 45:* 409 (1967).
3. Tennant, B., Reina-Guerra, M., Harrold, D., and Goldman, M., *J. Nutr. 97:* 67 (1969).
4. Yoshida, T., Pleasants, J. R., Reddy, B. S., *Br. J. Nutr. 22:* 732 (1968).
5. Fakambi, L., Flanzy, J., Francois, A. C., *C. R. Acad. Sc., Paris, Serie D 269:* 2233 (1969).
6. Flanzy, J., Rerat, A., and Francois, A. C., *Ann. Biol. Anim. Bioch. Biophys. 8:* 537 (1968).
7. Sacquet, E., Garnier, H., and Raibaud, P., *C.R. Soc. Biol. 164:* 532 (1970).

INTESTINAL STRANGULATION IN MONOCONTAMINATED RATS

Charles E. Yale and *Edward Balish*
Departments of Surgery and Medical Microbiology
University of Wisconsin Medical School
Madison, Wisconsin 53706, U.S.A.

Introduction

The bacteria in the intestinal tract are primarily responsible for the deaths of many patients with intestinal strangulation. Using the monocontaminated rat, we have found that the common intestinal bacteria vary considerably in their ability to cause death after intestinal strangulation (1-4). The present study summarizes the course of ischemic and hemorrhagic intestinal strangulation in rats monocontaminated with *Clostridium perfringens, Clostridium sporogenes, Lactobacillus bifidus, Citrobacter freundii, Enterobacter aerogenes,* or *Klebsiella pneumoniae.*

Materials and Methods

The bacteria were purchased from the American Type Culture Collection, Rockville, Maryland 20852, U.S.A. (Table I). The morphological and chemical characteristics of each species were verified before and after each experiment. A test inoculum of each type of bacteria was prepared in a manner similar to that described in a previously published study (3). The initial concentrations of the suspensions varied from 2.1 x 10^9 to 7.4 x 10^9 viable cells per milliliter (ml), and the final concentrations (after the last operation) had decreased by less than one log.

Eighty-four Sprague-Dawley germfree rats of each sex from our own breeding colony were used. The average weights and hematocrit values were, respectively: males, 451 g and 52.8%; and females, 287 g and 50.7%. Fourteen germfree rats of each sex were individually caged in each of 6 separate flexible film isolators. A separate operating chamber was attached to each isolator.

One of 4 separate operations was done on each animal. After the rat was anesthetized with pentobarbital sodium, intramuscularly, the abdominal cavity was opened through a midline incision. In the **first** type of operation, 1 ml of either normal saline (NS) or of the test suspension (TS) was injected into the

561

TABLE I. Characteristics of the Bacteria

Species	Strain (ATCC)	Gram Stain	Oxygen Requirements
C. perfringens	3624	+	Anaerobic
C. sporogenes	19404	+	Anaerobic
L. bifidus	11146	+	Anaerobic
C. freundii	8090	−	Aerobic
E. aerogenes	13048	−	Aerobic
K. pneumoniae	13883	−	Aerobic

lumen of the distal ileum, and the abdominal incision closed. In the **second** operation, a 20-cm segment of the distal ileum was isolated by ligating its distal and proximal ends with heavy silk. After dividing the bowel above the proximal and below the distal tie, the continuity of the intestinal tract was restored by an end-to-end anastamosis. Either 1 ml of NS or TS was injected into the isolated, bypassed, closed loop, and the abdomen closed. A 10-cm intestinal segment was isolated in the **third** operation, its venous return ligated, producing a hemorrhagic intestinal strangulation, and 1 ml NS or TS was injected into the closed loop. After restoring the continuity of the intestinal tract, the abdomen was closed. The **fourth** operation was identical to the second, except that both the arterial and venous blood supplies to the 20-cm test segment were ligated, resulting in an ischemic strangulation.

On the first operating day, in each isolator, 1 animal of each sex had 1 of each of the 4 types of operations. Only normal saline was used. On the second day, the test suspension was introduced into the isolator. Two rats of each sex had each of the first 2 types of operation, and 3 animals of each sex had the third and fourth types of operation.

Postoperatively, the animals were given feed and water *ad libitum.* They were closely observed to mark the time of death, and the survivors were killed and autopsied after 2 weeks. Additional details on similar types of experiments have been reported previously (3).

Results

All 168 rats were suitable for analysis (Table II). The sex of the animal did not appear to alter the results and monocontamination alone was without effect. Bacterial inoculation of the 20-cm long isolated, but not strangulated, test segment caused the death of only 5 of 24 animals. Four of these deaths occurred between 57 and 65 hours after operation, and the last 1 after 239 hours. None of the animals monoassociated with *E. aerogenes* or *K. pneumoniae* died.

Ischemic strangulation seemed to be as lethal as hemorrhagic strangulation, regardless of the bacteria present. Some organisms were much more lethal than

TABLE II. Intestinal Strangulation in Monocontaminated Rats

Type of Operation	Organism	No. of Animals	Survival time, hours*
No strangu-lation, no test segment	normal saline	12	(12)
	C. perfringens	4	(4)
	C. sporogenes	4	(4)
	L. bifidus	4	(4)
	C. freundii	4	(4)
	E. aerogenes	4	(4)
	K. pneumoniae	4	(4)
No strangu-lation, 20-cm test segment	normal saline	12	(10), 65, 116
	C. perfringens	4	(3), 65
	C. sporogenes	4	(2), 57, 62
	L. bifidus	4	(3), 60
	C. freundii	4	(3), 239
	E. aerogenes	4	(4)
	K. pneumoniae	4	(4)
Hemor-rhagic strangu-lation, 10-cm test segment	normal saline	12	(8), 74, 77, 82, 86
	C. perfringens	6	8, 8, 8, 9, 10, 11
	C. sporogenes	6	(2), 39, 42, 58, 63
	L. bifidus	6	(4), 51, 85
	C. freundii	6	(4), 32, 40
	E. aerogenes	6	(3), 9, 18, 21
	K. pneumoniae	6	(6)
Is-chemic strangu-lation, 20-cm test segment	normal saline	12	(9), 48, 64, 81
	C. perfringens	6	7, 7, 8, 8, 8, 8,
	C. sporogenes	6	(3), 26, 58, 62
	L. bifidus	6	(3), 48, 62, 78
	C. freundii	6	(3), 38, 38, 192
	E. aerogenes	6	(4), 84, 102
	K. pneumoniae	6	(6)

*No. in parentheses indicate animals killed two weeks after operation.

others. *C. perfringens* killed all the animals with ischemic or hemorrhagic strangulation between 7 and 11 hours after operation, while *K. pneumoniae* caused no deaths. *C. sporogenes* killed 7 of the 12 rats with ischemic or hemorrhagic strangulation, while *L. bifidus, C. freundii,* and *E. aerogenes* each killed 5 of the 12. Any animal that lived 3 days usually lived to the end of the experiment.

All initial cultures of the 168 rats and the 6 isolators were sterile. At the end of the experiment, each isolator and each animal was monocontaminated with the appropriate organism, and there had been no detectable accidental contamination. The morphological and chemical characteristics of each of the organisms were determined by single colony isolates at the end of the study, and found to be identical to those of the original species. Each organism was found throughout the gastrointestinal tract in concentrations of 10^5 to 10^9 viable cells per gram of contents (wet weight).

Discussion

The operations used in this study rarely cause the death of a germfree animal. However, in this experiment, 9 of 48 germfree (i.e., NS-injected) animals died. Four of these deaths occurred in the isolators monocontaminated with *C. perfringens* and *C. sporogenes*, the most lethal organisms in the study. Probably, monocontamination of the NS-injected animals approximately 24 hours after operation increased the severity of the insult.

In most of our studies with monocontaminated animals, ischemic strangulation has been about as lethal as hemorrhagic intestinal strangulation. Monoassociation with *Escherichia coli* (1) was the one exception to this generalization. The length of the test segment was purposely limited to 10 cm, to avoid the undue blood loss and death secondary to hemorrhagic shock alone.

The survival rates of rats with either ischemic or hemorrhagic intestinal strangulation and monocontamination with 1 of 14 different species of microorganisms is collected in Table III. This summary of our results to date (1-4)

TABLE III. Percent Survival of Monocontaminated Rats with Intestinal Strangulation

Germfree (144)	86
++*K. pneumoniae* (12) 100	++*E. aerogenes* (12) 58
B. fragilis (12) 92	++*L. bifidus* (12) 58
L. acidophilus (12) 92	++*C. sporogenes* (12) 42
S. faecalis (12) 92	*E. coli* (60)* 23
S. aureus 80/81 (12) 83	*P. vulgaris* (12) 8
C. albicans (49)* 78	++*C. perfringens* (120)* 1
++*C. freundii* (12) 58	*P. aeruginosa* (12) 0

( ) No. of animals tested.   * Several strains tested.
++ Reported in present study.

emphasizes that the various microorganisms found commonly in the intestinal tract have greatly different lethal potentialities in a rat with intestinal strangulation. As this work is expanded and repeated in other germfree animals, the relative importance of the intestinal microflora will be clarified. Hopefully, then, the septic processes in man and animals will prove to be similar enough to enable the clinician to choose rationally the antibiotics necessary to counteract the sepsis of intestinal strangulation.

Conclusions

The effect of monocontamination by each of 6 common bacteria was studied in germfree rats with an isolated closed intestinal loop, and similar loops with either ischemic or hemorrhagic intestinal strangulation. The results of this and previous studies emphasize that different organisms vary greatly in their ability to cause death. It is hoped that a better understanding of the toxicity of the intestinal bacteria will lead to better treatment of the septic phase of intestinal strangulation in man.

Acknowledgement

This research was supported in part by Public Health Service Grant AI 06956 from the National Institute of Allergy and Infectious Diseases.

References

1. Yale, C. E., and Vivek, A. R., *Infect. Immunity 1:* 195 (1970).
2. Yale, C. E., and Balish, E., *Infect. Immunity 3:* 481 (1971).
3. Yale, C. E., and Balish, E., *Arch. Surg. 104:* 438 (1972).
4. Yale, C. E., and Balish, E., *Canad. J. Microbiol. 18:* 1049 (1972).

STUDIES ON ENTEROPATHOGENIC *E. COLI* ENTEROTOXINS; MICROBIAL FLORA AND DISACCHARIDASE CONCENTRATION CHANGES IN LIGATED PIG INTESTINAL LOOP

Laszlo Pesti and *Gabor Semjen*
Veterinary Medical Research Institute
Hungarian Academy of Sciences
Budapest, Hungary

Introduction

American and English authors (1-4) have demonstrated by means of tests in ligated segments of pig small intestine that live cultures of *Escherichia coli* strains isolated from diarrhea-associated conditions possess "segment dilating activity" and the majority of them produce an exotoxin-like thermostable enterotoxin (ST) and a cell-bound thermolabile enterotoxin (LT) as well.

The present paper deals with the enterotoxins of enteropathogenic *E. coli* culture and the mechanism of action of these toxins.

Materials and Methods

Studies were made on the distribution of ST and LT enterotoxins (prepared according to Smith and Halls (1) and Gyles and Barnum (2)) among "Hungarian-born" strains of *E. coli* enteropathogenic for pigs and on the relationship of the former to one another. Enterotoxin neutralization was assayed by means of the loop test; changes of the intestinal bacterial flora (Pesti (5)) in the ligated segments and changes of disaccharidase enzyme activity (Dahlquist (6)) in differently treated walls of such segments were determined.

The 63 animals used in the experiment were 10 – 12 weeks old large white pigs, weighing an average of 12 – 15 kg. The loop test was carried out according to a modification of the method of Smith and Halls (1), which required the introduction of enterotoxin into ligated segments of the gut and the measurement of the accumulation of liquid in it. The animals were killed and examined 24 hours after the operation. "Segment dilating activity" was expressed by: weight of the full segment, minus empty weight of segment, divided by empty weight of segment ("wt/wt ratio"). Ratios of 1.00 or higher were regarded as positive loop test. The 83 *E. coli* strains used in the experiments originated from

567

47 swine farms from epidemiologically unrelated *E. coli* disease of swine.

Results

The greater part (80.3 per cent) of strains from diarrheal conditions possessed segment dilating activity. Thus, the great majority of *E. coli* diarrhea strains could be qualified as enteropathogenic. Of the strains examined serologically 84.8 per cent (piglet and post-weaning diarrhea strains) belonged to serotypes 0147 and 0149. Formerly no strains of these types were found in our country.

ST and LT enterotoxins were prepared from serologically typed strains; the strains were grouped according to the clinical pictures for which they had

TABLE I. Response of Ligated Intestinal Segments of the Pig to Injection of *E. coli* Live Cultures, Heat-Labile and Heat-Stable Enterotoxins

Source of strains	Antigenic formula	No. of strains tested	Ligated intestine test with live cultures		Type of enterotoxin produced Heat – Labile (LT)		Heat – Stable (ST)	
			Intestine dilating activity	wt/wt ratio*	Intestine dilating activity	wt/wt ratio	Intestine dilating activity	wt/wt ratio
Piglet diarrhea	0147, K88ac	3	+	4.16	+	3.24	+	4.63
	0149, K88ac	5	+	3.97	+	5.78	+	5.30
	014, K88ac	1	+	6.86	+	3.75	+	6.50
	0139	1	+	2.13	+	10.55	+	10.65
Post-weaning diarrhea	0147, K88ac	9	+	4.16	+	6.79	+	4.47
	0149, K88ac	11	+	3.80	+	6.01	+	4.79
	0115	1	+	2.99	+	3.09	+	3.90
Edema disease	0138	1	+	5.02	–	0.50	+	1.83
	0139	4	–	0.32	–	0.30	–	0.64
	0141	1	–	0.84	–	0.25	–	0.33

*Ratio of total segment weight minus empty wall weight to empty wall weight

been responsible (Table I). All strains originating from diarrheal conditions produced both ST and LT enterotoxin. The "edema disease" strains (showing no diarrhea) had no demonstrable LT toxin product. It appears that both kinds of toxins are required to elicit diarrhea-associated conditions.

TABLE II. Influence of Two Different Antiserum on the Ligated Intestines Response to Heat-Stable (ST) Heat-Labile (LT) Enterotoxins and *E. coli* Live Cultures

Inoculation of Ligated Segment	Response in Ligated Segment	
	Neutralization Effect	Weight/Weight Ratio*
0149 ST		2.57
0149 ST + Homologous Antiserum	+	1.30
0141 ST		1.83
0141 ST + Homologous Antiserum	+	1.22
0149 ST		10.89
0149 ST + 0141 Antiserum	+	3.90
0139 ST		1.33
0139 ST + 0141 Antiserum	+	0.30
0138 ST		8.12
0138 ST + 0141 Antiserum	+	1.87
0138 ST		9.30
0138 ST + 0149 Antiserum	+	3.15
0149 ST		9.44
0149 ST + Negative Serum	−	9.23
0141 LT		15.92
0141 LT + Homologous Antiserum	+	0.33
0149 LT		16.00
0149 LT + 0141 Antiserum	+	0.55
0141 LT		5.40
0141 LT + Negative Serum	−	3.20
0149 Live Culture 5 x 10^5 Germs		4.00
0149 Live Culture 5 x 10^5 + Homologous Antiserum	+	0.76
0149 Live Culture 5 x 10^4		3.16
0149 Live Culture 5 x 10^4 + Homologous Antiserum	+	0.40

*Ratio of Total Segment Weight minus Empty Wall Weight to Empty Wall Weight

The neutralization test evaluations (Table II) suggested two implications: 1) the antiserum prepared by us neutralized, not only the homologous and heterologous LT enterotoxin and the segment dilating activity of live homologous organisms, but also the loop dilating activity of the ST enterotoxin. It should be noted that the neutralization effect was not always complete, the wt/wt ratio remaining in some cases slightly above 1.00. Tests with negative serum showed, however, no neutralization effect at all. 2) Results of neutraliza-

TABLE III. Number of Bacteria in Treated and Untreated Ligated Loops of Small Intestine of 11 Pigs

		Live Culture of 13 Loop Test Positive Strains	Live Culture of 7 Loop Test Negative Strains	Heat-Stable Enterotoxin of 0141 Strain Loop Reaction Positive	Heat-Labile Enterotoxins of 6 Loop Test Positive and 7 Loop Test Negative Strains	Uninoculated Control Loops
No. of Loops Tested		27	19	15	13	33
No. Positive Loops		26	19	14	13	26
E. coli	Mean	4.2×10^8	9.3×10^9	3.4×10^8	7.4×10^8	5.9×10^8
	Range	$2.0 \times 10^7 - 1.0 \times 10^9$	$3.6 \times 10^7 - 2.0 \times 10^9$	$2.4 \times 10^7 - 1.4 \times 10^9$	$5.0 \times 10^7 - 1.6 \times 10^9$	$1.1 \times 10^7 - 1.1 \times 10^9$
No. Negative Loops		—	—	1	—	7
No. Positive Loops		13	3	7	13	15
Enterococci	Mean	2.6×10^7	2.9×10^5	4.4×10^7	1.4×10^8	3.5×10^7
	Range	$4.0 \times 10^5 - 1.0 \times 10^8$	$3.2 \times 10^4 - 8.0 \times 10^5$	$8.0 \times 10^6 - 1.2 \times 10^8$	$8.0 \times 10^5 - 5.2 \times 10^8$	$4.0 \times 10^4 - 1.7 \times 10^8$
No. Negative Loops		14	16	8	—	18

Aerobic Lactobacilli	No. Positive Loops	11	2	7	12	12
	Mean	1.5×10^8	6.2×10^5	2.2×10^7	2.8×10^7	3.5×10^7
	Range	$3.2 \times 10^5 - 8.0 \times 10^8$	$4.0 \times 10^4 - 1.2 \times 10^6$	$2.4 \times 10^6 - 1.4 \times 10^8$	$1.6 \times 10^5 - 1.6 \times 10^8$	$2.8 \times 10^5 - 3.0 \times 10^8$
	No. Negative Loops	16	17	8	1	21
Clostridia	No. Positive Loops	2	—	4	8	9
	Mean	1.4×10^7	—	2.0×10^6	3.1×10^6	9.6×10^6
	Range	$2.0 \times 10^6 - 2.6 \times 10^7$	—	$2.0 \times 10^5 - 4.0 \times 10^6$	$1.6 \times 10^4 - 8.0 \times 10^6$	$2.0 \times 10^3 - 5.0 \times 10^3$
	No. Negative Loops	25	19	11	5	24
Bacteroides	No. Positive Loops	—	2	2	1	—
	Mean		1.6×10^6	1.8×10^6	2.0×10^6	
	Range		$8.0 \times 10^5 - 2.5 \times 10^6$	$1.2 \times 10^6 - 2.4 \times 10^6$		
	No. Negative Loops	2	5	3	8	9

Staphylococci
Aerobic
Sporeformers
and Yeasts

Negative Results in the Tested Loops

tion tests performed with the ST enterotoxin and the two sera indicate that the latter could neutralize the ST enterotoxin not only of homologous, but also of heterologous strains. These findings suggest a great similarity between the ST and LT enterotoxins of different strains as well as the probable presence of anti-enterotoxic (anti-ST and anti-LT) antibodies in our antisera.

Microbial flora examinations (Table III) gave the following results: Loop test positive, E. coli treated segments had high E. coli counts. Inoculation of live cultures of no loop dilating activity also resulted in a marked increase of E. coli counts in the segment contents. Also, the uninoculated control loops contained high coli counts; these were, as a rule, non-hemolytic.

The germ count examinations suggest that the loop dilating activity of the examined enteropathogenic E. coli strains was due not only to multiplication, but also to enterotoxin production, because if multiplication alone were responsible, fluid accumulation would have taken place also in the control segments. No general rule or tendency could be inferred from the fluctuations of enterococcus, lactobacillus and clostridium counts. Multiplication very likely depended on their presence or absence in the loop at ligation.

Changes of maltase and invertase enzyme concentrations in differently treated walls of ligated segments are shown in Table IV. It can be seen that the concentrations of maltase and invertase decrease significantly compared to normal in the walls of dilated loops inoculated with live loop test positive E. coli organisms and ST enterotoxin, but the mural enzyme levels did not change in segments inoculated with loop test negative strains not causing a dilatation. The trehalase and lactase concentration changes showed the same phenomenon. In dilated loops the loop fluid disaccharidase activity was high, while the mural level of the enzymes was low. In undilated loops, neither the small amount (0 − 2 ml) of contents nor the rinsing fluid displayed any disaccharidase activity on assay. Apparently, extreme accumulation of fluid in the ligated loop, which is clearly a consequence of intestinal mucosa permeability disturbance, results in "washing" off of disaccharidase enzymes from their mucosal sites. Permeability disturbance, on the other hand, seems to depend exclusively on enterotoxin action, because loop test negative E. coli strains, which did not produce enterotoxin, did not effect a reduction of mural enzyme activity either.

Conclusions

It seems fairly certain from observations of others and from our own experience that E. coli strains develop diarrheal action through their entero-toxins, i.e., in the same manner as Vibrio cholerae. All enteropathogenic strains isolated from diarrheal conditions were found to produce both heat-labile and heat-stable enterotoxins. Both kinds of enterotoxins differ from the E. coli endotoxin. The enterotoxins seem to alter the permeability of the intestinal

TABLE IV. Effect of *E. coli* Live Cultures and Heat-Stable (ST) Enterotoxins on
Ligated Pig Intestinal Wall Maltase and Invertase Activities

Age and no. of animals	Inoculation of ligated segments	Loop reaction	Maltase activity[1]	Invertase activity[1]
15 weeks 5 animals	Untreated	−	8613 ± 899[2] /10/[3]	1793 ± 374 /10/
	0141 strain live culture	+	1897 ± 467 /5/	320 ± 102 /5/
	0141 strain, ST enterotoxin	+	2985 ± 356 /10/	463 ± 61 /10/
	4 different loop test negative strains, live cult.	−	7992 ± 2006 /8/	1895 ± 546 /8/
10 weeks 4 animals	Untreated	−	3714 ± 434 /22/	687 ± 118 /19/
	0141 strain live culture	+	1518 ± 603 /5/	124 ± 75 /5/
	12 different loop test positive strains, live cult.	+	1178 ± 234 /12/	98 ± 35 /12/

		Statistical significance	
		maltase activity	invertase activity
1st group	Untreated vs. 0141 ST and live culture	$P \langle 0.001$	$P \langle 0.01$ and $P \langle 0.02$
	Untreated vs. loop test neg. strains	NS	NS
2nd group	Untreated vs. 0141 strain live culture	$P \langle 0.05$	$P \langle 0.05$
	Untreated vs. loop test pos. strains	$P \langle 0.001$	$P \langle 0.001$

[1] enzyme activities are expressed as micromoles of respective disaccharide hydrolyzed /hour/ gram protein
[2] averages $\pm$ se of mean
[3] number of segments tested

mucosa and probably also of the intestinal vessels by a not yet fully understood
mechanism and the permeability change might well be held responsible for the
extreme accumulation of fluid in the intestinal lumen, which again results in

washing off of disaccharidases from their mucosal sites and in the consequent rise of these enzymes in the intestinal contents.

Apparently, a considerable rise of intestinal *E. coli* counts is in itself not pathogenic, unless the strain is an active producer of enterotoxin(s). The positive results of the enterotoxin neutralization tests are promising in respect to future control of the implicated disease.

References

1. Smith, H. W., and Halls, S., *J. Path. Bact. 93:* 531 (1967).
2. Gyles, C. L., and Barnum, D. A., *J. Infect. Dis. 120:* 419 (1969).
3. Nielsen, N. O., Ph. D. Thesis, Univ. Minnesota, (1963).
4. Smith, H. W., and Gyles, C. L., *J. Med. Microb. 3:* 387 (1970).
5. Pesti, L., *Zbl. fur Bakt. I. Orig. 189:* 282 (1963).
6. Dahlquist, A., *Anal. Biochem. 7:* 18 (1964).

THE GASTROINTESTINAL TRACT OF GNOTOBIOTIC PIGS

O. P. Miniats and *V. E. Valli*
Departments of Clinical Studies and Pathology
Ontario Veterinary College, University of Guelph
Guelph, Ontario, Canada

Introduction

Germfree and colostrum deprived contaminated pigs are being used for biomedical research, and gnotobiotic technology is applied for surgical delivery and rearing of Specific-Pathogen-Free (SPF) pigs for the establishment of minimal disease swine herds. As the pig is too large for prolonged maintenance in isolation, usually young pigs are used in gnotobiotic work. However, only limited data are available on the characteristics of the gnotobiotic pig (1, 2).

Comparative studies of germfree, colostrum deprived contaminated (SPF) and conventional pigs from birth to 8 weeks of age were undertaken at the Ontario Vetinary College. This is a report on the gross and microscopic morphology of the digestive (GI) tract and certain physical properties of its contents.

Materials and Methods

A total of 126 pigs were studied: 6 neonates, 48 germfree, 48 SPF, and 24 conventional pigs. The germfree and the SPF pigs were hysterectomy derived and reared in isolation (3) on one of two artificial diets: a special formula SF (SPF Lac, Borden Co., New York) or condensed cow's milk (CM) supplemented with iron. After delivery the SPF pigs were exposed to either accidental contaminants or to a limited defined bacterial flora consisting of Lactobacilli, fecal streptococci and non-virulent strains of *Escherichia coli* and *Clostridium perfringens*. The conventional pigs were being suckled by their dam in a normal swine barn environment. The data presented here are of 6 categories of pigs: 1) neonatal, 2) germfree pigs fed SF, 3) germfree pigs fed CM, 4) SPF pigs fed SF, 5) SPF pigs fed CM, and 6) conventional pigs. There were 6 animals within each category and age group (birth, 2, 4, 6 and 8 weeks old).

The histologic observations were made on hematoxylin-eosin stained sections of the mid jejunum and mid cecum of 2 animals within each category and age group. Linear measurements of the depths of the villous layer, the crypts, the lamina propria and the circular and longitudinal layers of the muscularis were performed using an ocular micrometer. The mean values were calculated from pooled samples of each of the germfree, SPF and conventional pigs regardless of their age or diet fed.

Results

Under the conditions of this investigation the conventional pigs grew at about twice the rate as did both groups of the hysterectomy derived pigs reared in isolation. Of the latter, germfree pigs made somewhat better gains than did the SPF pigs and the pigs fed CM grew faster than their counterparts fed the SF (Table I).

TABLE I. Body Weights of Germfree (GF), Colostrum Deprived Contaminated (SPF) and Conventional Pigs

| Category | Body Weight in Kilograms* | | | |
	2 weeks	4 weeks	6 weeks	8 weeks
GF fed SF[1]	2.37 + 0.24	4.86 + 0.37	7.14 + 0.51	9.53 + 0.80
GF fed CM[2]	2.23 + 0.27	4.79 + 0.17	7.43 + 0.50	9.56 + 0.44
SPF fed SF	2.30 + 0.43	4.14 + 1.04	6.26 + 1.26	8.69 + 0.75
SPF fed CM	2.45 + 0.46	5.14 + 0.43	7.71 + 0.53	9.32 + 0.28
Convent.	4.44 + 0.91	8.26 + 1.64	14.23 + 1.23	19.59 + 1.40

[1]SF — Special Formula   [2]CM — Condensed Cows Milk
*The values represent means and standard deviations of 6 pigs within each category and age group.

The digestive tract of conventional pigs increased in weight at a much greater rate than did the GI tracts of both groups of the colostrum deprived pigs, particularly after 4 weeks of age (Table II). Unlike the slower body growth of the SPF pigs, their digestive tracts were heavier than the GI tracts of germfree pigs, both in absolute terms (Table II) and expressed as a percentage of body weight (Table III). The variations in body and GI tract weights at a given age, as well as most of the other parameters studied, were smaller in germfree pigs than in the pigs exposed to a microflora.

Expressed as a percentage of body weight, the small intestine of germfree pigs was smaller than that of the other groups and its relative size decreased as the age of the animal increased. The opposite was true in the case of conventional pigs. The ceca and colons were the heaviest in SPF pigs ranging from 1.0 to 1.6 and 1.6 to 3 per cent of body weight respectively. The corresponding values for germfree pigs were: ceca 0.2 to 0.4%, colons 1.0 to

TABLE II. Weights of the Gastrointestinal Tracts of Germfree (GF), Colostrum Deprived Contaminated (SPF) and Conventional Pigs

Category of pig	Weight of Gastrointestinal Tract in Grams*			
	2 weeks	4 weeks	6 weeks	8 weeks
Neonatal	(Birth 60.15 + 6.95)			
GF fed SF[1]	200 + 38.8	360 + 24.7	407 + 42.8	606 + 96.4
GF fed CM[2]	177 + 28.8	387 + 95.8	397 + 23.1	604 + 47.1
SPF fed SF	251 + 49.7	411 + 134.4	547 + 117.5	697 + 122.1
SPF fed CM	170 + 46.5	454 + 63.5	590 + 98.7	950 + 136.4
Convent.	383 + 31.7	441 + 82.4	1286 + 292.7	1950 + 174.2

[1]SF − Special Formula   [2]CM − Condensed Cows Milk
*The values represent means and standard deviations of 6 pigs within each category and age group, after overnight fast, and included the stomach contents and pancreas.

2.2%. In conventional pigs ceca were 0.3 to 0.6% and colons 1.2 to 1.9% of total body weight.

The percentage distribution by weight of the different tubular organs as compared to the weight of the total GI tract (Table IV) indicates that in relation to the neonate, all parts of the digestive tract of conventional pigs became progressively larger with increasing age, none gaining a particular predominance. In the SPF pig there was a significant increase in the size and weight of the colon and particularly of the cecum, which occurred within the first 2 weeks of life and persisted up to 8 weeks of age. In germfree pigs the relative size of the colon increased as the pigs grew older, while no such increase could be observed in the size of the cecum.

The wall of the intestinal tract of conventional pigs appeared relatively thick throughout its length with well developed Peyer's patches and mesenteric lymph nodes. The small intestines of germfree and SPF pigs were essentially

TABLE III. Weight of the Gastrointestinal Tract of Germfree (GF), SPF, and Conventional Pigs Compared to Body Weight

Category of pig	G.I. Tract − % of Body Weight*			
	2 weeks	4 weeks	6 weeks	8 weeks
Neonatal	(Birth: 4.66 + 0.4)			
GF fed SF[1]	8.83 + 1.63	7.71 + 0.42	5.64 + 0.41	6.40 + 0.68
GF fed CM[2]	8.64 + 0.91	7.48 + 2.03	5.20 + 0.47	6.21 + 0.63
SPF fed SF	11.45 + 1.23	9.84 + 2.75	9.05 + 1.15	7.70 + 1.03
SPF fed CM	9.04 + 1.81	8.88 + 1.33	7.45 + 1.03	9.74 + 1.08
Convent.	8.91 + 1.49	6.25 + 1.28	9.34 + 2.09	9.78 + 1.17

[1]SF − Special Formula   [2]CM − Condensed Cows Milk
*Means and standard deviations from 6 animals in each category and age group.

TABLE IV. Distribution by Weight of Segments of the Digestive Tract of Germfree (GF), SPF and Conventional Pigs

Category of pig	Organ	% Weight of Total GI Tract*			
		2 weeks	4 weeks	6 weeks	8 weeks
Neonatal		(at birth)			
	GI Tract, g	56.00			
	Stomach, %	12.44			
	Small int., %	64.93			
	Cecum, %	4.09			
	Colon,%	18.54			
GF fed SF[1]	GI Tract, g	171.44	327.90	378.96	547.49
	Stomach, %	9.57	11.23	13.54	12.85
	Small int., %	72.91	68.74	57.68	47.11
	Cecum, %	3.44	3.87	3.92	5.34
	Colon, %	14.08	16.16	24.86	34.70
GF fed CM[2]	GI Tract, g	153.69	337.70	378.71	533.68
	Stomach, %	10.69	11.46	13.33	11.19
	Small int., %	58.88	63.96	55.06	43.81
	Cecum, %	5.05	3.26	4.78	4.84
	Colon, %	25.38	21.32	26.83	40.16
SPF fed SF	GI Tract, g	204.89	340.92	510.86	611.71
	Stomach, %	7.50	8.10	8.91	10.43
	Small int., %	50.90	55.98	44.00	48.26
	Cecum, %	10.84	12.13	12.93	8.24
	Colon, %	30.76	23.79	34.16	33.07
SPF fed CM	GI Tract, g	147.97	395.82	554.40	868.51
	Stomach, %	9.49	9.17	8.69	6.77
	Small int., %	57.32	53.27	49.15	57.36
	Cecum, %	9.88	17.28	14.48	11.28
	Colon, %	23.31	20.28	27.68	24.59
Conventional	GI Tract, g	301.49	407.35	1096.40	1667.26
	Stomach, %	9.04	10.10	9.83	9.10
	Small int., %	63.08	62.20	60.72	59.86
	Cecum, %	4.74	5.85	4.93	6.95
	Colon, %	23.14	21.85	24.52	24.09

[1]SF – Special Formula   [2]CM – Condensed Cows Milk
*The total GI Tract weights represent the means from 6 pigs in each category and age group with stomach empty and pancreas removed.

similar in appearance, but the lymphoid tissue was more prominent in SPF pigs. The walls of the ceca and colons of germfree pigs were thin and translucent, while those of SPF pigs appeared denser and were light brown in color. There was an indication of an increase in the dry matter content per unit weight of the GI tract wall in all groups of pigs with increasing age (Table V). In an early age there was generally more dry matter per unit weight of empty small intestine in pigs associated with a microflora than in germfree pigs, but the reverse was true

TABLE V. Percentage of Dry Matter in the Gastrointestinal Tract Wall of Germfree (GF), SPF and Conventional Pigs

Category of Pig	Age in Weeks	% of Dry Matter in GI Tract Wall*					
		Stomach	Duodenum	Jejunum	Ileum	Cecum	Colon
Neonatal	0	13.3	18.0	18.6	18.6	17.6	12.0
GF fed SF[1]	2	15.2	19.5	19.0	16.0	15.5	16.0
GF fed CM[2]		15.7	18.3	19.3	15.6	18.7	16.6
SPF fed SF		15.2	20.7	19.7	18.2	17.7	16.5
SPF fed CM		15.6	19.9	18.9	18.0	17.1	17.1
Convent.		16.0	21.0	21.6	18.0	19.0	15.6
GF fed SF	8	19.0	21.0	22.3	21.0	24.3	22.3
GF fed CM		19.8	21.0	21.0	21.2	22.0	20.6
SPF fed SF		20.8	21.0	21.2	21.0	18.2	22.0
SPF fed CM		18.7	20.2	19.2	20.0	18.2	20.5
Convent.		19.6	20.3	20.0	18.6	20.6	20.0

[1]SF — Special Formula   [2]CM — Condensed Cows Milk
*Mean values from 3 to 5 animals in each category and age group.

at 8 weeks of age. The wet weight per unit length of the small intestine was the lowest in germfree pigs, followed by SPF pigs, and the highest in conventional pigs.

In general, the germfree pigs had longer jejunal villi, less volume of lamina propria, fewer reticuloendothelial cells in the lamina propria and a thinner muscular wall than the conventional pigs. The same parameters for the SPF pigs tended to be intermediate between the latter groups (Table VI and Figs. 1, 2). The cecal measurements tended to give results similar to those of the jejunum except that the crypt depth in the conventional pigs was significantly greater than in both germfree or SPF pigs (Table VI and Figs. 3, 4).

The percentage of dry matter in the contents of the small intestines was variable, being comparable in all groups, regardless of their microbial status or age. The ingesta became increasingly liquid in the lower ileum. The cecal and

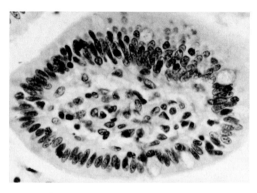

FIG. 1. Villus cross section, conventional pig 4 wks. Note reticuloendothelial (R.E.) cells in lamina propria (nuclei surrounded by granules are eosinophils) and in epithelium. X 200.

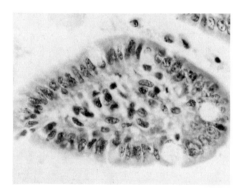

FIG. 2. Villus cross section, germfree pig 4 wks. Note reduction in area of lamina propria and in R.E. cells as compared to Fig. 1. X 200.

colon contents of germfree pigs were dark brown in color, became more liquid with increasing age and contained less dry matter than the light chocolate colored contents of SPF pig large intestines. The contents of the large intestines of conventional pigs had the highest percentage of dry matter (Table VII).

The pH values of the stomach contents of all groups of pigs regardless of age were about pH 4. The acidity gradually decreased along the small intestine being near the neutral point in the ileum. The contents of the ileum and of the large intestine were mildly alkaline in germfree pigs and near neutral or mildly acid in pigs exposed to bacteria (Table VII). Feeding of SF or CM to the germfree and SPF pigs resulted, in most instances, in only minor differences among the parameters studied.

TABLE VI. Mean Depths of Villus Layer, Lamina Propria and Smooth Muscle in the Intestine of Pigs

	Thickness of Layer in Microns:		
	Germfree	SPF	Conventional
		Jejunum	
Villus	640.0 + 118.4	656.8 + 213.6	472.8 + 162.4
Lamina propria	80.7 + 7.2	83.7 + 21.0	112.8 + 57.6
Muscularis (C)	84.7 + 24.0	108.0 + 27.2	168.0 + 63.2
Muscularis (L)	61.6 + 25.6	80.8 + 16.0	108.8 + 31.2
		Cecum	
Crypt	265.6 + 28.8	312.8 + 67.2	436.8 + 136.8
Lamina propria	27.0 + 6.9	26.1 + 9.6	54.0 + 28.5
Muscularis (C)	91.2 + 9.6	116.8 + 40.0	118.0 + 62.4
Muscularis (L)	53.6 + 14.4	48.8 + 18.4	86.4 + 26.4

C — Circular muscle layer   L — Longitudinal muscle layer

Conclusions

The digestive tract of germfree pigs differed from that of conventional pigs by its lower weight, reduced thickness and cellularity of the lamina propria and muscularis, poorer development of the associated lymph tissue, and by the liquid contents of the cecum and colon. These characteristics are essentially similar to those of other gnotobiotic animals with the notable exception of the cecum which was not enlarged as is the case with gnotobiotic rodents (1, 4, 5).

The digestive tract of colostrum deprived contaminated SPF pigs, although in some respects intermediate, resembled more closely the GI tract of germfree pigs than that of conventional pigs. Association with bacteria in the SPF pig stimulated the development of lymphoid tissue, and resulted in enlargement of the cecum and a reduced fluid content in the large intestine. While the latter may have occurred due to improved fluid absorption (1, 4) and due to bacterial cells forming part of the bulk of the contents, the cecal enlargement of the SPF pig remains unexplained.

The digestive tract of the SPF pigs was populated by the principal defined bacterial elements found in the intestines of young conventional pigs (6). It could be considered, therefore, that the development of the digestive tract and its function in the pig is influenced by its microflora, by circulating and local maternal antibody which was present only in the intestine of the conventional pig, and by nutritional factors which differed in colostrum deprived and conventional pigs.

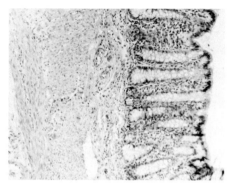

FIG. 3. Cecum, Conventional pig 4 wks. Note depth of crypts and muscularis and many R.E. cells in lamina propria. X 80.

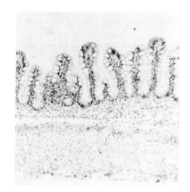

FIG. 4. Cecum, germfree pig 4 weeks. Note all layers of wall thinner than in Fig. 3 and fewer R.E. cells. X 80.

TABLE VII. Percentage of Dry Matter in the Contents of Colon of Germfree (GF), SPF and Conventional Pigs

Category of pig	Per cent of dry matter*			
	2 weeks	4 weeks	6 weeks	8 weeks
GF fed SF[1]	10.7 + 2.6	10.3 + 0.9	9.0 + 1.3	9.6 + 1.7
GF fed CM[2]	16.0 + 4.5	12.3 + 1.2	10.0 + 0.8	11.0 + 0.6
SPF fed SF	12.2 + 1.4	12.4 + 3.2	21.0 + 3.2	14.6 + 0.4
SPF fed CM	20.8 + 3.7	20.0 + 4.6	14.7 + 1.2	12.2 + 2.9
Convent.	24.3 + 3.8	24.6 + 3.7	25.3 + 6.2	21.0 + 1.6

[1]SF – Special Formula   [2]CM – Condensed Cows Milk
*Means and standard deviations from 3 to 5 animals in each category and age group.

TABLE VIII. pH Values of the Contents of Gastrointestinal Tract of 8 Week Old Germfree (GF), SPF and Conventional Pigs

Category of Pig	pH Values*					
	Stom-ach	Duo-denum	Jeju-num	Ileum	Ce-cum	Colon
GF fed SF[1]	4.06	6.24	6.16	7.16	8.35	7.67
GF fed CM[2]	5.34	6.43	6.33	7.33	8.07	7.05
SPF fed SF	3.82	6.50	6.59	6.34	6.77	6.69
SPF fed CM	3.90	6.32	6.37	6.67	7.30	6.96
Convent.	3.52	6.17	6.69	7.39	6.69	6.54

[1]SF — Special Formula   [2]CM — Condensed Cows Milk
*Mean values from 3 to 5 animals in each category.

Acknowledgement

Supported by MRC Grant 2082 and by the Ontario Department of Agriculture and Food.

References

1. Gordon, H. A., and Pesti, L., *Bact. Rev. 35:* 390 (1971).
2. Waxler, G. L., in "Diseases of Swine," (H. W. Dunne, ed.), Iowa St. Univ. Press, Ames, Iowa, 3rd ed., (1970).
3. Alexander, T. J., Miniats, O. P., Ingram, D. G., Thomson, R. G., and Thackeray, E. L., *Can. Vet. J. 10:* 98 (1969).
4. Luckey, T. D., *Germfree Life and Gnotobiology,* Acad. Press N.Y. and London, p. 283, (1963).
5. Gordon, H. A., Bruckner-Kardoss, E., Staley, T. E., Wagner, M., and Wostmann, B., *Acta Anat. 64:* 367 (1966).
6. Pesti, L., *Zentralbl. Bacteriol. Parasitenk, Infectionskr Hyg. Orig. 189:* 282 (1963).

EFFECTS OF GERMFREE RODENT'S CECAL CONTENTS ON SPONTANEOUS VILLUS MOVEMENT

E. Kokas

Department of Physiology, School of Medicine
University of North Carolina
Chapel Hill, North Carolina 27514

and

B. S. Wostmann* and *H. A. Gordon*
Department of Pharmacology, College of Medicine
University of Kentucky
Lexington, Kentucky 40506, U.S.A.

Introduction

It has been reported that the contents of the enlarged cecum of germfree rodents contain vasoactive substances which affect smooth muscle in a variety of preparations (1-3). Cecal contents from comparable conventional animals were either inactive or displayed activity in a very reduced form in these preparations. The present work concentrates on the effects of germfree and conventional rat cecal contents on the spontaneous motility of dog's intestinal villi, when topically applied to the mucosa. Villus activity consists of rhythmic contraction and relaxation of the fingerlike villi, whose movement can be well observed and quantitated. It has been known for some time that a number of vasoactive substances stimulate or depress this activity in a highly reproducible form (3).

Methods

Villus motility was observed on the exteriorized small intestinal mucosal surface in anaesthetized dogs (30 mg pentobarbital/kg bodyweight), with a stereomicroscope, under low power magnification (40X) (4). The rate of spontaneous contraction was counted in a quadrant of the visual field, before and after the topical application of the substance to be tested and the contraction index (CI) was computed:

*On sabbatical leave from Lobund Laboratory, Department of Microbiology, University of Notre Dame, Notre Dame, Indiana 46556, U.S.A.

$$CI = \frac{EC - BC}{BC}$$

(EC = experimental count; BC = basal count). The pH and osmolality of the substances were adjusted: pH 7.2, osmolality 0.9% NaCl equivalent (300 m Osm). Two drops of the test substances were applied on the mucosa and the dissipation of the sample from the visual area was prevented by a shallow cylindrical ring made of thin cardboard and placed on the mucosal surface. Counts were taken at 30 seconds after application, then at 2 minute intervals, each count lasting 30 seconds. Before application of a new substance, the mucosal surface was washed with 38°C saline and the basal level re-established. Basal villus contractions remained fairly steady in the individual animals during a 3 – 4 hour experiment. The stimulatory or depressant effects of a substance on villus motility is indicated by positive, negative or zero signs, depending on the contraction index.

Substances acting on villus contractility were isolated from rat cecal supernatant (15,000 g, 15 min) as follows. First, the supernatant was run through a cationic exchange column (Biorex 70, hydrogen form), using gradient elution with NaOH solution (0.01 to 0.25 N). This resulted in the separation to two pigmented fractions ("initial pool," negatively charged; "terminal pool," negatively charged to neutral). The terminal pool was further subjected to anionic exchange column chromatography (Bio-Rad AG 1-X4, hydroxyl form) using HCl solution as eluent (0.01 N). This caused the separation of the pigment into two fractions, named alpha and beta. Futher details of these procedures are given in one of our previous papers (3). Of these isolated fractions, initial pool depressed, alpha pigment enhanced villus motility. Beta pigment proved inactive. For further purification of the active fractions, gel filtration was used. In case of the initial pool, the gel of choice was Sephadex G 100, in case of alpha pigment, it was Sephadex G 50 (5, 6).

Cecal supernatants originating from germfree and conventional Fischer 344 (Charles River Breeding Laboratories, Wilmington, Mass.) rats fed diet L462 (7) were used as source material; similar to those studied in our previous work (3). In addition, the cecal supernatant derived from conventional rats treated orally for 42 days with antibiotics (bacitracin, streptomycin and nystatin) was used after similar chromatography and gel filtration. The latter were the same rats as described by Wiseman (8) in this publication.

Results

Alpha pigment. Table I lists substances occurring in the intestine which stimulate villus motility and which were tested in our previous work: alpha pigments isolated from germfree and conventional rats, ferritin, villikinin, bradykinin, serotonin, histamine and acetylcholine. The action of all these

586

TABLE I. Effects of Villus Stimulatory Agents[1]

	Germfree α-pigment	Conventional α-pigment	Ferritin	Villi-kinin	Brady-kinin	Serotonin	Histamine	Acetylcholine
No pretreatment	++	0, +	++	++	++	+	+	+
Pretreatment with blockers or degrading agents[1]	++[2-5]	.	++[2-5]	0[2]	0[2]	0[3]	0[4]	0[5]
O_2 atm, 6 hrs incub.	0	.	0	.	.	.	.	.
N_2 atm, 6 hrs incub.	++	.	++	.	.	.	.	.
Antiferritin serum, 2 hrs incub. N_2 atm	0	.	0	.	.	.	.	.
Trypsin, 12 hr incub. in N_2 atm	++	.	0	.	.	.	.	.
Trypsin, 12 hrs incub., then cecal flora in 48 hrs incub. in N_2 atm	0	.	0	.	.	.	.	.

1. For dosages and origin of stimulatory and blocking agents as well as for procedures mentioned in this Table, see ref. 3.
2. Carboxypeptidase B
3. d-Lysergic acid
4. Tripelenamine
5. Atropine

In this and subsequent Tables the following symbols are used for characterizing changes of the contraction index:

$$CI > 1.0 = {+}{+}$$
$$1.0 > CI > 0.3 = +$$
$$0.3 > CI > -0.2 = 0$$
$$-0.2 > CI > -0.5 = -$$
$$-0.5 > CI = -1.0 = --$$

No observation = .

agents could be neutralized by specific blockers or degrading enzymes. Germfree alpha pigment and ferritin were left unaffected by substances inactivating villikinin, bradykinin, serotonin, histamine and acetylcholine. The action of both these agents could be neutralized by oxygenation, while bioactivity was reestablished on removal of oxygen in nitrogen atmosphere. Both these agents were inactivated by incubation with antiferritin rabbit serum. Trypsinization was ineffective, while trypsinization followed by incubation with cecal flora inactivated both germfree alpha pigment and ferritin (3).

Ferritin is known to reach the intestinal lumen in sizable quantities on desquamation of the intestinal epithelium (Conrad *et al.* (9); Crosby (10)) where it is a protein involved in iron storage and/or transport. It was indicated by Mazur and Shorr (11) that ferritin exerts epinephrine inhibitory effects on smooth muscle. These findings are in accordance with our observations, since in lamina propria smooth muscle (which maintains villus movement), inhibition of exogenous or endogenous epinephrine has a stimulatory effect, whereas epinephrine activation has a depressant effect (12). Additional details on these issues, including aspects of dose and response quantitation, were given in our previous publication (3).

Table II shows the result of purification, and actions of alpha pigment and ferritin in further detail. Alpha pigment obtained from antibiotic treated conventional rats proved as effective a villus stimulant as germfree alpha pigment and ferritin. On purification by gel filtration, samples taken from the single peak of alpha pigments at molecular weight (MW) 4,800 (for additional details see

TABLE II. Effects of Native and Purified Alpha Pigment and Congeners

	Germfree rat α-pigment	Antibiotic treated rat[1] α-pigment	Conventional rat α-pigment	Ferritin
Derived by cationic and anionic chromatography	++	+,++	0,+	++ (native)[2]
Purified on Sephadex G 50	+,++[3]	+[4]	.	+ (digested)[5]
Approx. MW of compound	4800	4800	4900	3900[5]

[1]42 days antibiotic treatment (see text).

[2]Horse spleen, 2X cryst., Cd-free, GBI, Chagrin Fall, O. (MW 860,000, est.), 0.1 − 0.2 mg/ml.

[3]0.4 − 1.0 mg protein/ml

[4]0.2 mg protein/ml

[5]Digestion mix (ingredients, in mg): ferritin 25, glutahion 50, trypsin 20, chymotrypsin 20, Krebs-Henseleit solution to 10 ml; 5 hrs incubation at 37°C. In final dilution, 0.15 mg protein/ml.

Wostmann *et al.* (5)) originating from germfree or antibiotic treated conventional cecal supernatants, proved almost or as effective as the parent preparations. Ferritin when subjected to digestion by trypsin and chymotrypsin in the presence of sufficient glutathion, offered a MW peak at 3900 (5) which caused marked villus stimulation.

Summing up our findings on alpha pigment, the present data suggest a process in the course of which ferritin, a constituent of the intestinal epithelium, reaches the gut lumen in sizeable quantities. Here it is broken down by digestive enzymes to a smaller component of fairly uniform molecular weight, alpha pigment, which retains at the same time ferritin's epinephrine inhibitory, musculoactive property (i.e., it stimulates intestinal and depresses vascular smooth muscle). Though the molecular weight of alpha pigment is 4,800, some of it appears to reach the circulation. This is suggested by the following findings: a) the microvasculature in the germfree rat's mesentery is highly refractory to the vasoconstrictive effect of epinephrine (13); b) on surgical removal of the enlarged cecum in germfree rats (i.e., the large reservoir of cecal contents), the mesenteric vessel's epinephrine sensitivity is restored to normal (14); c) topical pretreatment of conventional rat's mesenteric vessels with germfree cecal supernatant renders them refractory to successively applied epinephrine (15). The congenerity of alpha pigment and ferritin is indicated also by the fact that the digestive degradation of ferritin of an unrelated source (horse spleen), resulted in a comparable, small molecular compound whose bioactivity was similar to from that of alpha pigment (5). In the gut of conventional rats the microflora appears to reduce the quantity and the activity of alpha pigment.

"Initial pool." To date only preliminary work has been done on the villus depressant (possibly epinephrine sensitizing) effect of initial pool fractions. Table III indicates that initial pools prepared from germfree or antibiotic treated conventional rat's cecal supernatants greatly depressed (often completely stopped) villus movement. Separation of initial pool by gel filtration resulted in a large molecular, muco-polysaccharide fraction (MW > 100,000 containing little pigment, and which was absent from initial pools prepared from conventional rat's cecal supernatant, see also ref. 6) which was devoid of any activity on the villus preparation. A "mucoprotein" fraction consisting of smaller molecular compounds (MW < 20,000 with a major component of approximately 6,000, which contained a sizable amount of pigment) markedly depressed villus motility. This fraction was present also in conventional controls but was not tested as yet on the villus preparation. Although in this context the term "mucoprotein" is used, this only indicates that the fraction contained protein and hexuronic acid, but these do not necessarily portray the villus active component. The nature of this component is unknown.

TABLE III. Effects of Native and of Purified Components of "Initial Pool"

| | Isolated from Cecal Supernatant of | |
	Germfree rat Initial Pool	Antibiotic treated rat Initial Pool
Derived by cationic chromatography	− −	− −
Fractions of gel filtration on Sephadex G 100		
(a) MW ⟩ 100,000 (mucopolysaccharide fraction)	0	.
(b) MW ⟨ 20,000 ("mucoprotein" fraction)	− −	.

[1]42 days antibiotic treatment (see text).

Conclusions

The indicated coexistence of epinephrine inhibitory and epinephrine sensitizing substances in the intestine, some of which presumably are more available for absorption than others, points to the possibility of a "metabolic imbalance" which may exist in germfree rodents. Such substances may be implicated in the depressed cardiovascular function (16) and in the maintenance of reduced intestinal muscle tone (17) which are found in these animals. In conventional counterparts the intestinal microflora appears to be engaged in the inactivation of some of these substances.

Acknowlegements

This work was supported by U.S. Public Health Service (Grants AM 04675 and AM 14621).

References

1. Gordon, H. A., *Nature (London) 205:* 571 (1965).
2. Gordon, H. A., *Ann. N. Y. Acad. Sci. 147:* 83 (1967).
3. Gordon, H. A., and Kokas, E., *Biochem. Pharmacol. 17:* 2333 (1968).
4. Kokas, E., and Johnston, C. J. Jr., *Am. J. Physiol. 208:* 1196 (1965).
5. Wostmann, B. S., Reddy, B. S., Bruckner-Kardoss, E., Gordon, H. A., and Singh, B., in "Germfree Research: Biological Effect of Gnotobiotic Environments," (J. B. Heneghan, ed.), Academic Press, New York, p. 261, (1973).
6. Gordon, H. A., and Wostmann, B. S., in "Germfree Research: Biological Effect of Gnotobiotic Environments," (J. B. Heneghan, ed.), Academic Press, New York, p. 593, (1973).

7. Wostmann, B. S., *Ann. N.Y. Acad. Sci. 78:* 175 (1959).
8. Wiseman, R. F., in "Germfree Research: Biological Effect of Gnotobiotic Environments," (J. B. Heneghan, ed.), Academic Press, New York, p. 441, (1973).
9. Conrad, M. E., Weintraub, L. R., and Crosby, W. H., *J. Clin. Invest. 43:* 963 (1964).
10. Crosby, W. H., *Blood 22:* 441 (1963).
11. Mazur, A., and Shorr, E., *J. Biol. Chem 176:* 771 (1948).
12. Kokas, E., and Gordon, H. A., *J. Pharmacol. & Exp. Ther. 180:* 56 (1972).
13. Baez, S., and Gordon, H. A., *J. Exp. Med. 134:* 846 (1971).
14. Baez, S., Bruckner, G., and Gordon, H. A., in "Germfree Research: Biological Effect of Gnotobiotic Environments," (J. B. Heneghan, ed.), Academic Press, New York, p. 527, (1973).
15. Bruckner, G., in "Germfree Research: Biological Effect of Gnotobiotic Environments," (J. B. Heneghan, ed.), Academic Press, New York, p. 535, (1973).
16. Wostmann, B. S., Bruckner-Kardoss, E., and Knight, P. L. Jr., *Proc. Soc. Exp. Biol. & Med. 128:* 137 (1968).
17. Gordon, H. A., Bruckner-Kardoss, E., Staley, T. E., Wagner, M., and Wostmann, B. S., *Acta Anat. 64:* 367 (1966).

CHRONIC MILD DIARRHEA IN GERMFREE RODENTS: A MODEL PORTRAYING HOST-FLORA SYNERGISM

H. A. Gordon and *B. S. Wostmann**
Department of Pharmacology, College of Medicine
University of Kentucky
Lexington, Kentucky 40506, U.S.A.

Introduction

Liquid contents of the lower bowel and diarrhea in germfree guinea pigs have been described by Nuttal and Thierfelder in 1896 (1). This observation, in varying degrees, has been repeated ever since in other germfree rodents throughout their life span. Meynell (2) has described similar conditions in antibiotic treated conventional mice. The occurrence of protracted diarrhea in orally antibiotic treated patients is commonly observed in clinical work.

The work of Beaver and Wostmann (3) on the dry matter of intestinal contents in germfree rats indicated an efflux of water into the cecum and possibly lower ileum of these animals. In the absorption of water from the lower small intestine, replacing the natural contents with saline, Csaky (4) found that in germfree rats there was an initial lag, but that the ultimate rate of water absorption was not different between germfree and conventional animals. Loeschke and Gordon (.5), working with the cecum of rats and replacing the contents with saline, observed that water absorption in germfree animals was sizably elevated in comparison to conventional controls. It was speculated that these phenomena in germfree animals can be explained by an accumulation of water attracting macromolecules in intestinal contents and that the intestinal mucosa in these hosts is unimpaired.

Lindstedt *et al.* (6) observed elevated fecal excretion of hexosamines in germfree rats. Combe and Pion (7) found in the lower bowel of germfree rats elevated levels of amino acids which are characteristic of mucoproteins. In the same animal material Loesche (8, 9) described elevated quantity of macromolecular mucopolysaccharides. Hoskins (10) described absence of mucinases in intestinal contents of germfree rats, while these enzymes were present in conventional controls. According to Gordon and Nakamura (11) the colloid

*On sabbatical leave from Lobund Laboratory, Department of Microbiology, University of Notre Dame, Notre Dame, Indiana.

osmotic pressure in the cecal supernatant from germfree rats and mice is considerably higher than in conventional controls or in the blood plasma of either germfree or conventional animals.

It appears that the impaired water absorption caused by the lack of the intestinal flora is conditioned also by another mechanism. Asano (12, 13) observed slightly reduced sodium and very low chloride ion concentrations in germfree rat cecal contents. Feeding chloride-yielding resin to these animals increased the chloride levels in the gut contents and considerably improved water absorption from the lower bowel. Qualitative similarity in intestinal constituents between germfree and antibiotic treated conventional rodents have been found by Wostmann et al. (14) and by Wiseman and Gordon (15).

The purpose of this work was to further elucidate the nature of the implicated components and the mechanism of water absorption inhibition which develop in the absence or modification of the intestinal flora.

Methods

Animals used in these studies were germfree and conventional young adult rats of both sexes (CDF, The Charles River Breeding Laboratories, Wilmington, Mass.) fed autoclaved L-462 diet. In addition, decontaminated conventional rats, which were fed bacitracin-streptomycin-nystatin in their drinking water as specified by Wiseman (16), formed another experimental group.

In the present work, the following parameters were studied in cecal supernatant (15,000 g, 10 min): a) Cl⁻, Chloridometer, Buchler Instruments, Fort Lee, N.J.; b) HCO_3 calculated from pH and pCO_2, determined in Gas Analyzer, Instrumentation Laboratory (IL), Boston, Mass.; c) Na^+, K^+, Flame Photometer, IL; d) Colloid osmotic pressure, method of Krogh and Nakazawa (17); and e) Colloid water attraction, using a flux-chamber, modified method of Ussing and Zerhan (18).

In addition, negatively charged colloids were partly purified and converted to acidic form by passing the cecal supernatant through a cationic exchange resin column (Biorex 70, Bio-Rad Labs, Richmond, Calif.). Their presence in the effluent fractions was ascertained by determinations of viscosity (Ostwald viscosimeter); titratable acidity also was determined in the same fractions.

Water absorption studies (5) from the ligated cecal sack in vivo were carried out as follows: The rats were anesthetized with urethane (150 mg/100 g bodyweight, sc.) and through an abdominal midline incision, the ileum and colon were ligated immediately at their emergence from the cecum; the major blood vessels of this area were left intact. Through a small opening cut into the apex of the cecum its contents were removed and the lumen was rinsed with isotonic saline. The body temperature of the animals was kept at $36 - 38°C$ by means of a heating pad and a lamp throughout the experiment. Volume changes of the cecal fluid were measured both volumetrically and with ^{14}C-polyethylene glycol (polyethylene-1,2-^{14}C-glycol, MW cca 4000, New England Nuclear Corp., Boston, Mass.). Dry weight determinations of the cecal wall were done after removal of all visible fat from the organ.

Results

Table I indicates that, in cecal supernatant prepared from conventional rats, the colloid osmotic pressure is essentially similar to that found in blood plasma. In comparison to this value, the levels observed in the germfree supernatant were considerably elevated. The colloid osmotic pressure of the cecal supernatant obtained from the antibiotic treated conventional rats indicated intermediate values. This table also indicates that, if germfree supernatant and a polyvinyl-pyrrolidone solution of plasma-like colloid osmotic pressure (or blood plasma) are placed respectively into either sides of a flux-chamber which is separated by a membrane impermeable for colloids, the germfree supernatant will draw liquid from the counter fluid at a sizable rate. Other characteristics of the negatively charged colloid fraction of germfree cecal

TABLE I. Characteristics of Colloids in Rat Cecal Supernatant (15,000 g, 10 min)

A. *Colloid Osmotic Pressure.* **Means and SD given for 4-11 rats/group
(Further characterized in Fig. 1; "Initial Pool" may not contain all COP-active material)**

Germfree	AT Conventional, 7 days* (bacitr-streptom-nystat)	Conventional
	mm Hg	
107 + 9	63 + 4	40 + 8

Prefiltration: 0.45 μ millipore; *Membrane:* pore r 24 Å, thickness 0.28 mm (Dialysis Membrane, Union Carbide, Chicago);
Counter liquid: 0.9% NaCl

*Length of antibiotic treatment

B. *Colloid Water Attraction.* Average from 0-4 hrs. observations

Germfree Cecal Supernatant *from* 2.5% PVP soln in saline (COP approx. 40 mm Hg)	4.4 + 1.0 μl/cm^2/hr

Measured in flux-chamber of approx. 8 ml volume, separated by same kind of membrane, 4.5 cm^2 area, atmospheric pressure maintained on either side of membrane, period of observation 3-4 hrs.

supernatant, purified by cationic chromatography ("initial pool") are illustrated in Figure 1. Here viscosity and hexuronic acid concentration showed two almost coinciding peaks, although in this and most other observations the highest viscosity value was found before hexuronic acid concentration was maximal. Titratable acidity values (H^+) were found more drawn out in the first few tubes, yet the highest ones appeared at the spot of the former two peaks. In the process of H^+ exchange by our resin, some sodium was retained by the material in this portion of the germfree cecal supernatant. Colloid osmotic pressure, in a somewhat delayed and drawn out form, showed an overall parallelism with the former characteristics.

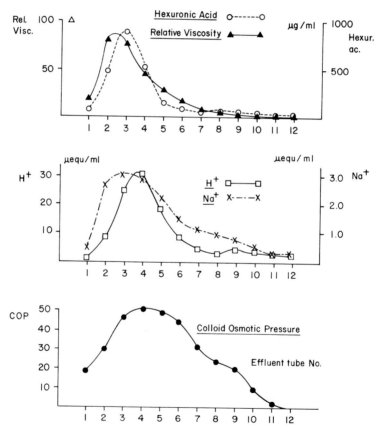

FIG. 1. Characteristics and solutes of effluent (first 12 tubes) from germfree rat cecal supernatant on cationic exchange resin column (Biorex 70, H^+). Gradient elution: 0.01-0.25 N NaOH. "Initial Pool"

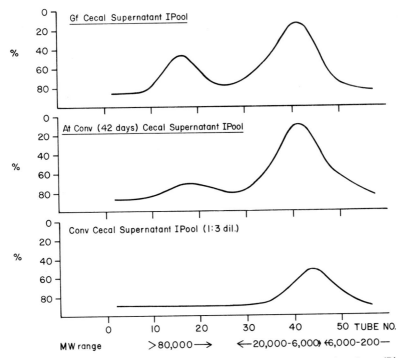

FIG. 2. Gel filtration (Sephadex 100) of effluent (tubes 3-4) from cationic column (Biorex 70, H⁺) (Maximum solute concentration in "Initial Pool"). Transmission at 253 mμ.

Figure 2 illustrates an attempt to establish by gel filtration the molecular weight of the substances that appear in the effluent at the peaks shown in the previous table. Two ranges were indicated. One range, which contained material with molecular weight higher than 80,000 and which showed little pigment, was clearly indicated in the germfree cecal supernatant and also was present in the supernatant of the antibiotic treated conventional rats. In conventional controls this part of the effluent was essentially "empty." A second group of substances showing less than 20,000 molecular weight and with a peak at approximately 6,000 and containing sizeable amounts of pigment, was about similar in all three investigated groups.

In Table II we have tried to draw an "ionic balance sheet" for the cecal supernatants of the three animals groups. Here we can not give numerical values for the macromolecular anions as yet, and their quantity is indicated only in approximation. The data show that no essential differences existed in cation concentrations among the three examined groups. Among anions, in the germfree supernatant, chloride and bicarbonate were very low, while muco-polysaccharide anions abounded. In conventional controls opposite conditions

597

TABLE II. Partial "Ionic Balance Sheet" of Cecal Supernatants (Undiluted)

	Cations		Anions		"Muco-	"Muco-
	Na$^+$	K$^+$	Cl$^-$	HCO$_3^-$	polysacch."	peptides"
		μequ/ml			)80,000	20,000-6,000
Germfree	61	17	0.6	8	+ + +	+ + +
At Conv (42 days)*	77	23	3.5		+ +	+ + +
Conventional	58	26	17	30	0	+ + +

*Length of antibiotic treatment.

existed. In the supernatant of antibiotic treated animals an intermediate state was indicated. In all cases, however, considerable and apparently comparable amounts of anions in the less than 20,000 molecular weight range were present.

TABLE III. Net Solute and Water Transport in Rat's Ligated Cecal Sack
(3 hr Experiment *in vivo*) When Natural Contents Are Replaced by Saline

	Na$^+$ absorption	K$^+$ efflux	Cl$^-$ absorption	HCO$_3^-$ efflux	Water absorption μl/0.1g dry wt./hr	Water absorption μl/100 μM Na$^+$
		μM/0.1g dry wt.*/hr				
Germfree	133 $\pm$ 25	14 $\pm$ 0	183 $\pm$ 24	63 $\pm$ 20	774 $\pm$ 145	581 $\pm$ 9
Conventional	41 $\pm$ 11	10 $\pm$ 2	95 $\pm$ 9	76?	190 $\pm$ 51	515 $\pm$ 20

*Dry weight of cecal wall
4 rats per group
Means and standard deviations

Table III illustrates an attempt to assay the ability of the cecal mucosa to transport ions and water when its contents were replaced by saline. Here it is indicated that the germfree cecal sack, when "relieved" from its natural contents and in conditions of isotonicity, showed elevated net transport of sodium, chloride and water per unit dry wall weight compared to conventional controls. However, when the amount of water was expressed per unit of transported sodium, then no sizable differences were found between the opposing groups. Figure 3 illustrates the relationship between net water transport from the cecum and the availability of diffusible ions and the presence of colloids, respectively. In case the supply of sodium and chloride were adequate and no colloids were present, water transport was at a high level. If the diffusible solute's concentration was equally adequate, but colloid was present (causing the colloid osmotic pressure to be equivalent to that of germfree cecal supernatant), water

NET WATER TRANSPORT IN GERMFREE RAT'S LIGATED CECAL SACK (3 hrs. experiment in vivo) WHEN NATURAL CONTENTS ARE REPLACED BY SIMILAR AMOUNTS OF:

	GF CECAL SUPERNATANT	10% PVP IN SALINE	SALINE
Na$^+$, µequ/ml $\rightarrow$	60	130	140
Cl$^-$, µequ/ml $\rightarrow$	1	130	140
Colloid osmotic pressure mm Hg $\rightarrow$	110	120	0

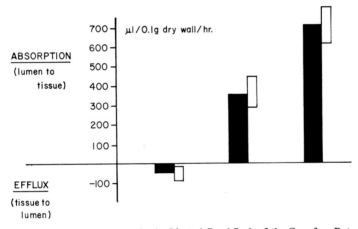

FIG. 3. Net Water Transport in the Ligated Cecal Sack of the Germfree Rat.

absorption from the cecum was considerably reduced. A complete stop of absorption, or even a slight efflux of water from the tissues to the lumen, could be achieved when natural colloid concentration was high and diffusible negative ion concentration inadequate (presently illustrated by placing germfree cecal supernatant into the cecal sack).

Discussion

This work in general confirms previous findings on the following characteristics of germfree rodent's cecal contents: a) considerably reduced concentration of chloride and essentially normal levels of sodium (12, 13); b) increased quantity of macromolecular compounds of mucopolysaccharide nature (6-9, 14); and c) elevated colloid osmotic pressure (11).

The reduced water absorption from the cecum of germfree rodents can be explained on the basis of the preponderance of water retentive force, colloid water attraction, in cecal contents and on the reduced availability of ions needed for mucosal solute coupled water absorption. Sodium, the principal ion needed in this process, though it is present in adequate amounts, is accompanied by low levels of diffusible anions (chloride, bicarbonate) and is thus not available in needed quantity. In addition, the data in Figure 1 suggest that the acidic colloids in cecal contents may sequester sizable amounts of sodium. The nature and role of macromolecular compounds in the less than 20,000 molecular weight range, which apparently occur in similar amounts in both germfree and conventional cecal contents, need further investigation.

At the root of water absorption inhibition from the lower bowel of germfree rodents appears to be the lack of mucinases in intestinal contents of these animals (10). These might act by both degrading water retentive colloids and indirectly, by thus "making more room" for, and possibly producing diffusible anions. In this light, elements of the intestinal flora supplying mucinases must be considered as true synergists of the host. The observations, that neutralization of the intestinal flora by antibiotics in conventional animals precipitates germfree-like conditions of water absorption inhibition, might explain the mechanism of diarrheas which are observed on oral antibiotic treatment in clinical work.

Summary

Conditions existing in the cecum of germfree and orally antibiotic treated conventional rodents inhibit water absorption at least on two counts: a) the accumulated colloids attract water into the cecal lumen with considerable force, and b) undegraded negatively charged colloids of mucopolysaccharide nature which are not available for absorption, sequester a large proportion of diffusible cations within the lumen. The diffusible anions and corresponding cations are insufficient for maintaining the active process of "solute coupled water transport" across the mucosal membrane. On replacing the cecum's natural contents with saline, normal or even elevated levels of water absorption have been observed. In conventional rodents the flora apparently degrades colloids to absorbable compounds, eliminating thus their water-retentive force and permitting the establishment of diffusible anion and cation concentrations conducive to the absorption of water.

Acknowledgements

This work was supported by U.S. Public Health Service (Grants AM 14621 and HD 00855).

We thank Messrs. B. F. Schwartz and R. W. Valentine for their help.

References

1. Nuttal, G. H. F., and Thierfelder, H., *Hoppe Seyler's Z. Physiol. Chem. 22:* 62 (1896).
2. Meynell, G. G., *Brit. J. Exp. Pathol. 44:* 209 (1963).
3. Beaver, M. H., and Wostmann, B. S., *Brit. J. Pharmacol. 19:* 385 (1962).
4. Csaky, T. Z., in "The Germfree Animal in Research," (M. E. Coates, ed.), Academic Press, Inc., New York, p. 151, (1968).
5. Loeschke, K. and Gordon, H. A., *Proc. Soc. Exp. Biol. Med. 133:* 1217 (1968).
6. Lindstedt, G., Lindstedt, S., and Gustafsson, B. E., *J. Exp. Med. 121:* 201 (1965).
7. Combe, E., and Pion, R., *Ann. Biol. Anim. Bioch. Biophys. 6:* 255 (1966).
8. Loesche, W. J., *Proc. Soc. Exp. Biol. Med. 128:* 195 (1968).
9. Loesche, W. J., *Proc. Soc. Exp. Biol. Med. 129:* 380 (1968).
10. Hoskins, L. C., *Gastroenterology 54:* 218 (1968).
11. Gordon, H. A., and Nakamura, S., 8th Annual Meeting Assn. Gnotobiotics, Oak Ridge National Laboratory, Oak Ridge, Tenn., Abtr. No. 3, (1969).
12. Asano, T., *Proc. Soc. Exp. Biol. Med. 131:* 1201 (1969).
13. Asano, T., *Amer. J. Physiol. 217:* 911 (1969).
14. Wostmann, B. S., Reddy, B. S., Bruckner-Kardoss, E., Gordon, H. A., and Singh, B., in "Germfree Research: Biological Effect of Gnotobiotic Environments," (J. B. Heneghan, ed.), Academic Press, New York, p. 261, (1973).
15. Wiseman, R. F., and Gordon, H. A., *J. Lab. Clin. Med. 78:* 834 (1971).
16. Wiseman, R. F., in "Germfree Research: Biological Effect of Gnotobiotic Environments," (J. B. Heneghan, ed.), Academic Press, New York, p. 441, (1973).
17. Krogh, A., and Nakazawa, F. *Biochem. Z. 188:* 240 (1927).
18. Ussing, H. H., and Zerhan, K., *Acta Physiol. Scand. 23:* 110 (1951).

601

SECTION XII

GNOTOBIOTIC TECHNOLOGY

A LIGHTWEIGHT STAINLESS STEEL ISOLATION SYSTEM FOR ADULT GNOTOBIOTIC DOGS

James G. Linsley and *Charles E. Yale*
Department of Surgery, University of Wisconsin Medical School
1300 University Avenue, Madison, Wisconsin 53706, USA

Introduction

The adult gnotobiotic dog is infrequently used in biomedical research because of the difficulties encountered in housing these animals for long periods of time. A previously reported isolation system (1) has been recently modified. This report describes these modifications and the results of a 168 day study on the efficiency and safety of four of these units.

Materials and Methods

Description of the isolation system. The modified isolation system (FIGS. 1 and 2) consists of the isolator, an inlet and an outlet air filter, a feed hopper, a water tank and roller pump, and a waste tank. The isolator is divided by removable metal doors into two cages, each 48 in. wide (W) x 36 in. deep (D) x 36 in. high (H), and a 96 in. W x 18 in. D work area along the front. The isolator is serviced by a pair of gloves on either side of an 18 in. diam entry port. The principal modifications in the isolator were a change in the shape of the work area, the installation of larger windows (now sealed with RTV-630A&B, General Electric Silicone Product) and the use of a new 18 in. diam inner door (2). The inlet filter was essentially unchanged, but the outlet filter was altered so that the air leaves the filter through a 3 in. diam orifice. The water and waste tanks were enlarged to hold 160 and 190 gallons of water, respectively. An internal heating-cooling coil was built into the water tank. A conical feed hopper, 28 in. H x 44 in. diam, was mounted on top of the isolator.

The isolator, with its attached filters, is sterilized in a large high pressure steam autoclave. The full water tank, and the empty waste tank and feed hopper are steam sterilized and connected to the isolator. Pelleted dog feed is autoclaved in a large cuboidal sterilizing chamber and pneumatically transferred to the feed hopper on top of the isolator (3).

Evaluation of the isolation system. Four isolation systems and four

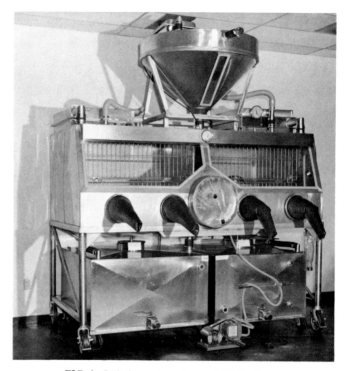

FIG. 1. Isolation system for gnotobiotic dogs.

Cesarean derived gnotobiotic dogs of each sex were used in the 168 day study. All animals had been reared in the isolation systems and were at least one year old at the start of the tests. The males weighed an average of 18.2 kg and the females, 17.0 kg.

Balance studies were done on the feed and water consumption and waste production occurring in each isolator by weighing these commodities in and out of the system.

Efficiency studies detailed the time needed to perform each step in the care of the animals and the isolation system. For example, the time necessary to clean the isolator, and feed and water the dogs once each day was recorded as the animal care time; and the man-hours necessary to remove, empty, clean, inspect, sterilize and reattach the waste tank was designated as the waste tank recycle time.

The safety of the system was evaluated by careful weekly inspections, and by composite cultures, every 28 days, of the surfaces and supplies within the isolator, and the animals' urine and feces. A variety of media was used to insure the growth of yeasts, and of aerobic and anaerobic bacteria.

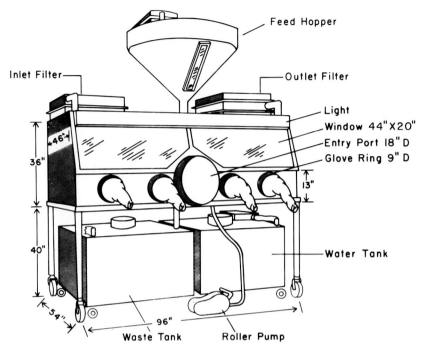

FIG. 2. Schematic drawing of the isolation system for gnotobiotic dogs.

Results

The *balance studies* (Table I) showed that each dog ate an average of 350 g of pelleted dog feed per day; that an average of 7.5 kg of water per dog per day were used to service and clean the isolator; and that the water tank needed recycling every 33 days (for the two dogs in each isolator).

The *efficiency studies* (Table II) indicate that it took an average of 4.8 min

TABLE I. Summary of Balance Studies.

	Feed used g/dog/day	Water used kg/dog/day	Waste produced kg/dog/day
No. of tests	9	19	12
Range	300-410	4.4-9.0	4.0-7.9
Average	350	7.5	6.6
Tank capacity, kg	100	500	700
Length of cycle, days/dog	286	67	106

TABLE II. Summary of Efficiency Studies.

	No. of Tests	Range	Average
Isolator sterilization & assembly, hr	4	15-20	18
Animal care, min/dog/day	672	3.3-5.5	4.8
Inspection, min/isolator	96	18-30	28
Water tank recycle, min	19	50-105	75
Waste tank recycle, min	13	89-150	115
Feed transfer, min	8	90-160	120
Total labor, min/dog/day	4	8.1-10.7	9.4

per dog per day to care for the animals in the isolator. When the time necessary to inspect and culture the isolator, sterilize and transfer the feed, and recycle the water and waste tanks was added to the in-isolator animal care time, the total labor required to maintain a gnotobiotic dog rose to 9.4 min per dog per day.

The *safety studies* (Table III) revealed that five breaks in isolation

TABLE III. Summary of Safety Studies.

No. of isolation systems	4
No. of adult dogs/isolator	2
	(1 of each sex)
Duration of study, isolator days	672
No. of paired glove entries	1695
No. of transfers	43
No. of isolator inspections	96
No. of breaks in isolation	5*
No. of cultures/isolator	7
Qualitative change in isolator flora	none

*2 equipment and 3 personnel.

occurred during the 672 isolator days of the study. Two breaks were due to equipment failures — one was a torn glove and the other, a tear in a small plastic bag attached to the isolator (used to pass out culture tubes). Three breaks were attributed to personnel failures — two were due to a loose connection between the feed hopper and the isolator, and the third was caused by a loose inspection door on a waste tank.

Two of the isolators contained bicontaminated dogs *(Candida albicans* and *Staphylococcus epidermidis)*, while the other two had animals contaminated with bacteroides, clostridia, lactobacilli, staphylococci, and *Escherichia coli.* The initial, interval, and final cultures from each isolator showed a constant, or unchanging, flora during the 24 weeks of the study.

Discussion

The University of Wisconsin Medical School Animal Care Unit has found that it takes 7.1 min per day to care for a conventional dog in a standard cage and 8.8 min per day in a metabolism cage. The daily care time (with once a day feeding and cleaning) for a dog in our isolator was 4.8 min. Even our total labor time of 9.4 min per dog per day compares favorably with the conventional care times.

The present dog isolation system has been under development since 1964. Some of the animals used in this study have lived in the system for more than four years. To all outward appearances, their health could not be better. During the present study, one female had two litters of pups. Without help or interference, she weaned two of the four pups of the first, and all four pups of the second litter. This is somewhat unscientific testimony to the quality of the environment provided by this safe and efficient dog isolation system.

Conclusions

A lightweight stainless steel isolation system for the long term housing of adult gnotobiotic dogs was described. This is a safe and efficient system which provides an environment conducive to the good health of the animals during growth, development, and reproduction.

Acknowledgements

This research was supported in part by Public Health Service Grant AI 06956 from the National Institute of Allergy and Infectious Diseases.

References

1. Yale, C. E., *Lab. Anim. Care 19:* 103 (1969).
2. Yale, C. E., *Lab. Anim. Sci. 21:* 588 (1971).
3. Yale, C. E., *Appl. Microbiol. 17:* 291 (1969).

RAISING GERMFREE BABOONS (*PAPIO CYNOCEPHALUS*)

S. S. Kalter, J. Eichberg and *R. L. Heberling*
Southwest Foundation for Research and Education
San Antonio, Texas 78284, U.S.A.

Introduction

A number of laboratories are currently engaged in the study of germfree life. Activities associated with the use of animals raised under germfree conditions involve different biologic areas. Perhaps most important consideration is rearing a "pure" animal under standardized conditions in a controlled environment. It should be recognized, however, that an animal living under such conditions must be considered as unique in the sense that the germfree state is not a normal manner for existence. Also antigenic stimulation does occur as a result of ingestion of food and the presence of dead bacteria and other organisms. Lastly, it must be recognized that vertical transmission of viruses through the placenta from mother to offspring occurs with regular frequency so that "germfree" should be construed as a relative term. A number of reviews are available providing general information and background material of interest for those desiring such material (1-4).

Rats, chickens and guinea pigs are the animals most commonly used in germfree research, although such animals as dogs, swine and even larger animals as the horse and cow have been raised under these conditions for a period of time. Use of germfree nonhuman primates has been extremely limited (5-8), however, Valerio *et al.* (9) have recently described rearing conventional rhesus infants in modified germfree isolators. It is the purpose of this report to provide information relating to our experiences in the maintenance of germfree baboons (*Papio cynocephalus*).

Results

General conditions. Probably the greatest limiting factor in raising germfree simians is the need for breeding facilities which are obviously necessary for the contemplation of this type of program. Existence of a number of centers for the breeding of monkeys and apes, therefore, permits the development of germfree colonies employing procedures currently in use for other animals. In addition to breeding facilities, laboratories capable of monitoring these animals, especially for bacterial and viral infections resulting from vertical transmission or a break in technique, is also essential. Thus, all animals (mothers as well as infants) are monitored for the presence or absence of microorganisms. Serologic surveillance for antibodies and procedures for the isolation of organisms from throat, rectal and tissue specimens are standard to most microbiological laboratories and are those used by us (10-11).

Rearing techniques. Germfree baboon infants were obtained by methods similar to those used for other species of animals. Cesarean sections as modified by Thimm *et al.* (12) for delivery of various species animals, were employed for deriving baboon infants. A polyvinylchloride (PVC) plastic film sealed to form a completely closed bag or an ordinary plastic sack fitted with surgical gloves and then sterilized with peracetic acid was used to facilitate germfree surgery. This sack was then placed over the prepared abdominal area of the pregnant anesthetized baboon and attached with adhesive spray. Because our isolators hold two animals comfortably, we generally do two sections simultaneously. The flexible surgical field offered a good visual perspective and permitted the surgeon to pass the infants into the attached isolator if there was no break in sterility technique during the operation. An assistant received the infant through the air lock of the isolator then obtained the various desired samples: blood was taken from the umbilical cord which was then clamped, rectal and throat swabs were then collected and the infant dried with a towel. At this stage it has been found that cord blood was more readily accessible than attempting venipuncture. The surgical sack is cut from the isolator air lock and the mothers are given conventional postoperative care.

Post delivery care of the infants may necessitate maintaining a temperature of approximately 85°F. This was safely accomplished by appropriately placing infra-red lamps outside the isolator. Infants were fed on SMA iron fortified (Wyeth Laboratories, Inc., Philadelphia, Pa.) diluted 1:1.1 with water prior to sterilization by autoclaving. Dilution of 1:1 resulted in a perineal rash, not seen when this same dilution was used with the regular SMA. Infants were given formula 4-5 times daily in ordinary baby bottles and nipples maintained in the isolator. At approximately 1-2 weeks the infants became capable of feeding themselves from a bottle, fixed to the cage. After two months the babies were offered autoclaved monkey chow pellets (Ralston-Purina Co., Fremont, Mich.) softened in milk. Weight gains have been comparable to conventional animals raised in incubators.

Summary of Data

The results to date suggest that the program described above may be successfully employed for raising germfree simians. Leucocyte counts were somewhat lower than conventional animals but this may be a reflection of a number of factors. Immunoglobulin in the form of IgG was present at birth but declined markedly within 3 weeks in contrast to that seen in conventional animals. IgM was not present at birth but a low level was apparent after approximately one week followed by a decline. IgA was not detected in sera of any of the animals up to 4-5 weeks following delivery. Eleven animals have been raised under these conditions, the oldest animal is now over 7 months of age. Most germfree baboons have been used for experimental purposes, details of these experiments have been reported elsewhere (13).

Acknowledgements

This study was funded in part by U.S.P.H.S. grant RR00361 and WHO grant Z2/181/27. This laboratory serves as the WHO Regional Reference Centre for Simian Viruses. Dr. Eichberg is a Visiting Scientist sponsored by the Deutsche Forschungsgemeinschaft, Bad Godesberg.

References

1. Reyniers, J. A., Editor, "Germfree Vertebrates: Present Status," *Ann. N. Y. Acad. Sci. 78:* 1 (1959).
2. Coates, M. E., Editor, "The Germfree Animal in Research," Academic Press, London (1968).
3. Gordon, H. A., and Pesti, L., *Bact. Rev. 35:* 390 (1972).
4. National Academy of Science, "Gnotobiotics," Natl. Acad. Sci., Washington, (1970).
5. Reyniers, J. A., *J. Bact. 43:* 778 (1942).
6. Reyniers, J. A., and Trexler, P. C., in "Micrurgical and Germfree Techniques: Their Application To Experimental Biology and Medicine," (J. A. Reyniers, ed.), C. C. Thomas, Springfield, p. 114, (1943).
7. Brant, H. G., Kundzines, N., Reese, W. H., and Keber, W. T., *Lab Anim. Care 13:* 557 (1963).
8. Wolfe, L., Griesemer, R., Rohovsky, M., *Lab. Anim. Care 16:* 364 (1966).
9. Valerio, D. A., Darrow, C. C. II, Martin, D. P., *Lab. Anim. Care 20:* 713 (1970).
10. Kalter, S. S., "Procedures for Routine Laboratory Diagnosis of Virus and Rickettsial Diseases," Burgess Publishing Co., Minneapolis, (1963).
11. Lennette, E. H., and Schmidt, N. J., Editors, "Diagnostic Procedures for Viral and Rickettsial Infections," 4th edition, American Public Health Assoc., New York, (1969).
12. Thimm, H. J., Hiller, H. H., Eichberg, J., and Juhn, N. C., *Z. Versuchsteirk 11:* 281 (1969).
13. Heberling, R. L., Eichberg, J., and Kalter, S. S., *Bact. Proc.,* (1972).

THE ESTABLISHMENT OF A DEFINED HAMSTER COLONY
UTILIZING GNOTOBIOTIC TECHNIQUES

Gilbert M. Slater and *Barbara J. Anastor*
Lakeview Hamster Colony
Newfield, New Jersey 08344, U.S.A.

Introduction

For the past year we have been involved in a full-time project to derive a germfree hamster. During this time we have made progress and have learned enough to be optimistic about our eventual success. However, it became obvious that the project would take time and that we should consider an interim technique to provide "clean" hamsters, free of internal and external parasites, common viruses, and "wet-tail."

We decided to attack the problem in five phases: Phase 1 — Eliminate PVM and SV-5, the two viruses for which conventional Lakeview hamsters have a positive titer, Phase 2 — Eliminate *Syphacia obvelata*, Phase 3 — Reduce and define gut flora, Phase 4 — Reduce surface bacteria, and Phase 5 — Establish a beneficial flora.

Results

Phase 1 — Eliminate PVM and SV-5 Viruses. Routine testing in our hamster colonies for 12 viruses indicates the presence of antibodies to PVM and SV-5. The incidence of these two is approximately 30-50%. Therefore, we felt that we could successfully select and isolate some animals that were free of both viruses (1, 2). We isolated a group of 25 female and 10 male hamsters in individual filtered cages. These hamsters were bled from the orbital sinus and serum samples were sent to our corporate virus diagnostic laboratory in Wilmington, Massachusetts. Two of the 25 females and two of the 10 males were negative for antibodies to PVM and SV-5. These four hamsters were moved to a laminar flow isolation area (Bio-Clean 100) and mated. During pregnancy, they were again tested and found to be negative for all viruses. Two resulting litters, totaling 16 males and 14 females, were then started on Phase 2.

Phase 2 — Eliminate *S. obvelata*. Dyrex (Fort Dodge Labs) has previously been proven effective in eliminating *S. obvelata* (3). Therefore, these 30 hamsters were given Dyrex in their drinking water at a level of 1.5 g/liter. At an average consumption of 10 ml of water per day, this provided 15 mg/day of Dyrex per hamster. In order to reduce coprophagy to a minimum, wire mesh inserts were placed in the bottom of standard polypropylene hamster cages. The inserts allowed about one inch of space at the bottom of the cage and this space was filled with a concentrated germicide solution. Medication with Dyrex was continued until two subsequent fecal samples were negative for *S. obvelata.*

Phase 3 — Reduce and Define Gut Flora. Lattuada (4) and Spaulding (5) described methods of intestinal asepsis, and Hagen (6) reported on the intestinal microflora of normal hamsters. As hamsters are rather sensitive to some types of antibiotics, we decided to simplify the technique and reduce the number of antibiotics to the minimum necessary to accomplish our objective. Neomix (neomycin sulfate — Upjohn Co.) was selected as the primary treatment and was added to the drinking water at a level of .02 mg/ml. After one week on Neomix, the hamsters were given four doses of 2.5 mg of Chloromycetin (chloramphenicol — Parke Davis Co.) by intubation. Thus, the hamsters received a total of 10 mg Chloromycetin over a period of 24 hrs. Immediately after the last dose, the hamsters were prepared for Phase 4.

Phase 4 — Reduce Surface Bacteria. A surgical and a holding isolator were set up and sterilized in preparation for Phase 4. Swabs taken at air inlets, outlets, gloves and several locations within the isolator bags verified the sterility of the two units. After the holding isolator was ventilated for 24 hrs, six Charles River CD-1 mice (Crl:CD-1 (ICR) BR) associated with Schaedler Flora were introduced. The surgical isolator was equipped with a 3 in. rigid plastic tube stoppered at both ends, generally used during Cesarean derivations. The outside end of this tube was immersed in a container of Wescodyne (West Chemical Company) and water, and both stoppers removed. The treated hamsters were then placed in the Wescodyne one at a time and allowed to swim for about 30 sec. At this time, the hamster was pushed under the surface, directed to the submerged end of the tube and allowed to swim up the tube. A second technician reached down the tube with long forceps, grasped the hamster and pulled it into the cage within the isolator. In this manner the Wescodyne penetrated the fur completely and covered all areas of skin. After a brief rest and drying period, the hamsters were placed in sterile plastic cups and passed via a transfer sleeve from the surgical isolator to the 5 ft holding isolator for Phase 5. Swabs taken from feces and the anal area indicated the presence of *Streptococcus faecalis* and an aerobacter species.

Phase 5 — Establish a Beneficial Flora. When the hamsters were settled in cages, fresh mouse feces were mixed in their drinking water. This "cocktail" was made fresh daily and continued for one week. Swabs of feces and isolator surfaces indicated the presence of *S. faecalis,* aerobacter, bacteroides, *Echerichia coli,* lactobacillus, streptococcus, and a fusiform bacillus. The enterococcus and clostridium from the original Schaedler Flora apparently did not establish themselves.

This nucleus was expanded within isolators to a group of 75 hamsters. To insure a broad gene pool, a series of 42 Cesarean derived litters was passed into isolators and foster nursed on associated mothers (7). The Cesareans resulted in a pool of 315 hamsters (143 males and 172 females). All of the females and 50 males were then prepared for transfer to a mobile laboratory. Transfer was accomplished by placing groups of 10 animals in sterilized paper bags which were passed out of the isolators. The bags were placed in plastic containers, which were then sprayed with peracetic acid and passed into the mobile laboratory through a port in the personnel lock.

The mobile laboratory is a windowless, 12 ft x 60 ft unit into which was built a series of personnel entry locks. The unit, with all equipment in place, was gassed with formaldehyde one week prior to entry of the hamsters by heating Formaldygen (Vineland Labs). Since the initial gassing, the mobile laboratory has been operated as a barrier building (8, 9). All personnel dress in full Dacron coveralls, masks and gloves. All entering material is either sprayed twice with peracetic acid or wiped down with a germicide.

The unit has been in operation for some 10 months. During this time approximately 20,000 hamsters have been born. At this time, the virus profile remains unchanged, *S. obvelata* is absent, and we have not observed clinical signs consistent with "wet-tail" or any similar disease problem.

Conclusions

While our objective continues to be the derivation of a germfree hamster, we feel that a suitable interim measure has been developed. A program of selection, chemotherapy, isolation, and association has produced a hamster free of all common hamster problems.

We have also proven to our satisfaction that mobile laboratories, properly equipped and operated, can provide quick space at a reasonable cost, and are secure enough for special animal projects.

References

1. Trentin, J. J., Van Hoosier, G. L. Jr., Shields, J., Stephens, K., Stenback, W. A., and Parker, J. S., "Viruses of Laboratory Rodents," (R. Holdenried, ed.), NCI Monograph 20: p.147, (1966).
2. Van Hoosier, G. L. Jr., Stenback, W. A., Parker, J. C., Burke, J. G., and Trentin, J. J., *Lab. Anim. Care 20:* 232 (1970).
3. Arthur, B. W., and Casida, J. E., *J. Agr. Food Chem. 5:* 186 (1957).
4. Lattuada, C. P., Schmidt, A. R., Paust, J., and Barmore, D. E., "Scientific Abstracts, Symposium on Gnotobiotic Research," p. 43, Madison, Wisconsin (1967).
5. Spaulding, E. H., Tyson, R. R., Harris, M. J., Jacobs, B., Wildrich, L., and Johnson, K.

O., Antibiotics Annual, p. 236, (1957).

6. Hagen, C. A., Shefner, A. M., and Ehrlich, R., *Lab. Anim. Care 15:* 185 (1965).
7. Burke, J. G., Van Hoosier, G. L. Jr., and Trenton, J. J., *Lab. Anim. Care 20:* 238 (1970).
8. Foster, H. L., Foster, S. J., and Pfau, E. S., *Lab. Anim. Care 13:* 711 (1963).
9. Foster, H. L., and Pfau, E. S., *Lab. Anim. Care 13:* 629 (1963).

STUDIES ON REARING THE HAMSTER GERMFREE

Howard J. Bohner
Division of Research Services, Veterinary Resources Branch
National Institutes of Health, Bethesda, Maryland 20014

and

Carl E. Miller
National Cancer Institute, National Institutes of Health
Bethesda, Maryland 20014, U.S.A.

Introduction

In the 1960's some of our associates at the National Institutes of Health (NIH) working with problems in biomedical research expressed interest in the germfree hamster (*Mesocricetus auratus*). Encouraged by development of successful techniques by J.R. Pleasants (1) and others for hand feeding of germfree mice and rats, a project to develop a method of rearing a germfree hamster was undertaken in the Germfree Unit, Veterinary Resources Branch, Division of Research Services at the NIH. More than 100 litters of hamsters have been used in an attempt to establish a germfree colony of this species. Studies were conducted in both the conventional and germfree environments. Attempts were made first in the conventional environment, and techniques developed were adapted for use in the germfree environment.

Materials and Methods

Equipment. Flexible plastic rearing isolators 24 in. x 24 in. x 60 in. were constructed on 1/2 in. transite bases. The temperature in the isolator was controlled by regulating steam flow through 1/4 in. i.d. coils located on the underside. Humidity was controlled by water in pans and restricting air flow through the isolator. Germfree animals were obtained by hysterectomy using Foster's method (2), except that we used 1:750 dilution of Zephiran in the dip tank. When possible, the hysterectomy was performed after the female had delivered one neonate, thus assuring maturity of the remaining fetuses.

Small colonies of conventional white tailed rats (*Mystromys albicaudatus*), spiny mice (*Acomys dimidiatus*), and mongolian gerbils (*Meriones unguiculatus*) were established to provide animals for trials as possible foster mothers for hamster pups.

Rearing Techniques. The non-inbred Sprague-Dawley rat (*Rattus norvegicus*) and the NIH Swiss mouse (*Mus musculus*) were used to cross-suckle the hamster in both environments. All pregnant hamsters for hysterectomy and newborn hamster pups (less than 24 hrs old) were obtained from the NIH colony. In cross-suckling studies, conventional females lactating less than 24 hrs were set up in cages in an open room. The natural litter was removed from the female and intermingled with the hamsters just prior to placing the newborn hamsters with the female. The technique was the same for placing the germfree hamsters with the dams in an isolator. To aid, if possible, in the acceptance of the hamster pups by the dam in foster-rearing, at times teeth of the young hamsters were clipped, tranquilizers may or may not have been used on the foster mother, cedar shavings to mask scent were sometimes employed, and removal of all or part of the natural litter was tried.

Hand Rearing. A variety of sizes and shapes of nipples made of latex (Lotol, Naugatuck Chemical Co.) and silicone were used. Stomach tubes were made of polyethylene tubing (PE No.20) on a 25 gauge needle. Hamster milk was collected from day 1 through 7 lyophilized and sterilized by radiation.

Hand feeding of newborn hamster pups was attempted in both environments. In conventional studies, hamsters were maintained in a pan with toweling or gauze in an incubator at 85°F - 90°F and approximately 80% relative humidity. They were placed on a heating pad on the laboratory bench while being fed. Various milk formulae, including hamster milk, were fed approximately every 2 hrs. The amount of milk fed each time varied from 0.01 ml - 0.02 ml. Elimination of feces and urine was aided by massaging the pups with cotton swabs moistened with warm water.

Results

Conventional Animals. More than 300 hamster pups less than 24 hrs old were used in the studies. Cross-suckling was attempted on over 50 different mice and rats. In general, pups were lost during the first 72 hrs; however, we did experience some success. In one study, nine golden hamsters less than 24 hrs old were obtained from the NIH conventional colony, and cross-suckled on three conventional Sprague-Dawley rats. All survived to day 5, and six survived to day 10. On day 11 three survivors were removed from the dams for hand-rearing. Hamster milk, including colostrum, was fed by intubation when the stomach appeared empty. Stomach tubes proved more effective in feeding than nipples. Intestinal gas was removed by direct puncture through the wall of the abdomen with syringe and needle. Amino Plus (Pitman-Moore Co.), and L356 vitamin concentrate (3) were administered per os daily. Fruits and vegetables were offered *ad libitum* beginning on the third day; whole and evaporated milk were used after day 21. Slivers of apple were forced into the mouth causing the infant to chew. The only surviving female was bred and raised 9 of 11 hamsters to weaning age. This animal lived 178 days and died of intussusception of the jejunum.

In other conventional studies, an NIH mouse cross-suckled Chinese hamsters (*Cricetulus griseus*) to weaning age on two separate occasions. A Chinese hamster fostered a golden hamster and a Mystromys cross-suckled a golden hamster to weaning age.

Germfree Animals. Approximately 300 Cesarean derived hamster pups were used in germfree studies in isolators. All attempts to hand feed or foster-nurse the golden hamster in the isolator beyond 96 hrs failed. The following animals, however, were successfully hand-fed or fostered through weaning age in the germfree isolators:

The African white tailed rat (*Mystromys albicaudatus*) was cross-suckled on germfree Sprague-Dawley rats. Since the length of the gestation period for Mystromys has been variously reported as being from 30 - 37 days (4), pregnant females were weighed daily prior to term. When the weight of the animal failed to increase for two consecutive days, the female was judged to be within 24 hrs of parturition, and the hysterectomy was performed. The animals appeared not to need colostrum, since three were successfully foster-nursed on Sprague-Dawley dams which had been lactating for three days. Numerous litters of Mystromys were weaned, and maintained germfree for as long as two years on L356 diet.

One germfree female Mystromys produced two litters. The first was ignored by the mother and died, but the second was accepted and nursed for 11 days, at which time the mother died from torsion of the cecum. Enlarged ceca (5) were common and quite often females died from torsion of the cecum before the age of six months. This was less evident in males.

Hysterectomy derived spiny mice (*Acomys dimidiatus*) were hand-reared to weaning age as well as cross-suckled on the Sprague-Dawley rat under germfree conditions. Three pups were hand-fed using Similac (Ross Laboratories) diluted 1:1 with water and fed every 4 hrs the first week. The pups lapped milk from the tip of polyethylene tubing on a 20 gauge needle and syringe. The feedings were reduced at about seven days, when they were able to eat wheat, oats, sunflower seed, pablum, and L356 diet, all of which were fed *ad libitum*. These mice were weaned in 37 days and maintained on L356 diet. Three spiny mice were also foster-nursed on the Sprague-Dawley rat. Thus a total of six animals (four females and two males) were reared germfree. Spiny mice were maintained germfree for 27 months, during which time the females were bred and produced three litters, all of which were weaned. The spiny mice, however, would not foster nurse the germfree hamster.

Although unrelated, but maybe of some interest, gerbils (*Meriones unguiculatus*) were foster-nursed on germfree NIH mice. Two pairs were maintained germfree for 22 months. No offspring were produced and the study was terminated when the animals became contaminated.

Conclusions

The hamster has been reared in the conventional environment by cross-suckling and hand-rearing. Similar success, however, has not been attainable in the germfree environment. There appears to be one or more unidentified requirements for the hamsters. The milk formula may be deficient or the hand-rearing technique may need improvement. Nevertheless, our work with Mystromys, which we have reared and bred in the germfree environment, has given us some encouragement. The fact that Mystromys will live up to six years in the conventional environment and will tolerate their pups, which affix themselves tenaciously to the nipple until about the third week, has provided a stimulus for additional investigation with this species.

References

1. Pleasants, J. R., *Ann. N. Y. Acad. Sci. 78:* 116 (1959).
2. Foster, H., *Lab. Anim. Care 9:* 135 (1959).
3. Larner, J., and Gillespie, R. E., *J. Biol. Chem. 225:* 279 (1957).
4. Hall, A. III, Persing, R. L., White, D. C., and Ricketts, R. T. Jr., *Lab. Anim. Care 17:* 180 (1967).
5. Phillips, B. P., Wolfe, P. A., and Gordon, H. A., *Ann. N.Y. Acad. Sci. 78:* 183 (1959).

RAISING SPECIFIED PATHOGEN-FREE GUINEA PIGS AND RABBITS BY USING GNOTOBIOTECHNIQUES

H. Haacks, Willi Heine and *Axel Thunert*
Zentralinstitut fur Versuchstierzucht
Hannover, Germany/BRD

Introduction

Reliable results in animal experiments can only be achieved if uncontrolled environmental factors are prevented from influencing the course of the experiment and its results. Part of the environmental factors which might interfere with the animal experiment are microorganisms, especially those which might be obligatory or facultative pathogens. From the microbiological viewpoint in laboratory animal science, a gnotobiotic animal with a totally known and balanced "normal" flora would be desired.

Because of the costs and the expensive maintenance methods of using isolators, the gnotobiotic animal remains a special tool. However, all laboratory animals should be at least free of interfering specified pathogenic microorganisms. Following a proposal of Reyniers (1), we have used gnotobiotechniques in our institute since 1964 to raise large numbers of specified pathogen-free rats and mice, approximately 500,000 mice and 150,000 rats per year.

Materials and Methods

As previously reported (2, 3), we associated germfree mice and rats of our animal strains with only three species of germs isolated from our conventional colonies, that is from healthy looking conventional animals which we had observed for one breeding period. This flora, consisting of only three species of microorganisms, caused considerable difficulties after transferring the animals from the isolator to the barrier type animal house (4). However, since 1967 we have not detected 23 specified species of microorganisms in our mice and rat colonies. We routinely examine our animals for the following microorganisms:

ectoparasites	ectromelia virus	Adeno virus of mice
endoparasites	pneumonia virus of mice	polyoma virus
Bartonella sp.	Sendai virus	SV-5 virus

Toxoplasma sp.	K-virus	LCM virus
Salmonella sp.	reo-3-virus	minute virus of mice
Pasteurella sp.	Theiler virus	Kilham's rat virus
Leptospira sp.	mouse hepatitis virus	Toolan's H-1 virus
Mycoplasma sp.	Corona rat virus	

Furthermore, we have not detected clinical signs of either enzootic pneumonia or infantile diarrhea. All examinations were negative with the exception of the detection of one flagellate.

Based on our experience with mice and rats, we tried to raise specified pathogen-free guinea pigs and rabbits. We started with conventional colonies of both species in order to obtain pregnant females for hysterectomy. In these conventional animals of both species we found the following flora:

streptococci group D	*Proteus vulgaris*	*Bacillus sphaericus*
streptococci group H	*Proteus mirabilis*	*Clostridia sp.*
Staphylococcus albus	pseudomonas	*Bacteroides sp.*
Sarcina lutea	*Lactobacilli sp.*	eimeria
Sarcina ureae	*Microbacterium flavum*	*Trichomonas sp.*
Escherichia coli	*Bacillus megatherium*	

From this flora we isolated the germs we intended to associate with the germfree guinea pigs and rabbits we had already developed in our Trexler-type isolators. The following microorganisms were used for association:

Lactobacillus bifidus	*Bacillus cereus*	*Micrococcus flavus*
Lactobacillus lactis	*Bacillus sphaericus*	*Escherichia coli*
Clostridium sp.	*Streptococcus faecalis*	(08:K-:H-)
Bacillus subtilis	*Staphylococcus albus*	

Guinea pigs and rabbits were associated with the same flora because we intended to maintain both species in the same barrier type animal house. This is similar to what we did with mice and rats.

The flora of guinea pigs and rabbits contains more anaerobic bacteria than that of mice and rats. Unfortunately, until recently we have not had the facilities and the equipment to cultivate anaerobic germs, e.g. clostridium and bacteroides. In connection with the postgraduate program in our institute, we have currently started some work along this line.

We associated guinea pigs and rabbits with the bacteria in the sequence listed above. During each of the first five days, we offered glucose broth with the lactobacilli to the animals. On each of the following days we gave one of the succeeding germs.

Results

Guinea pigs. We encountered no difficulties during the association of germfree guinea pigs inside the isolator, except we found it difficult to associate guinea pigs older than 3 − 4 weeks. Only a few of these older animals ingested the flora. Most of them died. However, we encountered considerable trouble with the guinea pigs when we passed germfree puppies by hysterectomy into an already associated isolator. All these young animals died of *E. coli* enteritis. In addition, several of the already associated older animals in the isolator died of enteritis. In all of the dead guinea pigs we found a pure Gram negative flora.

We transferred the associated guinea pigs which survived in the isolators into a barrier type animal room. After a time *E. coli* again caused difficulties and a number of the animals died.

We had associated the guinea pigs with an *E. coli* type 08:K-:H-. In the animal house the animals died of an enteritis caused by *E. coli* of type 015:K?:H14 and 0146:H21. Both types are known to cause severe enteritis in animals. We assume these coli types were brought into the animal house by the animal technician. In order to offer to the animals some other non-pathogenic germs, hoping to reduce the enlarged ceca, we brought rats of our SPF-colonies into the same animal room. The animals which survived the *E. coli* infection remained alive, as well as their progeny. However, to date, we have failed to introduce new associated animals into this animal house.

In raising the associated guinea pigs in the isolators, we have also found difficulties caused by inadequate diets. We tried different formulas according to the literature (5; Udes, H., pers. com.) and the Lobund diet L-477 (6). After having transferred the guinea pigs from the isolators to the animal room, we simultaneously exposed the animals to SPF-rats and introduced a new diet developed in our institute. Subsequently, the formerly enlarged ceca became normal. Although the guinea pigs came in contact with the rats and the new diet at the same time, we believe that the rats with their flora are responsible for the reduction of the size of the ceca.

Our efforts resulted in a small colony of SPF-guinea pigs. These animals were successfully propagated. Unfortunately, the entire colony died due to excessive temperature in the animal room caused by a technical failure of the air conditioning system.

Rabbits. The rabbits were successfully raised with the Lobund-diet L-499 GE1 (7). However, we encountered considerable difficulties in handfeeding the germfree puppies because of pneumonia caused by the aspirated milk and with enlarged ceca.

The association with the same germ species as used for the guinea pigs brought no difficulties. After being transferred from the isolators to the animal room, the rabbits were also exposed to the SPF-rats. In addition, we changed the food to our new formula. As in the guinea pigs, the ceca were reduced to normal size. Again we believe this is caused by the contact with the rat flora, because in a preliminary test in one rabbit, a reduction in the size of the cecum

625

was noticed after having exposed the animals to SPF-rats without changing the diet.

Today we are running a small colony of healthy rabbits. In this colony we have observed, as described by many authors, a delayed maturity in hand-fed animals. A certain percentage of the females raised under these conditions are bad breeders.

Conclusion

In general, it seems to us that the difficulties in raising SPF-guinea pigs are problems of the intestinal flora, especially of *E. coli*. In raising SPF-rabbits we only found complications in feeding techniques. We believe exposure to SPF-rats can help to establish a balanced flora in associated guinea pigs and rabbits outside the isolators. However, there are still many problems to be solved, and we have to repeat the whole procedure of raising guinea pigs and rabbits to gain more knowledge in this field. In order to get SPF-animal colonies of these species as quickly as possible, we were forced to neglect many connected questions.

References

1. Reyniers, J. A., *Proc. Anim. Care Panel 7:* 9 (1957).
2. Heine, W., and Thunert, A., in "Advances in Germfree Research and Gnotobiology," (M. Miyakawa and T. D. Luckey, eds.), CRC Press, Cleveland, Ohio, p. 9, (1968).
3. Thunert, A., and Haacks, H., "Observations made in starting and running SPF mice, rats, guinea pigs and rabbit colonies." In preparation.
4. Thunert, A., *Z. Versuchstierk. 13:* 87 (1971).
5. Hammerli, U., and Hurni, I., Symp. Schweiz. *Mikrobiol. Ges., Bibl. Microbiol. 7,* Karger, Basel/New York, p. 59, (1969).
6. Reddy, B. S., Wostmann, B. S., and Pleasants, J. R., "The Germfree Animal in Research," (M. Coates, ed.), Acad. Press, p. 87, (1968).
7. Wostmann, B. S., and Pleasants, J. R., *Proc. Anim. Care Panel 9:* 47 (1959).

OBSERVATIONS ON THE REPRODUCTIVE PERFORMANCE AND LABORATORY USE OF INBRED MICE WHOSE ANCESTORS WERE DERIVED VIA SURGICAL/ISOLATOR TECHNIQUES

Samuel M. Poiley
Mammalian Genetics and Animal Production Section
DR&D, Chemotherapy, National Cancer Institute
Bethesda, Maryland 20014, U.S.A.

Introduction

Our interest in isolator animal rearing systems is not primarily for the development of germfree colonies for research. We are concerned with the use of derived animals with defined microbial flora as progenitors of pathogen-free breeding animals. During the past several years, our efforts in this field have been continuously expanded. Although our final goal has not been attained, we feel that it can be achieved during the next several years.

The primary mission of the Mammalian Genetics and Animal Production Section is the provision of laboratory rodents for a variety of intra- and extramural research programs of the National Cancer Institute. It is dependent upon the maintenance of centers to produce breeding animals for large-scale production colonies and for special research projects. These animal resources are located in various geographic areas of the United States. Although these colonies are managed by contractors, they remain the property of the United States Government. The contractors include commercial organizations, commercial institutions, and universities. The major portion of the animals are transferred to diverse contract-supported laboratories for the performance of research and testing projects.

Methods

The details concerning the methods of inbred and outbred production have been reported previously (1, 2).

The derivation of laboratory animals by means of surgical intervention and the rearing of neo-natals in isolators have been described by Foster, Gustafsson, Luckey, Pleasants and Reyniers (3-9). Since our methods are similar, I will refrain from describing this phase of our activities. The isolators differ in certain

627

respects such as size and configuration. Germfree foundation colonies are kept in 5 ft long Trexler (10, 11) isolators. Expansion colonies with defined microbial flora are propagated in 6 ft Trexler isolators, 6 ft long Landy (12) rigid plastic isolators, and the ferris wheel and intermediate steel and plastic concepts by Lattuada (13).

During the initial phases of the isolator derivation program, it was our intent to follow the procedures suggested by predecessors in this field. These methods are based upon the development of germfree colonies whose offspring are infected with a small number of the organisms discussed by Schaedler and co-workers (14, 15). During the first year of effort, the rate of progress was unsatisfactory and the system was revised. Our current practices include derivation and rearing in isolators with defined flora. Germfree nuclei are subsequently derived in order to establish seed-stock colonies. In this manner, we have been able to markedly accelerate the output of breeding animals for the production colonies. The numbers of animals that are currently being produced are of sufficient magnitude for an evaluation of the efficacy of this scheme.

For purposes of comparison, 5 centers located in 5 different geographic areas of the United States were selected for this study. Each center is associated with unique characteristics, but they can be divided into 2 groups. Although ambient outdoor climates differ, these differences are minimized if air handling systems provide uniform conditions throughout the year. Lighting cycles are programmed and are controlled manually or by means of automatic timing devices. In general, a fairly constant period of approximately 10 hr per day is employed for illumination. Brief descriptions of the 5 centers are noted below.

Center A. Our colonies are housed in a building which also contains the contractor's commercial stocks. The staff members are assigned to specified locations, but central services are shared. The air handling system represents improvements over those commonly used for dwellings, industrial plants and public buildings. However, the filters are incapable of removing fine particles, and 50% of the air is recirculated. Temperature is maintained between 72-74°F, and relative humidity ranges between 40-65%. These colonies have never been associated with an isolator system. This management system is termed modified conventional.

Center B. Our colonies are produced in a specially constructed building located on a site at a distance of several miles from the contractor's principal plant. The air handling system provides 100% fresh air, and the filters are designed for approximately 80% efficiency. The temperature is maintained between 72-74°F, and the relative humidity ranges between 45-55%. This unit is self-contained and central services are not shared. The colonies did not originate from an isolator system, and the management method is termed modified conventional.

Center C. The colonies are propagated in a separate building on the premises of the contractor. Central services are shared with the manager's commercial colonies. Fine filtration is not available, and 30% of the air is recirculated. These colonies have been maintained in a modified conventional environment since their inception. The ancestors of the animals did not originate from an isolator system.

Center D. Our colonies are maintained in a building which also houses the contractor's stocks. The air handling system is based upon 25% return air, and the filtration activity is 99% efficient. Temperature is controlled between 72-74°F, and the relative humidity ranges between 45-60%.

This center includes isolators. Expansion colonies with defined flora furnish breeding animals for pedigreed colonies in bio-containment (SPF) environmentally controlled rooms. Husbandry methodology is achieved at maximal levels. These colonies furnish the animals for production colonies in this center. Husbandry practices in production rooms are termed modified conventional.

Center E. Our colonies are kept in zoned portions of buildings which also house the contractor's colonies, and in small isolated modular buildings. Each zonal and modular colony is self-contained. Central services are not shared. The air handling equipment furnishes 100% fresh air, with filtration efficiency at a level of 99%. Temperature range is held to 72-74°F, and the relative humidity ranges between 45-55%.

This center includes isolators which provide animals for bio-containment breeder producing colonies. The latter in turn furnish breeding animals for production colonies. All colonies are managed in accordance with maximal animal husbandry practices.

The colonies in all centers are routinely monitored for the presence or absence of Ectromelia, LCM, MHV, MAdV, K, Sendai, Reo 3, Theiler's GDVII, Toolan's H-1, PVM, Polyoma and SV 5 viruses (16, 17). The schedule requires the submission of 50 samples selected at random at intervals of 2 months. Colony managers submit monthly reports which contain the data listed in Tables 1 through 4. The data presented represents a summary of events for calendar year 1971. Raw data is collected by the respective animal technician staffs and summarized for reporting purposes by the individual colony managers. This information was extrapolated to uniform breeding populations of 1000 females each. In this manner, we have the ability to predict production levels based upon multiples or fractions of this baseline breeding population.

Strains BALB/cCr (BALB/c), C57BL/6CR (C57BL/6) and DBA/2Cr (DBA/2) were selected for this study because they are the most frequently used inbred mice.

Contact bedding is used for all centers, and we consider pine shavings with no resin content and maple chips to be equally acceptable. Bedding material is sterilized only for Centers D and E. Commercially prepared compressed block-type diets are used in all centers. Four different formulations, which we consider to be equally acceptable, are being used in all 5 centers. Not more than 2 and generally only 1 kind is used by an individual center. BALB/c and DBA/2 mice receive diets which contain 4-5% fat and 22-24% protein. C57BL/6 mice are offered diets which contain 10-11% fat and approximately 15-17% protein. The food is pasteurized for the mice reared only in Centers D and E.

Results

Table 1 compares production results based upon output of weanlings and weaned litter averages. The final results reflect a combination of facilities design, methodology, and animal husbandry practices. It would therefore appear to be incongruous that Center E, with the most advanced systems, yields the lowest weaned litter average. There are 2 reasons for this result. In the first place, we have observed that colonies emerging from an isolator system demonstrate reduced fecundity. Secondly, 1971 represented the first full year of experience with these colonies on a significantly large-scale production program. Center D, for example, has completed its second year of production, and has demonstrated improved reproductive activity.

TABLE I

PRODUCTION RATES PER 1000 BREEDING FEMALES

BALB/cAnCr

Production Center	A	B	C	D	E
Litters Weaned	4875	4370	4795	4841	3441
Males Weaned	17036	16286	14343	16003	9692
Females Weaned	16794	15631	13950	15449	9978
Total Mice Weaned	33830	31917	28293	31452	19670
Weaned Litter Average	6.9	7.3	5.9	6.5	5.7

C57BL/6Cr

Production Center	A	B	C	D	E
Litters Weaned	3452	3175	4261	3501	2650
Males Weaned	10940	10952	12887	13004	6976
Females Weaned	9748	12178	11529	11861	7033
Total Mice Weaned	20688	23130	24416	24865	14009
Weaned Litter Average	6.0	7.3	5.7	7.1	5.3

DBA/2Cr

Production Center	A	B	C	D	E
Litters Weaned	3976	3263	4271	4105	3451
Males Weaned	10480	10229	10209	11760	9388
Females Weaned	9491	9532	9127	11444	8995
Total Mice Weaned	19971	19761	19336	23204	18383
Weaned Litter Average	5.0	6.0	4.5	5.7	5.2

Although Centers A, B, and C are somewhat similarly managed, it does appear that physical separation from other colonies affords a better system for controlling environmental factors.

Culling rates, i.e., animals discarded for abnormal conditions, are shown in Table 2. It is quite obvious that the methodology applied in Center E is worthwhile. The excessive rates of culling reported for Center D are due to the hypercritical attitude of the colony manager, and in some manner is related to a sharing of central services. Culling rates for weanlings are generally highest because decisions are made at this point for the selection of animals for laboratory studies.

TABLE 2

CULLING RATES PER 1000♀♀ BREEDERS

STRAIN BALB/cCr

Production Center	Breeders ♂	Breeders ♀	Future Breeders ♂	Future Breeders ♀	Weanlings ♂	Weanlings ♀	Pre-Weanlings ♂ and ♀
A	95	460	36	49	359	327	1647
B	21	147	2	3	1	157	4
C	55	213	21	20	188	158	33
D	11	28	269	511	314	342	206
E	3	3	0	0	17	23	15

STRAIN C57BL/6Cr

A	137	427	7	30	163	183	335
B	33	176	7	17	162	177	26
C	22	32	8	13	163	150	84
D	110	329	80	194	485	672	179
E	16	29	0	0	21	21	23

STRAIN DBA/2Cr

A	132	422	50	75	110	108	101
B	22	77	20	29	18	33	67
C	83	136	41	55	106	120	80
D	16	69	129	127	229	285	133
E	8	31	0	0	29	66	56

Adult death rates reported in Table 3 adequately demonstrate the usefulness of our approach to improvements in laboratory animal colony management. The results obtained in Centers D and E confirmed our expectations. The unusually high rate of pregnant deaths in Center E for the DBA/2 strain is commonly encountered for a recently developed colony.

The miscellaneous losses shown in Table 4 are confined to age categories ranging from day 1 to weaning at 4 weeks. The results reported for the "cleanest" colonies maintained in Centers D and E, in general, reflect the usefulness of maximal environmental control. Specific reasons why mothers

TABLE 3

ADULT DEATH RATES PER 1000 BREEDING ♀♀

STRAIN BALB/cCr

Production Center	Pregnants	Family Groups	Lactating Females	Active Breeders ♂	Active Breeders ♀	Future Breeders ♂	Future Breeders ♀
A	22	64	46	15	43	28	21
B	12	41	25	10	52	9	17
C	11	35	34	19	30	10	17
D	8	20	10	21	60	4	3
E	18	5	5	8	24	1	0

STRAIN C57BL/6Cr

A	30	39	5	25	31	33	27
B	34	11	4	15	35	9	11
C	38	35	7	10	23	23	11
D	23	53	43	9	56	3	9
E	35	3	7	8	33	0	0

STRAIN DBA/2Cr

A	6	113	75	52	74	4	9
B	7	96	66	41	48	4	12
C	9	154	69	34	41	7	6
D	3	39	31	26	45	4	2
E	78	21	32	15	21	0	0

cannibalize litters continue to remain elusive. Based upon our experiences, the rates will vary in a colony throughout the year. We continue to attempt to diagnose each incident and institute indicated corrective procedures.

We evaluate management efficiency by means of the Production Efficiency Index (P.E.I.). This value represents the numbers of weanlings or fraction of a weanling produced per breeding female per week. Table 5 reports this information. The P.E.I. and weaned litter averages are generally lower for new colonies, and these facts are aptly demonstrated by the data reported for Center E.

Conclusions

The data reported in this review of one year of experience emphasizes the need for constant improvement in laboratory animal quality. It also demonstrates that current technology can be applied for this purpose if an appropriate program is pursued with vigor.

When culling and death rates are nominal in the colonies, one can expect equally favorable results in laboratory applications for these animals. The mice issued from Center E, for example, are deliberately assigned to projects which employ potentially carcinogenic materials and viral agents for long-term studies.

TABLE 4

MISCELLANEOUS LOSS CATEGORIES PER 1000♀♀ BREEDERS

STRAIN BALB/cCr

Production Center	Litters Cannibalized	Litters Died	Litters Culled	Weanlings Died ♂	Weanlings Died ♀	Pre-Weanlings Died ♂ and ♀
A	340	103	446	82	63	187
B	203	25	11	25	39	158
C	291	72	41	99	63	136
D	173	30	0	32	41	130
E	68	9	0	5	3	33

STRAIN C57BL/6

A	927	53	121	25	26	123
B	243	51	25	36	24	94
C	1533	89	67	35	33	108
D	669	35	10	69	85	129
E	81	20	3	15	13	89

STRAIN DBA/2

A	529	512	410	184	154	151
B	629	219	285	64	65	131
C	2182	489	311	281	321	298
D	1598	56	8	54	84	152
E	207	66	7	24	33	89

TABLE 5. Production Efficiency Indexes

Strain	Production Centers				
	A	B	C	D	E
BALB/cCr	.650	.614	.544	.605	.378
C57BL/6Cr	.398	.445	.469	.478	.262
DBA/2Cr	.384	.380	.372	.446	.354

Reports from the laboratories confirm our opinion that the mice have served to enhance the various investigations.

Physical separation of colonies is an important adjunct for the control of quality. This factor is aptly shown when Centers D and E are compared, and in the comparison of Center B with the results reported for Centers A and C.

It is our opinion that the availability of an isolator support system for mouse production colonies will ensure a continued supply of pathogen-free animals.

References

1. Poiley, S. M., *Proc. of the 8th Annual Technical Meeting of the American Assoc. for*

Contamination Control, p. 138, (1969).

2. Poiley, S. M., *Lab. Anim. Care 17:* 573 (1967).
3. Foster, H. L., *Proc. Animal Care Panel 9:* 135 (1959).
4. Foster, H. L., *Proc. 2nd Symposium on Gnotobiote Technol.*, p. 145, (1960).
5. Foster, H. L., *Ann. N.Y. Acad. Sci. 78:* 80 (1959).
6. Gustafsson, B. E., *Acta Pathol. Microbial. Scand.,* Suppl. No. 73: 1 (1948).
7. Luckey, T. D., in "Germfree Life and Gnotobiology," Academic Press, p. 171, (1963).
8. Pleasants, J. R., *Ann. N.Y. Acad. Sci. 78:* 116 (1959).
9. Reyniers, J. A., *Am. J. Vet. Res. 18:* 678 (1957).
10. Trexler, P. C., *J. Animal Care Panel 9:* 119 (1959).
11. Trexler, P. C., *Ann. N.Y. Acad. Sci. 78:* 29 (1959)
12. Landy, J. J., IX International Congress for Microbiology, Moscow, p. 383, (1966).
13. Lattuada, C. P., ARS/Sprague-Dawley Co., Madison, Wisc., (unpublished information).
14. Schaedler, R. W., Dubos, R. J., and Costello, R., *J. Exp. Med. 122:* 59 (1965).
15. Schaedler, R. W., Dubos, R. J., and Costello, R., *J. Exp. Med. 122:* 77 (1965).
16. Briody, B. A., Mouse Pox Service Laboratory, N. J. College of Med. & Dentistry, Newark, N. J.
17. Poiley, S. M., *Lab. Anim. Care 20:* 643 (1970).

TECHNOLOGY ADVANCEMENTS IN THE GROWTH OF GERMFREE PLANTS AT THE MANNED SPACECRAFT CENTER

C. H. Walkinshaw, B. C. Wooley and *G. A. Bozarth*
NASA Manned Spacecraft Center
Houston, Texas 77058, U.S.A.

Introduction

The quarantine program for the Apollo missions required the use of germfree plants in screening for possible pathogens of lunar origin. The advantages of using germfree plants in research had been emphasized before the Apollo missions (1-3). Previously, disinfected seeds and excised embryos had been used as starting materials for many investigations (4, 5). Recent technique improvements have made it possible to obtain germfree seedings from differentiated callus cultures (3) and dissected shoot tips (6). Plants initiated by these procedures grow and develop normally in sterile environments. Success with these techniques suggests that numerous germfree plants can be grown for quarantine investigations. If germfree plants are used, the problem of identifying a pathogen is simplified.

Materials and Methods

The major problems encountered in growing germfree plants for postflight lunar investigations were the lack of a source of germfree initiating material for economic crop plants, a means of certifying the material as germfree, and methods for maintaining the germfree plants within Class III biological cabinetry (7). After selecting seeds as initiating material for germfree plants, studies were conducted to establish the endogenous microflora of seeds and to define reliable methods for germination and growth of seedlings in sterile environments. Numerous problems were experienced in the standardization of the procedures, the detection of latent microorganisms, the residual toxicity of the disinfectants, and the control of environmental parameters. Balancing light intensity, air flow, temperature, and humidity was difficult in sterile chambers.

Before discussing these technical problems, several terms used to describe plants and their associations with microorganisms need to be defined. Conventional plants or plant parts are contaminated microbially so that the ecological

635

integrity of the population of microorganisms is maintained. Gnotobiotic plants grow in the presence of one or more types of microorganisms of known identity. This type of association is usually unbalanced ecologically. Suspected germfree plants are defined as those plants in which microbial contamination is not detected when tissue specimens are incubated in fluid thioglycollate and trypticase soy media at ambient temperature. Germfree plants are grown for several weeks in an environment that has been examined extensively for all forms of microorganisms, using a variety of media and different incubation conditions, without any signs of microbial growth. In addition, random pieces of actively growing tissue must be free of mycoplasma and viral contamination when examined by means of electron microscopy.

Results

Large variations in the internal microbial contamination occurred in seeds of different species, seed lots of the same species and variety, and seeds obtained from different companies. In many cases, commercially available seeds were unsuitable as a source of germfree plants regardless of the disinfection procedure. Seeds were disinfected with sodium or calcium hypochlorite (0.5%, pH 6-7 in potassium phosphate buffer) and were germinated on nutrient or trypticase soy agar. Representative findings from over 100 plant species are given in Table I. Seeds of certain varieties of cabbage, lettuce, and slash pine had no microbial contamination after surface disinfection. Variation in the microbial contamination of cabbage seeds obtained from different vendors was striking. Seed of the variety Red Acre from vendor A had 17% contamination, whereas that from vendor B had only 2%. When seeds from 6 other varieties were compared on Sabouraud dextrose, trypticase soy, fluid thioglycollate, potato dextrose, and nutrient agar, those from vendor B were uniformly lower in their endogenous microflora.

When seed from commercial sources is high in endogenous microflora, the microbial population might be reduced by manipulation of growing procedures. Both corn grown in nursery beds and hand-pollinated corn gave only 10% contamination compared with 90% for commercial seed. Spinach grown indoors produced uncontaminated seed in contrast to the highly contaminated seed from commercial sources (Table I).

Citrus, tomato, and watermelon seed have been obtained microorganism-free by aseptic removal from disease-free fruits. Tomato seed from 4 fruits was uncontaminated, whereas seed from 2 other fruits gave 20% and 54% contamination. A similar variation occurred for watermelon seed, whereas citrus seed was free of microbes in all cases. The most reliable method to obtain germfree seedlings is to use seeds produced on germfree plants. To date, soybean, lettuce, and tobacco seeds have been produced by means of this procedure.

TABLE I. Variation in Microbial Contamination of Commercially Available Seeds[a]

Scientific name	Common name	No. var. tested	Microbial contamination, %
Brassica oleracea L.	cabbage	5	0-22
Capsicum frutescens L.	pepper	3	21-45
Citrullus vulgaris Schrad.	watermelon	3	67-99
Cucumis sativus L.	cucumber	5	3-46
Lactuca sativa L.	lettuce	11	0-3
Lycopersicon esculentum Mill.	tomato	3	24-100
Pinus elliottii Engelm.	slash pine	2	0-6
Raphanus sativus L.	radish	3	2-13
Spinacia oleracea L.	spinach	5	92-100

[a]Seeds were disinfected with sodium or calcium hypochlorite and germinated on trypticase soy agar for 14 days at 22°C under continuous light of approximately 5,000 lux.

When seed disinfectants are required, sodium and calcium hypochlorite solutions (1, 8) appear to be the most useful. By comparison with other chemicals (formalin, peracetic acid, ethanol and 20% hydrogen peroxide), sodium hypochlorite was shown to be superior in most cases. In some cases, calcium hypochlorite was less inhibitory to seed germination and seedling development than was the sodium salt.

Seed germination was reduced at temperatures optimal for detection of bacterial contaminants (35-38°C). Furthermore, germination of cantaloupe, lettuce, pepper, and wheat seed was inhibited significantly on the following agars: blood, brain-heart infusion, chocolate, MacConkey, mannitol salt, Mitis Salivarius, Sabouraud dextrose, urea, and XLD. Detection of mycoplasma has been difficult because adequate media for their culture from plants are just now being evaluated (9).

The limited effectiveness of nutrient agar for detection of seed contamination was shown by dipping 500 7-day-old seedlings (cabbage, pepper, and radish) in tryptic soy broth. Of the seedlings that appeared clean initially on nutrient agar, 29% gave rise to microbial growth when dipped in broth. Although valuable for detecting microorganisms, this procedure was unsuitable because all seedlings died within 1 month. An alternative was to germinate seed on nutrient agar overlayed with tryptic soy broth. This alternative increased the efficiency of detecting soybean contaminants five-fold; however, this technique is detrimental to some species.

A medium that showed some promise for initiating germfree seedlings was prepared from equal parts of potato dextrose, nutrient, and Sabouraud dextrose agar. This medium limits growth, allows more time for microbial detection, and promotes root-hair development.

Transfer of transplanted seedlings into sterile chambers was accomplished by decontamination of transfer containers with formaldehyde or sodium hypochlorite (8, 10). Mason jars are the most economical and acceptable gas-tight containers for this transfer. After transfer into sterile environmental chambers, the standard metal insert cap can be replaced either by a transparent polypropylene film or by a flexible or hard plastic tubing which may be secured to the lids to increase aerial space for certain plants (Figs. 1A and 1B).

Seedlings transferred to sterile growth chambers can be maintained for extended periods within Mason jars (Fig. 1C), or they can be transplanted into plastic or clay pots. Seedlings for nutritional or root-exudate investigations can be transferred to specialized filter units so that samples of the soil solution could be analyzed (Fig. 1D).

Garden soil, peat, vermiculite, and mixtures of these have not been good substrates for germfree plants. Quartz sand, perlite, mixtures of these two, or the block form of BR-8 (American Can Corporation) were best for growing germfree plants.

Modifications of stainless-steel cabinetry used in this quarantine were published previously (7). Another modification is illustrated in Fig. 2A. Four Plexiglas boxes (30 x 30 x 60 cm) were placed in each steel chamber. Except when measurements are made on the germfree seedlings, each box contains a glove port capped with plastic film. Filtered and temperature-controlled intake air was provided through a manifold system. This system offers double protection against accidental contamination, insulates from heat, and increases the control of temperature and humidity. Also, germfree plants could be maintained at a positive pressure within Class III cabinetry that operated at negative pressure with respect to the room environment.

Two of the more useful designs of plastic glove boxes that have been constructed and tested are illustrated in Figs. 2B, 3A, and 3B. Large chambers are designed to grow plants to maturity, whereas small chambers are used for experiments. A decontamination entry box is attached to one end of each large chamber. The entry port of one of the chambers has an additional entry chamber equipped with a dunk tank and air-vent system for formaldehyde decontamination. A Plexiglas tunnel, with doors at each end, connects the two large chambers. This gas-tight transfer tunnel permits the use of the large chambers as either isolated or coupled units.

The smaller glove boxes are similar to the design of the flexible Trexler bag (11). Because the boxes are rigid, they offer protection against loss of germplasma when unscheduled electrical outages occur.

Another useful chamber, although expensive to purchase, is the rigid, cylindrical, vacuum glove box manufactured by Manostat Corporation. This unit has been tested successfully with germfree plants at 100 and 300 mm Hg pressure.

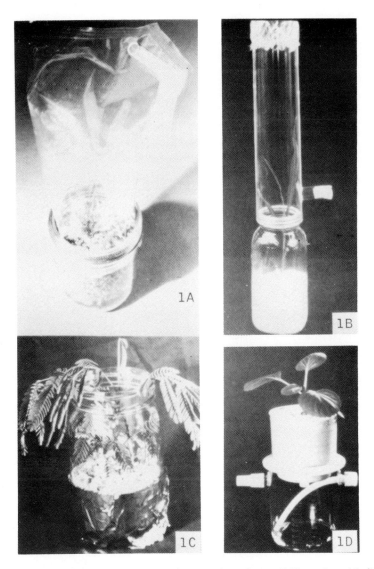

FIG. 1. Primary containers used for growing germfree plants. A) Mason jar with flexible plastic attachments; B) Mason jar with rigid Plexiglas attachment; C) mimosa seedling growing in BR-8 in Mason jar; D) cabbage seedling growing in root-exudate collection apparatus.

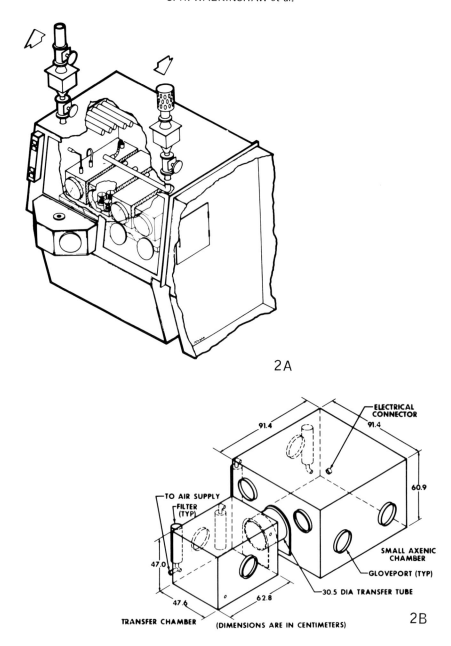

FIG. 2. Plexiglas chambers used for growing germfree plants. A) Class III cabinet cutaway showing Plexiglas boxes and manifold system; and B) small glove box and transfer chamber used for germfree passage of supplies into the chamber.

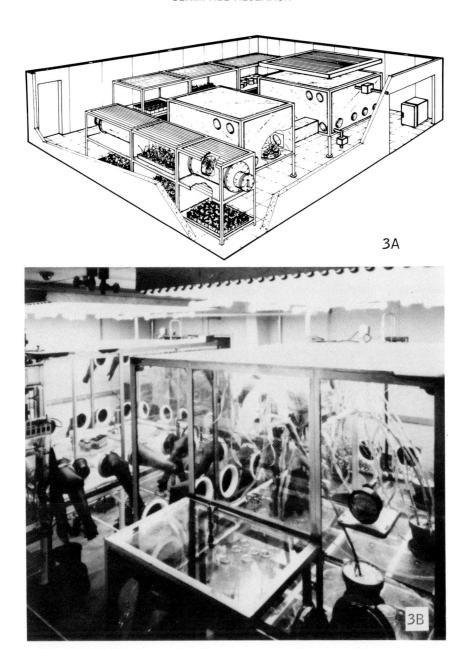

FIG. 3. Large Plexiglas glove boxes used to grow mature plants. A) plant growth room with chambers in center of room; B) view of chambers containing mature corn plants.

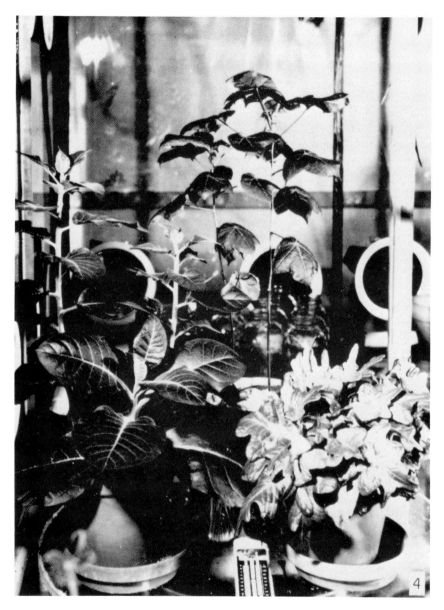

FIG. 4. Large plants of lettuce, tobacco, and cotton grown germfree for approximately three months.

The chambers have been used successfully for growing large numbers of germfree plants for periods of several months. Germfree plants of lettuce, cotton, soybeans, corn, and tobacco were grown to maturity simultaneously under germfree conditions in the large Plexiglas chambers (Fig. 4). Citrus and tomato plants have been kept germfree in a small Plexiglas chamber for 5 months. Also, germfree plants have been used in postflight investigations to detect any microorganisms in lunar materials, in nutritional studies with lunar materials and terrestrial basalts, and in comparative analytical experiments aimed at defining differences between germfree and conventional plants.

Subsequent to the elimination of quarantine (Apollo 14), a research program with germfree plants as material for biochemical and tissue-culture investigations has been implemented. In one set of experiments with soybeans grown under identical conditions (except that one group was inoculated with a mixture of soil microorganisms), the germfree plants yielded more dry weight and protein than did the contaminated plants. Also, elemental abundances in the germfree soybean plants were considerably different from conventional amounts. Of the elements determined, 70% (including iron, manganese, phosphorous, and silicon) existed in a higher concentration in the germfree plants.

The sterile growth chambers are proving to be valuable for root-exudate studies using the collection apparatus illustrated in Fig. 1D. Large amounts of sterile root exudates have been collected without affecting the sterility of the plants.

Conclusions

The propagation of large numbers of germfree plants from seed obtained from different sources has been shown. Microorganisms were not required for tobacco, lettuce, and soybeans to form viable seeds. Many difficulties have been encountered in the certification of plants as germfree, and propagation of these plants in sterile chambers. Movement of the large quantities of water into the chambers and the loss of numerous seedlings during certification were major difficulties. However, if the results of initial experiments on the analytical chemistry of germfree plants can be used as a guide, the scientific value of germfree botanical research will be significant.

Acknowledgements

We are grateful to Wade Bolton, Phillip Covington, Nina Gehring, Lecil Hander, and Pratt Johnson for their assistance.

References

1. Nilsson, P. E., *Arch. Mikrobiol. 26:* 285 (1957).

2. Lindsey, D. L., *Phytopathology 57:* 960 (1967).

3. Pillai, S. K., and Hildebrandt, A. C., *Plant Dis. Reptr. 52:* 600 (1968).

4. White, P. R., in "Micrurgical and Germfree Techniques," (J. A. Reyniers, ed.), Charles C. Thomas, Springfield, Illinois, p. 188, (1943).

5. Gawel, L. J., and Bollen, W. B., *Agron. J. 52:* 718 (1960).

6. Baker, R., and Phillips, D. J., *Phytopathology 52:* 1242 (1962).

7. Walkinshaw, C. H., Sweet, H. C., Venketeswaran, S., and Horne, W. H., *BioScience 20:* 1297 (1970).

8. Sykes, G., "Disinfection and Sterilization," 2nd Ed., J. P. Lippincott Co., Philadelphia, Pennsylvania, (1965).

9. Chen, T., and Granados, R. R., *Science 167:* 1633 (1970).

10. Taylor, L. M., Barbeito, M., and Gremillion, G., *Appl. Microbiol. 17:* 614 (1969).

11. Trexler, P. C., and Reynolds, L. I., *Appl. Microbiol. 5:* 406 (1957).

PLANT GNOTOBIOTIC RESEARCH IN PLANT PATHOLOGY AND PLANT PHYSIOLOGY

Maynard G. Hale, Khalid M. Hameed, and *Houston B. Couch*
Department of Plant Pathology and Physiology
The Virginia Polytechnic Institute and State University
Blacksburg, Virginia 24061, U.S.A.

Introduction

A certain amount of expertise and knowledge has been developed in the last six years by a research group at the Virginia Polytechnic Institute and State University working in the areas of root exudation, axenic plant culture, plant gnotobiotics and ecology of root diseases. The axenic culture of peanuts, *Arachis hypogaea* L.; of tobacco, *Nicotiana tabaccum* L.; of marigolds, *Tagetes erecta* L.; of corn, *Zea mays* L.; and of some grasses is routine (1-5). Pine has also been used. A facility for plant gnotobiology has been built and includes temperature and light controls in two plant growth rooms, each housing six isolator chambers.

Materials and Methods

In the preparation of germfree plants, seeds are surface sterilized, usually with 20% commercial bleach solution or with hydrogen peroxide, and incubated on an agar solidified nutrient medium for several days to check for sterility before they are introduced into the isolator chambers. After introduction into the chambers, periodic sterility checks are made, using five different nutrient media, and the final check is made just before termination of an experiment. It has become necessary to remove the cotyledons from peanut embryos to obtain sterile plants (1). The embryos are cultured on an inorganic salts medium with 2% sucrose added. Plants are grown in a hydroponic system in various types of containers, dependent upon the plant species used and the conditions of the experiment. Organic compounds released by the roots (exudates) are extracted from lyophilized nutrient solution in which roots have been growing, and the compounds present are measured by chromatography (1, 2, 4, 6).

The use of these techniques in plant research can be illustrated by two examples; one involves an analysis of organic compounds released from roots, and factors affecting the exudation; and the second involves investigations of the colonization of roots by fungi and their effects on physiological processes in the plant as well as on root exudation.

Results

Calcium content of the nutrient solution bathing the roots of axenic peanut plants was found to affect exudation of sugars (4, 5, 7). When peanut plants were grown under light intensities of 1.59×10^3 lux at $30\pm 0.5°C$, calcium concentrations of 10, 20, 35 and 50 mg/liter had a varying effect on the amount of sugar exuded, as shown in Table I. There was a four-fold increase in total sugars exuded at 10 mg Ca/liter compared to 50 mg Ca/liter. The sugars and sugar derivatives separated by gas chromatography (6) consisted of five unidentified compounds plus arabinose, ribose, xylose, fructose, mannose, glucose, galactose, mannitol, galacturonic acid, inositol and sucrose.

TABLE I. **Micrograms of Sugars* Exuded at Four Calcium Concentrations**

	10 mg Ca/liter	20 mg Ca/liter	35 mg Ca/liter	50 mg Ca/liter
1st week	33	34	20	15
2nd week	49	40	24	8
3rd week	69	53	29	20
4th week	69	62	31	15
Total	220	189	104	58

*Trimethyl silyl derivatives of sugars were measured on a temperature programmed, gas-liquid chromatograph (4, 6).

When 38-day-old, axenic marigold plants were inoculated with washed conidia of *Penicillium simplicissimum* (Oud.) Thom., a fungus generally considered to be saprophytic in soil, the roots became colonized. There was a change in the concentration of carbohydrates, reducing sugars, and fructose in the leaves (Table II) of inoculated plants when compared with axenic plants. Root-colonized plants had greater growth and flowered earlier. There was also an effect of colonization on exudation (Table III). Exudation was more pronounced at 34 days after inoculation than at 20 days after inoculation (2, 3, 8).

Conclusions

Calcium may be affecting sugar exudation from peanut roots by changing permeability of cell membranes. The use of gnotobiotic techniques has enabled the quantitative measurement of the organic exudates which would otherwise have been altered by microorganisms colonizing the roots or in the rhizosphere

TABLE II. Total Water Soluble Carbohydrates, Reducing Sugars, and Fructose in Leaves of 58 and 72 Day Old Plants, 20 and 34 Days After Inoculation with *Penicillium simplicissimum**

	Days after inoc.	Dry wt. shoots g	H$_2$O sol. CH$_2$O μg/g	Red. sugars μg/g	Fructose μg/g
Axenic	20	7	65	17	10
	34	13	77	32	21
Inoc.	20	9†	74	24††	13†
	34	15†	88††	33	19

*Data is average of ten plants.
†, †† Indicates statistically significant difference from corresponding value for axenic plants at the 1% and 5% level of confidence, respectively.

TABLE III. Chemical Composition (Per Plant, Average of 10 Plants) of Root Exudates of 58 and 72 Day Old Plants, 20 and 34 Days After Inoculation with *Penicillium simplicissimum*

	Days after inoc.	H$_2$O sol. organic matter mg	H$_2$O sol. CH$_2$O mg	Red. sugars μg	Proteins mg	Amino acid (valine eq.) μm
Axenic	20	410	2.49	270	4.02	1.63
	34	462	1.36	225	2.77	2.42
Inoc.	20	362††	2.07	265	3.39†	2.15
	34	419	3.80††	665††	4.19†	3.02†

†, †† Indicates statistically significant difference from corresponding value for axenic plants at the 1% and 5% level of confidence, respectively.

(9). Plant gnotobiotics has been used for studies on seedlings in test tubes and small chambers for many years. The advantage of the isolator system is that whole plants can be used and studies made throughout their life cycle. The difference in the nature of exudation from colonized roots and from axenic roots needs further investigation because significant quantitative differences were demonstrated for marigold plants. Colonization also affects physiological processes within the plant, as shown by alteration of foliar components and the timing sequence in development.

Acknowledgements

This research was supported, in part, by Plant Sciences Division, Agricultural Research Service, U.S. Department of Agriculture under cooperative agreement 12-14-100-9711 (34); and in part by a fellowship to K. M. H. by the Iraqi government.

References

1. Hale, M. G., *Plant Soil. 31:* 463 (1969).
2. Hameed, K. M., Ph.D. Dissertation, Virginia Polytechnic Institute and State University, (1971).
3. Hameed, K. M., and Couch, H. B., *Phytopathology 59:* 1556 (1969).
4. Shay, F. J., Ph.D. Dissertation, Virginia Polytechnic Institute and State University, (1971).
5. Shay, F. J., and Hale, M. G., *Proc. South. Agric. Workers Conf. 68:* 205 (1971).
6. Shay, F. J., Young, R. W., and Hale, M. G., *Va. J. Sci. 22:* 85 (1971).
7. Shay, F. J., and Hale, M. G., *Va. J. Sci. 22:* 82 (1971).
8. Hameed, K. M., and Couch, H. B., *Phytopathology 62:* 669 (1972).
9. Hale, M. G., Foy, C. L., and Shay, F. J., *Adv. in Agron. 23:* 89 (1971).

BACTERIAL GROWTH, GLUCIDIC AND NITROGENOUS METABOLISM IN GNOTOXENIC ENSILAGES OF LUCERNE, RAY GRASS, AND FESCUE

Ph. Gouet, M. Contrepois, N. Bousset-Fatianoff and *J. Bousset*
Laboratoire de Microbiologie
I.N.R.A. — 63 — St. Genes Champanelle — France

Introduction

The metabolic changes occurring during the ensiling of forages are due to simultaneous development of several bacterial species, facultative or strict anaerobes, sporulated or not, as well as to the action of some plant enzymes. The fermentation pattern and intensity depend on the microflora of the forage at the moment of harvesting (1), on the biochemical composition of the forage species constituting the substrate, on its dry matter content (2), as well as on the temperature (3-5), the pH, and the anaerobiosis in the silo. Losses of nutrients, mainly in the form of gas, the silage quality and palatability directly depend on the proliferation of bacterial species during the ensiling process.

The *in situ* analysis of the bacterial development in a naturally contaminated "holoxenic" (conventional) silage has remained incomplete until now, because of the absence of techniques allowing selective count of the species belonging to the same physiological group or to the same family, but whose metabolic products differ by their nature and (or) their concentration. This study can only be performed with "axenic" (germfree) forages which can be inoculated with a known, simple or complex microflora, the development of which can be subjected to analytic investigation. This presupposes production of a germfree plant (6, 7) in amounts large enough to allow realization of all the biochemical and microbiological analyses or it presupposes sterilization (8, 9) of a forage harvested in the field without affecting its biochemical composition and enzyme equipment. The advantage of the last method is that the results can easily be extrapolated to silages produced in practice. We have already shown (10) that gamma irradiation does not change very much either the composition of the forage or the proteolytic activity of its enzymes, although its sterilization is assured. By means of this method it is thus possible to separate, in the silage, the bacterial enzymatic activity from that of the plant. The aim of the present study was the following: 1) to investigate the kinetics of the development, the

649

persistency and eventual antagonistic effects of some dominating bacterial species from "holoxenic" silages inoculated separately or combined in "axenic" silages of Lucerne, Fescue and Raygrass; 2) to define the role of plant and bacterial enzymes in the catabolism of the different N-fractions; and 3) to analyze the contribution of the enzymes of the plant and those of some bacterial species respectively as regards catabolism of the carbohydrates into acids and alcohols as well as the resulting losses of gas.

The present report only deals with part of the results that we have obtained in this field.

Materials and Methods

Three forages were harvested in the field at the moment of their first growth cycle: a Lucerne variety (Flemish) at the bud stage, a variety of Raygrass (RINA) and a meadow Fescue at the early earing stage. These forages were rapidly ground and distributed into large jars (400 g per bottle of 0.7 liters) or into small jars (20 g per jar of 50 ml). The contents of the large jars allowed the analysis of carbohydrate or nitrogen fractions as well as that of the fermentation metabolites.

The contents of a series of jars were used as "holoxenic" controls; another series was irradiated (2 Mrad): one part was kept as "axenic" control samples and the rest were inoculated with one or several bacterial strains. The "monoxenic" silages were inoculated with *Enterobacter sp. (Ent.), Lactobacillus plantarum (L. pl), Lactobacillus brevis (L. br),* "branching" *Lactobacillus ("br" L.), Pediococcus sp. (Pe), Streptococcus faecalis (S. f), Clostridium butyricum (C. b), Clostridium tyrobutyricum (C. t),* and *Clostridium proteolytique (C. p).* The "polygnotoxenic" silages were inoculated with 3 to 6 of these strains. All silages were placed in an incubator at $22 \pm 1°C$ and counted on days 2, 5, 8, 15, 30, 50, 90, and 150 of storage. In the large jars, the bacteria were only counted at the end of the storage period (100 days).

In the "polygnotoxenic" silages *L. pl, L. br, Pe* and *S. f* were counted on the M.R.S. agar-agar medium (11). Differentiation was obtained as follows: *L. pl* resisted to 100 μg/ml bacitracine and *L. br* was insensitive to 2 μg/ml penicillin. *Pe* grew selectively in Petri dishes (pH 5 and 42°C) and *S. f* at pH 9.6 and 37°C. In "monoxenic" silages *"br" L.* was counted in Petri dishes on a M.R.S. medium at 30°C and in "polygnotoxenic" silages, it was counted by means of immunofluorescence (Breed's method). *Ent.* was counted selectively on Violet Red Bile (Difco).

Lactic acid was determined according to the method of Barnett (12) and volatile fatty acids (V.F.A.) by gas-liquid chromatography. Total soluble carbohydrates were determined according to the methods of Somogyi (13) and Nelson (14) and the oses of the different fractions by gas-chromatography (15).

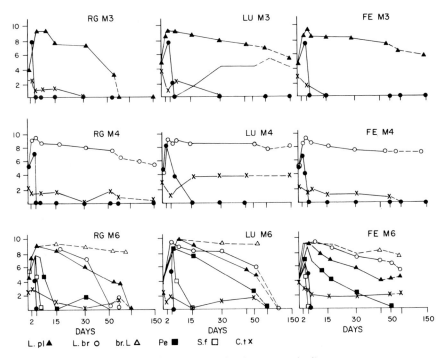

FIG. 1. Microbial evolution in gnotoxenic silages.

Non-protein nitrogen (non-precipitable by trichloracetic acid at 5 percent) was determined by Micro Kjeldahl, NH$_3$ —N by the method Conway (16), nitrates according to Fatianoff and Gouet (17). Amino acids were analyzed by column chromatography according to Moore and Stein.

Results

Kinetics of the bacterial development (Figure 1). The kinetic study carried out for 150 days showed that all non-sporulating species, in monoxenic silages, exhibited rapid and identical growth phases and reached 10^9 to 5.10^9/g after 24 to 48 hours. On the contrary, the persistence was variable according to strains and forages; thus, the phase of decline was generally more rapid in Raygrass.

In combined cultures (polygnotoxenic silages) *L. pl* and *L. br* showed identical development, but the latter had a higher longevity, especially in Lucerne. *Pe sp* multiplied rapidly, but remained sub-dominating compared with the two previous ones, whereas *S. f* and *Ent.* were rapidly eliminated by *Lactobacilli* and *Pe*.

Among the sporulated anaerobes, the proteolytic *Clostridium* never developed, probably because of a too low incubation temperature. In monoxenic

651

silages, *C. b* multiplied in Fescue and Raygrass, but not in Lucerne. On the other hand, *C. t* (in mono or polygnotoxenic silages) developed nearly always on Fescue and never on Raygrass and Lucerne. The germination phase in Fescue was situated between 5 and 10 days after ensiling. This phenomenon is clearly demonstrated in Figure 1, which shows a reduction of the number of spores during this interval.

Nitrogen metabolism. Silages always contain a very large fraction of soluble nitrogen, which leads to an insufficient metabolic efficiency. Are the solubilization of nitrogen and the ammoniogenesis of vegetable plant or bacterial origin?

TABLE I. Ammonia, Non Proteic Nitrogen, Nitrate Nitrogen in Green Forage and Silages

	NH_3*	NPN*	NO_3**
GREEN	0.6	19.1	12.4
Silage:			
AXEN	3.6	72	13.4
HOLO	16.1	75	0.1
GNOT	5.4	55	—
L. PL	2.2	58	0.1
L. br	5.5	64	11.4
br. L	2.3	58	10.8
Pe	3.7	49	11.0
En	13.5	69	0.2
C. b	5.3	77	11.3
C. t	2.1	57	0.2
C. p	3.2	67	10.6
S. f	4.2	58	0.1

*(% TOTAL − N)   ** mg % DM

Table I shows that this proteolysis, independent of the variations related to the forage species, was maximum in axenic silages and minimum in polygnotoxenic silages. It was generally reduced by nearly all the strains, but especially by the acidifying species *L. pl* (final pH 3.8 − 4.1), *L. br* (4.1 − 4.6), *"br." L.* (3.7 − 4.4), *Pe* (3.9 − 4.4), *S. t* (4.6 − 4.8). As regards the ammoniogenesis, a small part depended on the action of the plant enzymes, but the main part was caused by *Enterobacter sp.* Among the *Clostridium, C. b* and *C. t* did not produce any ammonia; however, if the proteolytic *Clostridium* had developed it would have brought about an intense ammoniogenesis.

Study of the nitrogen fraction, carried out on Lucerne silages only, very clearly shows that the free and non-metabolized amino acids (except arginine) accumulated in the axenic control samples. Among the gnotoxenic silages, the smallest metabolic changes were observed in the presence of *L. pl, "br" L.* and *Pe*: non-protein nitrogen content lower than 60 per cent of the total nitrogen,

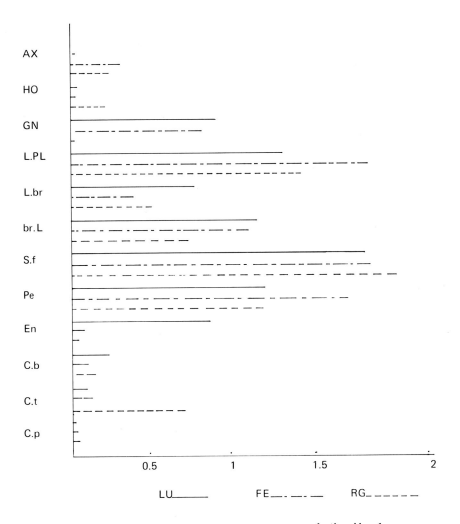

FIG. 2. Transformation factor for lactic acid. "F" = $\dfrac{\text{lactic acid carbon}}{\text{soluble carbohydrates carbon}}$

high proportions of combined amino acids and low proportions of free amino acids. In addition, no amino acids were subjected to degradation except arginine in the case of *Pediococcus sp.*

Which is then the origin of the large metabolic changes of the amino acids and the ammonia concentrations observed in holoxenic silages?

It was observed that *L. br* may have some action on these changes, but *Ent.* played the main role; in fact, it massively degraded arginine, serine,

TABLE II. Soluble Carbohydrates, Lactic Acid, Acetic Acid Concentrations
in Green Forage and Silages (% corrected dry matter)

Dry matter (D.M.) losses in different silages (gas)
(% ensiled dry matter)

	Solub. carbo.			Lactic acid			Acetic Acid			D.M. Losses		
	Lu	Fe	RG	Lu	Fe	RG	Lu	Fe	RG	Lu	Fe	RG
GREEN	8.5	14.4	25.8	0.1	0.1	0.1	0.1	0.0	0.0			
Silage:												
Axenic	12.0	13.8	23.9	0.2	0.2	0.4	0.2	0.2	0.2			
Holoxenic	1.9	4.2	9.5	0.1	0.2	3.1	2.2	0.7	0.2			
Gnotoxenic	0.6	2.1	—	10.5	9.3	—	2.6	1.9	—	9.1	4.0	—
L. plantarum	3.4	7.1	15.3	11.2	12.1	12.1	0.7	1.2	0.6	1.1	2.9	2.6
L. brevis	1.9	1.8	6.4	7.7	4.7	9.0	2.3	3.9	2.5	2.5	7.0	3.3
"branching" *L.*	4.2	4.2	13.9	9.2	10.5	8.2	0.5	0.6	0.4	3.8	0.7	3.3
S. faecalis	8.0	9.8	22.4	7.2	7.2	6.9	1.4	0.2	0.2	4.4	6.0	0.1
Pediococcus	4.0	6.4	15.0	9.6	12.7	10.8	0.6	0.4	0.3	1.3	7.6	2.0
Enterobacter	1.9	4.7	9.1	0.9	0.7	0.4	2.2	0.8	1.3	4.5	7.7	22.0
C. butyricum	1.4	10.5	14.9	0.2	0.2	1.2	0.6	0.6	0.8	6.6	4.4	10.2
C. tyrobutyricum	9.8	10.1	23.4	0.1	0.2	0.3	0.1	0.0	0.0	5.8	5.9	1.9
C. proleolytique	13.9	14.3	23.9	0.2	0.3	0.3	0.3	0.2	0.2	-1.8	0.2	0.8

Lu = Lucerne   Fe = Festuca   RG = Ray Grass

threonine, aspartic acid and asparagine and it accumulated ammonia as well as large amounts of undetermined non-protein nitrogen probably mainly composed of amines. However, our results were incomplete since the proteolytic *Clostridium* did not develop in monoxenic silages, whereas it probably brought about the total disappearance of lysine and histidine in the holoxenic control silage.

The microflora also played a fundamental role in the metabolism of nitrates. Forage plants contain variable amounts of nitrates depending on the cultural conditions. In the silo, they are reduced into nitrites and then into nitrogen dioxide, which is particularly toxic for humans and animals (methemoglobinemia). It was shown (Table I) with Lucerne and Raygrass that the reduction of nitrates was total in the presence of *L. pl, "br." L., Ent., C. t,* whereas the other species as well as the plant enzymes did not have any effect on this reaction.

Carbohydrate and fermentation metabolism (Table II and Figure 2). Among the results obtained, the following points can be emphasized: a) the plant enzymes played a much smaller role in carbohydrate metabolism than in nitrogen metabolism. They acted by hydrolizing, on the one hand, the disaccharides, oligosaccharides, fructosanes into oses, and, on the other hand, a fraction of non-cellulose membrane polyhosides releasing, especially, xylose and arabinose. This phenomenon was very marked in Lucerne where the increase of soluble carbohydrates reached 42 per cent in the axenic control silage. b) The "transformation factor" (F) (developed lactic acid carbon weight/disappeared carbohydrate carbon weight ratio, expressed as glucose or fructose) definitely exceeded the unit for *L. pl, S. f, Pe,* whereas it was lower in the case of the heterofermentative strains: *L. br, Ent., C. b, C. t* (Figure 2). This fact shows that the first three species did not only use carbohydrate as energy source and their metabolism did not cause any loss of gas. This result was confirmed by the lactic acid concentrations obtained in the different forages (Table II) allowing classification of the "lactic species" and estimation of the most useful ones: 1 — *L. plantarum,* 2 – *Pediococcus sp.,* 3 – "branching" *Lactobacillus,* 4 – *L. brevis.* The gas losses considerably varied (1.1 to 22 per cent of the ensiled dry matter) from one bacterial species to another (Table II) and from one forage to another. *L. plantarum* was still the most interesting species and Fescue led to higher losses than Lucerne and Raygrass.

Discussion and Conclusions

The bacterial strains used in these trials certainly do not represent all the strains that may be present in holoxenic silages: *L. casei, L. arabinosus, Leuconostoc mesenteroides* and *Str. liquefaciens* should also be taken into account. However, the persistence of these four strains is often ephemeral and their role, in a first approach, may be considered as secondary.

The associations used constitute some of the main combinations that can be imagined between the three dominating lactic species (*L. pl, L. br, Pe.*) and the two species whose development has to be inhibited (*C. t* and *Ent.*). In fact, the latter are gas producing and their metabolism causes the most important losses of nutrients (18) by diverting part of the fermentative carbohydrates from the lactic acidification. In addition, the butyric fermentation, by raising the pH, allows the development of putrefactive bacteria. The temperature used in these trials was 22° C because, by favoring the lactobacilli growth, it generally permits achievement of moist "holoxenic" silages of better quality. However, the role of the temperature, the importance of which is known (3, 4), has to be studied.

The results obtained during this first study confirm the observations made from holoxenic silages. Thus, the gram negative microflora develops as quickly as the lactic microflora, but the former rapidly disappears, whereas the latter develops as a dominating flora (19).

All these analytical studies carried out by means of axenic or gnotoxenic silages gave, for the first time, the possibility of dissociating the actions of bacterial enzymes and plant enzymes.

These investigations have shown the unfavorable role of some dominating species such as *Enterobacter sp.* and even *L. brevis* and have pointed out the unsuspected efficiency of species such as "branching" *Lactobacillus* or *Pediococcus sp.*

Finally, the perfect and rapid lactic acidification of *L. plantarum,* its interesting consequences as regards protection of nitrogen, sparing of soluble carbohydrates, decrease of losses, emphasize the interest of controlling the development of the silage microflora. Even though the extrapolation of these results to "holoxenic" silages is not possible yet, one may think that judiciously chosen bacterial associations, different according to forages, could probably inhibit the butyric fermentations and, consequently, reduce the losses of nutritive substances and improve the palatability of moist silages.

References

1. Langston, C. W., *J. Dairy Sci. 43:* 1575 (1960).
2. Gouet, Ph., Fatianoff, N., Zelter, S. Z., Durand, M., Chevalier, R., *Ann. Biol. Anim. Bioch. Biophys. 5:* 79 (1965).
3. Lanigan, G. W., *Austr. J. Biol. Sc. 16:* 606 (1963).
4. Lanigan, G. W., *Austr. J. Biol. Sc. 18:* 555 (1965).
5. Gibson, T., Stirling, A. C., Keddie, R. M., Rosenberger, R. F., *J. Gen. Microbiol. 19:* 112 (1958).
6. Mabbitt, L. A., *Proc. Soc. Appl. Bact. 14:* 147 (1951).
7. Luckey, T. D., *Germfree Life and Gnotobiology,* Acad. Press, New York and London, (1963).
8. Huhtanen, C. N., Pensack, J. M., *Appl. Microbiol. 11:* 529 (1963).
9. Gouet, Ph., Fatianoff, N., *Ann. Inst. Pasteur,* 711 (1964).
10. Gouet, Ph., Fatianoff, N.,, and Bousset, J., *C. R. Acad. Sci. 270:* 1024 (1970).
11. DeMan, J. C., Rogosa, M., and Sharpe, E., *J. Appl. Bact. 23:* 130 (1960).
12. Barnett, A. S. G., *Silage Fermentation,* Butherworths Sc. Publ., London, (1954).
13. Somogyi, M., *J. Biol. Chem. 195:* 19 (1952).
14. Nelson, W. L., *J. Biol. Chem. 153:* 375 (1944).
15. Bousset, J. A., Fatianoff, N., and Gouet, Ph., *C. R. Acad. Sci. 270:* 1174 (1970).
16. Conway, E. J., *Microdiffusion Analysis and Volumetric Error,* Crosby, Lockwood, and Son, Ltd., London, (1957).
17. Bousset-Fatianoff, N., and Gouet, Ph., *Ann. Biol. Anim. Bioch. 11:* 705 (1971).
18. Bousset, J., Bousset-Fatianoff, N., Gouet, Ph., and Contrepois, M., *Ann. Biol. Anim. Bioch. Biophys. 3:* (1972).

STUDIES ON THE NUTRITION OF THE SNAIL *BIOMPHALARIA GLABRATA* UNDER AXENIC CONDITIONS

Enio C. Vieira, Ioni A. Senna, Sonia Maria G. Rogana and *Maria Luiza V.C. Tupynamba,*
Departamento de Bioquimica, Instituto de Ciencias Biologicas, Universidade Federal de Minas Gerais, Belo Horizonte, MG. Brasil

Introduction

Snail nutrition is not well known. These mollusks have been reared in the laboratory on artificial diets containing the following organic nutrients: powdered milk, wheat germ, and lettuce (1-3). The ideal system for studying the nutrition of aquatic animals is the "germfree system." In this field, very little has been done, according to recent reviews (4-7).

In 1957, Chernin described a method of securing axenic snails (8). Later, growth of axenic *Biomphalaria glabrata* on a medium consisting of *Escherichia coli* and yeast was reported (9). This paper describes some results obtained in our laboratory, besides those previously reported (10, 11).

Results

Growth and reproduction of axenic snails were obtained for the first time on a medium consisting of powdered milk, wheat germ, dried lettuce, starch, salt mixture, yeast extract, α-tocopherol, water-soluble vitamins, and spring water (10). This artificial diet was used as the standard medium. In order to transform this medium into a chemically defined one, we successively omitted nutrients and replaced them with pure substances. We also attempted to enrich the medium with the addition of cod liver oil. The results of these experiments are shown in Table I. Based on the results summarized in Table I, a diet consisting of casein, lettuce, salt mixture, α-tocopherol, water-soluble vitamins, and distilled water was found adequate to maintain snail culture (11). A purified medium was also reported, with the following composition: casein, cellulose, pectin, starch, glucose, sucrose, salt mixture, α-tocopherol, ascorbic acid, cysteine, water-soluble vitamins, and distilled water (11). This purified medium represents a step forward towards the chemical definition of snail needs, even though snail growth and reproduction are much lower in this medium than in the standard one.

657

TABLE I. Summary of the Results from Experiments with Standard Media

	Effect on growth	Effect on reproduction
Addition of:		
cod liver oil	none	none
Omission of:		
yeast extract	none	negative
wheat germ	none	none
powdered milk	negative	—
starch	positive	none
vitamins	negative	—
Exposure to light	negative	—
Substitution of:		
distilled for spring water	none	none
casein for powdered milk	positive in early age	negative

Lately, we have studied several aspects of snail nutrition, such as: the vitamin needs, the chemical definition of the protein needs, the α-tocopherol effect on reproduction, and the lipid nutrition.

The vitamin needs. Vitamins were omitted one by one from the vitamin solution, and the effect of this omission on snail growth was compared to the medium with the complete vitamin solution. Table II shows the results of these experiments.

TABLE II. Vitamin Needs of Snails

Essential	Non-essential
folic acid	inositol
calcium pantothenate	choline
pyridoxine	biotin
thiamine	ascorbic acid
niacin	riboflavin
vitamin B_{12}	

The chemical definition of the protein need. Casein is not a chemically defined protein (12). Neither casein hydrolyzate nor an amino acid mixture works as a casein substitute, probably due to their solubility. Apparently, snails need to eat solid food.

We tried to replace casein with several other proteins whose amino acid sequences have been worked out, such as: ovalbumin, lactalbumin trypsin, chymotrypsin, human globin A, or lysozyme. These proteins, used in the medium in the same amount as casein, were enriched with amino acids, in an attempt to mimic the amino acid composition of casein, as indicated in Table III.

TABLE III. Amino Acid Fortification of Proteins Used as Casein Substitutes

Protein	Amino acid added (mg) per g of protein
Ovalbumin	none
Lactalbumin	none
Human globin A	tyrosine (30), proline (25), methionine (25), glutamic acid (125), isoleucine (60).
Trypsin	phenylalanine (35), leucine (30), proline (90), glutamic acid (75), arginine (15), histidine (10), methionine (15).
Chymotrypsinogen	phenylalanine (16), lysine (13), tyrosine (38), leucine (10), proline (80), histidine (21), methionine (24), glutamic acid (75), arginine (17), isoleucine (18).
Lysozyme	phenylalanine (19), lysine (28), tyrosine (28), leucine (28), proline (99), histidine (21), methionine (15), valine (30), glutamic acid (179), isoleucine (13).

None of these amino acid fortified proteins were able to replace casein with the same efficiency.

The α-tocopherol effect. As reported previously (10), α-tocopherol has a remarkable effect on snail reproduction. We used N,N'-diphenyl-1,4-p-phenylenediamine (DPPD) and 1,2-dihydro-6-ethoxi-2,2,4-trimethylquinoline (EMQ) as vitamin E substitutes. Snail survival was much lower when either DPPD or EMQ was used. The survivors did not lay eggs.

Lipid nutrition. The purified medium contains no lipid. We enriched the medium with a lipid mixture consisting of: triolein (4.4 g), vitamin A acetate (20 mg), vitamin E (400 mg), and linoleic acid (100 mg). Snail growth on a diet containing 10% of this lipid mixture was the same as in the purified medium.

Conclusions

We were able to obtain reproduction of axenic snails. Vitamin E was shown to be essential for reproduction. A purified medium was developed, and it is not very far from being chemically defined. Casein in the medium could not be replaced by any of the proteins tried. We do not know whether this is due to better digestibility, to amino acid composition, or to contaminants of casein. The vitamin needs of the snails were traced. Some were shown to be essential vitamins for them. It remains to be determined whether the nonessential nutrients are present in minute amounts in the medium.

α-Tocopherol could not be replaced by either DPPD or EMQ. In rats,

DPPD is substituted for vitamin E (13).

The purified diet contains no lipid except for vitamin E. Enrichment of the diet with essential lipids did not improve it. This is unusual, since vitamin A has been detected in the eyes of a pulmonate snail (14).

The culture of axenic snails on a chemically defined diet will help us comprehend their nutritional needs, digestive processes, and metabolic transformations.

Acknowledgement

This work was supported by United States Public Health Service grant AI-08245, and by Conselho Nacional de Pesquisas grant TC-7853. Part of the permanent equipment was a gift of the Rockefeller Foundation.

References

1. Noland, L. E., and Carriker, M. R., *Am. Midland Nat. 36:* 467 (1946).
2. Standen, O.D., *Ann. Trop. Med. Parasitol. 45:* 80 (1951).
3. Moore, D. V., Thillet, C. J., Carney, D. M., and Meleney, H. E., *J. Parasitol. 39:* 215 (1953).
4. Whitelock, O. V. St., *Ann. N.Y. Acad. Sci. 77:* 25 (1959).
5. Luckey, T. D., *Germfree Life and Gnotobiology,* Academic Press, N.Y., (1963).
6. Teah, B. A., *Bibliography of Germfree Research, 1885-1963,* (1964). Annual Supplements have been published through the 1969 Supplement (1970).
7. Weyer, E. M., *Ann. N.Y. Acad. Sci. 139:* 1 (1966).
8. Chernin, E., *Proc. Soc. Exp. Biol. Med. 96:* 204 (1957).
9. Chernin, E., and Schork, A. R., *Am. J. Hyg. 69:* 146 (1959).
10. Vieira, E. C., *Am. J. Trop. Med. Hyg. 16:* 792 (1967).
11. Senna, I. A., and Vieira, E. C. *Am. J. Trop. Med. Hyg. 19:* 568 (1970).
12. Dougherty, E. C., *Ann. N.Y. Acad. Sci. 77:* 27 (1959).
13. Draper, H. H., Bergan, J. G., Chiu, M., Csallany, A. S., and Boaro, A. V., *J. Nutr. 84:* 395 (1964).
14. Eakin, R. M., and Brandenburger, J. L., *Proc. Natl. Acad. Sci. 60:* 140 (1968).

PARTICIPANTS

Abelseth, M. K.
New York State Health Dept.
Albany, New York 12201

Alam, Syed
LSU Medical Center
1542 Tulane Avenue
New Orleans, Louisiana 70112

Alpert, S.
2 East 86th St.
New York, New York 10028

Aranki, A.
Univ. of Michigan
Ann Arbor, Michigan 48104

Athey, W. L.
Microbiological Associates Inc.
Walkersville, Maryland 21793

Baez, Silvio
Albert Einstein College of Medicine
1300 Morris Park Avenue
Bronx, New York 10461

Balish, E.
Univ. of Wisconsin Medical School
185 Med. Sci. Bldg.
Madison, Wisconsin 53706

Barney, George
Vanderbilt University
Nashville, Tennessee 37202

Bealmear, Patricia
Division of Experimental Biology
Baylor College of Medicine
Texas Medical Center
Houston, Texas 77025

Bickers, J. N.
LSU Medical Center
1542 Tulane Avenue
New Orleans, Louisiana 70112

Bienvene, Alice
LSU Medical Center
1542 Tulane Avenue
New Orleans, Louisiana 70112

Blackmore, D. K.
M.R.C. Lab. Animals Centre
Woodmansterne Road, Carshalton,
Surrey, England

Boeckmann, R.
LSU Medical Center
1542 Tulane Avenue
New Orleans, Louisiana 70112

Bohner, Howard J.
National Institutes of Health
Bldg. 14G, Room 101
Bethesda, Maryland 20014

Bornside, Bette
Dept. of Surgery
LSU Medical Center
1542 Tulane Avenue
New Orleans, Louisiana 70112

Bornside, George H.
Dept. of Surgery
LSU Medical Center
1542 Tulane Avenue
New Orleans, Louisiana 70112

Bradley, Richard E.
Dept. of Veterinary Sci.
Univ. of Florida
Gainesville, Florida 32601

Brick, J. O.
Director of Quality Assurance
Carworth, Inc.
New City, New York 10956

Bruckner-Kardoss, Edith
Lobund, Dept. of Microbiology
University of Notre Dame
Notre Dame, Indiana 46556

Bruckner, Geza
Dept. of Pharmacology
Univ. of Kentucky Med. Center
Lexington, Kentucky 40506

Bruun, Johan N.
Graduate Hospital of Univ. of Pa.
Philadelphia, Pennsylvania 19104

Calderbank, F. J.
The BioClean Division
Fieldstone Corp.
W. Conshohocken, Pennsylvania
19428

Carter, Joan
Trudeau Institute
P. O. Box 59
Saranac Lake, New York 12983

Carter, P. B.
Trudeau Institute
P. O. Box 59
Saranac Lake, New York 12983

Chakhava, Otar V.
The Gamaleya Institute
Gamaleya Str. 18
Moscow, D-98
U.S.S.R.

Chorpenning, Frank W.
Ohio State University
Columbus, Ohio 43210

Clapp, H. W.
The Upjohn Co.
301 Henrietta Street
Kalamazoo, Michigan 49001

Clark, J. Derrell
Tulane Medical School
1430 Tulane Avenue
New Orleans, Louisiana 70112

Coates, Marie E.
National Institute for Research
in Dairying
Shinfield, Reading,
RG2-9AT, England

Cohn, Isidore, Jr.
Head, Dept. of Surgery
LSU Medical Center
1542 Tulane Avenue
New Orleans, Louisiana

Collister, R.
Royal Vet. College
Royal College Street
London, N.W.1
England

Combe, Etiennette
Institut National de la
Recherche Agronomipue
63 St. Genes, Champanelle,
France

Contrepois, M.
I.N.R.A.
Clermont Ferrand
France

Coriell, L. L.
Institute for Medical Research
Copewood Street
Camden, N. J. 08103

Dankert, J.
Lab. Medical Microbiology
Oostezsingel 59
Groningen
The Netherlands

Dascomb, H.
Charity Hospital
New Orleans, Louisiana 70112

Decuypere, Jaak
Univ. of Ghent
9230 Melle
Ghent, Belgium

Deerberg, F.
Zentralinstitut for Versuchuterrucht
3 Hannover, Germany

Demarne, Yves
I.N.R.A. – C.N.R.Z.
78 Jouy-en-Josas
France

DeSomer, Pieter
Rega Institute for Medical Research
Minderbroederstraat 10
B-3000 Leuven, Belgium

Dietrich, Manfred
University of Ulm
(Zimk) Steinhoevelstr. 9
D 79 Ulm (Donau), Germany

Diluzio, N.
Tulane Medical School
1430 Tulane Avenue
New Orleans, Louisiana 70112

Ducluzeau, Robert
I.N.R.A. – C.N.R.Z.
78 Jouy-en-Josas
France

Edstrom, William E.
Edstrom Industries, Inc.
Route 1, Box 4
Waterford, Wisconsin 53185

Eichberg, J.
Southwest Foundation for Research
P. O. Box 28147
San Antonio, Texas 78228

Elmofty, S.
University of Alabama
Birmingham, Alabama 35223

Eyssen, H.
Rega Institute for Medical Research
Minderbroederstraat 10,
B – 3000 – Leuven
Belgium

663

Finerty, J. F.
Vice-Chancellor,
LSU Medical Center
New Orleans, Louisiana 70112

Fitzgerald, Robert J.
V. A. Hospital
1201 N.W. 16th Street
Miami, Florida 33134

Fitzgerald, Dorothea
V. A. Hospital
1201 N.W. 16th Street
Miami, Florida 33134

Foster, Henry L.
The Charles River Breeding Labs
251 Ballardvale St.
Wilmington, Mass. 01887

Frederick, G. Thomas
Ohio State University
484 W 12th Ave.
Columbus, Ohio 43210

Freter, Rolf
University of Michigan
6722 Med. Sci. Bldg. No. 2
Ann Arbor, Michigan 48104

Gabriel, G.
635 Midland Avenue
Garfield, New Jersey 07026

Garcia, Sirio
Tulane Medical School
1430 Tulane Avenue
New Orleans, Louisiana 70112

Garlick, Norman L.
Dept. of Lab. Animal Medicine
Medical University of So. Carolina
80 Barre St.
Charleston, South Carolina 29401

Geissinger, H. D.
Department of Biomed. Science
University of Guelph
Guelph, Ontario, Canada

Gibson, Don C.
N.I.H.
9000 Wisconsin Avenue
Bethesda, Maryland 20014

Gordon, Helmut A.
University of Kentucky
College of Medicine
Lexington, Kentucky 40506

Gouet, P.
Centre de Recherches
Zootechniques, Champanelle 63,
France

Griesemer, Richard
Nat. Ctr. for Primate Biology
Univ. of Calif.
Davis, California 95616

Gustafsson, Bengt E.
Karolinska Institutet
Stockholm 60, Sweden

Hale, M. G.
Virginia Polytechnic Institute
Blackburg, Virginia 24061

Hara, Noriyoshi
Keio University School of Med.
Shinjuku-ku Tokyo, Japan

Harris, A. S.
Head, Dept. of Physiology
LSU Medical Center
New Orleans, Louisiana 70112

Harrison, G. F.
NIRD
Shinfield, Reading,
RG 2-9 AT, England

Hashimoto, Kazuo
Department of Microbiology
Keio University School of Med.
35 Shinanomachi Shinjuku-ku
Tokyo, Japan

Hegner, James R.
NCDC
1600 Clifton Road
Atlanta, Georgia 30304

Heine, Willi
Zentralinstitut fur Versuchstierzucht
Lettow-Vorbeck Allee 57
3 Hannover, Germany

Henderickx, H. K.
Dept. of Nutrition and Hygiene
Bosstraat I, B. 9230
Melle, Belgium

Heneghan, J. B.
Dept. of Surgery
LSU Medical Center
1542 Tulane Avenue
New Orleans, Louisiana 70112

Hentges, David J.
Univ. of Missouri
School of Medicine
Columbia, Missouri 65201

Herman, Robert H.
U.S. Army Medical Research
& Nutrition Laboratory
Fitzsimons General Hospital
Denver, Colorado 80240

Herman, Yaye F.
U. S. Army Med. Res. & Nutr.
Lab. Fitzsimons Gen. Hospital
Denver, Colorado 80240

Herrell, Wallace
Emeritus Professor
445 Central Avenue
Northfield, Illinois 60093

Hohage, R.
Dept. of Clinical Physiology
Center for Basic Research
Univ. of Ulm
Ulm/Donau, Germany

Holman, John E.
N.I.H.
Bethesda, Maryland 20014

van Hoosier, G. L.
Washington State University
Pullman, Washington 99163

Hull, Edgar W.
LSU Medical Center (Medicine)
1542 Tulane Avenue
New Orleans, Louisiana 70112

Ichihashi, Yasuo
Keio University School of Med.
35 Shinjuku-ku
Tokyo, Japan

Ito, Yasuo
National Tokyo Gen. Hospital
2-5-1 Higashigaoka-Meguro K4
Tokyo, Japan

Iwata, Kazuo
Dept. of Microbiology
Faculty of Medicine,
Univ. of Tokyo
7-3-1 Hongo Bunk-ku
Tokyo, Japan

Iyaki, Tsuneo
Dept. of Microbiology
Faculty of Medicine,
Univ. of Tokyo
7-3-1 Hongo Bunk-ku
Tokyo, Japan

Jeansonne, E.
Dean, LSU School of Dentistry
1100 Florida Avenue
New Orleans, Louisiana 70119

Johnson, Joyce
Poultry Dept.
Univ. of Georgia
Athens, Georgia 30601

Jorgensen, Gary
Filtek Div. Appleton Wire Works, Inc.
Appleton, Wisconsin 54911

Joyce, Jeanne
University of Southern California
Medical Center
2025 Zonal
Los Angeles, California 90033

Kallman, R. F.
Department of Radiology
Stanford Univ. Med. Sch.
Stanford, California 94305

Kalter, S. S.
Southwest Foundation for Res.
and Education
P. O. Box 28147
San Antonio, Texas 78228

Kamei, Hideo
The 2nd Dept. of Surgery
Nagoya, Japan

Kaufman, H.
LSU Medical Center
1542 Tulane Avenue
New Orleans, Louisiana 70112

Kawai, T.
LSU Medical Center
1542 Tulane Avenue
New Orleans, Louisiana 70112

Kellogg, T. F.
Mississippi State Univ.
P. O. Drawer BB
State College, Miss. 39762

Kenworthy, R.
Unilever Research, Colworth House
Sharnbrook, Bedfordshire
England

Khelghati, A.
LSU Medical Center
1542 Tulane Avenue
New Orleans, Louisiana

Kikuchi, T.
Keio Univ. School of Med.
Shinjuku-ku, Tokyo
Japan

Kline, B. F.
WARF Institute Inc.
Madison, Wisconsin 53705

Kobayashi, I.
Sugiyama Univ. Chikusaku
Nagoya, Japan

Köhle, K.
ZIMK Steinhoevelstr. 9D79
Ulm, Germany

Kokas, E.
Dept. of Physiology
UNC School of Medicine
Chapel Hill, North Carolina 27515

Kovar, E. W.
Kansas State University
Rossville, Kansas 66533

Landy, J.
Germfree Labs, Inc.
2600 SW 25th Avenue
Miami, Florida 33133

Lattuada, C. P.
ARS/Sprague Dawley
2801 Industrial Drive
Madison, Wisconsin 53713

Legler, D. W.
Dept. of Oral Biology
Univ. of Alabama
Birmingham, Alabama 35333

Levenson, S.
Albert Einstein College of Medicine
1300 Morris Park Ave.
Bronx, New York 10461

Linsley, James G.
Dept. of Surgery
University of Wisconsin
Medical School
1300 Univ. Ave.
Madison, Wisconsin 53706

Listgarten, M.
Dept. of Periodontics
Univ. of Pennsylvania
4001 Spruce St.
Philadelphia, Pennsylvania 19104

Longoria, S.
Dept. of Surgery
LSU Medical Center
1542 Tulane Avenue
New Orleans, Louisiana 70112

Loosli, C.
USC School of Medicine
2025 Zonal Ave.
Los Angeles, California 90033

Lowthian, J.
Environmental Engineer
Charity Hospital
New Orleans, Louisiana 70112

Luckey, T. D.
University of Missouri
School of Medicine
Columbia, Missouri 65201

Lukemeyer, J. W.
Indiana University Sch. of Med.
Indianapolis, Indiana 46202

Maley, M.
Shrine Burns Institute
Cincinnati, Ohio 45219

Mandel, A.
N.A.S.A. Ames Research Center
Moffett Field, California

Maki, T.
Lab. of Germfree Life Research
Kawaschima, Japan

McCullough, B.
Ohio State University
1425 Coffey Road
Columbus, Ohio 43210

McGarrity, G.
Institute for Medical Research
Copewood St.
Camden, New Jersey 08103

Meyer, H.
University of Ulm
Parkstave II
Ulm, Germany

Miller, Carl
N.I.H.
Bldg. 37, Room 5E-12
Nat. Cancer Inst.
Bethesda, Maryland 20014

Miniats, O. P.
Ontario V.C., Univ. of Guelph
Guelph, Ontario, Canada

Mirand, E. A.
666 Elm Street
Roswell Park Mem. Inst.
Buffalo, New York 14203

Miyakawa, Masaumi
Lab. of Germfree Life Research
Eisai-Campus, Kawashimacho
Hajima-Gun, Gifu-ken, Japan

Nance, F. C.
Dept. of Surgery
LSU Medical Center
1542 Tulane Avenue
New Orleans, Louisiana 70112

Nelson, J.
Charity Hospital
New Orleans, La. 70112

Nelson, Norman
Dean, LSU Medical Center
1542 Tulane Avenue
New Orleans, Louisiana 70112

Nielsen, A.
Dept. of Microbiology
Univ. of Kansas Sch. of Med.
Kansas City, Kansas 66103

Nomura, Tatsuji
The Central Institute for
Exp. Animals
17-2, Aobadai-2, Meguro
Tokyo 135, Japan

Oestreicher, E. J.
Shrine Burns Institute
202 Goodman Street
Cincinnati, Ohio 45219

Orcutt, R.
Charles River Breeding Labs.
251 Ballardvale St.
Wilmington, Massachusetts 01887

Ozawa, Atsushi
2nd Tokyo Nat. Hosp.
2-5-1, Meguro, Higashigaoka
Tokyo, Japan

Perrot, A.
Iffa-Credo
Lyon (69)
France

Pesti, L.
Hungarian Acad. of Science
XIV Hungaria Korut 21
Budapest, Hungary

Phillips, Bruce P.
N.I.H., Bldg. 8 — Room 320
Bethesda, Maryland 20014

Pilcher, M. F.
Bethnal Green Hospital
London, England

Pleasants, J.
Lobund Labs
University of Notre Dame
Notre Dame, Indiana 46556

Poiley, S. M.
National Cancer Institute
Bldg. 37 Rm. 5E12
9000 Wisconsin Avenue
Bethesda, Maryland 20014

Pollard, M.
Lobund Labs.
University of Notre Dame
Notre Dame, Indiana 46556

Przyjalkowski, Z. W.
Institute of Parasitology
Polish Acad. of Sci.
Pasteur-3, S.P. 153
Warszawa 22, Poland

Pugh, N. O.
LSU Medical Center
1542 Tulane Avenue
New Orleans, Louisiana 70112

Radhakrishnan, C. V.
Dept. of Veterinary Science
Univ. of Florida
Gainesville, Florida 32601

Raibaud, P.
I.N.R.A. — C.N.R.Z.
78 Jouy-en-Josas
France

Rasche, H.
ZIMK University of Ulm
Steinhoevelstr. 9
Ulm/Darustr, Germany

Regan, D. L.
Plas Labs, 917 East Chilson St.
Lansing, Michigan 48906

Reid, M. W.
University of Georgia
Athens, Georgia 30601

Rice, J.
University of Georgia
Athens, Georgia 30601

Riedel, Gunther
I.E.T.F.
Universitat Munchen
8 Munchen 22, Veterinarstrasse 13
Germany

Robie, D. M.
Roswell Park Memorial Institute
666 Elm St.
Buffalo, New York 14203

Rodriguez, V.
M.D. Anderson Hospital
Houston, Texas 77025

Rommel, Karl
Universitat Ulm
ZIMK 79 Ulm/Donau,
Germany

Rosen, S.
Ohio State University
305 West 12th Ave.
Columbus, Ohio 43210

Rovelar, P.
Charity Hospital
New Orleans, Louisiana 70112

Rovin, Sheldon
College of Dentistry
University of Kentucky
Lexington, Kentucky 40506

Rovira, B. A.
Tahoe Forest Hospital
Box 2177
Truckee, California 95734

Rozmiarek, H.
Biomedical Lab
Edgewood Arsenal
Maryland 21010

Russel, J.
ARS/Sprague Dawley
Madison, Wisconsin 53711

Sacksteder, Miriam
Germfree Life Research Center
3301 College Avenue
Fort Lauderdale, Florida 33314

Sacquet, Edmond
CNRZ
Gif-sur-Yvette 91
France

Sanchez, R.
LSU Medical Center
1542 Tulane Avenue
New Orleans, Louisiana 70112

Sasaki, Shogo
Dept. of Microbiology
Keio University
35 Shinanomachi, Shinjuku-ku
Tokyo, Japan

Savage, D. C.
Department of Microbiology
University of Texas
Austin, Texas 77025

Schulz, K. D.
c/o Dr. Thomae, K. GmbH
795 Biberach/Riss
Germany

Sharon, Nehama
Lobund Labs.
Dept. of Microbiology
Univ. of Notre Dame
Notre Dame, Ind. 46556

Silence, T.
Paxton Processing Company
P. O. Box 120
Paxton, Illinois 60957

Silverberg, E.
635 Midland Avenue
Garfield, New Jersey 07026

Simmons, M. L.
216 Congers Road
Carworth
New City, New York 10956

Slater, Gilbert M.
Lakeview Hamster Colony
P. O. Box 85
Newfield, New Jersey 08344

Smith, J. Cecil, Jr.
Vet. Administration Hosp.
50 Irving St. N.W.
Washington, D. C. 20422

Springer, W. T.
Dept. Vet. Science
Louisiana State University
Baton Rouge, Louisiana 70821

Stewart, W.
Chancellor
LSU Medical Center
1542 Tulane Avenue
New Orleans, Louisiana 70112

Stout, R.
LSU Pediatrics
1542 Tulane Avenue
New Orleans, Louisiana 70112

Sumi, Yukiko
Institute of Germfree Life Research
Nagoya University School of Med.
Tsurumai-cho, Showa-kur
Nagoya, Japan

Szal, J. M.
Marketing Director
Plas-Labs, Scientific Div.
917 East Chilson Avenue
Lansing, Michigan 48906

Ivorec-Szylit, O.
CNRZ – INRA
78 Jouy-en-Josas, France

Tashirocho, K.
Chikusaku, Nagoya City
Japan

Thompson, Linda
LSU Medical Center
1542 Tulane Avenue
New Orleans, Louisiana 70112

Tornyos, K.
VA Hospital
1601 Perdido Street
New Orleans, Louisiana 70112

Treveiler, R.
Standard Safety
Equipment Co.
431 N. Quentin Road
Palatine, Illinois 60067

Trexler, P. C.
Royal Vet. Coll.
Royal College Street
London, NW1, O.T.U.
England

Ukai, Mitsuo
Nagoya University School
of Medicine
65 Tsuruma-cho Showa-ku
Nagoya, Japan

Valentine, R.
Univ. of Kentucky
Albert B. Chandler
College of Medicine
Lexington, Kentucky 40506

Vela, Richard
Dept. of Surgery
LSU Medical Center
1542 Tulane Avenue
New Orleans, Louisiana 70112

Vieira, E. C.
University Minas Gerais
Caiza Postal 2486 Belo Horizonte
M.G., Brazil

Vossen, J. M.
Dept. of Pediatrics,
Univ. Hospital
Leiden, The Netherlands

van der Waaij, D.
Radiobiological Institute
TNO, 151 Lange Kleiweg
Rijswijk, (Z.H.)
The Netherlands

Wagner, Morris
Lobund
University of Notre Dame
Notre Dame, Indiana 46556

Walburg, H. E., Jr.
Oak Ridge National Lab.
P. O. Box Y
Oak Ridge, Tennessee 37831

Walkinshaw, C. H.
NASA Manned Spacecraft Center
Route 1
Houston, Texas 77058

Walter, R. G.
Brooks AFB
127 Thornell
San Antonio, Texas 78205

Washington, J. L.
LSU Medical Center
1542 Tulane Avenue
New Orleans, Louisiana 70112

Werder, Alvar
Department of Microbiology
University of Kansas School of Med.
Kansas City, Kansas 66103

Wescott, R. B.
Dept. of Veterinary Pathology
Washington State Univ.
Pullman, Wash. 99163

White, E.
University of Southern California
925 W. 34th
Los Angeles, California 90007

Wiles, Linda
University of Southern California
925 W. 34th
Los Angeles, California 90007

Jayne-Williams, D.
National Institute for Research
in Dairying
Reading, Shinfield, Berkshire
United Kingdom

Wilson, Raphael
Baylor College of Medicine
Texas Medical Center
Houston, Texas 77025

Wiseman, R. F.
Dept. of Microbiology
University of Kentucky
Lexington, Kentucky 40506

Wostmann, B. S.
Lobund Laboratories
University of Notre Dame
Notre Dame, Indiana 46556

Yale, C. E.
University of Wisconsin
1300 University Avenue
Madison, Wisconsin 53706

Yates, J. W.
Roswell Park Memorial Inst.
666 Elm Street
Buffalo, New York 14003